17971

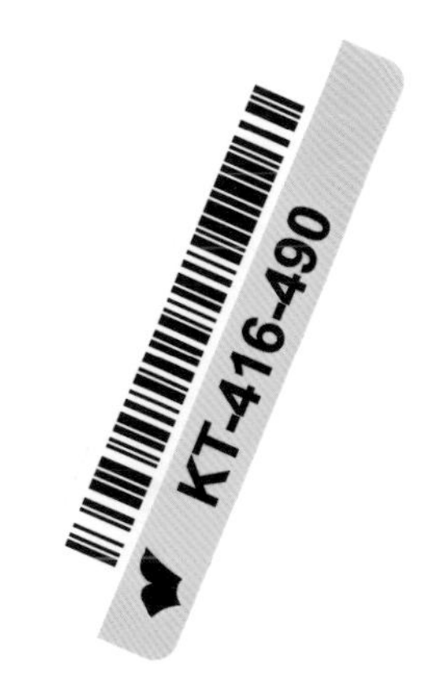
KT-416-490

Nursing Care of WOMEN WITH CANCER

Nursing Care of WOMEN WITH CANCER

KAREN HASSEY DOW, PHD, RN, FAAN
Professor, School of Nursing;
Beat and Jill Kahli Endowed Chair in Oncology Nursing
College of Health and Public Affairs
University of Central Florida
Orlando, Florida

MOSBY

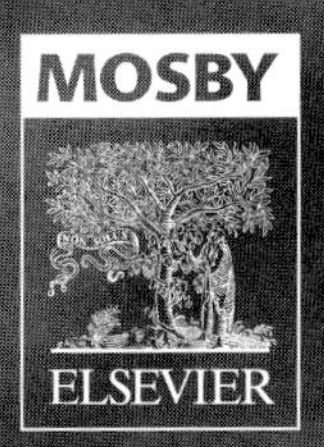

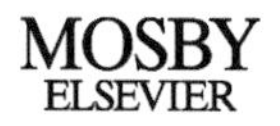

11830 Westline Industrial Drive
St. Louis, Missouri 63146

Nursing Care of Women with Cancer

ISBN-13: 978-0-323-03639-9
ISBN-10: 0-323-03639-2

Notice

Knowledge and best practice in this field are constantly changing. As new research and experience broaden our knowledge, changes in practice, treatment and drug therapy may become necessary or appropriate. Readers are advised to check the most current information provided (i) on procedures featured or (ii) by the manufacturer of each product to be administered, to verify the recommended dose or formula, the method and duration of administration, and contraindications. It is the responsibility of the practitioner, relying on their own experience and knowledge of the patient, to make diagnoses, to determine dosages and the best treatment for each individual patient, and to take all appropriate safety precautions. To the fullest extent of the law, neither the Publisher nor the [Editors/Authors] [delete as appropriate] assumes any liability for any injury and/or damage to persons or property arising out or related to any use of the material contained in this book.

The Publisher

FIRST EDITION

ISBN-13: 978-0-323-03639-9

ISBN-10: 0-323-03639-2

Executive Publisher: Barbara Nelson Cullen
Acquisition Editor: Sandra Clark Brown
Senior Developmental Editor: Sophia Oh Gray
Publishing Services Manager: Deborah L. Vogel
Senior Project Manager: Steve Ramay
Designer: Jyotika Shroff

Printed in the United States of America
Last digit is the print number: 9 8 7 6 5 4 3 2 1

This book is dedicated to women with cancer who enrich our understanding about surviving cancer, to nursing colleagues who share that wisdom with others, and to my daughter Lauren and my family for always being there.

Acknowledgments

It takes patience, perseverance, pride, and plain hard work to bring a book to publication. I wish to gratefully acknowledge all who have contributed their time, resources, energy, and insights into the writing, editing, and publishing of this text. A special thanks to our expert contributors who graciously gave up their meager free time to write and submit their chapters, to Sophia Oh Gray at Elsevier who guided us through the entire project, to Patrick McNees and Victoria Loerzel who are generous to a fault; and to Sharon Austin, Thalia Basora Montes, and Lauren Hassey for their good humor and endurance in coordinating the enormous number of letters, e-mails, and telephone calls during the entire project.

Contributors

Jane M. Armer, PhD, RN
Professor
Sinclair School of Nursing
University of Missouri at Columbia
Columbia, Missouri;
Director
Nursing Research
Ellis Fischel Cancer Center
Columbia, Missouri
12. Lymphedema

Lisa Begg, DrPH, RN
Director of Research Programs
Office of Research on Women's Health
Office of the National Institute of Health Director
National Institutes of Health
Bethesda, Maryland
1. Women's Health and Cancer

Ann M. Berger, PhD, RN, AOCN
Associate Professor and Niedfelt Nursing Professor;
Advanced Practice Nurse
University of Nebraska Medical Center
College of Nursing
Omaha, Nebraska
19. Sleep and Wakefulness

Cheryl Brohard-Holbert, MSN, RN, AOCN
Clinical Integration Plan Coordinator
M.D. Anderson Cancer Center Orlando
Orlando, Florida
23. Work Considerations

Linda Burhansstipanov, MSPH, DrPH, CHES
Executive Director
Native American Cancer Research
Pine, Colorado
27. American Indian and Alaska Native Women and Cancer

Angeline Bushy, PhD, RN, FAAN
Professor and Bert Fish Chair
Community Health Nursing
University of Central Florida
School of Nursing—Daytona Regional Campus
Daytona Beach, Florida
29. Rural Women and Cancer

Kristin L. Campbell, BSc, PT, MSc, PhD(c)
Physical Therapist
Cross Cancer Institute
Edmonton, Alberta, Canada
20. Physical Activity in Women Cancer Survivors

Patricia A. Carter, PhD, RN, CNS
Assistant Professor
The University of Texas at Austin
School of Nursing
Austin, Texas
15. Anxiety and Depression

Carol Cherry, MSN, RNC, OCN
Project Manager
Family Risk Assessment Program
Fox Chase Cancer Center
Philadelphia, Pennsylvania
7. Ovarian Cancer

LYNN CLOUTIER, RN, MSN, AOCN, ACNP
Inpatient Nurse Practitioner
M.D. Anderson Cancer Center
Houston, Texas
8. Endometrial, Vulvar, and Vaginal Cancers

KERRY S. COURNEYA, PHD
Professor and Canada Research Chair in Physical Activity and Cancer
Faculty of Physical Education
Edmonton, Alberta, Canada
20. Physical Activity in Women Cancer Survivors

REGINA S. CUNNINGHAM, PHD, RN, AOCN
Assistant Professor Family Medicine—Research Division
Robert Wood Johnson Medical School
Piscataway, New Jersey;
Chief Nursing Officer
The Cancer Institute of New Jersey
New Brunswick, New Jersey
5. Breast Cancer

GEORGIA M. DECKER, RN, MS, CS-ANP, CN, AOCN
Founder and Nurse Practitioner
Integrative Care, NP, PC
Albany, New York
21. Complementary and Alternative Medicine (CAM)

LISA HOLLAND DOWNS, MSN, RN, CPNP
Nurse Practitioner
Hospital of the University of Pennsylvania
Philadelphia, Pennsylvania
10. Non-Hodgkin's Lymphoma

MARGARET I. FITCH, RN, PHD
Assistant Professor
Faculty of Nursing
University of Toronto
Ontario, Canada;
Head Oncology Nursing and Support Care
Toronto Sunnybrook Regional Cancer Centre
Sunnybrook and Women's Health Science Centre
Toronto, Canada
22. Spouse and Family Considerations

TRACY K. GOSSELIN-ACOMB, RN, MSN, AOCN
Clinical Associate
Duke University School of Nursing
Durham, North Carolina;
Director
Department of Radiation Oncology
Duke University Health System
Durham, North Carolina
9. Colorectal Cancer

MARILYN L. HAAS, PHD, RN, CNS, ANP-C
Nurse Practitioner
Mountain Radiation Oncology
Asheville, North Carolina
4. Lung Cancer

MAUREEN B. HUHMANN, MS, RD
Instructor
University of Medicine and Dentistry of New Jersey
Newark, New Jersey;
Clinical Dietitian
The Cancer Institute of New Jersey
New Brunswick, New Jersey
18. Nutrition

DIANNE N. ISHIDA, PHD, APRN
Associate Professor
University of Hawaii at Manoa
School of Nursing and Dental Hygiene
Honolulu, Hawaii
26. Asian Women and Cancer

JEAN F. JENKINS, PHD, RN, FAAN
Senior Clinical Advisor
Office of the Director
National Human Genome Research Institute
National Institute of Health
Bethesda, Maryland
3. Genetic and Genomic Information

KRISTINA H. KARVINEN, BA, MA, PHD(C)
Faculty of Physical Education and Recreation
University of Alberta
Edmonton, Alberta, Canada
20. Physical Activity in Women Cancer Survivors

JUNG-WON LIM, MSW, PHD(C)
Doctoral Student;
Research Assistant
University of South California
Los Angeles, California
2. Advocacy for Women with Cancer

VICTORIA WOCHNA LOERZEL, MSN, RN, OCN
Instructor;
Project Director, Breast Cancer Education Intervention
University of Central Florida
School of Nursing
Orlando, Florida
24. Hidden Populations of Women

SUZANNE M. MAHON, RN, DNSC, AOCN, APNG
Assistant Clinical Professor
Department of Internal Medicine
School of Medicine;
Associate Clinical Professor
Adult Nursing
Edward and Margaret Daisy College of Health Sciences
Saint Louis University
St. Louis, Missouri
11. Osteoporosis and Cancer

VIRGINIA R. MARTIN, RN, MSN, AOCN
Clinical Director
Ambulatory Care
Fox Chase Cancer Center
Philadelphia, Pennsylvania
7. Ovarian Cancer

MARGARET L. MCNEELY, BSC, PT, MSCPT, PHD(C)
Sessional Instructor
Therapeutic Exercise
Department of Physical Therapy
Rehabilitation Medicine Faculty
University of Alberta
Edmonton, Alberta, Canada;
Physical Therapist
Cross Cancer Institute
Edmonton, Alberta, Canada
20. Physical Activity in Women Cancer Survivors

PATRICK MCNEES, PHD
Research Project Consultant, Breast Cancer Education Intervention
Co-investigator, Fertility in Young Breast Cancer Survivors: A Web-based Study;
Research Associate, Doctoral Program in Public Affairs
University of Central Florida
Orlando, Florida
14. Chronic Wounds

JUDITH KEHS MUCH, CPNP, APRN-BC, MSN
Oncology Nurse Practitioner
The Cancer Institute of New Jersey
New Brunswick, New Jersey
13. Aches, Pain, and Neuropathy

RITA MUSANTI, MSN, APRN-BC, AOCN
Advanced Practice Nurse
Cancer Institute of New Jersey
New Brunswick, New Jersey
17. Fatigue

LUTCHMIE NARINE, PHD, MSC, BSC
Associate Professor and Director of the Master of Health Administration Program
University of North Carolina at Charlotte
Charlotte, North Carolina
25. African American Women and Cancer

JUDITH A. SHELL, RN, PHD, AOCN
Medical Family Therapist;
Marriage and Family Therapist
Osceola Cancer Center
Kissimmee, Florida
16. Body Image and Sexual Functioning

ALICE SPINELLI, MSN, AOCN
Gynecologic/Oncology Nurse Practitioner and Clinical Nurse Specialist
Holmes Regional Medical Center
Melbourne, Florida
6. Cervical Cancer

CARRIE TOMPKINS STRICKER, MSN, CRNP, AOCN
Oncology Nurse Practitioner
Hospital of the University of Pennsylvania
Philadelphia, Pennsylvania
10. Non-Hodgkin's Lymphoma

GLORIA VELEZ-BARONE, ARNP, MSN, AOCN
Clinical Nurse Specialist
Oncology and Pain Management Services
Parrish Medical Center
Titusville, Florida
28. Latino Women and Cancer

MARGARET CHAMBERLAIN WILMOTH, PHD, MSS, RN
Professor
Department of Adult Health Nursing
School of Nursing
College of Health and Human Services
University of North Carolina at Charlotte
Charlotte, North Carolina
25. African American Women and Cancer

BRAD ZEBRACK, PHD, MSW, MPH
Assistant Professor
University of Southern California
School of Social Work
Los Angeles, California
2. Advocacy for Women with Cancer

Reviewers

Mary Magee Gullatte, MN, RN, AANP, AOCN
Director of Nursing
Oncology and Transplant Services
Emory University Hospitals and Winship Cancer Institute
Atlanta, Georgia

Maureen E. O'Rourke, RN, PhD
Associate Clinical Professor of Nursing
University of North Carolina—Greensboro
Greensboro, North Carolina;
Adjunct Assistant Professor of Medicine, Hematology/Oncology
Wake Forest University School of Medicine
Winston-Salem, North Carolina

Noemi Salcido, RN, BSN
Oncology Clinical Research
El Paso Cancer Treatment Center
El Paso, Texas

Patti Simmons, RN, MN, CHPN
Assistant Professor of Nursing
North Georgia College and State University
Dahlonega, Georgia

Preface

Typically, when we talk about women and cancer, we most often consider women with breast and/or gynecologic cancer. Less often do we consider how women are affected by other common cancers such as lung or colorectal cancer or lymphoma. The purpose of the first edition of this textbook is to address other cancers affecting women and to explore the larger framework of women's health and women's cancers.

The book is organized into six sections. The first section places women and cancer within the global perspective of women's health, advocacy for women with cancer, and changes in our genomic era. The second section reviews and provides an update on the pathophysiology, diagnosis, and treatment for nine major cancers affecting women including lung, breast, cervical, ovarian, endometrial, vulvar, vaginal, colorectal cancer, and non-Hodgkin's lymphoma. The third section examines common physical and psychosocial effects of cancer treatment paying particular attention to current evidence-based interventions and explores research directions. With the larger number of cancer survivors, the fourth section explores ways to maintain health after cancer with regards to sleep and rest, physical activity, and complementary and alternative therapies. The fifth section examines the impact of cancer in women on family and social lives. Family concerns, work, finances, and insurance issues have a major impact on women with cancer. Our final section focuses on ways to reach culturally and ethnically diverse women with cancer.

The appendices contain additional resources, including a drug index of the major agents used in treatment of the aforementioned cancers, assessment tools for evaluating symptoms and quality of life, and a listing of national and community agencies dedicated to helping women with cancer.

We are most fortunate to have an impressive group of contributing authors representing a wide range of experts in practice, education and research who have generously shared their wisdom in practice, pearls in education, and research findings.

-KHD

Contents

VI. Reaching Culturally and Ethnically Diverse Women

Appendix

UNIT I

Women and Cancer: A Global Perspective

CHAPTER

1 Women's Health and Cancer

Lisa Begg

INTRODUCTION

Women's health as a global concept includes many different disorders in addition to cancer. For example, although tuberculosis (TB) is essentially controlled within the United States, it represents 2% of all deaths in women worldwide, more than any maternal cause or even breast cancer mortality.[1] It should be noted that TB kills more young women than any other disease.[1] Of interest is that there is variation in detection rates between men and women, because case detection through sputum microscopy appears to be less sensitive in detecting TB in women compared to men. Malaria is another major cause of morbidity and mortality throughout the world, with over 50% of the world's population being exposed to this disease.[2]

The worldwide face of human immunodeficiency virus/acquired immunodeficiency syndrome (HIV/AIDS) is also changing, with women increasingly at risk for acquiring and dying from this disease. Globally, slightly less than half of all people living with HIV/AIDS are female, and the percentage continues to increase. Major increases in cases are being observed in Eastern Europe, Asia, and Latin America, and the association between class inequality, gender, violence and HIV has prompted policy-makers and governmental officials to conclude that different prevention programs must be devised and undertaken to stem this epidemic.[3]

The global burden of cancer is now receiving major attention as countries around the world seek to form innovative partnerships to address their specific needs as well as respond to those of the international community. The World Health Organization (WHO) estimates that more than 10 million people are diagnosed with all forms of cancer each year, and it is projected that this number will increase to 15 million annual new cancer cases by the year 2020.[4] Currently, cancer causes over 6 million deaths annually, or about 12% of the total deaths worldwide. The human and economic burden of cancer is expected to grow substantially in the next 20 years, with the total cancer deaths increasing to 10 million a year.[4]

These trends for women's health and cancer have major implications for nurses, for it has been stated that nursing is key to accomplishing almost anything related to the needs of cancer patients.[5] To advance the discussion of ways that nursing can substantially contribute, this chapter will provide a historical perspective of cancer globally and a discussion of the impact that it is having on international women's health, the current issues of importance, and the implications for nursing practice, research, and education. Internationally there is much discussion about the status of women's health in general, especially as it relates to several contexts: the cultural milieu that is affecting the HIV/AIDS pandemic, violence against women, the interplay between women's health and poverty, women's acknowledged lack of control in decision-making, and the overall health status of girls and women globally.[6]

Consistent with the figures cited above, cancer in women is a major cause of morbidity and mortality across the globe. In describing international rates for cancer incidence and mortality, most references use the terms "developing" countries versus "developed" countries. The former term describes "resource-poor" countries such as those found in Eastern Europe, sub-Saharan Africa, Latin America, and parts of Asia. The latter term, developed countries, includes the United States, Western Europe, Canada, and Australia.[7] Countries in this latter category have established health care infrastructure at all levels of the population and possess sufficient resources with which to develop a variety of cancer programs for their citizens.

Internationally, the five most common types of cancer in women are breast, cervix, stomach, lung, and colorectal.[8] There is considerable international variation in incidence for these five sites, a fact that can provide clues into the underlying etiology of these different forms of cancer. For example, breast and cervical cancers are more common in Europe and South America, in part because women in these countries have adopted more westernized lifestyles in terms of dietary consumption patterns, reproductive factors, and levels of physical activity.[8] Within Europe, breast cancer is the most common cancer in women, accounting for 27.4% of all female cancer cases. It also leads in cancer mortality in women, with 130,000 deaths per year.[9] In contrast, stomach cancer, whose incidence is declining in European countries, is still predominant in Asian populations, including in women.[9] Lung cancer is increasingly seen in women worldwide, based on their increased use of tobacco products. There are more than 1 million people dying of lung cancer worldwide, almost half of them in developing countries. Overall, women accounted for slightly more than 25% of all lung cancer deaths.[10] Since most of these deaths are directly attributable to tobacco use, it is estimated that the number of tobacco-related deaths, including lung cancer, will approach 10 million deaths annually by the year 2030. The largest increases will come from the less developed countries.[11] In addition to providing etiologic clues, these international variations in cancer incidence also provide opportunities to undertake global cancer control interventions.

There is general agreement that the purpose of cancer control is to reduce the burden of cancer. Cancer control consists of a broad range of interventions, including primary prevention, early detection and screening, treatment, palliative care and quality of life.[5] Because of the underlying importance of research, the National Cancer Institute (NCI) defines cancer control science as "the conduct of basic and applied research in behavioral, social, and population sciences to create or enhance interventions that, independently or in combination with biomedical approaches, reduce cancer risk, incidence, morbidity and mortality, and improves the quality of life."[12]

On a global level, cancer control uses public health approaches that are aimed at reducing the causes and subsequent consequences of cancer through a variety of translational efforts, such as chemoprevention for high-risk populations and targeted communication for smoking cessation. Two examples included now….

HISTORICAL PERSPECTIVE

The International Agency for Research on Cancer (IARC) was established in May 1965 through the XVIIIth World Health Assembly, as an extension of the WHO.[13] IARC's founding members were the Federal Republic of Germany, France, Italy, the United Kingdom, and the United States. The current IARC membership numbers 16 countries, including the original five countries and Australia, Belgium, Canada, Denmark, Finland, Japan, Norway, Spain, Sweden, and Switzerland. IARC coordinates and conducts both epidemiologic and laboratory research into the causes of cancer; its activities include monitoring global cancer occurrence, identifying the causes of cancer, elucidating mechanisms of carcinogenesis, and developing scientific strategies for cancer control.

Using these 15 global leaders, additional infrastructure has been established within each of these countries as well as among them that facilitates the training of international health ministry officials and providers, together with the coordination of alert/reporting systems so that strategic information can be shared quickly and efficiently. Two notable examples are the Centers for Disease Control and Prevention (CDC) and the National Institutes of Health (NIH), two agencies within the U.S. Department of Health and Human Services. Both of these agencies have substantial cancer-related programs and distinguished track records in training cadres of international health officials and scientists and generally advancing the global health network.

The IARC programs are aimed at finding global approaches to preventing cancer, including both primary prevention and the early detection methods. WHO and IARC seek to promote and strengthen comprehensive national cancer control programs throughout the world. These two organizations focus on building and expanding international networks and partnerships for cancer control, and especially to create low-cost approaches to respond to global needs for pain relief and palliative care.

Employing the WHO terminology, the current framework for global cancer services is expected to include primary prevention, secondary prevention or screening, and improved diagnosis, treatment, and palliative care.[13] Examples of each of these areas will be described later in the chapter. Within this global approach, however, is the recognition of a problem that is more crucial for those governing in developing countries. For those officials, initiating cancer detection and screening programs must be undertaken within the context of *comprehensive* cancer control programs. Specifically, the health care providers in each country must be able to follow up on any suspicious findings in order to obtain truly beneficial screening outcomes. It has come to be recognized that well-meaning efforts to screen citizens in developing countries are deprived of any beneficial outcomes if the interventions are not part of a continuum of care.[13]

CURRENT ISSUES OF MAJOR IMPORTANCE

Global Health Partnerships

Most of the major international issues regarding cancer revolve around increased public health cooperation among the IARC sponsor countries and their health agencies, the globalization of commerce, the increasing interdependency of countries including those of the European Union (EU), trends in cancer incidence and mortality, and common risk factors such as tobacco use. For example, tobacco use is associated with numerous cancers and other adverse outcomes, from premature or underweight births to cardiovascular disease, and curbing the use of tobacco products has been the object of unprecedented international efforts.[14] Thus tobacco use broadly affects women's health across the life span and the health-illness continuum. It also holds a unique place in terms of preventive health behaviors, which have the potential for reducing the number of new cancers worldwide. The cooperation achieved through stewarding international efforts to reduce tobacco use has translated into innovative partnerships across the health care and research continuum.[14]

In the late 1990s, and then after the terrorist attacks of September 11, 2001, countries and their health agencies increased their formal and informal country-to-country linkages in order to investigate and combat a new array of emerging infections that have the potential to devastate entire regions of the world or to interfere with global travel and commerce.[15] An additional motivation for these key countries was the recognition that they needed to construct real-time networks that incorporated health surveillance and law enforcement in order to prevent, or respond to, global bioterrorism threats. The growing pandemic that HIV/AIDS has become has also necessitated the expansion of surveillance and treatment systems worldwide.[3] One good example of these partnerships is the role that the Pan American Health Organization (PAHO) is playing by partnering with a variety of governmental agencies to combat HIV/AIDS in Latin American and the Caribbean, which has also benefited international cancer control efforts.[16]

International commerce has undergone significant changes in the last two decades with the increased number of multinational corporations, the trans-shipment of food products from distant locations and the mass production of foods outside of traditional country borders. In addition, the emergence of a strong and expanded EU has brought uniformity across most of Europe, including in programs focusing on health and health care. The expanding role of the World Bank in addressing poverty and supporting the advancement of developing countries is also being used to upgrade the capacity of these countries to create viable cancer control programs.[17] All of these global trends and developments set the stage for the adoption of the *WHO Framework Convention on Tobacco Control (FCTC)*.[18]

WHO Framework Convention on Tobacco Control

The 2003 FCTC was the first treaty negotiated under the auspices of the WHO.[18] In the making for many years, the FCTC was developed in response to the globalization of the tobacco epidemic and an acknowledgment that tobacco use caused numerous adverse health outcomes to people of all ages, races, and socioeconomic levels. Evidence against tobacco use had been building, including its cross-border effects, the effect of trade liberalization on tobacco use, the global marketing of tobacco products and the transnational nature of tobacco advertising, promotion, and sponsorship, and the direct foreign investment in the international manufacture of cigarettes and other tobacco products. To date, shared responsibility for ratifying this treaty has yielded 168 signatories who are members of WHO or the United Nations.[18]

Tobacco As a Risk Factor. Over the past 40 years, a tremendous amount of research has been conducted and reported on tobacco use that demonstrates the variety of adverse health outcomes in both men and women, related both to cancer and to other conditions, that are directly due to tobacco products.[21] In the American Cancer Society *Cancer Facts and Figures 2005*, it is clearly stated that "all cancers caused by smoking can be prevented completely."[19] Over forty years ago, the U.S. Surgeon General's (SG) report indicated that cigarette smoking was deleterious to a person's health.[20] In the ensuing years, each SG report has expanded on the impact of tobacco use on a variety of cancers, along with how it affects cardiovascular and pulmonary diseases; the evidence is incontrovertible that preventing the onset of smoking, or facilitating the quitting of smoking, will reduce tobacco-related deaths by substantial numbers worldwide.[21] WHO estimates that tobacco kills nearly 5 million people in the world every year, a figure that includes cancers as well as pulmonary and cardiac-related conditions.[22] In terms of sex differences, it is estimated that men account for 1 billion smokers, and women for 250 million smokers worldwide. More worrisome, the rates of tobacco use continue to increase in developing countries so that by the year 2025, 500 million women are expected to be active cigarette smokers.[19]

Women and Smoking. To address the issue of women's health and its connection to tobacco use, the NCI, other federal partners and private foundations hosted a working group meeting in February 2003. The 2003 meeting was a follow-up to the 2001 report of the Surgeon General, *Women and Smoking*, which identified several strategies to reduce smoking among women.[23] The 2003 NCI report, entitled *Women, Tobacco and Cancer: An Agenda for the 21st Century*,[24] identified gaps and research priorities in this area. Specifically, the 2003 report seeks to (1) increase understanding of sex and gender differences* across the broad range of research on women, tobacco, and cancer; (2) develop new and more effective interventions to prevent and treat the effects of tobacco use and environmental tobacco smoke (ETS) exposure especially among women and girls, the populations at greatest risk; (3) ensure the widespread delivery of these interventions; (4) harness and expand partnerships, networks, and innovative research platforms to design and launch board-based strategies to eliminate the harms of tobacco use and ETS exposure; and (5) improve national and global evaluation and surveillance of the harms of tobacco use and ETS exposure and of women's and girls' knowledge, attitudes, and behaviors

*Sex and gender differences are defined as follows, based on the 2001 IOM report:[46] The definition of sex is the classification of living things, generally as male or female, according to their reproductive organs and functions assigned by the individual's gender presentation. Gender is shaped by environment and experience.

related to tobacco use and harms.[24] The NCI continues to implement a variety of programs and policies related to the recommendations from this meeting.

Obesity

Obesity, once thought to be prevalent only in developed countries, is now being recognized as a global epidemic and related to many adverse health outcomes including a variety of cancers.[25] Obesity is defined by using body mass index (BMI), which is calculated by taking a person's weight in kilograms and dividing it by the square of the height in meters (kg/m2). A person whose BMI is over 30 is defined as obese. One whose BMI falls between 25 and 30 is considered overweight.[26] Within the United States, obesity has developed into a true epidemic, with resulting adverse health outcomes such as type 2 diabetes, in both adolescents and adults, and heart disease, and is a strong risk factor for certain cancers such as breast and endometrial cancers in women, and kidney, gallbladder, and colon cancers in both women and men.[27] Women exhibit higher rates of obesity than do men.[28] Obesity is also associated with depression, stigma, and discrimination. WHO has now begun to publicize global data that indicate more than 1 billion overweight adults and at least 300 million others who are considered clinically obese.[26] As shown by the U.S. data, obesity and overweight also contribute to several other chronic diseases such as stroke and hypertension and disability. Ironically, obesity has even been observed to coexist in developing countries with undernutrition.[26] In a 2002 WHO report, the presence of multiple risk factors such as obesity, smoking, high blood pressure, and high blood cholesterol was estimated to contribute to 58% of the diabetes observed, 21% of ischemic heart disease cases, and 8% to 42% of certain cancers.[29] Closely related to obesity are physical activity and dietary consumption patterns. Most global reports focus on body weight rather than on physical activity patterns. The recent IARC report concentrates on evaluating all three dimensions, in a further effort to reduce cancer risk, incidence, and mortality.[30]

Palliative Care

The Institute of Medicine (IOM) defines palliative care in a broad sense as the total care of the body, mind, and spirit; it also involves giving support to the entire family, basically from the time of diagnosis onward.[31] The IOM statement indicated that the purpose of palliative care is to prevent or lessen the severity of pain and accomplish symptom management for a range of problems to maximally improve the person's quality of life. The Oncology Nursing Society (ONS) has focused on a broader range of symptoms that nurses can seek to alleviate with palliative care, including chemotherapy-induced nausea and vomiting, hematologic toxicities, cancer therapy–induced diarrhea, oral mucositis, anorexia, fatigue, depression, sleep disturbance, and cognitive dysfunction.[32-36]

In 2002, the NIH contributed guidance when it issued a "State-of-the-Science" statement on three key cancer-related symptoms: pain, depression, and fatigue.[37] The NIH statement acknowledged that numerous scientific advances have led to cancer becoming increasingly a chronic condition. This change, positive as it may be, raises important issues about the quality of life and quality of care for those persons surviving their initial diagnosis and the impact of cancer on the family unit. The expert panel charged with evaluating the current research base for these three symptoms found definitive data lacking in all three areas, and proposed that more research be funded by NIH to improve the basic descriptive epidemiology of pain, depression, and fatigue. They also concluded that too many cancer patients with pain, depression, and fatigue receive inadequate treatment for their symptoms.[37]

Because chronic pain secondary to cancer is now recognized as a global problem, WHO is leading additional efforts to address this issue in many countries.[38] In addition, some chronic pain conditions are now being recognized as occurring more often in women than in men.[39] Treatments for chronic cancer pain can include medication, acupuncture or relaxation techniques, local electrical stimulation or brain stimulation, psychotherapy or behavior modification therapies, surgery, or combinations of any of these modalities.

Survivorship

Based on NCI definitions, an individual is considered a cancer survivor from the time of diagnosis through the balance of his or her life.[40] Research into this area encompasses the short- and long-term physical, psychosocial, and economic consequences of cancer from diagnosis and treatment onward. Survivorship also includes care provided in a variety of settings and at all levels of health. Ultimately, the goal of cancer survivorship research is to improve the quality of life for the survivor and family, and to provide guidelines for optimal follow-up care. In addition to the areas cited above, survivorship research also evaluates whether health disparities exist in the form of socioeconomic factors such as minority status and geographic location.[40]

The President's Cancer Panel of the NCI issued a report in 2004 that presented issues affecting cancer survivors across the life span entitled, *Living Beyond Cancer: Finding a New Balance.*[41] This report cited several additional areas needing evaluation, such as complications and side effects on the heart and damage on other organs, infertility secondary to treatment, the development of second cancers, cognitive dysfunction, employment issues, and difficulties with health, disability, and life insurance eligibility. The report also included a commentary on unique aspects of European-based cancer care compared to the health care provided to cancer patients in the United States. Based on regional interviews, it appears that certain European countries are now including rehabilitation services as a standard part of cancer treatment, and expanded resources for families of children undergoing cancer treatment (Sweden), integrated psychosocial programs after treatment that last 3 to 6 months (the Netherlands), and paying family members to provide hospice care to their loved ones (Denmark). Northern Ireland established a 6-week post-treatment rehabilitation program for breast cancer patients to aid them in making the transition from acute care to life after cancer diagnosis.[41] It should be noted that all of these reports acknowledge the important role of the caregiver and the need for all health providers to work in partnership with the patient and family to maximize long-term quality of life.

Cervical Cancer and Human Papillomaviruses

Cervical cancer, one major cancer with a worldwide impact on women's health, causes more than 200,000 deaths annually around the globe, making it the second most common cause of cancer mortality in women worldwide.[42] A wealth of scientific evidence has shown that virtually all cases of this cancer are attributable to cervical infection by a subset of human papillomaviruses (HPV). About one half of cervical cancer is attributable to HPV-16 infection. The second most frequent type, HPV-18, accounts for another 10% to 20% of these cancers. HPV infection, predominantly HPV-16, also appears to cause most anal cancers, as well as a proportion of vulvar and head and neck cancers.[43,44]

An effective HPV vaccine should be able to reduce the incidence of cancers attributable to HPV infection.[45] Further evidence of the role that HPV plays in humans is the decision in 2004 by the National Toxicology Program to classify HPV strains 16 and 18 as carcinogenic to humans based on sufficient evidence in humans.[46] Vaccine clinical trials are currently underway, and if these clinical trials prove effective, there would be a reduction in deaths secondary to this cancer of approximately 150,000 women each year.[45] There is also growing evidence of the link between HIV/AIDS and HPV infections.[47] Globally, HIV/ AIDS is a major health problem for women. Recent research reports confirm that women who are HIV-positive are often coinfected with HPV. In these women, the HPV infection is more likely to be persistent and less likely to regress.[47]

In terms of a unifying theory, research on cervical cancer was further advanced by the 2004 SG report,[21] indicating there was sufficient current evidence to support a causal link between smoking and cervical cancer. This documented linkage has proven to be a motivator to the partner IARC nations, because it has spurred renewed efforts to prevent cervical cancer through vaccine development and clinical trials of vaccines.

Vaccines have been shown to prevent precancers.[45] HPV, a sexually transmitted disease, is documented in countries where cervical cancer is common, like Costa Rica. Researchers have created formal partnerships between government officials and researchers to evaluate ways to prevent cervical cancer.[44] Other areas of the world where the rate of cervical cancer remain high are South America, Eastern Africa, and India, and slightly lower rates are observed in Mexico.[42]

There are other examples of infections leading to various cancers, especially internationally. Two such examples include the association between *Helicobacter pylori* infection and stomach cancer, which is the fourth most common cancer worldwide.[4] The American Cancer Society estimates that about 60% of gastric cancers in developing countries are related to *H. pylori* infection.[19] Another example of a relationship between infections and cancer incidence is the association between chronic infection with hepatitis B virus and primary liver cancer[48] that accounts for fully 35% of all hepatocellular carcinoma (HCC) worldwide.

IMPLICATIONS FOR NURSING

Cancer is increasingly a global health problem that intersects with multiple conditions that affect women. Moreover, the world's peoples are becoming more and more interdependent in terms of international commerce, travel, lifestyle factors, and health outcomes. The U.S. Department of State now considers the health aspects to many of its foreign policy initiatives because of the increasing importance of health to international issues. The global use of tobacco products is just one example of how these factors intersect and the economic and health impact on diverse populations.

While infectious diseases such as malaria, TB, and HIV/AIDS are still widespread throughout many areas of the world, chronic diseases such as cancer are becoming more common in the developing world. The international health agencies such as WHO and its affiliates are now forming country-to-country networks to address these trends and to establish appropriate surveillance and care delivery systems.

For some health behaviors such as smoking, the contribution from the developing countries is becoming a significant proportion of the total global numbers. What does this mean for nurses who are working with women and men at risk for cancer, or who are caring for patients already diagnosed with cancer? In many respects, the world has come to America. The U.S. population is increasingly diverse in terms of country of origin, race, and ethnicity. Because of the chronic shortage of registered nurses in the United States, the nurse workforce is becoming increasing diverse as health care employers recruit nurses from overseas to meet their staffing needs. There appears to be a freer flow of information back and forth, as evidenced by the international contributions to complex subjects as palliative care, pain control, and tobacco control. Fortunately, there are now nursing organizations across the globe so that any nurse can establish ties with her counterparts anywhere in the world. The expanded use of the Internet and the global networks are making it more efficient and easier for nurses to communicate with one another to educate women and girls about cancer, its risk factors, and ways to prevent cancer or to detect it at the earliest stage, and to enhance care and quality of life for patients and their families.

REFERENCES

1. Maher D, Raviglione M. Global epidemiology of tuberculosis, *Clin Chest Med* 26:167-182, 2005.
2. Breman JG, Alilio MS, Mills A: Conquering the intolerable burden of malaria: what's new, what's needed: a summary, *Am J Trop Med Hyg* 71:1-15, 2004.
3. The Joint United Nations Programme on HIV/AIDS (UNAIDS): *2004 Report on the global HIV/AIDS epidemic: 4th global report*, Geneva, 2004, World Health Organization.
4. World Health Organization: *Global Action Against Cancer Now—Updated edition*, Geneva, 2005, World Health Organization.
5. Alliance for Global Cancer Control: *June 3, 2003 Meeting summary,*— Joint Report, World Health Organization and International Union Against Cancer. World Health Organization, Geneva, and the International Union Against Cancer, Lyon, France.
6. Ogden L and others: Impact of HIV on women internationally, *Emerg Infect Dis* 10:2032-2033, 2004.

7. World Health Organization: *National cancer control programmes: policies and managerial guidelines,* ed 2, Geneva, 2002, World Health Organization.
8. Boyle P, Ferlay J: Cancer incidence and mortality in Europe, 2004, *Ann Oncol* 16:481, 2005.
9. Parkin DM and others: Global cancer statistics, 2002, *CA Cancer J Clin* 55:74-108, 2005.
10. Mathers CD and others: Global patterns of healthy life expectancy in the year 2002, *BMC Public Health* 4:66, 2004.
11. Mathers CD and others: Counting the dead and what they died from: an assessment of the global status of cause of death data, *Bull World Health Organ* 83:171-177, 2005.
12. Best A, Hiatt RA, Cameron R, Rimer BK, Abrams DB. The Evolution of cancer Control Research: An International Perspective from Canada and the United States. *Cancer Epidemiol Biomarkers Prev.* 12(8):705-712, 2003.
13. International Agency for Research on Cancer: On the Web at www.iarc.fr/ENG/General/membership.php; accessed 3/31/2005.
14. Shafey O, Dolwick S, Guindon GE, editors: *Tobacco control country profiles 2003,* Atlanta, 2003, American Cancer Society.
15. Epstein, Daniel: September 11: everything changed, *Mag Pan Am Health Org* 6(2):2002.
16. Hitt E: Cancer in the Americas, *Lancet Oncol* 4:9, 2003.
17. Levine R, Schneidman M, Glassman A: *The health of women in Latin America and the Caribbean,* The International Bank for Reconstruction and Development, World Bank headquartered in Washington, D.C., 2001.
18. World Health Organization: *WHO Framework Convention on Tobacco Control,* Geneva, Switzerland, 2003, updated reprint 2004.
19. American Cancer Society: *Cancer facts and figures 2005,* Atlanta, 2005, American Cancer Society.
20. U.S. Department of Health, Education, and Welfare, Public Health Service: *Smoking and health: report of the Advisory Committee to the Surgeon General of the Public Health Service,* 1964, Public Health Service Publication No. 1103.
21. U.S. Department of Health and Human Services: *The health consequences of smoking: a report of the Surgeon General—Executive Summary,* 2004, U.S. Department of Health and Human Services, Centers for Disease Control and Prevention, National Center for Chronic Disease Prevention and Health Promotion, Office on Smoking and Health.
22. Tobacco Free Initiative and the Global Tobacco Research Network*: The tobacco atlas,* produced by the World Health Organization, Geneva, 2002.
23. U.S. Department of Health and Human Services: *Women and smoking,* 2001, U.S. Department of Health and Human Services, Centers for Disease Control and Prevention, National Center for Chronic Disease Prevention and Health Promotion, Office on Smoking and Health.
24. U.S. Department of Health and Human Services: *Women, tobacco, and cancer: an agenda for the 21st century,* 2004, U.S. Department of Health and Human Services, National Institutes of Health, National Cancer Institute (NIH Publication No. 04-5599).
25. Vainio H, Kaaks R, Bianchini F: Weight control and physical activity in cancer prevention: international evaluation of the evidence, *Eur J Cancer Prev* 11:S94-S100, 2002.
26. Bray GA: Evaluation of obesity. Who are the obese? *Postgrad Med* 114:19-27, 38, 2003.
27. Pender JR, Pories WJ: Epidemiology of obesity in the United States, *Gastroenterol Clin North Am* 34:1-7, 2005.
28. Centers for Disease Control and Prevention: Overweight and obesity: obesity trends: U.S. obesity trends 1985–2003. CDC on the Web at http://www.cdc.gov/nccdphp/dnpa/obesity/trend/obesity_trends_2003.pdf), 2003.
29. World Health Organization: *The world health report 2002 – reducing risks, promoting healthy life,* Geneva, 2002, World Health Organization.
30. World Health Organization: Process for a global strategy on diet, physical activity and health, Geneva, 2003, World Health Organization.
31. Foley KM, Gelband H, editors: *Improving palliative care for cancer,* Institute of Medicine and National Research Council, National Cancer Policy Board, Washington, D.C., 2001, National Academy Press.
32. Ropka ME, Spencer-Cisek P: PRISM: Priority symptom management project: Phase 1 Assessment, *Oncol Nurs Forum* 28(10), 1585-1594, 2001.
33. Barsevick AM, Sweeney, C, Haney, E, Chung E: A systematic qualitative analysis of psychoeducational interventions for depression in patients with cancer, *Oncol Nurs Forum* 29(1), 73-87, 2002.
34. Brown, JK: A systematic review of the evidence on symptom management of cancer-related anorexia and cachexia, *Oncol Nurs Forum* 29(3), 517-532, 2002.
35. Nail, LM: Fatigue in patients with cancer, *Oncol Nurs Forum* 29(3), 537-546, 2002.
36. Shell, JA: Evidence-based practice for symptom management in adults with cancer: Sexual dysfunction, *Oncol Nurs Forum* 29(1), 53-69, 2002.
37. National Institutes of Health State-Of-The-Science Statement on symptom management in cancer: Pain, depression and fatigue, July 15-17, 2002, Final Statement October 26, Bethesda, MD, 2002, National Institutes of Health.
38. World Health Organization, *Cancer pain release.* On the Web at www.whocancerpain.wisc.edu.
39. Dionne RA and others: Individual responder analyses for pain: does one pain scale fit all? *Trends Pharmacol Sci* 26(3):125-130, 2005.
40. Office of Cancer Survivorship: *About survivorship research: survivorship definitions,* National Cancer Institute, on the Web at http://dccps.nci.nih.gov/ocs/definitions.html; accessed on Oct 5, 2005.
41. Reuben SH, preparer for the President's Cancer Panel: *Living beyond cancer: finding a new balance, President's Cancer Panel 2003-2004 Annual Report,* Bethesda, MD, 2004, Department of Health and Human Services, National Institutes of Health, National Cancer Institute.
42. Bosch FX, de Sanjose S: Chapter 1: Human papillomavirus and cervical cancer—burden and assessment of causality, Monograph, *J Natl Cancer Inst* 31:3-13, 2003.
43. Schiller JT, Lowy DR: Papillomavirus-like particle based vaccines: cervical cancer and beyond, *Expert Opin Biol Ther* 1(4):571-581, 2001.
44. Lowy DR, Howley PM: Papillomaviruses. In Knipe DM, Howley PM, editors: *Fields Virology,* vol. 2, ed 4, Philadelphia, 2001, Lippincott Williams & Wilkins.

45. Pastrana DV and others: Reactivity of human sera in a sensitive, high-throughput pseudovirus-based papillomavirus neutralization assay for HPV 16 and HPV 18, *Virology,* 321:205-216, 2004.
46. National Toxicology Program: *Report on carcinogens,* ed 11, Research Triangle Park, NC, 2005, U.S. Department of Health and Human Services, Public Health Service.
47. Massad LS and others: HPV testing for triage of HIV-infected women with papanicolaou smears read as atypical cells of uncertain significance, *J Women's Health* 13(2):147-153, 2004.
48. Pan CQ, Zhang JX: Natural history and clinical consequences of hepatitis B virus infection, *Int J Med Sci* 2(1):36-40, 2005.

CHAPTER

2 Advocacy for Women with Cancer

Brad Zebrack and Jung-Won Lim

INTRODUCTION

In 1998, *Time* magazine profiled 100 of the most influential people of the twentieth century. Among 20 identified "leaders and revolutionaries," including Martin Luther King, Ghandi, and Ronald Reagan, were just three women: Margaret Sanger, Eleanor Roosevelt, and Margaret Thatcher.

In a testament to Margaret Sanger, Gloria Steinem[1] wrote in *Time*:

> While working as a practical nurse and midwife in the poorest neighborhoods of New York City in the years before World War I, Margaret Sanger saw women deprived of their health, sexuality and ability to care for children already born. Contraceptive information was so suppressed by clergy-influenced, physician-accepted laws that it was a criminal offense to send it through the mail. Yet the educated had access to such information and could use subterfuge to buy "French" products, which were really condoms and other barrier methods, and "feminine hygiene" products, which were really spermicides. It was this injustice that inspired Sanger to defy church and state. In a series of articles and finally through neighborhood clinics that dispensed woman-controlled forms of birth control (a phrase she coined), Sanger put information and power into the hands of women.

As for Eleanor Roosevelt, historian Doris Kearns Goodwin[2] wrote:

> She gave a voice to people who did not have access to power . . . Nowhere was Eleanor's influence greater than in civil rights. Long before the contemporary women's movement provided ideological arguments for women's rights, Eleanor instinctively challenged institutions that failed to provide equal opportunity for women. Through her speeches and her columns, she was instrumental in securing the first government funds ever allotted for the building of child-care centers. And when women workers were unceremoniously fired as the war came to an end, she fought to stem the tide. She argued on principle that everyone who wanted to work had a right to be productive, and she railed against the closing of the child-care centers as a shortsighted response to a fundamental social need. What the women workers needed, she said, was the courage to ask for their rights with a loud voice.

Although *Time* magazine saw fit to identify only three women as the most influential leaders of the twentieth century, women have contributed immensely to causes related to the alleviation of suffering for women and for all of civil society. At the turn of the twentieth century, Alice Paul and Lucy Burns fought alongside thousands of women to achieve the right to vote in the United States. For Candy Lightner, the experience of her 13-year-old son's tragic death at the hands of a drunk driver mobilized her to found the enormously popular and effective advocacy organization Mothers Against Drunk Driving. After actress Elizabeth Glazer's child was diagnosed with AIDS, she organized the Pediatric AIDS Foundation as a means of advocating on the behalf of children who rarely, if ever, have a voice to advocate for themselves.

The work of these twentieth-century advocates, along with others, represents social movements. They were activists attempting to change the physical, environmental, social, and economic conditions that contributed to the causes and exacerbations of women's suffering and oppression as well as the suffering and oppression of others.

WHAT IS ADVOCACY?

Generally speaking, advocacy may be characterized as efforts of people to come together in groups in order to resolve mutual individual needs, and may consist of individuals sharing concerns about personal, emotional, health or family problems.[3] It can be defined as the act of directly representing, defending, intervening, supporting, or recommending a course of action on behalf of one or more individuals, groups or communities.[4] This action can involve the assessment and identification of individual, group, or community characteristics that, when supported, enhanced or reversed, result in better quality of life.

> Advocacy also may involve the identification and transformation of social and/or environmental conditions that obstruct or preclude necessary and vital changes in people's lives. Furthermore, an important component of advocacy is empowerment the process whereby individuals, communities and groups increase their own capacity to influence other people and organizations that affect their lives.[5,6] These change efforts may involve pleading or speaking on behalf of others, representing another, taking action, promoting change, accessing rights and benefits, serving as a partisan, and empowering clients.

CANCER ADVOCACY

Cancer has extraordinary circumstances that affect ordinary people throughout a survivorship continuum that spans cancer prevention and screening to diagnosis and treatment and on into long-term survival or the end of life. As a result, advocacy efforts occur throughout this continuum. They involve individual interventions and family-focused support, public and professional education, and the promotion of institutional or governmental programs and policies that enhance cancer care and quality of life. Whether at the individual, professional, or community/societal level, advocates and activists in both professional and lay realms have been busy developing programs, organizing community-based patient/survivor groups and professional associations, and rallying for the implementation of laws and policies that protect the public interests where cancer and health care are concerned. Advocacy efforts can involve enhancing the awareness and ability of individuals to improve their own conditions and become advocates on their own behalf. These efforts also may involve individuals active on the behalf of others to offer support or assistance. Or, the sharing of concerns may evolve into a political awareness and coordinated action to change or influence hospital or government policies.

A Historical Perspective on Advocacy for Women with Cancer

Women's involvement in cancer advocacy may be seen as having developed in conjunction with a broader feminist movement of the 1960s, with women publicly questioning the limitations and inadequacies of a male-dominated institution of medicine. Historically, many normal physiologic conditions experienced by women (pregnancy and childbirth, premenstrual syndrome and menopause) have been medicalized and defined as health problems.[7] Recall an era when "hysteria" was a diagnosable psychiatric condition associated with menstruation. Enter thus the advocates who question these medical presumptions and pave the way for change.

Margaret Sanger's work at the turn of the twentieth century is an example of how one individual questioned societal norms and medical practices that precluded women's liberty, freedom, and access to health care information that could influence their lives and the quality of their lives. At the time, Sanger was and perhaps still is considered a radical espousing an extreme viewpoint on birth control, family planning, and abortion, and one who upset the moral and ethical underpinnings of a democratic society.

Yet, many women responded to Sanger's message. They banded together to share information, trade mutual experiences, and discuss their feelings (including the ethics and morality) about previously unspoken but very real social issues.

Radical or extreme thinking or action is only perceived as radical or extreme when compared to the current contemporary and sometimes narrow norms for appropriate social behavior. One can argue that "extreme," confrontational, or even unlawful activities like chaining oneself to a redwood tree or distributing clean syringes to injection–drug users to prevent the spread of Human Immunodeficiency Virus (HIV) and Aquired Immunodeficiency Deficiency Syndrome (AIDS) only alienate the mainstream, including those in positions of power who are the gatekeepers for change. However, it also may be true that articulating contrary positions or acting-out extends the level of public debate, making previously "liberal" or "progressive" suggestions for change seem moderate when compared or contrasted to new and "extreme" positions that get captured by the media.

Breast cancer advocates in the 1990s demonstrated that they had learned from HIV/AIDS activists, including those "extreme" approaches used by AIDS activists as part of the Act-Up (AIDS Coalition to Unleash Power) civil uprisings in the 1980s. The media coverage of this civil disobedience resulted in the extension of discussion and debate about HIV and AIDS that arguably would not have occurred without street-centered made-for-television protest. Throughout most of the 1960s, articles addressing issues related to women with breast cancer took a reassuring rather than controversial approach, making no attempt to suggest that there might be alternative treatment options and instead focusing mainly on the ways that a woman could adjust physically, psychologically, and even sexually after losing her breast.[8] Similar to AIDS activists, it took breast cancer advocates challenging the status quo before changes in breast cancer treatment and research were seen. Not until activists like Rose Kushner challenged the status quo for treatment options did things begin to change.

In 1975, journalist and cancer survivor Rose Kushner published *Why Me? What every woman should know about breast cancer to save her life.* The book represents a profound and pivotal milestone in feminist history in that Kushner's impassioned voice provoked action on a number of policy-related issues, in particular ethical problems related to cancer treatment such as the limits of mammography in detecting cancer, the dangers of irradiation, and the medical establishment's expressed need for a woman to undergo mutilating surgery.[9]

Until the 1970s, surgery was the only treatment for breast cancer. William S. Halsted (1852-1922), the first Chief of Surgery at the Johns Hopkins Hospital and School of Medicine, developed the radical mastectomy for the surgical treatment of breast cancer in the 1890s, and his theories about the spread of breast cancer and its surgical treatment were standard in the United States for at least 70 years.[10] Yet Rose Kushner confronted the medical and scientific rationale for a standard, one-step medical procedure that involved simultaneous biopsy and mastectomy. Kushner argued for a two-step process that separated biopsy results from surgical treatment, thereby allowing women to receive information about their disease in order to make an informed decision about surgery. Kushner's argument arose not so much out of a challenge to science as out of a concern for a woman's right—and, by extension, the right of everyone—to have all the information about one's disease before electing a course for treatment. Kushner's argument resonated with many women, who organized and lobbied to change the customary treatment. Thus her efforts resulted in a change of standard clinical procedure to a two-step process.[9]

Now, multimodal and diverse treatments including surgery, chemotherapy, and/or hormone therapy are being used for most women. Moreover, these changes to treatment of breast cancer gave women time to consider and investigate their options for breast reconstruction. The increasing use of reconstruction has positive impact on improving self image for patients with breast cancer.[11] Kushner's advocacy efforts are meaningful in that patients now play an active role in deciding upon optimal treatment options and in improving the quality of their care.

The social eruption of the 1960s provided women an opportunity to band together in a collectivist orientation to share feelings, information, and skills as a means of supporting one another through adverse times and to address their collective perceptions of the inadequacies of the existing health care system. Like Margaret Sanger, Rose Kushner's point of view represented a radical or extreme perspective. By challenging the status quo, Kushner contributed to an increased awareness of breast cancer and more than likely accelerated progress in the surgical treatment of this disease.[8] Her efforts, and those of her descendents-in-advocacy such as Fran Visco, Nancy Brinker, Amy Langer, and Susan Love, represent the establishment of political advocacy in that they challenged and confronted conventional notions about the adequacy and efficacy of cancer treatment and the nation's minimal investment in breast cancer research.[12] By articulating what were considered at the time to be controversial points of view, these advocates extended the level of debate, challenged doctors and scientists to reexamine their behaviors and practices with regard to cancer treatment, and stirred the public into questioning the contemporary approach to breast cancer treatment.

So why does this chapter focus on women and their involvement in advocacy? Why take a gendered approach that examines the role of women only? Perhaps women's involvement in advocacy has been and is what radical sociologist Mary Daly[13] once termed "a journey of exorcism and ecstasy," a voyage of women confronting male-dominated institutions (hospitals, government) and forcing those institutions to be responsive to the distinct needs of women in the development of clinical care and health care policies. In a historical and cyclical fashion, women have once again come together to confront a common adversary—breast cancer. They are mobilizing against a common affliction to change society's attitudes, behaviors, and investments when it comes to cancer prevention, treatment, research, and public policy.

Cancer Advocacy Today: Advocating for Self, for Others, for Society

Changes in the current organization of the U.S. health care system—one in which private health insurance companies carry out a primary and obligatory responsibility to their stockholders and a secondary responsibility to patient care—is limiting individuals' time with and access to health care professionals. The merging and reorganizing of health insurance companies is resulting in both patients and providers changing health care plans, thereby threatening continuity of care and survivors' and families' ability to remain with a doctor or medical group of their own choosing and over an extended period of time. As a result, today's health care consumers, particularly those with limited or no insurance, have to make many of their own critical decisions around a number of issues. These issues include where to go for cancer prevention, screening, and *reimbursed* postscreening follow-up if necessary; diet/nutrition information and counseling; psychosocial support; and long-term medical follow-up. These decisions require access to information about appropriate care for long-term survivors.

Feeling empowered to act on one's own behalf is the first step toward self-advocacy, and information seeking, communication, problem-solving ability, and negotiation skills have been identified as a set of skills that facilitate individuals' abilities to cope with the challenges of cancer.[6] Clinicians and researchers have noted the importance of these skills and have developed products, such as the Cancer Survival Toolbox,[14] to promote these abilities. Another product developed by the National Cancer Institute, entitled *The Cancer Journey: Issues for Survivors*,[15] represents a collaborative effort to educate health care professionals about the psychosocial and quality of life issues faced by cancer survivors, and trains them to address survivors' clinical concerns.

Health care providers have an important role in informing patients about treatment options and opportunities to participate in the decision making process.[16-20] Efforts to assist in this regard include the development of decision aids that improve communication and enable women to make a choice regarding treatment, because attention to patient preference increases satisfaction regarding treatment.[21] The notion of a partnership relationship between doctors and patients, and the participation of patients in decision making, has the potential to enhance the quality of care and treatment outcomes.

As part of a patient/consumer "movement" dating to the mid-1980s, cancer survivors themselves are playing an important role in patient support and in the development of cancer support organizations.[22] A "new breed of cancer survivors"[23] are volunteering in hospitals, sharing experiences with patients in treatment, working for cancer support organizations, participating in research projects and reviewing scientific research proposals, and raising funds and awareness for cancer by participating in walk-a-thons, bike-a-thons, and "extreme" sports like climbing to the tops of the world's tallest mountain peaks. They also are organizing community forums to express concerns and contribute to the development of state and federal action plans to improve the delivery of cancer care,[24] as well as continuing to form cancer survivors groups and networks of support for patients, survivors, and their families.[25]

Individuals involved in advocating for others have found it to be an empowering experience particularly because involvement offers survivors an opportunity to experience a sense of "giving back" to a medical community that survivors often feel saved their lives. Their involvement also offers an opportunity to connect with other cancer survivors and to share experiences with others who "have been there." In the process of helping others, cancer survivors help themselves.

The goals of early breast cancer groups were primarily to provide social support and draw attention to the need for information, research, or services. Yet many of these grassroots groups organized by women with breast cancer and breast cancer survivors through the 1970s have since transformed into highly organized and professionalized national interest organizations. For instance, as a breast cancer support group, Y-ME National Breast Cancer Organization, founded in Chicago in 1979, has provided support and information for women with breast cancer (www.y-me.org/). Today Y-ME champions chapters around the country and is involved in ventures ranging from making information available to providing testimony before governmental bodies. The Susan G. Komen Breast Cancer Foundation, founded in Texas in 1982, is another broad-based organization that has evolved to now sponsor its own research program as well as programmatic initiatives that support education, screening, and treatment projects in communities around the world.[26]

In some cases, targets for change are extending beyond mutual support to broader public policy issues affecting quality of life and quality of care for cancer survivors. The National Breast Cancer Coalition (NBCC) is an advocacy organization that has been described as "perhaps the world's most influential medical consumer lobby group."[27] The NBCC, formed in 1991, now comprises more than 600 groups and 70,000 individuals. Its main goals are to increase federal funding for breast cancer research and collaborate with the scientific community to implement new models of research, to improve all women's access to high-quality health care and breast cancer clinical trials, and to expand the influence of breast cancer advocates in all decisions that affect breast cancer research and policy. In particular, the most notable achievement of the coalition was in increasing the amount of grant funding for breast cancer research. Since NBCC's inception, federal funding for breast cancer has increased by 700% as a result of advocates lobbying the U.S. Congress over the past 10 years. In addition, as a means for developing and empowering a cadre of informed advocates, NBCC developed Project LEAD (Leadership, Education, and Development) to prepare breast cancer patients and survivors to partner with scientists and policymakers and influence their agendas. This project has provided a foundation of scientific knowledge and empowered advocates to contribute to breast cancer research and to educate their communities about breast cancer issues.[28]

THE FUTURE OF ADVOCACY—TAKING ADVOCACY MAINSTREAM

Today, cancer is a personal, tangible, powerful, and public issue for millions of Americans who want doctors, hospitals, and political leaders to implement policies that will combat this disease, ensure the delivery of quality cancer care, and provide necessary supports to enhance the quality of life for cancer patients and survivors. As more Americans are diagnosed with cancer, and as more are living longer after a cancer diagnosis, more than 800 cancer organizations in the United States are mobilizing efforts to address concerns and bring them to the forefront of mainstream attention.

Just as early advocacy efforts initiated by Terese Lasser, a breast cancer survivor and volunteer for the American Cancer Society, resulted in the establishment of the Reach to Recovery program in 1952,[29] today's advocates must continue to provide much-needed information and support. The tremendous amount of information made available through books, magazines, and the Internet makes it necessary for patients to have the skills to critically evaluate this information and use it to meet their needs. Patient advocates, working alone or in patient education/information centers located within cancer centers or in the community, will play a key role in this regard.

Increased public awareness about cancer screening and early detection, as well as about advances in knowledge, is necessary for enhancing patients' access and intent to use medical services. The development and promotion of a national cancer program or campaign will contribute to attract public interest. For example, the Lance Armstrong Foundation "LiveStrong" campaign represents an effort by a national nonprofit organization to raise public attention about the needs of cancer patients and survivors. These efforts emphasize the need for a coordinated national cancer program that produces more effective treatments (through clinical trials) and reduces disparities in cancer incidence, mortality, and long-term survival.

Advocacy efforts intent on delivering supportive interventions and recommendations for treatment guidelines and public policy must be driven by sound, credible scientific data and analysis. Until now, most organizations involved in these efforts have focused on calling for increases in government commitments to funding research, although several larger national organizations such as the Susan G. Komen Foundation and the Cancer Research Foundation of America have established their own budgets for sponsoring research. However, as evidenced by the work of Rose Kushner, more than solid scientific evidence is needed to develop appropriate and effective treatment and care for people with cancer.

Attending to the personal rights, desires, choices, values, and beliefs of individual patients in determining policy and research priorities is imperative. Thus there is value to incorporating advocates in research and policy-making enterprises. The National Institutes of Health, particularly the National Cancer Institute, along with other large nonprofit organizations like the American Cancer Society, have recognized the value of incorporating informed patient and survivor advocates in the scientific peer review process to determine the quality of scientific research proposals. As governments are responsible to citizen taxpayers and nonprofit organizations to their donors, the inclusion of patient advocates in the determination of scientific research agendas permits decision makers to learn from the population what it is they value and support. Their inclusion holds a mirror up to bureaucracy, allowing agency representatives to evaluate the extent to which they have been successful in communicating the message of the value of research. Advocates often educate and inform elected officials as to the value of and imperative for research aimed not only at improving effective treatments but also the quality of life for cancer patients, survivors, and their families.

It is important to note that the needs of women vary based on diverse social, cultural, and economic factors. For instance, advocates representing African American women are aware of the disproportionately higher mortality rates, lower long-term survival rates, and younger age distributions for breast cancer among African

Americans.[30] These advocates argue that the differences in the presentation of breast cancer among African American women influence how they respond to prevention efforts and screening and detection opportunities, as well as to treatment recommendations, including participation in clinical trials. The National Institutes of Health is now in the process of establishing initiatives and offices intent on reducing health disparities in ethnic minority and underserved populations (including those of lower socioeconomic status).[31] Thus it is important to identify and attend to the unique cultural values, beliefs, and insights of various subpopulations in the United States in the development of culturally sensitive and appropriate screening programs and clinical trials. One way of doing this is by developing partnerships between the medical and advocacy communities.

Finally, advances in genetic testing are producing new information and recommendations by means of which women are better able to make informed health care decisions, and current studies have demonstrated a strong desire for testing, even among women who are not members of high-risk groups.[32,33] However, the potential of genetic testing is tempered by a lack of legal protections against insurance agencies or employers that may discriminate against individuals whose genetic make-up may predispose them to higher risks for cancer. Until women can make their own choices about prevention, precautionary measures must be in place to assure women that the medical information regarding their genetic susceptibility, or their choices to act (or not) on that information, will remain confidential and not become fodder for health insurance industry representatives who determine who may get health insurance and what cost.

CONCLUSION

So why this chapter on women and advocacy? Over the past 100 years, and especially over the past 20 years, the U.S. medical system has become a vast industry, tied closely to a myriad of businesses in a profit-oriented system that positions health care as a privilege, as opposed to a right, bestowed upon each and every American. Rich and poor receive different levels of care and services, as do men and women. As evidenced by the work of Margaret Sanger, Rose Kushner, Eleanor Roosevelt and others, when citizens claim and reclaim the democratic principles upon which this country was founded—rights to due process, equal protections and the freedom to define their lives for themselves—profound social change results.

The women's movement in cancer represents the emergence of an organized and collective power to change the status quo and oppose the commodification of health care. Its grassroots origins represent a progressive politics intent on applying democratic principles to the organization of the U.S. health care system. As suggested by the Boston Women's Health Book Collective in its production and revisions of the seminal *Our Bodies, Ourselves*,[34] women have been claiming and reclaiming an important part of their heritage by coming together and exchanging collective experiences and wisdom with one another throughout the twentieth and now into the twenty-first century.

In her essay on the historical roots of self-help and advocacy, Ann Withorn[3] quotes feminist Elizabeth Somer, who defined the notion of advocacy as "both a philosophy and a practice through which we become active creators of our destinies." Inherent in notions of advocacy is the attempt to "systematically influence decision making in an unjust or unresponsive system."[35] Thus cancer advocacy is in essence a civil rights issue, a women's rights issue, and a human rights issue. It requires an acknowledgement that the norms, needs, and expectations for women in general, and for women with cancer in particular, are distinct. A health care system intent on delivering quality cancer care to a diverse population must acknowledge the diversity of need and plan accordingly. Women with cancer are best-positioned to articulate their own experiences and needs, and thereby enhance health care for all.

REFERENCES

1. Steinem G. Margaret Sanger: Her crusade to legalize birth control spurred the movement for women's liberation, *Time* April 13, 1998.
2. Kearns-Goodwin D: Eleanor Roosevelt: America's most influential first lady blazed paths for women and led the battle for social justice, *Time* April 13 1998.
3. Withorn A: Helping ourselves: the limits and potential of self-help. In Conrad P, editor: *The sociology of health and illness: critical perspectives,* ed 7, New York, 2005, Worth.
4. Mickelson JS: Advocacy. In Edwards RL, Hopps JG, editors: *Encyclopedia of social work,* ed 19, Washington, DC, 1995, NASW Press.
5. Clark EJ, Stovall EL: Advocacy: the cornerstone of cancer survivorship, *Cancer Practice* 4(5):239-244, 1996.
6. Gray RE, Doan B, Church K: Empowerment issues in cancer, *Health Values: J Health Behav Education Promotion* 15(4):22-28, 1991.
7. Conrad P: The social and cultural meanings of illness. In Conrad P, editor: *The sociology of health and illness: critical perspectives,* ed 7, New York, 2005, Worth.
8. O'Shea JS: The power of social change: the women's movement and breast cancer, *Breast J* 9(5):347-349, 2003.
9. Sharf B: Out of the closet and into the legislature: breast cancer stories, *Health Affairs* 20(1):213-218, 2001.
10. Fischer B and others: Twenty-year follow-up of a randomized trial comparing total mastectomy, lumpectomy and lumpectomy plus irradiation for the treatment of invasive breast cancer, *N Engl J Med* 347:1227-1232, 2002.
11. Noda S, Eberlein TJ, Eriksson E: Breast reconstruction, *Cancer* 74:376-380, 1994.
12. Stabiner K: *To dance with the devil: the new war on breast cancer politics, power, people,* New York, 1997, Bantam Doubleday Dell Publishing Group.
13. Daly M: Gyn-Ecology: The meta-ethics of radical feminism, Boston, 1978, Beacon Press.
14. Walsh-Burke K, Marcusen C: Self-advocacy training for cancer survivors: The cancer survival toolbox, *Cancer Pract* 7(6):297-301, 1999.
15. National Cancer Institute. *The cancer journey: issues for survivors. a training program for health professionals,* Bethesda, 1998, National Institutes of Health. NIH Publication No. 98-4259.
16. Wolf L: The information needs of women who have undergone breast reconstruction. Part I: decision-making and sources of information, Eur J Oncol Nurs 8(3):211-223, 2004.
17. Kronowitz S, Robb GL: Breast reconstruction with postmastectomy radiation therapy: current issues, *Amer Soc Plast Surg* 114(4):950-960.
18. Reaby LL: Breast restoration decision making: enhancing the process, *Cancer Nurs* 21(3):196-204, 1998.
19. Maly RC and others: Determinants of participation in treatment decision-making by older breast cancer patients, *Breast Cancer Res Treatment* 13(58):1-9, 2004.
20. Whelan T and others: Effect of a decision aid on knowledge and treatment decision making for breast cancer surgery, *JAMA* 292(4):442-496, 2004.
21. Janz NK and others: Patient-physician concordance: preferences, perceptions, and factors influencing the breast cancer surgical decision, *J Clin Oncol* 22(15):3091-3098, 2004.
22. Leigh S: Cancer survivorship: a consumer movement, *Semin Oncol* 21:783-786, 2004.
23. Spingarn ND: *The new cancer survivors: living with grace, fighting with spirit,* Baltimore, 1999, Johns Hopkins University Press.
24. Johnson J, Blanchard J, Harvey C: American's view of cancer, *Supportive Care Cancer* 8:24-27, 2000.
25. Chesler MA, Etheridge S: You are not alone: a sourcebook for support groups for families of children with cancer, Kensington, MD, 2000, Candlelighters Childhood Cancer Foundation.
26. Kasper AS, Ferguson SJ: *Breast cancer: society shapes and epidemic.* New York: St. Martin's Press; 2000.
27. Editorial, How consumers can and should improve clinical trials, *Lancet* 357:1721, 2001.
28. Platner JH and others: The partnership between breast cancer advocates and scientists, *Environmental Molec Mutagenesis* 39:102-107, 2002.
29. Morra M: Patients as citizen advocates, *Cancer Pract* 5(1):55-57, 1997.
30. Lythcott N, Green BL, Kramer Brown Z: The perspective of African-American breast cancer survivor-advocates, *Cancer* 97(1 Suppl):324-328.
31. Moy E, Dayton E, Clancy CM: Compiling the evidence: the national healthcare disparities reports, *Health Affairs* 24(2):376-387, 2005.
32. Lerner BH: Great expectations: historical perspectives on genetic breast cancer testing, *Am J Pub Health* 89(6): 938-944, 1999.
33. Tambor ES, Rimer BK, Strigo TS: Genetic testing for breast cancer susceptibility: awareness and interest among women in the general population, *Am J Med Genet* 68:43-49, 1997.
34. Boston Women's Health Book Collective: *The new our bodies, ourselves,* New York, 1992, Simon and Schuster.
35. Schneider RL, Lester: *Social work advocacy: a new framework for action,* Toronto, 2001, Brooks/Cole.

CHAPTER

3 Genetic and Genomic Information

Jean F. Jenkins

INTRODUCTION

A comprehensive and successful plan of care for the woman with cancer must include consideration of genetic and genomic information.[1] By using genetic and genomic information in the design of cancer interventions, oncology professionals are redefining the options available along the continuum of cancer care. Genetics is the study of individual genes and their impact on relatively rare single gene disorders.[2] Genomics is the study of all the genes in the human genome together, including their interactions with each other and the environment, and the influence of other psychosocial and cultural factors.[2] It is virtually certain that new knowledge produced by genome and cancer research will create an ongoing need to assess and revise our understanding of the influence of genetic and genomic factors influencing individual health outcomes. Options will increasingly include both genetic and genomic information along the pathway for care of all persons, including prevention, screening, diagnostics, prognostics, selection of treatment, and monitoring of treatment effectiveness. Ultimately, the knowledge gained from basic scientific research has the potential to improve outcomes through personalized care for the woman at risk or diagnosed with cancer.

IMPLICATIONS

Implications for the Individual

Health care in the twenty-first century will be influenced by three forces: information, choice, and control.[3] The pace of genomic discovery is exceeding the understanding of both consumer and health care professional. Use of genetic and genomic information challenges the individual patient to translate and extract what is crucial for her to facilitate decision making, often during a time of crisis. The choices about when to use screening tests, what drugs to take, and how to pay for care are all affected by genetic and genomic information. Individuals have increased personal responsibility to use this information to guide their personal healthy behavior strategies. Assuming control for choices about use of genetic and genomic information also has implications for more than just the individual. For example, details learned from genetic testing for risk of breast cancer have implications for other family members, who may also learn of their increased risk for cancer.[4]

Implications for the Family

A genetic diagnosis often indicates that other family members may also be at risk for the same condition.[5] Family relationships and dynamics and gender of the relative may influence an individual's communication to the rest of the family about genetic health information. For example, one study showed that the method of communication about a positive breast-ovarian (*BRCA*) genetic mutation differs by the gender of the relative.[6] Female mutation carriers thought it was important to notify at-risk relatives of the test result, with 88% notifying first-degree relatives. However, most subjects informed female relatives of the test result in person, with males being contacted over the phone or by letter. Different topics were presented to the male as opposed to the female relatives, more female relatives were likely to pursue testing, and feelings about the test result were more often discussed with female relatives. Such variation in communication of genetic information because of gender has implications for the design of genetics counseling strategies to assist the individual when considering how to approach family members about sensitive yet crucial health information.

Implications for Society

Genetic and genomic information is indeed sensitive information. Many individuals struggle with the decision about accessing genetics services because of their concern that genetic information may be used by insurers and employers to deny, limit, or cancel their health insurance (see www.genome.gov/11510227). There is not yet full legal protection that prevents genetic discrimination, although many states have passed legislation (see www.genome.gov/PolicyEthics/LegDatabase/pubsearch.cfm). Attention to how specific information about genetics services and test results is recorded, stored, and released will have to be addressed so as to ensure that genetic information becomes a routine but confidential component of cancer care.[7]

Implications for Oncology Professionals

Organizing a health care system that incorporates genetic and genomic information as an integral component of care requires knowledgeable and skilled providers. Existing practice recommendations are limited by the unavailability of research data that include genetic and genomic factors in the study design. For instance, any research exploring the biologic contributions to human health and disease, including cancer, should consider sex differences at the cellular and molecular level.[8] Interdisciplinary research that considers sex differences in physiologic and behavioral responses to environmental exposures across multiple generations is also recommended.[9] A recently published report making recommendations to improve the quality of care and life for women with breast cancer[10] fails to consider the implications of using genetic information for the psychosocial needs of the woman and her family. Knowledgeable oncology professionals can partner with policy-setting organizations and advocacy groups to help them recognize the needs of patients and communities when faced with decisions about using genetic and genomic information to decide on screening practices or treatment interventions.

EXEMPLARS OF ADVANCES AND CHALLENGES ACROSS THE CANCER CONTINUUM

All women with cancer will eventually be challenged to apply genetic and genomic information when deciding about their course of cancer care. The individual examples in each category of care described in the following material detail a single experience with only one type of cancer. Recognize that essentially all cancers fit into this paradigm with advances for that specific cancer occurring across this cancer continuum, from knowing at-risk status, to selecting interventions, to monitoring response. The challenge is to be able to know where to find information about the latest advances that can make a difference for patients and making referrals as needed for specialized services such as genetic testing (see www.cancer.gov).[11]

Predisposition Testing

Cancer predisposition in some women is known to result from a hereditary germ-line mutation. A possible genetics contribution to breast and ovarian cancer risk can be tested in women who are experiencing cancer and who are assessed as having an increased risk of cancer in their families compatible with autosomal inheritance of cancer susceptibility (Table 3-1). Hereditary mutations account for about 5% to 10% of breast cancer cases overall and when identified offer information for unaffected family members (see www.cancer.gov/cancertopics/pdq/genetics/breast-and-ovarian/healthprofessional). Diet, endocrine, reproductive, and environmental

Table **3-1** RISK ASSESSMENT CRITERIA IN BREAST-OVARIAN CANCER

Risk Level	Any of the Following Criteria:
	Non-Jewish Families
High risk	1 case of breast cancer ≤40 y in any FDR or SDR 1 FDR or SDR with both breast and ovarian cancer, at any age ≥2 cases of breast cancer in FDRs or SDRs if 1 is diagnosed at ≤50 y or is bilateral 1 FDR or SDR with breast cancer diagnosed at ≤50 y or bilateral and 1 FDR or SDR with ovarian cancer 3 cases of breast and ovarian cancer (at least 1 case of ovarian cancer) in FDRs and SDRs 2 cases of ovarian cancer in FDRs and SDRs 1 case of male breast cancer in an FDR or SDR if another FDR or SDR has (male or female) breast or ovarian cancer
Moderate risk, breast	2 FRDs if both diagnosed between 51 and 60 y 1 FDR and SDR (mother or sister and maternal aunt or maternal grandmother), if sum of their age is ≤118 y
Moderate risk, ovarian	1 FDR with ovarian cancer
	Jewish Family
High risk, breast-ovarian	1 case of breast cancer ≤50 y in an FDR or SDR ≥1 case of ovarian cancer at any age in an FDR or SDR ≥1 FDR or SDR with breast cancer at any age if another FDR or SDR has breast and/or ovarian cancer at any age ≥1 case of male breast cancer in an FDR or SDR

FDR, First-degree relative; *SDR*, second-degree relative; y, years of age.
Modified from Hampel H et al: Referral for cancer genetics consultation: A review and compilation of risk assessment criteria, *J Med Genet* 41:81-91, 2004.

factors play an important role in those identified through predisposition testing as being at an increased risk for cancer.[12] Breast cancer screening behaviors may also be influenced by results of genetic tests that predict an increased cancer predisposition. Ongoing research is evaluating the influence of perceived breast cancer risk on initiation and maintenance of health-protective behaviors.[13] Women who perceived that they had a higher breast cancer risk were more likely to pursue genetic testing or undergo prophylactic surgery. Clinicians can use these research findings to understand how risk-related messages are interpreted and how genetic information facilitates or hinders cancer-screening behaviors.

Risk Reduction

Women should be encouraged to develop a comprehensive family history. Accuracy and completeness of this information is valuable for review and discussion with health care providers and may be the first step in assessment of increased risk for cancer in a family. An on-line family history tool to facilitate discussion is now available at www.hhs.gov/familyhistory.

Colorectal cancer (CRC) is commonly diagnosed in women. A small percentage of those at risk or experiencing CRC (25%) have a family history that suggests a genetic contribution, common environmental exposures, or both (www.cancer.gov/cancertopics/pdq/genetics/colo

Table 3-2 Risk Assessment Criteria for Colon Cancer

Risk Level	Any of the Following Criteria:
High risk, HNPCC	3 FDRs or SDRs affected with any HNPCC cancers*, all cases can occur in 1 generation, no age restriction
	1 FDR or SDR with 2 or more HNPCC-associated cancers*
	1 FDR with CRC <50 y
Moderate risk, CRC	1 FDR with CRC ≥50 and one SDR with CRC at any age
	2 FDRs with CRC ≥50 at any age

*Colorectal cancer, endometrial, stomach, ovary, small bowel, pancreas, ureter, or renal pelvis
HNPCC; hereditary nonpolyposis colorectal cancer; FDR, first-degree relative; SDR, second-degree relative; y, years of age.
Modified from Hampel H et al: Referral for cancer genetics consultation: A review and compilation of risk assessment criteria, *J Med Genet* 41:81-91, 2004.

rectal/healthprofessional). An inherited CRC risk is less common (5% to 6%) and results from genetic changes or mutation. When a family history includes two or more relatives with CRC, the possibility of an inherited autosomal dominant cancer syndrome increases (Table 3-2). Several key features indicate the need for further evaluation, which may include referral to genetic nurses for consideration of genetic testing. Red flags include cancer occurring across multiple generations of the family and at younger ages than sporadic cancer, unusual presentation (right-sided CRC), and occurrence of multiple primary cancers in the individual and/or the family (e.g., colon, ureter, endometrial).

When assessment of the family health history indicates the need for genetic testing of the woman, she may be asking questions about the benefits and risks of having a genetic test for CRC mutations. One of the benefits of knowing her mutation status includes the opportunity for personalized recommendations based on genetic test results. For example, if she is identified as carrying a hereditary nonpolyposis colorectal cancer (HNPCC) genetic mutation in the *MSH2* or *MLH1* genes, her absolute risk of colorectal cancer is 80% by age 75 (www.cancer.gov/cancertopics/pdq/genetics/colorectal/healthprofessional/). However, in women with an HNPCC genetic mutation in the *MSH6* gene, the risk of colorectal cancer is lower (25% to 30% by age 75) than in a man (69% by age 75).[14] This information has implications for both counseling and surveillance recommendations. The identification of HNPCC can be life-saving if the individualized screening recommendations result in earlier detection and treatment of cancer.[15]

Diagnosis

Once cancer is detected, molecular technologies are helping rewrite disease classifications, often affecting the diagnosis and treatment decisions. For example, the diagnosis of hematologic cancers such as leukemia is now confirmed through analysis of molecular markers.[16] Chronic lymphocytic leukemia (CLL), morphologically once thought to be one disease, is now known to have two molecularly and clinically distinct subtypes.[17] *ZAP70* is one gene from roughly 160 genes analyzed that permits accurate distinction between the subtypes. This gene expression signature for CLL differentiates this form of leukemia from other lymphoid cancers. The future of molecular oncology is one in which once homogenous diseases are defined in more precise terms, which will allow tailored treatment based on the improved understanding of the individual's actual cancer molecular pathway.

Treatment Selection

Clinically tailored treatments offer a theoretical advantage because it is widely observed that individuals often respond differently to the same intervention. A study of large B-cell lymphoma patients identified two subgroups that had different outcomes after multiagent chemotherapy.[16] Identification of individual tumor biology through gene expression analysis revealed clinically distinct subgroups of tumors that had all been diagnosed as diffuse histiocytic lymphoma. Molecular profiling to predict survival after chemotherapy in these patients was used to identify those individuals needing more aggressive chemotherapy.[18] Improved survival for the poor-risk group, at the same time the favorable-risk group was spared from toxic drugs, resulted in improved clinical outcomes for the individual. Extensive efforts will be needed to validate basic research results and to verify molecular profiles, while taking into consideration multiple variables affecting outcomes, including gender.

Targeted Treatment

The National Cancer Institute (NCI) is collaborating with the National Human Genome Research Institute (NHGRI) to expand efforts to identify major genetic mutations in the 50 most common types of cancer.[19] A goal of this initiative is to improve treatment interventions with the development of targeted drugs based on an improved understanding of the genetic changes that occur in the cancer genome. Targeting therapy based on genetic changes in the cancer cell has already been successfully implemented in several cases including chronic myelogenous leukemia (Gleevec [Novartis, East Hanover, NJ]),[20] breast cancer (Herceptin [Genentech, San Francisco, CA]),[21] and lung cancer (gefitinib).[22] Persons with each of these cancers who exhibit a certain genotype may respond to medications targeting their specific gene products.[23] Drug development of the future will be based on an increasing knowledge of genetic variation. It will be an ongoing challenge to allocate resources and cope with economic implications. More research is needed to identify how to assess patient preferences and willingness to pay for these personalized services.[24]

Treatment Response

It is estimated that genetics can account for a large percentage of variability in drug disposition and effectiveness.[25] Pharmacogenomics uses a genome-wide focus to elucidate factors that are useful in guiding personalized drug selection and dosage. An example is an expanding awareness of how certain enzymes influence the metabolism of pain medications and antidepressants.[26] It is unclear whether the polymorphisms that influence the rate of drug metabolism are different in women when compared with men. However, chronic pain has been found to have greater severity and duration in women.[27] Genotyping and phenotyping as a method to improve the care of women is likely to have a significant effect on the ability to meet the supportive care needs of women with cancer.

Monitoring Response

Use of biomarkers such as molecular profiles in cancer clinical trials is a goal of the Food and Drug Administration (FDA) and the NCI (www3.cancer.gov/prevention/cbrg). A meeting was held to design a plan that included strategies, resources, and actions needed to enable and accelerate cancer biomarker discovery and validation. These efforts will enhance individualized treatment through use of new biomarkers for detecting, predicting, and monitoring response to cancer interventions. An example of using molecular profiling to monitor cancer response follows.

Individuals with follicular B-cell lymphoma commonly have a rearrangement of the *BCL2* gene that can be assayed for using polymerase-chain-reaction (PCR). The t (14;18) translocation disregulates *BCL2*, a key gene in the regulation of cell death.[28,29] This molecular marker was used as a tool to monitor response of patients to a monoclonal antibody labeled with a radionucleotide that binds specifically to CD20, a typical immunophenotype found on the surface of malignant B cells. In this study, bone marrow cells were assayed at baseline and at 6, 12, and 25 weeks after treatment to measure molecular response. Following treatment, a molecular remission was found (undetectable *BCL2* translocation) in 80% of patients assayed, which correlated well with clinical remission. Molecular markers such as these may be more sensitive and specific and less invasive than other methods of monitoring disease response and relapse.

EXEMPLARS OF ADVANCES AND CHALLENGES ACROSS THE LIFE CONTINUUM

Women with cancer will eventually be faced with challenging issues resulting from the potential use of genetic and genomic information, perhaps at several points within their lifetimes. The following individual examples detail a single experience illustrative of issues and challenges that women may face during a particular life stage. Oncology nurses have an important responsibility to present information and resources to assist the woman, her family, and society to consider the options. Not all the options that are technologically feasible may be the best choice. Recognize that essentially all cancers fit into this paradigm, with the potential of clinical genomics applications creating new opportunities, as well as dilemmas, throughout the lifecycle and challenging our physical, emotional, moral, and economic perspectives.

Prenatal Period

Prenatal genetic testing for adult-onset cancers is technologically possible.[4] Many individuals desire to avoid the trauma of bearing children with a predisposition to a cancer, if avoidable. A survey done by the Genetics and Public Policy Center (www.dnapolicy.org) found that a majority of Americans believe it is appropriate to use reproductive genetic testing to avoid having a child with a life-threatening disease. More than 67% of Americans, across gender and ethnic groups, approve of genetic testing of embryos during in vitro fertilization (IVF) procedures to select those embryos free of a fatal disease caused by a gene mutation when selecting the embryo to transfer to a woman's uterus. Quality and accuracy of test results, knowledge of influencing factors other than genetics that affect health outcomes, and societal values all have the potential to influence public policy and individual decisions related to embryo genetic testing.

Infancy

Newborn screening is a public health genetics screening program aimed at early detection and treatment of presymptomatic children affected by genetic conditions or birth defects whose effects may be mitigated by early diagnosis and intervention. The specific conditions to be included in each newborn screening panel are currently determined by the individual state (http://genes-r-us.uthscsa.edu). The advent of DNA microarray technology and multiplex gene analysis will lead to improved efficiency, but also has the potential to create more information than is helpful toeither health care providers or consumers.[30] Screening panels currently performed on newborns do not identify individuals who may have a genetic mutation that increases the risk of developing a specific cancer. Future technology and scientific knowledge may make this a realistic expectation. A partnership between women concerned about their children and knowledgeable clinicians will help to ensure the development of public health policies that take into consideration the clinical value of predictive rather than only diagnostic genetic tests.[31,32]

Adulthood

Genetic interventions have significant implications for the individual adult. Often the ramifications of newly designed interventions may be unknown. For example, gene therapy is currently offered for treatment of cancer (www.cancer.gov/cancertopics/Factsheet/Therapy/gene). Reproductive guidelines for a woman of child-bearing age who is undergoing gene therapy or gene-targeted interventions are not currently available. The hypothetical reproductive risks would depend on the type of gene therapy vector, the method of administration, and what other chemotherapy was received. The individual receiving a gene therapy intervention may question the nurse about what precautions must be taken. Further research is required to assess the short- and long-term effects of therapies that use genetics technology.

Adult Parents

Adult parents are often the first in the family approached by their children to consider initiation of collecting health information and to pursue genetic testing for a potential hereditary condition. In a study assessing reasons for pursuing genetic testing for HNPCC, more than half the responders believed that the most important reason for undergoing genetic testing was to learn about their children's risk.[33] Because genetic testing is initially done on an affected individual, adult parents may feel coerced into providing details about health information that influences their own sense of well-being. Parents often express remorse if they are found to carry a deleterious mutation that they have passed down to their children and, potentially, their grandchildren. Although the ability to select genes is not currently available, adult parents often express guilt and emotional anxiety about passing the increased risk of cancer throughout the generations.[4] As technology facilitates the clinical value of DNA, adult parents may feel additional pressure to bank blood or tissue for future use. If they do not want to participate in providing information or a blood sample, they may feel the emotional consequences of denying their family information that is perceived as valuable. Women are often gatekeepers of health information and utilization of health services and may play a key role in whether or not the family accesses genetic and genomic information.[34] It is important for nurses to consider the many complex issues raised by communication or noncommunication of genetic information among families.

CONTROVERSIAL ISSUES

Genome research will change the world as it is known, creating controversial issues as emerging knowledge challenges the current comprehension of interrelationships and interactions at the biologic and psychosocial levels. The expansion of genetics services will challenge resources: personal, professional, financial, and political. The choices made today about how to use this knowledge will have implications for future generations. There is much to learn so that genomics can be safely integrated into the foundation of nursing care for the twenty-first century. Technology will permit faster access to test results, but will the understanding of how to use that information keep pace? Will individuals be able to access and afford genetics services? Will oncology nurses have sufficient awareness and understanding of the power, possibilities, and limitations of genomics breakthroughs in the field of cancer care? With an increasing awareness of the possible magnitude of the approaching change, nurses can envision the personal and professional ramifications of these scientific advances. There are many steps that can be taken by oncology nurses to prepare for the potential opportunities, to head off dangers, and to be active in the design of infrastructure for health care delivery that makes a difference for the health and well-being of our patients.

Use of Technology

Advances in biotechnology have the potential to transform health care during the coming decade.[35] The value of understanding the human genome to be able to forecast, prevent, and manage cancer cannot be fully achieved without consideration of the many factors influencing the speed of discovery and application to practice, including leadership by nurses. Consequences, both negative and positive, must be considered in terms of short- and long-term benefits and costs for the individual, their families, and society.[36] Nursing research is needed to be able to identify outcomes of such interventions. The promise versus the reality of biotechnology is an important concept for nurses to understand and educate others about, if they are to provide assistance to individuals facing a life-threatening illness and help them have realistic expectations. Creating realistic expectations while maintaining hope will be an important role for nurses providing care in the genomics era.

CULTURE AND ETHNIC DIVERSITY

Women are disproportionately affected by some conditions in terms of incidence, diagnosis, course, response to treatments, and outcomes. Culture and ethnic diversity does matter in health outcomes, but how much of this is due to genetics is controversial. Factors such as poverty or low socioeconomic status, access to care, education, environmental exposures, and other modifiers should also be considered when assessing health disparities (http://orwh.od.nih.gov/research/05priorities.html). Recommendations from the Office of Research on Women's Health (ORWH) do include the need for increased research emphasis on sex as a modifier of gene function and response to treatment. Researchers are grappling with the concepts of race and ethnicity and how to construct research that adequately captures the true influence of biologic variation.[37]

ONCOLOGY NURSING LEADERSHIP

Leadership by oncology nurses has the potential to advance options of care for all patients. As one of the first specialty groups to be able to apply genetics and genomics advances to clinical care, oncology nurses have an opportunity to model for other nurses how to develop, integrate, and apply genomic-based health care. Consideration of the scope of practice and the role of the oncology nurse in taking research advances to the bedside is essential. Acquiring sufficient knowledge to be competent in providing quality genomic-based health care is necessary. Only then can the design of quality nursing care and services be safe as well as effective.

Role

The oncology nurse's role requires integration of cancer-related genetic and genomic information into both general and advanced oncology nursing practice.[1] For more information about core competencies in genetics identified as essential for all health care professionals,[38] visit www.nchpeg.org. Use of these identified competencies to develop nursing education model programs provides a basic foundation of genetics and genomics knowledge for all nurses. Building upon this foundation, specialty oncology nurses can then focus on the specific knowledge required to meet the needs of their patients. Three levels differentiate the scope of oncology nursing practice in genetics: that recommended for the general oncology nurse, the advanced practice oncology nurse, and the advanced practice oncology nurse with a subspecialty in genetics.[1] The Oncology Nursing Society (ONS) has published position statements detailing the role of the nurse in cancer predisposition genetic testing and risk assessment counseling.[39,40] The ONS has a special interest group of nurses interested in genetics offering a network of valuable resources. The ONS also offers workshops, a genetics toolkit, Internet resources, and publications that provide knowledge needed by all oncology nurses.

Knowledge

Genetic cancer-risk assessment is an emerging interdisciplinary practice that requires specialized knowledge, clinical abilities, and counseling skills. Studies to date indicate that nurses receive limited genetics and genomics information in their basic nursing programs.[41,42] A small expert group has plans to build upon past efforts of nurse leaders and design a competence-based education framework for U.S. nurses in the genomics era. There are many publications, including the Health Resources and Service Administration (HRSA)–sponsored Expert Panel Report on Genetics and Nursing,[43] that encourages the integration of genomics into nursing education, certification, and licensure. The foundation is now in place, but creating the building blocks that facilitate integration of genomics into education and practice to improve health outcomes is required. A plan has been developed to hold at least three meetings over the next 2 years with the goal of working with stakeholders to set an agenda for nursing education. Invited meeting participants will contribute to the endorsement of minimum common core competencies in genetics and genomics for nurses in the United States. Efforts are continuing to create national standards and exemplars that will be presented for consideration by representatives of education, licensing, and credentialing bodies and that may be useful for redesigning curricula. Models of specialty skill building have been implemented to improve upon such basic training through workshops, web-based courses, and intensive interdisciplinary courses.[44-46] Practicing nurses will have an ongoing need for continuing education programs that integrate genetic and genomic information targeted for specialty nurse education.

Services

New service delivery models may require consideration. Decisions about who should provide genetic information, and how they should do it, require careful consideration. The expanded use of genetics services may offer many potential clinical benefits. Access to specialized genetics services, such as hereditary cancer testing, may occur through innovative models of care such as telegenetics service delivery.[47] However, the economic challenges may be limiting if reimbursement and efficient resource utilization cannot be achieved.

Ethics

As genome research unravels the mysteries associated with cancer, the boundaries associated with utilization of this knowledge will be challenging. Focus on ethical issues that accompany the design of cancer services is essential, including confidentiality of patient information; access to genetics and genomics services; and implications for patients and families.[48] A story shared by someone experiencing these issues firsthand highlights the concerns best.

Box 3-1 Sharing the Gift of Medical Information

After being diagnosed with breast cancer at age 33, and after learning I carried a *BRCA2* genetic mutation, which put me at risk for further breast cancer and also ovarian cancer, my initial thoughts were concern for myself. But soon after receiving this news, my thoughts turned toward the implications that my diagnosis had for my family. At the time of my diagnosis, I had scant information about my family's medical history. We were never a close family, and on both sides of my family, there were few women. I was the only daughter of an only daughter, and my father had three brothers and only one sister. What I did know is that my paternal grandmother died young of "kidney" cancer back in the 40s. My mother died young of an aneurism, and her parents out-lived her and both died well into their 80s. My father remains healthy and alive to this day. I was never considered at high risk for any type of cancer. I was fortunate that I took exemplary care of my health, and found a benign lump on my first breast self-exam. At age 33, a follow-up mammogram found my cancer. My physicians had always questioned me about family history of cancer, but seemed to lose interest when told that the only cancer in my family was my paternal grandmother, and that she had died of "kidney cancer."

Even after my diagnosis of breast cancer, none of my physicians seemed to take note of the fact that I was 33 with breast cancer, and that my paternal grandmother had died young of cancer. I never made any connection with my grandmother's cancer, until I stumbled upon an article in a journal about 8 months after my diagnosis. The article highlighted the connection between hereditary breast cancer and ovarian cancer, and also mentioned certain populations that were at particularly high risk for carrying a genetic mutation, which could cause both cancers. It went on to explain the genetic test that was available to determine if someone carried one of these mutations.

Continued

Box 3-1 Sharing the Gift of Medical Information—cont'd

Several thoughts immediately hit me when I read the article. The first was that back in the 40s when medicine was not as sophisticated, it might have been quite easy to mistake advanced ovarian cancer for kidney cancer. The second was that I might be at high risk for further cancer. The third was that I wanted to have the test.

After much research I learned that before having a genetic test, I should see a specialist called a genetic counselor, who would detail at great length the benefits and risks of a predictive test. One of the first things the counselor did was ask me to research my family history both of cancer and of other diseases. I was dismayed to realize exactly how little I knew about my family's medical background, and how little detail the relatives with whom I was in contact could add. I did find the genetic counseling very helpful and informative, and afterwards decided that I wanted the test. I tested positive for a *BRCA2* mutation, which put me at extremely high risk for further breast cancer and also ovarian cancer.

After absorbing the shock of my results, I decided that I must inform the rest of my family. Issues of privacy and possible genetic discrimination were a concern, but not enough to keep me from notifying those who might be at risk as well. As my genetic counselor put it, I "was the red flag for hereditary cancer in my family." I used the Internet to find as many family members as I could, including cousins I hadn't spoken to in over 20 years. The phone calls weren't particularly easy to make, but I felt I had an obligation to let them know information that I would want to know in their position. Along with my genetic test results, I told them how they might find a genetic counselor in their area with whom they might discuss their options.

Through the nonprofit organization FORCE: Facing Our Risk of Cancer Empowered, which I founded, I've been able to advocate for the high-risk community. The issue of who should be told about genetic test results comes up periodically. I know of many young cancer patients who were never told about their relatives' cancer, even though multiple family members had similar diagnoses, which might have foreshadowed a family cancer syndrome. I also know of survivors who had very compelling reasons not to discuss their medical information with other family members. But the days when a cancer diagnosis is shrouded in shame and embarrassment and whispered among certain family members who are sworn to secrecy are hopefully a thing of the past. In my case there was no doubt that the important and unfortunate information that I was in possession of needed to be shared with my family.

Cancer is one of a number of diseases that can have a hereditary component. We don't know all the causes of cancer, and it is believed that most cancer is not hereditary. Certainly having a family member who has had cancer doesn't automatically confer a high risk for cancer on other family members. Nevertheless, medical information such as who has been diagnosed with cancer, at what age, and their relationship within the family tree can be an important and life-saving piece of medical history. Although my cancer diagnosis could hardly be called a positive thing, my sharing of medical information is a gift that I give to my relatives willingly, and I hope that the information is received and shared with other family members in this spirit.

Sue Friedman, DVM. *Dr. Friedman is executive director of the organization FORCE: Facing Our Risk of Cancer Empowered and is employed as a patient advocate at the H. Lee Moffitt Cancer Center, an NCI-designated comprehensive cancer center. She is serving a second 3-year volunteer appointment to the National Cancer Institute's Consumer Advocates in Research and Related Activities (CARRA) Program.*

Table **3-3** GENETIC INFORMATION RESOURCES

Resource	URL	Content
American College of Medical Genetics	www.acmg.net	Information and policy statements about medical genetics
American Society for Human Genetics	www.ashg.org	Information about human genetics
Centers for Disease Control and Prevention	www.cdc.gov/genomics	Genetics and public health concerns, family history
Cincinnati Children's Hospital-Faculty Education	www.gepn.cchmc.org	On-line courses and materials for nurses
Department of Energy	www.doegenomes.org	Multiple genetics educational resources
Genetics and Molecular Medicine (American Medical Association)	www.ama-assn.org/ama/pub/category/1799.html	Links to current articles and other resources
Health Resources and Services Administration-Genetics Services Branch	www.mchb.hrsa.gov	Multiple genetics educational resources
International Society of Nurses in Genetics	www.isong.org	Information about genetics in nursing; annual meeting
National Cancer Institute's CancerNet	www.cancer.gov/cancerinfo/prevention-genetics-causes	Authoritative information about cancer genetics
National Coalition for Health Professional Education in Genetics	www.nchpeg.org	Core competencies in genetics and reviews of education programs
National Human Genome Research Institute	www.genome.gov	Research, health, policy, ethics, education, and training information and resources
National Institute of Nursing Research-Summer Genetics Institute	http://fmp.cit.nih.gov/ninr	Summer genetics program that is designed to provide training in molecular genetics for use in research and clinical practice
National Society of Genetic Counselors	www.nsgc.org	Information about genetic counseling
Oncology Nursing Society	www.ons.org	Position statements, workshops, publications
The President's Council on Bioethics	www.bioethics.gov	Information on current bioethics issues
Secretary's Advisory Council on Genetics, Health, and Society	www4.od.nih.gov/oba/sacghs.htm	Policy issues regarding the impact of genetic technologies on society
U.S. Surgeon General's Family History Initiative	www.hhs.gov/familyhistory	Downloadable family history form

RESOURCES

Professionally, most practitioners have not been prepared in academic programs to understand the science of genetics. This limits the ability to educate and provide information to individuals and families to facilitate their decision making. Even the pace of discovery challenges the ability to remain knowledgeable about the implications of the science for the care of patients. Currently some continuing education programs, CD-ROM materials, and academic programs are beginning to offer genetics content. Professional societies such as the ONS are recognizing the need to offer ongoing genetics education to their membership. Organizations and other sources that can provide the most up-to-date information and materials are listed in Table 3-3. For an up-to-date listing of links to genetics information sources, visit www.genome.gov/11510197.

SUMMARY

The attainment of the dreams stimulated by inspiring genome technology and research and advancing our understanding of health and disease will only be realized if appropriate protections, incentives, and knowledge are achieved. Oncology nurses are among the first specialists touched by the scientific advances that are offering tremendous possibilities for those who care for women touched by cancer. The benefits and limitations of these advances are integral to the daily decision making already occurring in practice. Leadership by oncology nursing in translating genomics to health care practice will result in the design of comprehensive and successful plans of care that advance women's health and well-being. Only then can these discoveries make a difference for those individuals living with the risk of cancer, the diagnosis of cancer, or dying from cancer.

REFERENCES

1. Strauss Tranin A, Masny A, Jenkins J, editors: *Genetics in oncology practice,* PA, 2003, Oncology Nursing Press.
2. Guttmacher A, Collins F: Genomic medicine: a primer, *N Engl J Med* 347:1512-1520, 2002.
3. Frist W: Health care in the 21st century, *N Engl J Med* 352:267-272, 2005.
4. Patenaude A: *Genetic testing for cancer. Psychological approaches for helping patients and families,* Washington, D.C., 2005, American Psychological Association.
5. Burke W: Genetic testing, *N Engl J Med* 347:1867-1875.
6. McGivern B and others: Family communication about positive *BRCA1* and *BRCA2* genetic test results, *Genet in Med* 6:503-509, 2004.
7. Khoury M: Genetics and genomics in practice: the continuum from genetic disease to genetic information in health and disease, *Genet in Med* 5:261-268, 2003.
8. Institute of Medicine: *Exploring the biological contributions to human health: does sex matter?* Washington, D.C., 2001, National Academy Press.
9. Keitt S, Fagan T, Marts S: Understanding sex differences in environmental health: a thought leaders' roundtable, *Environmental Health Perspective* 112:604-609, 2004.
10. Institute of Medicine: *Meeting the psychosocial needs of women with breast cancer,* Washington, D.C., 2004, National Academy Press.
11. Hampel H and others: Referral for cancer genetics consultation: a review and compilation of risk assessment criteria, *J Med Genet* 41:81-91, 2004.
12. Lynch H, Casey J, Shaw T, Lynch J: Hereditary factors in gynecologic cancer, *The Oncologist,* 3:319-338, 1998.
13. Katapodi M and others: Predictors of perceived breast cancer risk and the relation between perceived risk and breast cancer screening: a meta-analytic review, *Prevent Med* 38:388-402, 2003.
14. Hendriks Y and others: Cancer risk in hereditary nonpolyposis colorectal cancer due to *MSH6* mutations: impact on counseling and surveillance, *Gastroenterology* 127:17-25, 2004.
15. Lynch H, De La Chapelle A: Hereditary colorectal cancer. In Guttmacher A, Collins F, Drazen J, editors: *Genomic Medicine,* Maryland, 2004, The Johns Hopkins University Press.
16. Staudt L: Molecular diagnosis of the hematologic cancers, *NEJM* 348:1777-1785, 2003.
17. Staudt L: Gene expression profiling of lymphoid malignancies, *Annu Rev Med* 53:303-318, 2002.
18. Rosenwald A and others: The use of molecular profiling to predict survival after chemotherapy for diffuse large B-cell lymphoma, *N Engl J Med* 346:1937-1947, 2003.
19. Kaiser J: NCI gears up for cancer genome project, *Science* 307:1182.
20. Mauro M and others: STI571: A paradigm of new agents for cancer therapeutics, *J Clin Oncol* 20:325-334, 2002.
21. Kaklamani V, Regan R: New targeted therapies in breast cancer, *Semin Oncol* 31:20-25, 2004.
22. Lynch T, Bell D, Sordella R: Activating mutations in the epidermal growth factor receptor underlying responsiveness of non-small cell lung cancer to gefitinib, *N Engl J Med* 350:2129-2139, 2004.
23. Prows C, Prows D: Medication selection by genotype, *Am J Nurs* 104:60-70, 2004.
24. Phillips K and others: Genetic testing and pharmacogenomics: issues for determining the impact to healthcare delivery and costs, *Am J Manag Care* 10:425-432, 2004.
25. Evans W, McLeod H: Pharmacogenomics-drug disposition, drug targets, and side effects, *N Engl J Med* 348:538-549, 2003.
26. Caraco Y: Genes and the response to drugs, *N Engl J Med* 351:2867-2869, 2004.

27. Davis R: Understanding pain: gender, genetics, and treatment, *University of Maryland Research and Scholarship*: 2-6, 2005.
28. Dave S and others: Prediction of survival in follicular lymphoma based on molecular features of tumor-infiltrating immune cells, *N Engl J Med* 351:2159-2169, 2004.
29. Kaminski M and others: ^{131}I-tositumomab therapy as initial treatment for follicular lymphoma, *N Engl J Med* 352:441-449, 2005.
30. Green N, Pass K: Neonatal screening by DNA microarray: spots and chips, *Nature Reviews Genetics* 6:147-151, 2005.
31. Burke W, Zimmern R: Ensuring the appropriate use of genetic tests, *Nature Review Genetics* 5:955-959, 2004.
32. Committee of bioethics: Ethical issues with genetic testing in pediatrics, *Pediatrics* 107:1451-1455, 2001.
33. Hadley D and others: Genetic counseling and testing in families with hereditary nonpolyposis colorectal cancer, *Arch Intern Med* 163:573-582, 2003.
34. Wilson B and others: Family communication about genetic risk: the little that is known, *Community Genet* 7:15-24, 2004.
35. Zajtchuk R: New technologies in medicine: biotechnology and nanotechnology, *Disease-a-month* 45:452-495, 1999.
36. Jenkins J, Lea D: *Nursing care in the genomic era: a case-based approach*, Boston, 2005, Jones and Bartlett.
37. Collins F: What we do and don't know about "race," "ethnicity," genetics and health at the dawn of the genome era, *Nature Genetics Suppl* 36:S13-S15, 2004.
38. Jenkins J and others: Recommendations of core competencies in genetics essential for all health professionals, *Genet in Med* 3:155-158, 2001.
39. Oncology Nursing Society: Cancer predisposition genetic testing and risk assessment, *Oncol Nurs Forum* 27:2, 2000.
40. Oncology Nursing Society: The role of the oncology nurse in cancer genetic counseling, *Oncol Nurs Forum* 27:1, 2000.
41. Monsen R: Genetics in basic nursing program curricula: A national survey, *Maternal-Child Nurs J* 13:177-185, 1984.
42. Hetteberg C and others: National survey of genetics content in basic nursing preparatory programs in the United States, *Nursing Outlook* 47:168-180, 1999.
43. Expert Panel Report on Genetics and Nursing: *Implications for education and practice*, Washington, D.C., 2000, BHP00177. Available on the Web at www.ask.hrsa.gov/
44. Blazer K and others: Outcomes from intensive training in genetic cancer risk counseling for clinicians, *Genet in Med* 7:40-47, 2005.
45. Prows C and others: Development of a web-based genetics institute for a nursing audience, *J Contin Ed Nurs* 35: 223-231, 2004.
46. Masny A and others: A training course for oncology nurses in familial cancer risk assessment: evaluation of knowledge and practice, *J Cancer Ed* 18:20-25, 2003.
47. Lea D and others: Telegenetics in Maine: successful clinical educational service delivery model developed from a 3-year pilot project, *Genet in Med* 7:21-27, 2005.
48. Cassells J and others: An ethical assessment framework for addressing global genetic issues in clinical practice, *Oncol Nurs Forum* 30:383-390, 2002.

UNIT II

Major Cancers Affecting Women

CHAPTER

4 LUNG CANCER

Marilyn L. Haas

INTRODUCTION AND OVERVIEW

In the United States and across the world, lung cancer is the "unspoken" or ignored cancer.[1] Clear ribbons are the new symbols for lung cancer, signify the almost invisible status of this devastating and stigmatized disease. Social stigmas are associated with this disease. Tobacco, a well-known carcinogen, is the main cause of lung cancer.[2]

Lung cancer is the most significant health problem in the United States. While incidence has decreased in men, it has increased among women. Forty percent of women in the United States report that they smoke, thus affecting the development of lung cancer.[3] Although the dangers of smoking are well documented, the risks for developing lung cancer remain controversial. Some researchers speculate that women are at higher risk than men; others report no statistical difference.[4]

While activists are working hard to influence the tobacco industry, pessimism continues to exist regarding prevention and treatment of lung cancer. Unlike screening for breast cancer (i.e., mammography) and cervical cancer (i.e., pelvic exams and PAP smears), there is no proven lung cancer screening test available. At present, the American Cancer Society does not recommend testing with computed tomography for early lung cancer detection in asymptomatic persons.[5] Unfortunately, when lung cancer is discovered, the cancer is already in the late stages for the vast majority of patients.[6,7] Treatment of late-stage disease is usually noncurative and palliative.

Lung cancer remains underfunded when compared with other female cancers. Breast cancer ranks number one in terms of medical expenditures. The 2003 reported expenditures show that $1,740 was spent per person per lung cancer death compared to $13,649 per person per breast cancer death.[8]

EPIDEMIOLOGY

In the United States, the American Cancer Society reports that lung cancer is the second most common cancer diagnosed in men and women.[7] The American Cancer Society (ACS) estimates there will be 172,570 new cases of lung cancer diagnosed in 2005, of which 79,560 will be in women (see Figure 4-1). One in seventeen women will develop lung cancer.[9] African-American females have higher incidence rates for lung cancer than any other ethnic group.[7,10] Lung cancer has become a full-blown epidemic among women throughout the United States (see Figure 4-2).

Lung cancer mortality rose among women between 1950 and 1997. Death rates from lung cancer among American women increased by more than 600%.[11] In 1987, female lung cancer deaths surpassed those from breast cancer, with the gap growing progressively larger over time. Today, lung cancer kills more women each year than breast cancer, ovarian, and uterine cancer combined,

The author would like to acknowledge the review and support of Tina M. St. John, MD, Medical Director, Caring Ambassadors Program and author of *With Every Breath: A Lung Cancer Guidebook,* Vancouver, WA, which can be found at www.lungcancerguidebook.org.

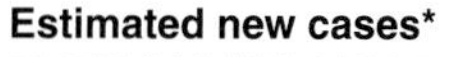

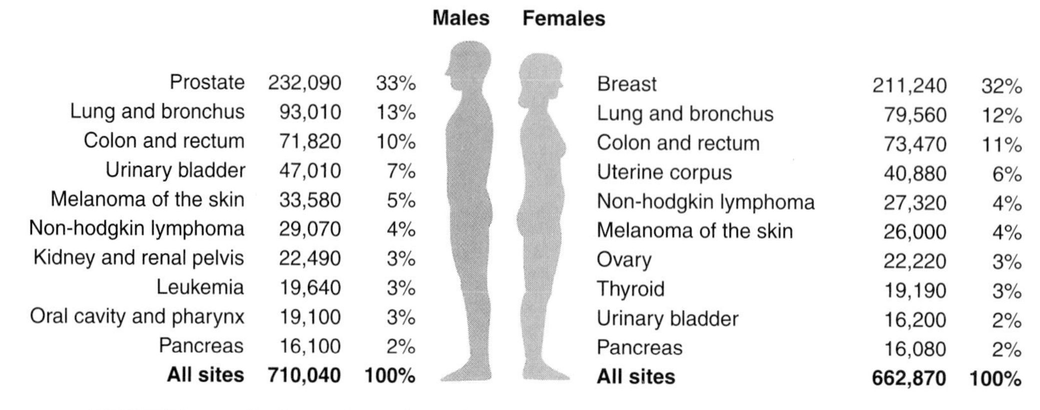

FIGURE 4-1 Estimated number of new lung cancers. (From *CA: A Cancer Journal for Clinicians*, 2005, American Cancer Society.)

claiming an estimated 73,020 women for 2005[7] (Figure 4-3). African American women have high death rates from lung cancer.[7,10] Unfortunately, few American women realize these devastating facts.

Internationally, lung cancer death rates among women have also risen. In 1990, 10% of all cancer deaths worldwide were due to lung cancer. Rates were even higher (20%) for developed countries, partly due to the increasing popularity of cigarette smoking.[9]

Lung cancer survival rates are shockingly low, in stark contrast to other common female cancers. The overall 5-year survival rate for lung cancer is only 15%, as compared to an 87% overall survival rate for breast cancer.[9] Survival rates decline with increasing age and stage at diagnosis for all histologic lung cancer cell types. Although overall survival rates are low, women typically have a better prognosis than do men with lung cancer.[12,13]

ETIOLOGY AND RISK FACTORS

Researchers are evaluating biologic differences between females and males in terms of the relative risk of developing lung cancer.[7,14-16] Some studies suggest that, given equal smoking histories, women may be more susceptible to lung cancer than men.[17-21] Some research has shown that women are 1.5 times more likely to develop lung cancer than men.[9] However, researchers[22] analyzed prospective data from former and current smokers in two large cohorts: the Nurses' Health Study of women and the Health Professionals Follow-up Study of men. Adjusting for age, number of cigarettes smoked per day, age of smoking initiation, and time since smoking cessation, their conclusions did not support the hypothesis that women are at higher relative risk of developing lung cancer than men. Researchers continue to explore the possibility of gender differences in the development of lung cancer.

Tobacco exposure via smoking is the primary identifiable risk factor associated with lung cancer, although it is not the only risk factor. Evidence suggests that lung cancer develops in a multistep carcinogenic process wherein genetic damage accumulates over time with ongoing carcinogenic exposure.[23-25] The incidence of lung cancer is related to tobacco quality, duration of tobacco use, and the daily dose/intensity of nicotine.[9,26] Approximately 80% to 90% of people who develop lung cancer are current or former smokers.[27,28] The risk of dying from lung cancer is 20 times higher among women who smoke two or more packs of cigarettes per day than among women who do not smoke.[9]

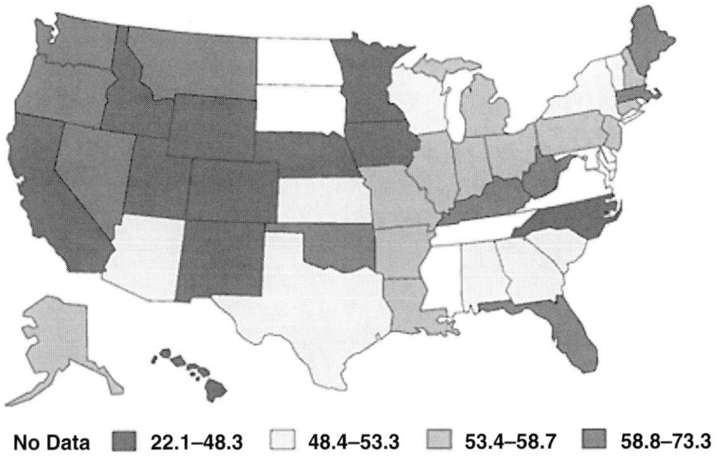

No Data 22.1–48.3 48.4–53.3 53.4–58.7 58.8–73.3

No Data	Delaware, Maryland, Mississippi, North Dakota, South Dakota, Tennessee, Virginia
22.1-48.3	California, Colorado, Hawaii, Idaho, Iowa, Wyoming, Minnesota, Nebraska, New Mexico, North Carolina, Utah
48.4-53.3	Alabama, Arizona, District of Columbia, Georgia, Kansas, New York, Rhode Island, South Carolina, Texas, Vermont, Wisconsin
53.4-58.7	Alaska, Arkansas, Connecticut, Illinois, Indiana, Louisiana, Michigan, Missouri, New Hampshire, New Jersey, Ohio, Pennsylvania
58.8-73.3	Florida, Kentucky, Maine, Massachusetts, Montana, Nevada, Oklahoma, Oregon, Washington, West Virginia

*Rates are per 100,000 persons and are age-adjusted to the 2000 U.S. standard population. Source: United States Cancer Statistics, 2001

FIGURE 4-2 Rates of developing lung cancer among women by state. (From United States Cancer Statistics, 2001.)

Women started openly smoking in significant numbers during and following World War II; smoking prevalence among American women peaked in the 1960s.[29] At first, many women did not inhale cigarette smoke. Cigarettes were seen as ornamental objects rather than nicotine devices. Over time, more women adopted the smoking style of men, and it became the norm for female smokers.[30] Today, over one quarter of women in the United States smoke.[11] Although lung cancer risk slowly decreases over time after smoking cessation, women currently smoking will remain at a significantly increased risk for lung cancer for at least 20 years even if they stop smoking immediately.[31]

Smoking affects women differently than it does men. Smoking has been linked to impaired female fertility, cancer of the cervix, osteoporosis, and menstrual and menopausal problems.[32] Further, Dr. David Satcher's Surgeon General's Report clearly states that women who smoke while pregnant have babies with lower birth weight.[32]

Women also suffer the effects of second-hand smoke, commonly referred to as passive smoke. Each year, 20,000 to 25,000 people who never were smokers are diagnosed with lung cancer, with the majority being women.[16,33-35] Each year in the United States, approximately 3,000 men

Estimated deaths

Males			Females		
Lung and bronchus	90,490	31%	Lung and bronchus	73,020	27%
Prostate	30,350	10%	Breast	40,410	15%
Colon and rectum	28,540	10%	Colon and rectum	25,750	10%
Pancreas	15,820	5%	Ovary	16,210	6%
Leukemia	12,540	4%	Pancreas	15,980	6%
Esophagus	10,530	4%	Leukemia	10,030	4%
Liver and intrahepatic bile duct	10,330	3%	Non-hodgkin lymphoma	9,050	3%
Non-hodgkin lymphoma	10,150	3%	Uterine corpus	7,310	3%
Urinary bladder	8,970	3%	Multiple myeloma	5,640	2%
Kidney and renal pelvis	8,020	3%	Brain and other nervous system	5,480	2%
All sites	**295,280**	**100%**	**All sites**	**275,000**	**100%**

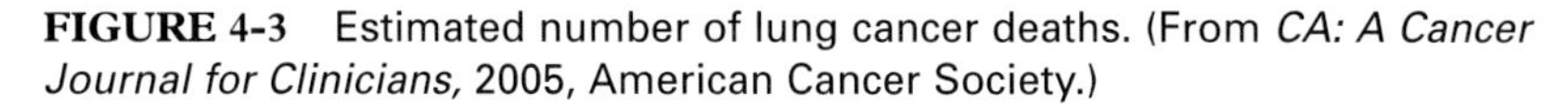

FIGURE 4-3 Estimated number of lung cancer deaths. (From *CA: A Cancer Journal for Clinicians,* 2005, American Cancer Society.)

and women die of lung cancer related to secondhand smoke, 65% of whom are women.[36]

Most of the attention and numerous epidemiologic studies have focused on active smoking as the primary risk factor for lung cancer. However, there are other risk factors that contribute to the development of lung cancer. These risks include both occupational and environmental exposures.[6,37,38] Radon contributes 10% of lung cancer risk, occupational exposures to carcinogens accounts for approximately 9% to 15%, and even outdoor air pollution 1% to 2% of the risk in all cases of lung cancer.[6] Add to the equation the interactions among all of these exposures, and the combined population attributable risk for lung cancer well exceeds 100%.[6] There are other risk factors for developing lung cancer: included are low socioeconomic status, lifestyle and behavioral factors such as poor diet and lack of exercise,[39,40] tuberculosis and other chronic pulmonary diseases, African-American ethnicity (e.g., lifetime smoking patterns),[26] and nutrition (e.g., lack of fresh fruits and vegetables and nutrients [carotenoids, Vitamins C and E and selenium]).[41-43]

Recently, interest has surfaced regarding the female hormone estrogen and a possible role it might play in the development of lung cancer. Lung tissue is known to have estrogen receptors. Higher circulating levels of estrogen could potentially affect the activity of the lung cells.[30] Although most studies are speculative, evidence is building that exogenous and endogenous estrogens may be involved in the development of lung cancer, specifically adenocarcinoma.[44] The Iowa Women's Health case-control study revealed an increased risk of lung carcinoma in women with a family history of female reproductive cancer.[45] Genetic susceptibility with special emphasis on *CYP1A1 (cytochrome P450)* and *GSTM1* (genotype of glutathione transferase class μ) metabolism in women has also been associated with increased lung cancer risk.[46] DNA mutations that activate oncogenes or inactivate tumor suppressor genes (p53 or K-*ras*) are also thought to be important in the development of lung cancer. However, additional research is needed to help clarify and elucidate lung cancer carcinogenesis and possible gender-related differences in these processes.

PREVENTION, SCREENING, AND DETECTION RELATING TO WOMEN

No other malignancy demonstrates a stronger epidemiologic relationship between prevention and incidence than that between smoking and lung cancer. Despite antismoking efforts, 20% of

Americans continue to smoke, with some not fully understanding the full dangers to their health.[47] Unfortunately, smoking rates remain high in women, especially among young girls and women with less education.[27] There would be a dramatic decline in incidence and mortality rates if women, as well as men, could be persuaded to stop smoking. Prevention and smoking cessation programs, along with institutional policies that discourage smoking, are essential tools in reducing the number of lung cancer cases and deaths. The challenge is to provide counseling at every health care visit. Popular Internet resources are free of charge and could help women who are interested in smoking cessation (see www.cancer.org/quittobacco).

Additional cancer prevention steps can be taken by women to lower their risk for developing cancers: for example, limiting fats in the diet, increasing intake of fruits and vegetables, avoiding excessive alcohol consumption, maintaining a healthy body weight, getting adequate daily exercise, and protecting the skin from sunlight. Again, this information on prevention could be conveyed during routine health prevention visits.

Various risk assessment screening tools can be located on several different Internet sites. One educational Internet site to help women understand their cancer risks can be found at Harvard's Center for Cancer Prevention (www.yourdiseaserisk.harvard.edu/hccpquiz.pl?quiz=lung&func=start). The site has a risk questionnaire that includes age, dietary habits, previous cancers, environment risks, and occupational risks. This is an initial step that can be included in any nursing assessment.

As with most cancer, early detection is crucial with lung cancer. The earlier that lung cancer is discovered, the better the chance for a cure. Unfortunately, the role of radiographic lung cancer screening remains controversial. While there is strong evidence to suggest that computed tomography screening detects lung cancer at much earlier stages than is the case without screening, a proven benefit in terms of decreased lung cancer mortality has yet to be firmly established.[48] More specifically, lung cancer screening to detect early lung cancer among women has not been researched and requires further investigation.

DIAGNOSIS AND STAGING

There are two major types of lung cancer: non–small cell lung cancer (NSCLC) and small cell lung cancer (SCLC). NSCLC accounts for approximately 80% of all lung cancer cases in the United States.[49] There are three histopathologic subtypes classified within NSCLC: adenocarcinoma, squamous cell carcinoma, and large cell carcinoma. Adenocarcinoma represents approximately 40% of all lung cancers in the United States. Nonsmokers are frequently diagnosed with adenocarcinoma and have lesions that are often located peripherally to the bronchi. These tumors frequently metastasize to the brain, adrenal glands, and bones. Proportionally, women also tend to develop adenocarcinomas more than men.[3] Some researchers have speculated that there is a reduced capacity in women to repair DNA in these tumors, thus suggesting that estrogen may have a role.

Squamous cell carcinoma, representing 30% to 35% of lung cancers, usually occurs centrally, near the main stem bronchi.[50] Proportionally, squamous cell carcinoma is associated more with persons who smoke. Large cell carcinoma, which represents 5% to 15% of lung cancer cases, is often located peripherally to the bronchi. These tumors grow and spread quickly.

The criteria of the Tumor, Node, Metastasis (TNM) staging system, which assists in accurately and concisely describing the tumor and extent of disease, were developed for NSCLC. The American Joint Committee on Cancer (AJCC) staging changed these in 1997 to reflect more detailed descriptions. Also, the stage groupings of the TNM subsets for lung cancer were revised based on treatment implications and survival differences (see Tables 4-1 and 4-2 (AJCC, 1997). Obviously, early stages (I and II) have better prognoses and outcomes than later-stage disease. Briefly, the major classification changes are:

- Stage I-tumors were further subdivided as IA and IB

Table 4-1 AJCC Staging of Lung Cancer

PRIMARY TUMOR (T)	
TX	Primary tumor cannot be assessed, or tumor is proven by presence of malignant cells in sputum or bronchial washings but cannot be visualized by imaging or bronchoscopy
T0	No evidence of primary tumor
T*is*	Carcinoma *in situ*
T1	Tumor 3 cm or less in greatest dimension, surrounded by lung or visceral pleura, without bronchoscopic evidence of invasion more proximal than lobar bronchus (i.e., not in main bronchus)
T2	Tumor with any of the following features of size or extent: More than 3 cm in greater dimension Involves main bronchus, 2 cm or more distal to the carina Invades the visceral pleura Associated with atelectasis or obstructive pneumonitis that extends to the hilar region but does not involve the entire lung
T3	Tumor of any size that directly invades any of the following: chest wall (including superior sulcus tumors), diaphragm, mediastinal pleura, parietal pericardium; or tumor in the main bronchus less than 2 cm distal to the carina but without the involvement of the carina; or associated atelectasis of obstructive pneumonitis of the entire lung
T4	Tumor of any size that invades any of the following: mediastinum, heart, great vessels, trachea, esophagus, vertebral body, carina; separate tumor nodule(s) in the same lobe; or tumor with a malignant pleural effusion
REGIONAL LYMPH NODES (N)	
NX	Regional lymph nodes cannot be assessed
N0	No regional lymph nodes metastasis
N1	Metastasis to ipsilateral peribronchial and/or ipsilateral hilar lymph nodes and intrapulmonary nodes involved by direct extension of the primary tumor
N2	Metastasis to ipsilateral mediastinal and/or subcarinal lymph node(s)
N3	Metastasis in contralateral mediastinal, contralateral hilar, ipsilateral or contralateral scalene or supraclavicular lymph node(s)
DISTANT METASTASIS (M)	
MX	Distant metastasis cannot be assessed
M0	No distant metastasis
M1	Distant metastasis present (includes synchronous separate nodule[s] in a different lobe)

Used with the permission of the American Joint Committee on Cancer (AJCC), Chicago, Illinois. The original source for this material is the *AJCC Cancer Staging Manual*, sixth edition (2002), published by Springer-Verlag, New York, www.springer-ny.com.

- Stage II-tumors were further subdivided as IIA and IIB
- Stage IIIA-tumors were classified differently into IIIA and IIIB groupings
- Stage IIIB and IV remain unchanged except for expansion of descriptors

SCLC represents 20% of all lung cancer cases and has a higher incidence rate proportionally in women.[27,51] The three subtypes within SCLC are oat cell (lymphocytic), intermediate, and combined (small cell combined with squamous or adenocarcinoma). All SCLC subtypes proliferate rapidly and are more likely to spread to other organs of the body than NSCLC. SCLC often starts in the main bronchi near the center of the lung. Staging for SCLC differs from that used for NSCLC. SCLC disease is typically classified as limited- and extensive-stage. Limited-stage refers to tumors that are confined to one hemithorax without pericardial or pleural effusion, and are encompassable in a single radiation therapy field.[52] Extensive disease applies to all other

Table 4-2 Stage Grouping

STAGE GROUPING OF THE TNM SUBSETS HAS BEEN REVISED AS FOLLOWS. TNM REFERS TO: PRIMARY TUMOR (T), REGIONAL LYMPH NOTE (N), AND DISTANT METASTASIS (M).			
Occult Carcinoma	TX	N0	M0
Stage 0	T*is*	N0	M0
Stage IA	T1	N0	M0
Stage IB	T2	N0	M0
Stage IIA	T1	N1	M0
Stage IIB	T2	N1	M0
	T3	N0	M0
Stage IIIA	T1	N2	M0
	T2	N2	M0
	T3	N1	M0
	T3	N2	M0
Stage IIIB	Any T	N3	M0
	T4	Any N	M0
Stage IV	Any T	Any N	M1

Used with the permission of the American Joint Committee on Cancer (AJCC), Chicago, Illinois. The original source for this material is the *AJCC Cancer Staging Manual,* sixth edition (2002), published by Springer-Verlag, New York, www.springer-ny.com.

presentations, which often includes distant metastases. Approximately one third of reported SCLC cases have limited disease at diagnosis, with the other two thirds first being seen with demonstrable distant metastases.[53,54]

The overwhelming majority of lung cancers are diagnosed in late stages: 15% are localized to a small area, 24% have regional disease involving lymph nodes, and 48% have distant metastases.[9] Reviewing the distribution between 1995 and 2000, 55% of SCLC cases were diagnosed with distant metastases, as compared to 36% for NSCLC. Very few SCLC and NSCLC were diagnosed early, without metastases (6% and 18%, respectively).[6] Stage of disease is the most important prognostic factor related to lung cancer survival. Other factors such as performance status, age, weight loss, and mutations in *ras* proto-oncogenes may also influence clinical outcomes.[1] Gender plays a small part in survival as well. Numerous clinical studies have shown that women survive longer than men.[12,13,27] Survival is based on treatment regimens and tolerability.

CLINICAL SYMPTOMS

Symptoms of lung cancer may be ignored by many women. Clinical manifestations for women do not differ from those experienced by men and may include a new and persistent cough, a change in a previously chronic cough, chest pain, hoarseness, weight loss, loss of appetite, bloody or rust-colored phlegm, shortness of breath, repeated bouts of pneumonia or bronchitis, lethargy, fatigue, intermittent fevers, and weakness.[55] Symptoms suggestive of advanced disease include superior vena cava syndrome, anorexia, unintentional weight loss, and pain from bony metastases. These symptoms are dependent on location and extent of disease.

TREATMENT AND SYMPTOM MANAGEMENT

Cancer treatment modalities (e.g., surgery, radiation, and chemotherapy) may be used to treat lung cancer, either alone or in combination. Treatment choices are based primarily on cancer type and stage of disease, and to a lesser extent on factors such as performance status and comorbidities. Treatment guidelines do not differ by gender. All patients are potential candidates for clinical trials; such options are best investigated thoroughly before treatment begins.

Presentations at diagnosis typically differ between NSCLC and SCLC. NSCLC is usually less aggressive and presents peripherally, but can also be located centrally in the chest. Progression of the disease is by the lymphatic system or invasion into the chest wall or diaphragm. Treatment choices are based on presentation, surgical candidacy, and the clinical stage. For stage 0, the cancer is limited to the lining layer of air passages and has not extended into the nearby lung tissues. Hence NSCLS is curable by surgery alone, and no chemotherapy or radiation is recommended (NCCN, version 1.2005). Surgical removal is done in wedges (wedge resection) or segments (segmentectomy). Stage I usually requires more extensive surgery, a lobectomy if the patient can tolerate it. Recent studies suggest that adjuvant chemotherapy for those with Stage IB improves the clinical outcome and survival.[49] Radiation therapy may be recommended if surgical margins were close. In stage II NSCLS, surgery is recommended with lobectomy or pneumonectomy, depending upon what is required to obtain clear surgical margins. Radiation therapy may be used after surgery to destroy occult cancer cells. Many clinical trials include chemotherapy in addition to surgery, to reduce recurrence.[49]

For stage IIIA, treatment depends on the location of the cancer and the extent of lymph node involvement. Chemotherapy plus radiation therapy is the standard of care when there is lymph node involvement. The role of surgery after chemotherapy (with or without radiation therapy) is controversial. Optimal clinical guidelines have yet to be established for stage IIIA disease, but clinical trials are ongoing.[56] Women tend to have better survival rates than do men when undergoing resection for NSCLC.[12] Survival rates are dramatically apparent in early-stage disease, and when adjusting for other factors such as extent of pulmonary resection and histopathologic features. Stage IIIB lung cancer describes cancerous spread within the chest but without evidence of distant metastases. Combined chemotherapy and radiation therapy is recommended. Surgical resection is sometimes performed after these modalities.

Stage IV NSCLC has spread beyond the chest to distant nodes or organs. Cure is not usually possible. Chemotherapy and/or radiation therapy are palliative in intent with an eye toward prolonged survival time and symptom control. Treatment may be used to open blocked airways, control bleeding, and palliate pain. New targeted drugs, such as gefitinib (Iressa) or erlotinib (Tarceva) may improve quality of life. However, current data suggest that gefitinib does not improve survival as second- or third-line therapy in treating adenocarcinoma.[57] When additional data become available, different treatment combinations may be recommended and guidelines may change.

SCLC is typically considered an aggressive cancer. Unfortunately, by the time it is diagnosed, SCLC has often spread to distant sites (e.g., brain, liver, and bones) even if the spread is undetectable by imaging or other diagnostic studies. Surgery is used with limited-stage disease if the person has a single nodule without evidence of disease elsewhere. Patients who undergo surgery after a mediastinoscopy are treated with postoperative chemotherapy. Patient who are not candidates for surgery are treated with chemotherapy and/or radiation.[58] If the SCLC is advanced, yet still classified as limited SCLC, and the individual is in reasonably good health, combined chemoradiation may be recommended. Chemotherapy or radiation alone is used in people with poor performance status. The most common chemotherapy combinations are either cisplatin or carboplatin plus etoposide, usually given for approximately 4 to 6 months. Other initial agents may include irinotecan (also known as CPT-11), ifosfamide, cyclophosphamide, vincristine, and doxorubicin. The best strategy is to review the most current clinical trials data and proceed with the best evidence. Since intracranial metastases occurs in 39% of patients with SCLC, randomized and nonrandomized studies have shown prophylactic cranial irradiation (PCI) is effective in preventing cerebral metastases (6% vs. 20%).[58] For patients diagnosed with limited-stage SCLC and complete response to therapy, PCI provides a 4% survival advantage.[59]

As with treatment, there are no sex differences when treating lung cancer symptomatology. Of lung cancer patients, 75% have a cough prior to treatment and 40% have a severe cough.[60] Simple over-the-counter cough suppressants may provide some relief, but a narcotic cough suppressant may be required.[61-63] Decreased activity with frequent rest periods, use of supplemental oxygen, avoiding pollutant irritants, and maintaining adequate food and fluid intake will help reduce or manage coughing.[64] Dyspnea, another common symptom, is frightening and unpleasant. Simple breathing exercises, supplemental oxygen, relaxation strategies, and/or pharmaceutical steroids may help alleviate this symptom.[65,66] Weight loss and anorexia are often experienced 6 months before diagnosis and occur in 60% of patients undergoing treatment. Over-the-counter (e.g., Eldertonic) or prescription appetite stimulants are recommended before or at the beginning of treatment.[55,67] Other treatment-related symptoms may occur from chemotherapy, radiation therapy or a combination thereof. These symptoms include esophagitus, pharyngitis, fatigue, skin changes, or pneumonitis. Resources for specific interventions can be located in the *Manual for Radiation Oncology Nursing Practice and Education.*[1,68,69]

PATIENT AND FAMILY EDUCATION

Despite the known addictive qualities of nicotine and the health consequences, women are still smoking. Female smokers aged 35 years and older are 12 times more likely to die prematurely of lung cancer, and 10.5 times more likely to die of emphysema or chronic bronchitis than their nonsmoking female counterparts.[9] Prevention of the initiation of smoking behavior, given the addictive characteristic of nicotine, should be the number one focus of patient education. The second priority should be smoking cessation.[11] Smoking cessation should focus on the young girl or woman, who might be persuaded to believe that smoking can control weight, or on pregnant women, because research has proven the harmful effects of tobacco on the fetus.[32] In addition to teaching about smoking cessation, the nurse should assess secondary risk factors. Women who live in areas with high levels of radon exposure should be tested for radon exposure, and abatement measures should be taken. The third priority is for women to avoid second-hand smoke (i.e., smoke from others' cigarettes and/or cigars).

Numerous Internet resources are available that provide information about lung cancer; they are listed in Table 4-3. One that has drawn attention to women is Women Against Lung Cancer (WALC). WALC is a nonprofit organization that was formed in 2001 and officially incorporated in 2003. The group is comprised of leading scientists, physicians, nurses, and advocates dedicated to eliminating lung cancer as a public health threat to women. Their mission is to decrease deaths due to lung cancer and to increase longevity through research, awareness, and advocacy.[70]

Special Considerations Among the Elderly

Lung cancer incidence increases with age. Most new cases of lung cancer are diagnosed in the elderly; 70 is the average age at diagnosis.[9] The risk of death from lung cancer also increases with age and is greater for men than women. In Table 4-4 the percentage of women dying from lung cancer is shown over different time periods extrapolated from the person's current age. For example, 1.4% of women who are 60 years old will die from lung cancer during the next 10 years (i.e., die by the age of 70 years). Translating this percentage to figures, for every 100 women currently 60 years old, one to two will die of lung cancer within 10 years.

Further, smoking affects the risk of dying from lung cancer as women age. A 50-year-old woman who smokes has a 4 in 1,000 chance of dying of breast cancer within the next 10 years, but a 10 in 1,000 chance of dying of lung cancer.[70]

IMPLICATIONS FOR PRACTICE, EDUCATION, AND RESEARCH

Health care professionals need to educate the public about the magnitude of the lung cancer threat to women. Education can enlighten women and men about the disease prevalence, risk factors, disease progression, treatment options, and quality of life for individuals with lung cancer and their families. Hopefully, this will bring a public outcry and the attention it needs and deserves to raise awareness about lung cancer.

Table 4-3 INTERNET RESOURCES FOR HEALTH PROFESSIONALS, INDIVIDUALS WITH LUNG CANCER, AND FAMILIES

ORGANIZATION	URL (WEBSITE)	MISSION
Alliance for Lung Cancer Advocacy, Support, and Education (ALCASE)	www.alcase.org	Dedicated solely to helping persons with lung cancer and those who are at risk for the disease, and to improving the quality of their lives through advocacy, support and education
American Cancer Society (ACS)	www.cancer.org	Includes specific Lung Cancer Resource Center, which describes lung cancer, its risk factors, prevention, causes, detection, symptoms, diagnosis, staging, and treatment
American Lung Association (ALA)	www.lungusa.org	Focuses on lung disease prevention, advocacy group; attention given to lung cancer and other lung diseases
Lung Cancer Online Foundation (LCOF)	lungcanceronline.org	Dedicated to improving the quality of care and the quality of life for persons with lung cancer by funding lung cancer research and providing information to patients and families
Cancer Care, Inc.	www.cancercare.org	Includes a Lung Cancer Support Program; site also provides extensive assistance to people with lung cancer including counseling services, information about cancer and treatment, referrals to other support services (home care, child care, transportation, pain management, entitlements), educational seminars and materials, and financial planning
International Association For the Study of Lung Cancer (IASLC)	www.iaslc.org	Promotes the study of the etiology, the epidemiology, the prevention, the diagnosis, the treatment and all other aspects of lung cancer and disseminates information about lung cancer to the members of the association, to the medical community at large, and to the public
National Familial Lung Cancer Registry (NFLCR)	www.path.jhu.edu/nfltr	Conducts research with families, studying DNA repair capacity and genetic markers and their relationship to environmental factors; goals of the registry are (1) to further understanding of the causes of lung cancer (beyond smoking), and (2) to serve as an educational resource for persons at risk for lung cancer

Table 4-4 SURVIVAL PREDICTIONS FOR MEN AND WOMEN WITH LUNG CANCER

Percent of Men And Women Who Die from Lung Cancer over 10-, 20-, and 30-Year Intervals According to Their Current Age						
	Men			Women		
Current Age	10 yrs	20 yrs	30 yrs	10 yrs	20 yrs	30 yrs
30	0.0	0.2	1.0	0.0	0.1	0.7
40	0.2	1.0	3.1	0.1	0.6	1.9
50	0.8	3.0	5.9	0.5	1.9	3.6
60	2.4	5.5	7.3	1.4	3.3	4.4

From Center for Disease Control (CDC); retrieved November 5, 2004, from www.cdc.gov/cancer/lung statistics.htm.

Because research is lagging behind in the lung cancer arena, support and encouragement for research regarding gender-related differences in the etiology, treatment, and prevention of lung cancer must become a top priority. Although numerous clinical studies have already identified smoking as the predominant risk factor in the development of lung cancer, there is still a need to advocate for increased funding for lung cancer research. Women should be actively recruited for clinical trials and protocols developed specifically for women.

If funding is low, so too is the direct involvement of women physicians and scientists studying lung cancer. The Council on Graduate Medical Education (COGME) provides ongoing assessments of physician workforce trends and recommends appropriate federal and private sector efforts to present identified needs to the government.[71] Summary findings show that women are underrepresented in higher academic and leadership positions, that women tend to cluster in primary care disciplines, and that the gender ratio should continue to be monitored in the physician workforce. This report validates a relationship between women in academic leadership positions and those involved in the health care of women. While only an advisory group, the panel of experts reported that in order to improve the health care of women, more equality and equity in the status of women physicians is needed before significant improvements can be made. Therefore encouraging and mentoring female health care professionals to pursue careers in lung cancer research is of utmost importance.

SUMMARY

Lung cancer is a major public health problem in the US. Lung cancer is most certainly not "just a man's disease." While the incidence of lung cancer among men is leveling off, the incidence of lung cancer among women is rapidly increasing. Research suggests that women may have a greater susceptibility to carcinogens than men do, but more research is needed to effectively intervene in the carcinogenic process.

Lung cancer is the number one cause of cancer mortality in women, and this tragic trend, primarily related to tobacco use, is expected to continue growing. Debates are likely to continue about the development and natural history of lung cancer among women and men as practitioners strive to sort theory from reality. However, let there be no debate about the cause of lung cancer. Smoking does lead to lung cancer. Curtailing smoking in the United States and internationally is the greatest challenge that faces women.

REFERENCES

1. Haas, M. *Contemporary issues in lung cancer: A nursing perspective.* Sudbury, Massachusetts, 2003, Jones and Bartlett.
2. Chapple A, Ziebland S, McPherson A: Stigma, shame and blame experience by patients with lung cancer: qualitative study, *BMJ* 328:1470, 2004.
3. Twombly R: New studies fan controversy over gender risk in lung cancer, *J Nat Cancer Inst* 96: 898-900, 2004.
4. Risch HA, et al: Are female smokers at higher risk for lung cancer than male smokers? A case-control analysis by histologic type, *Am J Epidemiol* 138: 281-293, 1993.
5. Smith R, Cokkinides V, Eyre H: American Cancer Society Guidelines for the early detection of cancer, *CA Cancer J Clin* 55:31-44, 2005.
6. American Lung Association: Trends in lung cancer morbidity and mortality, *American Lung Association Epidemiology and Statistic Unit Research and Scientific Affairs,* Birmingham, Alabama.
7. Jemal A and others: Cancer Statistics, 2005, *CA Cancer J Clin* 55(1):20-26, 2005.
8. National Cancer Institute: Lung cancer, on the Web at www.nci.nih.gov/cancertopics/types/lung, accessed on October 6, 2005.

9. American Cancer Society: Cancer facts and figures, Atlanta, Ga., 2004, The Society.
10. Centers for Disease Control and Prevention: Health, United States, National Center Health Statistics,. Hyattsville, MD, 2003, Centers for Disease Control and Prevention, www.cdc.gov/nchs/.
11. Patel J, Bach P, Kris M: Lung cancer in U.S. women: a contemporary epidemic, *JAMA* 291 (14):1763-1768, 2004.
12. Alexiou C, Onyeaka C, Beggs D: Do women live longer following lung resection for carcinoma? *Eur J Cardio-thorac Surg* 21(2):319-325, 2002.
13. De Parrot M: Sex differences in presentation, management, and prognosis of patients with non-small cell lung carcinoma, *J Thorac Cardiovasc Surg* 119(1):21-26, 2000.
14. Thun M, Henley S, Calle E: Tobacco use and cancer: an epidemiologic perspective for geneticists, *Oncogene* 21:7303-7325, 2002.
15. Peneger T: Sex, smoking and cancer: a reappraisal, *J Nat Cancer Inst* 93:1600-1602, 2001.
16. Zang E, Wynder E: Differences in lung cancer risk between men and women: examination of the evidence, *J Nat Cancer Inst* 88(3-4):183-192, 1996.
17. Dresler CM: Gender differences in genetic susceptibility for lung cancer, *Lung Cancer* 30(3):153-160, 2000.
18. Fasco M, Hurteau G, Spivack S: Gender-dependent expression of alpha and beta estrogen receptors in human nontumor and tumor lung tissue, *Mol Cell Endocrinol* 188(102):125-140, 2002.
19. Mollerup S and others: Sex differences in lung CYP1A1 expression and DNA adduct levels among lung cancer patients, *Cancer Res* 59(14):3317-3320, 1999.
20. Mooney LA and others: Gender differences in autoantibodies to oxidative DNA base damage in cigarette smokers, *Cancer Epidemiol Biomarkers Prev* 10(6):641-648, 2001.
21. Tang DL and others: Associations between both genetic and environmental biomarkers and lung cancer: evidence of a greater risk of lung cancer in women smokers *Carcinogenesis* 19(11):1949-1953, 1998.
22. Bain C and others: Lung cancer rates in men and women with comparable histories of smoking, *J Nat Cancer Inst* 96(11):826-834, 2004.
23. Brennan J and others: Association between cigarette smoking and mutation of the p53 gene in squamous-cell carcinoma of the head and neck, *N Engl J Med* 332(11):712-717, 1995.
24. Mao L and others: Clonal genetic alterations in the lung of current and former smokers. *J Nat Cancer Inst* 89 (12):857-862, 1997.
25. Wistuba, I and others: Molecular damage in the bronchial epithelium of current and former smokers, *J Nat Cancer Inst* 889(18):1366-1373, 1997.
26. Schottenfield D: Epidemiology of Lung Cancer. In: Pass H and others, editors: *Lung cancer: principles and practice,* New York, 1996, Lippincott-Raven.
27. Baldini E, Strauss G: Women and lung cancer: waiting to exhale *Chest* 112(4 Suppl):229S-234S, 1997.
28. Koyi H, Hillerdal G, Branden E: A prospective study of a total material of lung cancer from a county in Sweden 1997-1999: gender, symptoms, type, stage, and smoking habits, *Lung Cancer* 36(1):9-14, 2002.
29. Chollat-Traquet C: *Women and tobacco,* Geneva, 1992, World Health Organization.
30. Siegfried J: Women and lung cancer: does oestrogen play a role? *Lancet Oncol* 2:506-513, 2001.
31. Ebbert J and others: Lung cancer risk reduction after smoking cessation: observations from a prospective cohort of women, *J Clin Oncol* 21(5):921-926, 2003.
32. Satcher D: Women and smoking: A Report of the Surgeon General-2001. U.S. Department of Health and Human Service, Centers for Diseases Control and Prevention, National Center for Chronic Disease Prevention and Health Promotion Office on Smoking and Health. On the Web at www.cdc.gov/tobacco.
33. Hu J and others: Risk factors for lung cancer among Canadian women who have never smoked, *Cancer Detect Prevent* 26(2):129-138, 2002.
34. Nordquist LT and others: Improved survival in never-smokers vs. current smokers with primary adenocarcinoma of the lung, *Chest* 126(2):347-351, 2004.
35. Radzikowska E, Glaz P: Lung cancer—differences of incidence between the sexes, *Pneumonol Alergol Pol* 68 (9-10):417-424, 2000.
36. Environmental Protection Agency: Respiratory health effects of passive smoking: lung cancer and other disorders, Washington, D.C., 1992, The Agency.
37. Armstrong J: Tumors of the lung and mediastinum. In Leibel S, Phillips T editors: *Textbook of radiation oncology,* Philadelphia, 1998, WB Saunders.
38. Reddy A: Non-small cell lung cancer: imaging and staging, American Society for Therapeutic Radiology and Oncology 42nd Annual Meeting, Oct 22, 2000, on the Web at www.astro.org/, accessed on October 6, 2005.
39. Pearce N, Bethwaite P: Social class and male cancer mortality in New Zealand, 1984-7, *N Z Med J* 110(1045), 200-202, 1997.
40. Vagero D, Persson G: Occurrence of cancer in socioeconomic groups in Sweden: An analysis based on the Swedish Cancer Environment Registry, *Scand J Social Med* 14:151-160, 1986.
41. Alavanja M and others: Lung cancer risk and red meat consumption among Iowa women, *Lung Cancer* 34(1): 37-46, 2001.
42. Feskanich D And others: Prospective study of fruit and vegetable consumption and risk of lung cancer among men and women, *J Nat Cancer Inst* 92:1812-1823, 2000.
43. Ginsberg R, Vokes E, Rosenzweig K: Non-small cell lung cancer. In: DeVita VT, Heilman S, Rosenberg SA, editors: *Cancer: principles and practice of oncology* Philadelphia, Pa., 2001, Lippincott Williams & Wilkins.
44. Taioli E, Wynder E: Endocrine factors and adenocarcinoma of the lung in women, *J Nat Cancer Inst* 84:869-870, 1994.
45. Sellers T, Potter J, Poisom A: Association of incident lung cancer with family history of female reproductive cancers: the Iowa Women's Health Study, *Epidemiology* 8:199-208, 1991.
46. Alexandrie K and others: Genetic susceptibility to lung cancer with special emphasis on CYP1A1 and GSTM1: a study of host factors in relation to age at onset, gender, and histological cancer types, *Carcinogenesis* 15(9):1785-1790, 1994.
47. Bilello K, Nurin S, Matthay R: Epidemiology, etiology, and prevention of lung cancer, *Clin Chest Med* 23(1):1-25, 2002.
48. Elliott V: Chest CT scans detect early-stage lung cancer, American Medical Association (amednews.com), Dec 27, 2004.

49. American Cancer Society: Treatment choices by stage for non-small cell lung cancer, 2004, on the Web at www.cancer.org/docroot/CRI/content/CRI_2_4_4X_Treatment_Choices_by_Stage_for_Non-Small_Cell_Lung_Cancer_NSCLC_26.asp?sitearea.
50. American Cancer Society: Treatment Choices by Stage for Small Cell Lung Cancer, 2004, on the Web at www.cancer.org/docroot/CRI/content/CRI_2_4_4X_Treatment_Choices_by_Stage_for_Small_Cell_Lung_Cancer_SCLC_26.asp?sitearea=.
51. Murren J, Glatstein E, Pass H: Small cell lung cancer. In: DeVita VT, Heilman S, Rosenberg SA, editors: *Cancer: principles and practice of oncology,* Philadelphia, Pa., 2001, Lippincott Williams & Wilkins.
52. Kristjansen P, Hansen H: Management of small cell lung cancer: A summary of the Third International Association for the Study of Lung Cancer Workshop on Small Cell Lung Cancer, *J Nat Cancer Inst* 82:263-266, 1990.
53. Jeremic B and others: Initial versus delayed accelerated hyperfractionated radiation therapy and concurrent chemotherapy in limited small cell lung cancer: A randomized study. *Int J Radiation Oncol Biol Phys* 50(1): 19-25, 1997.
54. Detterbeck F: Diagnosis and staging of non-small cell lung cancer. Diagnosis and treatment of lung cancer: an evidence-based guide for the practicing clinician *Chest* 1(2):1-13, 2000.
55. Moore-Higgins G: Lung cancer outcomes in radiation therapy. In Watkins-Bruner, D, Moore-Higgins, G. and Haas, M, editors, *Outcomes in radiation therapy: multidisciplinary management,* Sudbury, Mass., 2001, Jones and Bartlett.
56. Robinson L, Wagner H, Ruckdeschel J: Treatment of stage IIIA non-small cell lung cancer, *Chest* 123(supp 1): 202S-220S, 2003.
57. AstraZeneca: Iressa shows no overall survival advantage as second- or third-line therapy. On the web at www.astrazeneca.com/ pressrelease/4245.aspx. Press release Dec 17, 2004.
58. National Comprehensive Cancer Network: Small cell lung cancer. Clinical Practice Guidelines in Oncology-Version 1. 2005, on the Web at www.nccn.org/professionals/physician_gls/PDF/sclc.pdf. (prev published 2002).
59. Auperin A And others: Prophylactic cranial irradiation for patients with small-cell lung cancer in complete remission. Prophylactic Cranial Radiation Overview Collaborative Group, *N Engl J Med* 341:476-484, 1999.
60. Chao K. Perez C, Brady L: *Lung cancer. Radiation oncology: Management decisions,* Philadelphia, 1999, Lippincott-Raven.
61. Haas M: *Pocket guide to lung cancer,* Sudbury, Massachusetts, 2004, Jones and Bartlett.
62. Kvale P, Simoff M, Prakash U: Palliative care, *Chest* 123(suppl 1):284s-311s, 2003.
63. McDermott K: Cough. In D. Camp-Sorrell and R. Hawkins, editors: *Clinical manual for the oncology advanced practice nurse,* Pittsburgh, 2000, Oncology Nursing Society.
64. Ingle R: Lung cancers. In Yarbro C and others, editors: *Cancer nursing: principles and practice,* Sudbury, Mass., 2000, Jones and Bartlett.
65. Chandler S: Nebulized opioids to treat dyspnea, *Am J Hospice and Palliat Care* 16(1):418-422, 1999.
66. Dudgeon D and others: Dyspnea in cancer patients: prevalence and associated factors, *J Pain Symptom Manage* 21(2):95-102, 2001.
67. Brown J: Systematic review of the evidence on symptom management of cancer-related anorexia and cachexia, *Oncol Nurs Forum* 29:517-532, 2002.
68. Watkins-Bruner D, Haas M, Gosselin-Acomb T, editors: *Manual for radiation oncology nursing practice and education,* Pittsburgh, 2004, Oncology Nursing Society.
69. Yarbro C, Frogge M, Goodman M: *Cancer symptom management,* ed 3, Sudbury, Mass., 2004, Jones and Bartlett.
70. WALC: Women Against Lung Cancer, 2004, on the Web at www.4walc.org.
71. COGME (Council on Graduate Medical Education): Fifth Report: women and medicine. U.S. Department of Health and Human Services Public Health Service, Health Resources and Services Administration, July:1-61, 1995.

CHAPTER

5 Breast Cancer

Regina S. Cunningham

INTRODUCTION AND OVERVIEW

EPIDEMIOLOGY

Invasive breast cancer is expected to occur in 211,240 women in the US in 2005.[1] Breast cancer will remain the leader in new cancer cases and be the second most common cause of cancer-related death in women. Breast cancer incidence has risen consistently over the past 25 years. This increase is due in part to more precise diagnostic methods that enable earlier detection of smaller tumors, but may also be related to the increased use of hormone replacement therapy and the increased prevalence of obesity in women.[1] Although rare, breast cancer does occur in men. It is estimated that 1,690 new cases will be diagnosed in men in 2005, accounting for less than 1% of all breast cancer cases.[1,2]

Breast cancer occurs most frequently in Caucasians, followed by African Americans, Asian Americans/Pacific Islanders, Hispanic/Latinos, and American Indian/Alaskan Natives. The increased incidence among whites is attributed to more frequent mammography, delayed age at first birth, and historically greater use of hormone replacement therapy. Mortality also varies by racial groups, with the highest rate found among African American women. Increased mortality among African Americans has been ascribed to limited access to regular screening, leading to more advanced disease at the time of presentation, and less access to timely, high quality treatments.[1]

A trend toward decreased breast cancer mortality has been observed in developed nations in recent years. In 1990, for the first time in 25 years, breast cancer mortality rates in the US began dropping slowly; by 1999 the age-adjusted mortality rate was 27 per 100,000 population, the lowest rate it had been since 1973.[3] Overall decreases in mortality rates have been attributed to increased use of effective screening strategies such as mammography, earlier detection, and improved therapeutic options that are based on evolving understanding of the biology of the disease.

ETIOLOGY

Breast Cancer Biology

The elucidation of the human genome has facilitated developments in molecular biology that have advanced our fundamental understanding of disease. It is now recognized that the initiation, progression, and metastases of human cancers are driven by genetic changes. Fundamentally, breast cancer is a genetic disease that occurs when a series of molecular and genetic aberrations result in a malignant phenotype. Newly developed technologies, such as microarray-based gene expression profiling, have helped to enhance our knowledge of the genetic basis of breast cancer and have shown promise in predicting clinical outcomes in this population. Microarray technology has enabled the identification of specific genetic patterns in breast cancer specimens, the detection of breast tumor cells in peripheral blood, the prediction of neoadjuvant chemotherapy response from fine needle aspirates, and the identification of disease-free surgical breast specimens and thus the prediction of overall survival.[4] This knowledge is translating clinically into improvements in our ability to prevent, detect, and treat breast cancers.

BREAST ANATOMY

Breasts are tear-shaped glands attached to the chest wall by ligaments (Figure 5-1). The glands are surrounded by fat, giving the breasts their size and shape. Each breast is comprised of 15 to 20 lobes that contain multiple smaller lobules. The terminal portion of each lobule contains sacs where

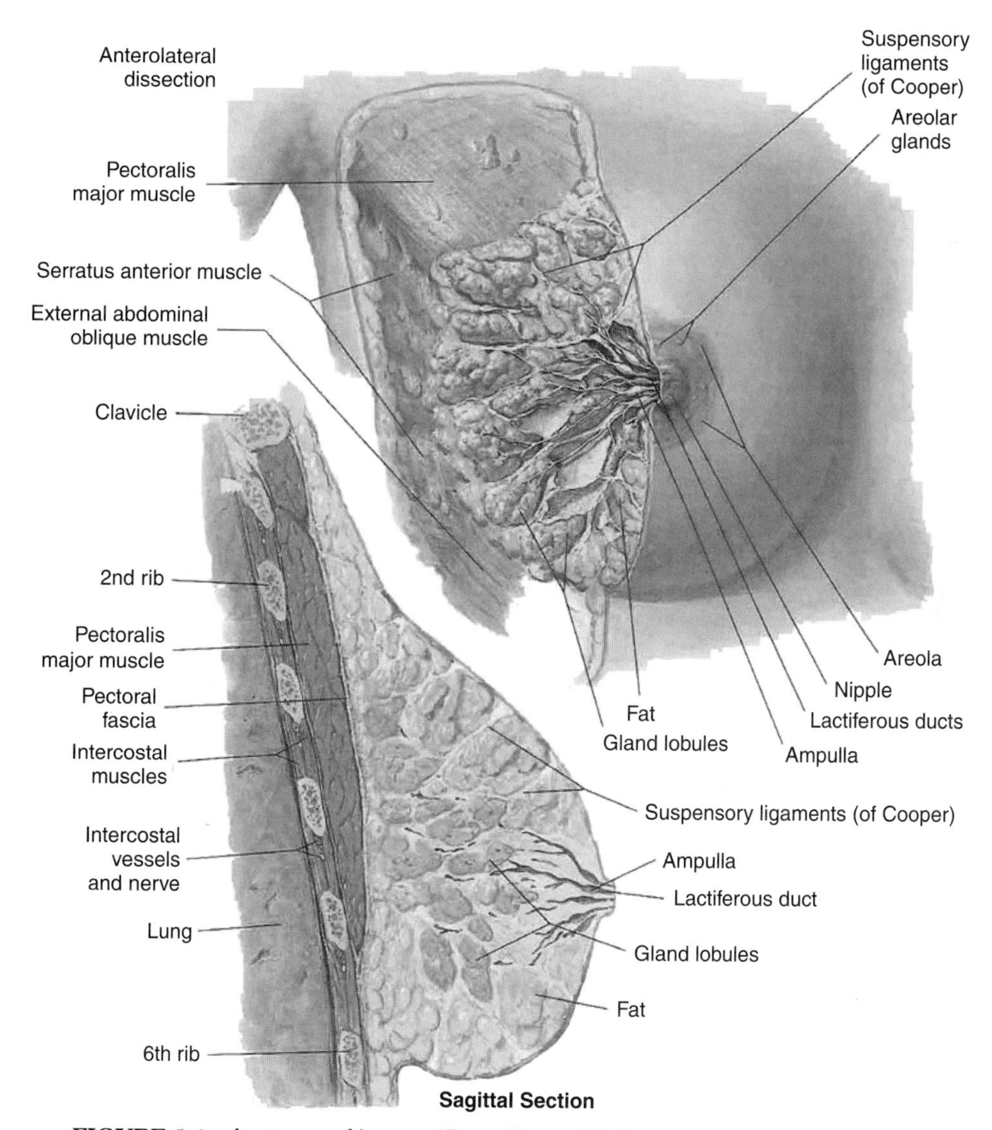

FIGURE 5-1 Anatomy of breast. (From Netter FH, Dalley II AF: Atlas of Human Anatomy, East Hanover, NJ, 1997, Novartis.)

milk production occurs under the direction of hormonal stimuli. Breast development, enlargement, and milk production are primarily controlled by the interplay of three hormones: estrogen, progesterone, and prolactin.

The breast is divided into four relatively symmetric quadrants that emanate from the nipple-areolar complex. These four quadrants are depicted in Figure 5-2. The most frequent location for the development of breast cancer is the upper outer quadrant.[5] Blood and lymph are drained from the breast area by a series of lymphatic channels that lead to axillary and internal mammary nodes (Figure 5-3); transmission of breast cancer often occurs through these lymphatic channels. Sentinel lymph node (SLN) mapping is a procedure used to identify the first node in the lymphatic basin; this node is at the highest risk for metastases. SLN biopsy provides accurate nodal staging for breast cancer with less morbidity than traditional nodal sampling procedures. SLN procedures will be discussed in detail later in the chapter.

RISK FACTORS FOR THE DEVELOPMENT OF BREAST CANCER

Epidemiologic studies have established a number of risk factors (Box 5-1) for the development of breast cancer. With the exception of female gender and age however, the majority of breast cancers occur in women with no identifiable risk factors. Breast cancer risk assessment is designed to calculate an individual woman's degree of risk and to personalize surveillance and management strategies based on this risk. The overall goal is to improve survival in women who are at high risk and to decrease costs and complications in women at low risk.[6]

Family History

Cross-sectional and case-control studies have clearly demonstrated that women who have one or more first-degree relatives with breast cancer have a twofold to fourfold increase in their risk to develop the disease.[7] Additional factors that contribute to increased risk include the number of relative(s) affected, the closeness of the relationship, and the age of disease onset in the affected relative, with younger age being associated with greater risk.[8] When conducting a family history it is essential to remember that there is an equal potential for maternal and paternal susceptibility transmission. As such, data from both lineages must be obtained.

Several models using family history data for estimating breast cancer risk have been developed. The most commonly used of these are the Gail and Claus models, which were derived using large population–based data sets. Using statistical methods applied to data from the Breast Cancer Detection and Demonstration Project, scientists at the National Cancer Institute (NCI) and the National Surgical Adjuvant Breast and Bowel Project (NSABP) developed the Gail model. This model uses current age, history of first-degree relatives with breast cancer (up to two relatives), number of previous breast biopsies (and whether they revealed atypical hyperplasia), age at menarche, and age at first delivery to project a woman's risk of invasive breast cancer over a 5-year period and over her lifetime. The Gail model is available on the NCI website (http://bcra.nci.nih.gov/brc/q1.htm).[9] The Gail model may not be as useful in the setting where there is a potentially strong

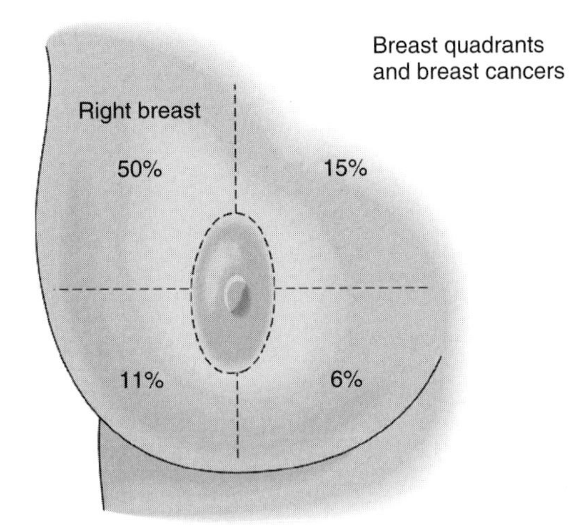

FIGURE 5-2 Breast quadrants and breast cancers. (From Byer CO, Shainberg LW, Galliano G: Breast quadrants and breast cancers. In Byer E, Shainberg LW, Galliano G, editors: *Dimensions in human sexuality*, New York, 1999, McGraw Hill.)

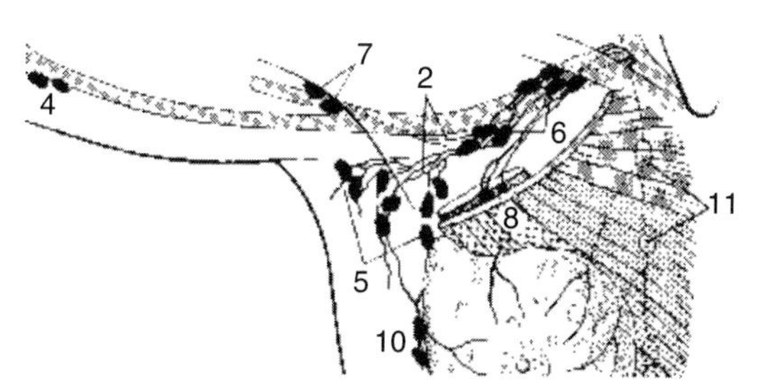

FIGURE 5-3 Lymphatic drainage of the breast. (From U.S. National Cancer Institute's Surveillance, Epidemiology and End Results (SEER) Program with Emory University, Atlanta SEER Cancer Registry: Figure 3. Regional Lymph Nodes of the Breast, 2000. Retrieved from http://training.seer.cancer.gov/ss_module01_breast/unit02_sec03_lymph_nodes.html.)

influence of paternal genes. In such cases, it may be more effective to employ the Claus model. The Claus model includes information about the number of breast cancers and the age at onset of breast cancers within a family. The Claus model accounts for both paternal and maternal relatives and is useful for women with a strong family history of breast cancer whose *BRCA1/2* status is unknown.

Box 5-1 RISK FACTORS FOR THE DEVELOPMENT OF BREAST CANCER

- Gender
- Age
- Family history of breast cancer
- Breast cancer susceptibility genes
- Hormonal factors
  - Early age at onset of menses
  - Nulliparity
  - First child birth after 30 years of age
  - Early or late menopause
  - Hormone replacement therapy
  - Obesity
- Alcohol consumption
- Radiation exposure
- Breast biopsies/benign breast disease

Breast Cancer Susceptibility Genes

Advances in molecular genetics have led to the identification of specific genes that confer an increased susceptibility to developing cancer of the breast. Although inherited forms of breast cancer represent a small portion of the total number of breast cancer cases, this knowledge is providing a means of identifying individuals who are at increased risk to develop the disease.[10,11] Two genes associated with hereditary forms of breast cancer have been identified: these include *BRCA1*, which is located on chromosome 17, and *BRCA2*, located on chromosome 13.[12] Other susceptibility alleles have been identified, but these are associated with the development of an even smaller number of breast cancer cases (Figure 5-4). For example, mutations in the cell cycle checkpoint kinase gene (*CHEK2*), account for approximately 5% of all familial cases of breast cancer, and mutations in *TP53* account for less than 1% of cases. The search for additional breast cancer susceptibility genes is an area of current research focus.[10]

Mutations in either the *BRCA1* or the *BRCA2* genes confer an increased lifetime risk of the development of both breast (60% to 85%) and ovarian (15% to 40%) cancers.[10] Both *BRCA* mutations are associated with the development of breast cancer at an early age.[13] *BRCA*-mutation carriers are also at increased risk to develop cancer in the contralateral breast[14,15] as well as ovarian cancer, fallopian tube cancer, and primary peritoneal cancers.[16]

In their nonmutated forms, *BRCA1/2* function as tumor suppressor genes. Both proteins participate in DNA repair and chromatin remodeling as well as other cellular processes. *BRCA1* has specific functions with regard to estrogen receptor activity and estrogen-induced proliferation of breast tissue. *BRCA2* is involved in cell cycle checkpoint control.[17] When *BRCA1* or *BRCA2* mutations occur, the functions of these proteins are lost. Cells have reduced ability to perform DNA repair and exhibit multiple chromosomal aberrations. Analysis of gene expression profiles have demonstrated that tumors associated with *BRCA1* or *BRCA2* mutations differ significantly from sporadic tumors.[18]

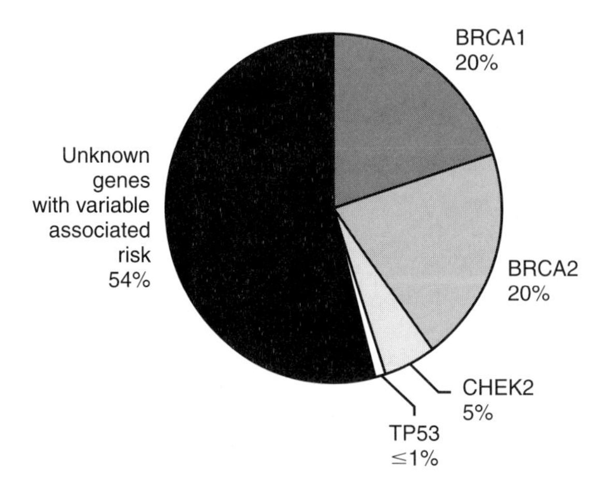

FIGURE 5-4 Breast risk wheel. (From Wooster, R. & Weber, B.L. (2003). Breast and Ovarian Cancer. The New England Journal of Medicine, 348(23), 2339-2347. Copyright© 2003 Massachusetts Medical Society. All rights reserved.)

Specific pathologic features have been identified in breast cancers associated with *BRCA1/2* mutations; typically, these tumors are aneuploid, are of a high nuclear grade with a high mitotic index, are frequently ductally invasive with "pushing" margins (a pathologic description of the pattern of invasion seen at the tumor edge), and have multiple lymphocytic infiltrates. *BRCA1* tumors are generally larger in size than sporadic tumors and are negative for estrogen and progesterone receptors. *BRCA2* mutations are heterogeneous and often high-grade and exhibit less tubule formation, but their mitotic count and cellular pleomorphism do not differ significantly from sporadic tumors. The majority of *BRCA2* tumors are positive for hormone receptors.[18-20]

Probability models that estimate the likelihood of detecting *BRCA1/2* mutations have been developed. Such models provide complementary information that can be used, along with clinical judgment, to inform a comprehensive approach to surveillance and management. There are currently four widely used probability models: these include Couch, Shattuck-Eidens, Frank, and BRCAPRO. Each of these has advantages and disadvantages and must be considered within the context in which it is applied, so that the most accurate information can be obtained.[6] BRCAPRO is a Web-based program that estimates the risk of *BRCA1/2* genetic mutations for women who have a strong family history of breast or ovarian cancer (or both); BRACPRO is available at http://astor.som.jhmi.edu/BayesMendel/brcapro.html.[21]

Genetic testing for mutations in *BRCA1/2* has become relatively common in oncology practice. The purpose of this testing is to provide appropriate recommendations for care of patients and families affected by hereditary cancer syndromes. The American Society of Clinical Oncology (ASCO) has outlined specific indications for genetic testing for cancer susceptibility. In the setting of breast cancer, these include the following: the individual is first seen with a personal or family history that is suggestive of a genetic cancer susceptibility; the test can be adequately interpreted; and the results will aid in diagnosis or management of a patient or family at risk for a hereditary breast cancer.[22] ASCO also recommends that genetic testing be done only in the setting of precounseling and postcounseling so that the results are adequately interpreted and the meaning of those results to the individual are addressed. Genetic testing optimally occurs within the context of a comprehensive cancer risk assessment and counseling program. Such programs enlist the aid of multidisciplinary experts, including physicians, nurses, genetic counselors, and social workers who have training and expertise in assessing and managing familial cancers. Patients who are suspected of having a genetic predisposition to breast cancer should undergo a comprehensive family history with completion of a pedigree and determination of candidacy for genetic testing so that familial risk can be accurately determined. These data should then be used to inform a risk-counseling plan. Guidelines for Genetic/Familial High-Risk Assessment for Breast and Ovarian Cancer have been developed by the National Comprehensive Cancer Network (NCCN) and are available at www.nccn.org.[8]

Nurses working in cancer risk assessment and counseling programs must be knowledgeable about breast cancer risk, be prepared to educate patients and families about the appropriateness and interpretation of genetic testing, and be aware of the psychosocial issues encountered by patients undergoing such testing. In carrying out these activities, nurses have the potential to maximize opportunities for breast cancer prevention and detection and healthy coping.[23]

Hormones

Many of the established risk factors for the development of breast cancer are mediated through hormonal activity.[24,25] In experimental models, estrogen is required for the optimal development of breast tumors. Moreover, epidemiologic studies have demonstrated decreased risk of breast cancer in women who have undergone ovarian ablation. Risk reduction in this population is inversely correlated to age; the younger the age of the woman at the time of ablation, the greater the risk reduction. Other hormonal factors also influence breast cancer risk. The number of years of ovulatory cycles for example, is an influencing factor. Higher incidence of the disease is found in women who experience early menarche or late menopause, as well as in those who are nulliparous. Women who begin menses before 12 years of age or who experience menopause after age 54 have twice the incidence of breast cancer.[26]

The role of exogenous hormones, including the use of hormone replacement therapy (HRT) and oral contraceptives has been a focus of study for several decades. Studies of oral contraceptives have demonstrated that there is a small increase in relative risk of breast cancer in current or recent users; however, this risk disappears within 10 years of discontinuing oral contraceptive use. In one study, women who began using oral contraceptives before the age of 20 had a greater relative risk of developing breast cancer.[26] For many years, estrogen was commonly prescribed to menopausal women to preserve bone strength, lower cholesterol, and provide cardiovascular protection. Over time, concerns about increased risk of breast and endometrial cancers among women taking these supplements were raised. These concerns led to the use of combined estrogen/progestin formulations of hormone therapy.[27] A large metaanalysis conducted by the Collaborative Group on Hormonal Factors in Breast Cancer found that the use of hormone replacement therapy was associated with a moderate increase in the risk of breast cancer; the relative risk was 1.35 for women who used HRT for a period of at least five years.[28] This increased risk for breast cancer in women taking HRT must be considered within the context of the health benefits provided by these agents in a given individual. Recently, new evidence has called into question some of the protective benefits of HRT. While early reports from the Heart Estrogen/ Progestin Replacement Study did document decreases in serum lipoproteins in women receiving hormone replacement, long-term follow-up showed no differences in coronary disease between women who received HRT and those who did not. Moreover, there was an increase in the incidence of thromboembolism, gall bladder disease, and risk for hip fractures.[29-31] In addition, results from the more recent women's health initiative study have demonstrated that cardiovascular risk reduction was not uniformly achieved in women receiving HRT. In this investigation, combined HRT increased the risk of coronary artery disease, stroke, and blood clots by 29%, 41%, and 26% respectively.[32]

Obesity

Height and body mass index (BMI) can influence the risk of breast cancer in women.[33,34] A number of case-control and prospective cohort studies have demonstrated an inverse relationship between weight and breast cancer. Most large epidemiologic studies have found that overweight or obese women are at greater risk of developing postmenopausal breast cancer.[35] Moreover, greater BMI is associated with more advanced disease at presentation. The increase in breast cancer risk associated with increasing BMI among postmenopausal women is largely the result of an increase in estrogens, particularly bioavailable estradiol.[36] Obese women are also at high risk to develop a metabolic syndrome that induces insulin resistance and hyperinsulinemia. In postmenopausal women, elevated insulin levels are associated with an increased risk for breast cancer as well as cardiac disease.[37]

A recent retrospective study investigated the association between growth during childhood and the risk of breast cancer in a cohort of over 117,000 Danish women. In this investigation, high birth weight, height stature at 14 years of age, low body mass index at 14 years of age, and peak growth at an early age were identified as independent risk factors for development of the disease. Authors concluded that birth weight and growth during childhood and adolescence influenced the risk of breast cancer.

Obesity may also have an adverse effect on treatment outcomes. The outcomes of surgery, chemotherapy, radiation therapy, and hormonal therapy can all be negatively influenced by obesity.[38]

The role of exercise and physical activity on the risk of developing breast cancer has also been investigated. Evidence supporting the role of exercise in reducing risk for breast cancer is evolving. The amount and type of exercise (aerobic versus or combined with progressive resistance training) are being studied, but at the present time there are not adequate data to formulate specific recommendations.

Alcohol

Several studies have investigated the relationship between consumption of alcohol and the development of breast cancer. An early metaanalysis and several subsequent studies suggested a dose-response relationship between alcohol consumption and risk, with the greatest risk occurring in women who consumed two or more drinks per day.[28,39-43] Results were less consistent for women who consumed small to moderate amounts of alcohol.[39] Ellison, Zhang, McLennan, and Rothman[44] performed a more recent metaanalysis of epidemiologic studies conducted through 1999 and found a monotonic increase in the risk for breast cancer in women who consumed an average of 12 g of alcohol per day (approximately one drink) compared to nondrinkers, but the magnitude of the effect was small. Menopausal status and type of alcoholic beverage consumed did not influence findings. Authors concluded that although a number of studies have investigated the relationship between alcohol and breast cancer risk, a definitive causal relationship between these variables has not yet been clearly established. Alcohol use has been identified as a modifiable behavior; as such, education and counseling may be of benefit to patients who report higher levels of consumption.

Radiation Exposure

Previous radiation therapy has been identified as a risk factor for the development of secondary breast cancers. The Childhood Cancer Survivor Study evaluated women with secondary breast cancer from a large cohort of cancer survivors who lived more than 5 years after being diagnosed with a childhood cancer between 1970 and 1986. This study considered a number of variables among these women: these included the influence of primary cancer, previous treatment, family cancer history, and menstrual and reproductive history. Data analysis indicated that survivors who had chest radiation therapy for Hodgkin's disease, bone sarcoma, soft-tissue sarcoma, sarcoma, non-Hodgkin's lymphoma, and Wilms' tumor were at increased risk for breast cancer compared with age-matched general population controls. In childhood survivors of Hodgkin's disease, the cumulative incidence of breast cancer was 12.9% at 40 years of age; the risk continues to increase dramatically over the next decade. A family history of breast cancer in first-degree relatives and a history of thyroid disease were also associated with increased risk of developing breast cancer. When assessing survivor's risk, oncology nurses should consider the previous cancer diagnosis, prior treatment with radiation therapy, family history of cancer, and a history of thyroid disease.[45]

Benign Breast Disease/Breast Biopsy

Benign breast disease includes a number of pathologic conditions. Several studies have suggested that the presence or history of benign breast disease increases risk for breast cancer. Other studies have demonstrated a relationship between breast biopsy for benign disease and breast cancer; however, this relationship appears to be limited to lesions that are proliferative (atypical ductal or lobular hyperplasia) or those that demonstrate atypia. When compared with women who never underwent breast biopsy, women with benign breast disease without hyperplasia had an odds ratio of 1.5 of developing breast cancer; women with hyperplasia had an odds ratio of 1.8, and women with hyperplasia and atypia had an odds ratio of 2.6 to 4.3 of developing breast cancer.[46,47] Women with adenosis, apocrine changes, ductal ectasia, or mild epithelial hyperplasia are not at increased risk to develop breast cancer. Moreover, no characteristic molecular abnormalities for various benign breast syndromes have been identified.[26]

PREVENTION, SCREENING, AND EARLY DETECTION

Chemoprevention

Tamoxifen citrate (Nolvadex) is the only agent that has been approved by the Food and Drug Administration for reduction of breast cancer risk. Tamoxifen is a selective estrogen receptor modulator (SERM) that produces potent antiestrogenic effects. Tamoxifen exerts its action by competing with estrogen for binding sites in target tissues such as breast. As a chemopreventive agent, tamoxifen is indicated in women who are 35 or more years of age who have a 1.66% or greater risk (calculated using the Gail model) of developing breast cancer.[48]

Tamoxifen's effect on breast cancer incidence was first observed when the agent was being tested as an adjuvant therapy. Early studies indicated that it reduced the risk of new cancers in the opposite breast by 47% among women who took the drug for a period of 5 years. Several large, randomized controlled trials investigating the effects of tamoxifen as a chemopreventive agent have now been completed. Early studies conducted in England and Italy did not demonstrate a reduction in overall breast cancer risk. In contrast, the National Surgical Adjuvant Breast and Bowel Project (NSABP) P-1 Study, which was also known as the Breast Cancer Prevention Trial, demonstrated substantial differences in the incidence of breast cancer between tamoxifen and placebo groups. The P-1 trial enrolled over 13,000 women aged 35 or greater who were identified as being at high risk. Eligibility criteria defined risk as having a 5-year predicted risk of breast cancer of 1.66% using Gail model criteria. Tamoxifen was found to reduce the risk of invasive estrogen receptor (ER)-positive breast cancer and noninvasive ER-positive breast cancer by 49% and 50% respectively. In women with lobular carcinoma in situ or atypical hyperplasia, the risk reduction was even greater. Adverse events related to tamoxifen use included an increased relative risk of endometrial cancer and thromboembolic disease.[49] Tamoxifen should be used with caution in patients who have a history of deep vein thrombosis, pulmonary embolism, thrombotic stroke, transient ischemic attacks, pregnancy, or pregnancy potential without an effective method of contraception.[50]

The NSABP P-2 Study of Tamoxifen and Raloxifene (STAR) was designed as an equivalency trial to compare tamoxifen with raloxifene in preventing breast cancers. Raloxifene, a later-generation SERM, was found to decrease the incidence of breast cancer in a study investigating its effect on osteoporosis in postmenopausal women. It is anticipated that raloxifene will be effective in reducing breast cancer incidence without the carcinogenic effects on the endometrium. The accrual target for the P-2 trial is 19,000 women; at the time of this writing, the accrual has been completed and enrolled patients continue to be followed.

Aromatase inhibitors are also being investigated for their efficacy in reducing the risk of breast cancer. Recent results from the Anastrozole, Tamoxifen Alone or in Combination (ATAC) trial demonstrated a significant reduction in the incidence of primary contralateral breast cancers in women who received anastrozole alone. Results from two additional adjuvant trials, demonstrating benefits of letrozole and exemestane over tamoxifen, have led to interest in designing trials to test the use of these agents as chemopreventives in women who are at increased risk to develop breast cancer.[51] Several other international trials are underway to investigate the effects of aromatase inhibitors on the prevention of breast cancer.[52,53]

Strong evidence supports the use of SERMs as a chemopreventive strategy for women who have ER-positive disease or who are at increased risk to develop breast cancer; however, the incidence of ER-negative cancers is not influenced by SERMs.[54] The development of chemopreventive strategies for women who are hormone receptor-negative remains a significant challenge. A number of other chemopreventive agents have been investigated in the context of breast cancer. Retinoids and their derivatives for example, have demonstrated the ability to inhibit mammary carcinogenesis in preclinical models. Retinoids play a critical role in cellular proliferation and differentiation. The X receptor-selective retinoid LGD1069 has been found to down-regulate cyclooxygenase-2 expression in human breast cancer cells through transcriptional cross-talk.[55] Fenretinide is a synthetic derivative of all-trans-retinoic acid. In a phase III trial, fenretinide showed a trend toward a reduction in second breast malignancies in women who were premenopausal; however, additional evidence is needed before recommendations about this agent can be made.[56] The administration of retinoids is associated with a number of untoward effects. Although these events may be acceptable to patients in a therapeutic setting, it is unlikely that many women would be willing to tolerate significant side effects in a chemopreventive context.

The role of Vitamin E, isoflavins, grape seed extract, and other micronutrients has been investigated in terms of their preventive activity in breast cancer. Additional research is warranted before any conclusive recommendations can be made about the role of these substances. Vaccines have also been investigated for their potential role in prevention. Clinical trials investigating the effects of vaccines in breast cancer are ongoing.[57]

Prophylactic Surgery

Primary prevention of breast cancer in women who are at high risk may be accomplished with prophylactic mastectomy. This intervention should be reserved for carefully selected women who have undergone a thorough multidisciplinary evaluation and are fully cognizant of the implications.[50,58] The effectiveness of prophylactic mastectomy in preventing breast cancer has been studied in several nonrandomized trials. In one observational study where women were identified through family history as being at moderate or high risk for the development of breast cancer, risk reduction following prophylactic mastectomy was 89.5% and 90% to 94.3% in the moderate- and high-risk groups, respectively.[59] A more recent multinational study compared women who were known BRCA mutation carriers and underwent prophylactic bilateral mastectomy (n = 105) to mutation status- and age-matched controls (n = 384) over a 6-year period. Breast cancer occurred in two of the subjects who underwent prophylactic mastectomy and in 184 of the controls.

Women who undergo prophylactic mastectomy do not require an axillary node dissection unless breast cancer is noted on the pathologic analysis of the mastectomy specimen. Follow-up for women who undergo prophylactic surgery includes close monitoring. Specific recommendations can be viewed on the NCCN website (www.nccn.org).[8]

Women who carry BRCA mutations are at risk to develop ovarian cancer as well as breast cancer. Due to its frequently obscure presentation, ovarian cancer is often diagnosed in the advanced stages when it is very difficult to treat. Women who are at known risk may choose to have prophylactic oophorectomy after they have completed childbearing to prevent ovarian cancer. Surgical removal of the ovaries does not eliminate the risk of primary peritoneal cancers, which have been reported up to 15 years after removal of the ovaries.[8] Prophylactic oophorectomy offers a reduction of risk for both ovarian and breast cancer. This effect appears to be most significant in women who have prophylactic oophorectomy before 35 years of age.[60]

Breast Duct Visualization and Epithelial Cell Sampling

Advanced technology has made direct visualization and biopsy of mammary ducts a new option to aid in the diagnosis of breast cancer. Ductoscopy involves the insertion of flexible microendoscope into a mammary duct for the purpose of visualization and specimen retrieval. Newer instrumentation has been designed with an outer air channel on the fiberscope to allow for instillation and aspiration of saline and collection of ductal cells. Breast massage is performed prior to the procedure to promote the expression of fluid from the nipple; this aids in the identification of a ductal orifice for cannulation. Topical lidocaine cream may be used to anesthetize the area prior to the procedure. Ductoscopy is still being evaluated and is available only on a limited basis. Current research is focusing on evaluation of the modality to investigate pathologic nipple discharge and high-risk patients, and to determine the extent of intraductal disease in women with breast cancer.[61]

Ductal Lavage

Ductal lavage is a relatively new and promising method of obtaining breast epithelial cells for cytologic analysis from high-risk women. Ductal lavage involves obtaining washings of cells aspirated from ducts in the nipple. The first step in this process involves applying mild suction to the nipple to identify fluid yielding ducts. Once a duct has been identified, an anesthetic is applied and a very thin flexible catheter is inserted into the duct opening. The catheter and duct are then irrigated with a saline solution. The solution is subsequently aspirated and sent for cytologic analysis. Side effects of ductal lavage are reported to be minimal. The majority of women who have undergone this procedure have indicated that it is no more uncomfortable than a mammogram. Ductal lavage is available at selected centers around the country.[62]

Ductal lavage can be used to improve risk stratification for women who have already been defined as being at risk and may be considered when additional information on cellular atypia will enlighten the risk reduction strategy.[63] In a recent investigation, Fabian and others demonstrated that cytologic atypia determined on periareolar fine needle aspirates was predictive of additional risk, independent of Gail model factors. Although results of this procedure may provide additional information in specific cases, it is important to note that the negative predictive value of normal cytology with ductal lavage has not been described. As such, normal cytology in ductal lavage aspirates in a high-risk woman does not reduce her already greater risk for developing breast cancer.[64] The role of ductal lavage in specific groups of high-risk women, such as those who are BRCA1-positive or BRCA2-positive or who have a strong family history of breast cancer has not yet been investigated.

Mammography

Mammograms are x-rays of the breast that are used to detect and diagnose breast disease in both asymptomatic and symptomatic women. Mammography is currently the most effective screening modality available for breast cancer. Although there may be variation in the specifics, all major medical organizations in the US recommend screening mammography for women who are 40 years of age or above.

Eight randomized clinical trials have been conducted to assess the effectiveness of mammography in detecting early breast cancers. While these trials varied in a number of ways, for women between 50 and 69 years of age, all reports of studies comparing screening with no screening demonstrated protective effects of screening, and metaanalyses that incorporated the findings of all trials showed statistically significant reductions in mortality.[65] Conclusions about the benefits of mammography were brought into question in two relatively recently published metaanalyses that reported that several of the screening trials had substantial methodologic flaws.[66,67] These publications raised questions about the efficacy and overall benefit of mammography in terms of cancer mortality. The criticisms raised in the metaanalyses have been thoroughly investigated in independent reviews; these reviews concluded that the use of mammography is effective, particularly in women who are 50 years of age or older.[3,68] In a February 2002 press release, the Department of Health and Human Services affirmed the value of mammography for detecting breast cancer. After careful deliberation, the National Cancer Institute continues to recommend that women in their 40s and older should be screened every 1 to 2 years with mammography, and women who are at increased risk should seek medical advice about individualized surveillance plans.[69] Additional recommendations on breast cancer screening are presented in Table 5-1. Breast image reporting criteria are identified in Table 5-2.

Digital Mammography

Full-field digital mammography captures x-ray images digitally (these images can either be printed for viewing or be viewed directly on a computer screen). Screen-film mammography captures x-ray images on film. Benefits of using digital images include the ability to manipulate the image while on the computer screen (e.g., to change the level of brightness or enlarge the field of view) and the ability to engage computer-assisted diagnostic tools.[70] Moreover, in an increasingly digital world there may also be logistical advantages to using images that can be viewed, stored, and retrieved very efficiently; health care providers and patients can easily maintain files of their digital images on a compact disk.

Several small trials have not produced conclusive data on the advantage of full-field digital as compared to screen-film mammography. A large, randomized controlled clinical trial investigating cancer detection rates among four manufacturers of full-field digital mammography and screen-film has completed accrual of 49,520 women and is currently under analysis (Digital versus film-screen mammography [ACRIN Protocol 6652]).[71] Results of this trial should provide important information on the role of these diagnostic interventions.

Screen-film mammography and full-field digital mammography are the only imaging procedures currently approved by the Food and Drug Administration (FDA) for the purposes of breast cancer screening. According to a recent

Table 5-1 Breast Cancer Screening and Testing Guidelines from the American Cancer Society (ACS) and the National Cancer Institute (NCI)[69]

ACS recommendations	Continuing NCI recommendations:
Mammography annually starting at age 40. Clinical breast exam (CBE) every 3 years for women 20-39; annually for women 40 and older. Breast self-exam (BSE) monthly starting at age 20.	Mammography every 1-2 years starting at age 40.
	Women aged 50 and older should be screened every 1-2 years.
Women with a family history of breast cancer should discuss guidelines with their doctors.	Women who are at higher than average–risk of breast cancer should seek expert medical advice on whether they should begin screening before age 40 and on the frequency of screening.

Table 5-2 American College of Radiology (ACR) Breast Imaging Reporting and Data System (BIRADS)[69]

Category	Finding
0	Assessment is incomplete and additional imaging evaluation is needed.
1	Normal: in this case, there is no significant abnormality to report. The breasts are symmetrical without masses, architectural distortion, or suspicious calcifications.
2	Benign (non-cancerous) finding. This is also a normal mammogram.
3	Probably benign finding – follow-up in a short time frame is suggested.
4	Suspicious abnormality – biopsy should be considered.
5	Highly suggestive of malignancy – appropriate action should be taken.

review of the literature on breast cancer screening methods, mammography remains the main screening tool for the diagnosis of breast cancer. While many newer modalities are being investigated, it is unlikely that any of them will replace mammography in the near future.[72]

Computer-Aided Detection

Computer-aided detection (CAD) uses computer programs to identify areas of concern on mammograms. The device scans the mammographic image using a laser beam and converts it into a digital image that is displayed on a video monitor, with any suspicious areas highlighted for the radiologist to review. Several breast imaging devices that use CAD are under development. The *ImageChecker* device is shown in Figure 5-5. This technique allows the radiologist to compare findings with the manual read to determine if any suspicious areas have been overlooked. The first breast imaging device that used CAD was approved by the FDA in 1998. The role of CAD in breast cancer screening is currently under investigation.

Scintimammography

Scintimammography refers to a noninvasive imaging technique that uses a radioisotope (Tc-99 tetrofosmin) to aid in the diagnosis of breast cancer. Breast malignancies typically demonstrate increased uptake of the Tc-99 tetrofosmin when compared to benign growths. This technique enhances breast visualization and is particularly helpful in the evaluation of women who have dense breasts. Scintimammography has been approved by the FDA as an adjunct diagnostic tool for breast cancer. A recent metaanalysis pooled data from four studies that reported on a total of 5340 subjects assessed for breast cancer using scintimammography. The overall sensitivity and specificity associated with this technique was 85.2% and 86.6% respectively; sensitivity and specificity were slightly higher for patients who presented with a palpable mass at 87.8% and 87.5% respectively. Researchers concluded that scintimammography is an effective adjunct to mammography in the diagnosis of breast cancer.[73]

Ultrasound

Ultrasound is an imaging technique that uses high-frequency sound waves that echo to create sonographic pictures. Ultrasound is most frequently used to differentiate between lesions that are solid and those that are cystic. It may also be used to further examine lesions that are difficult to characterize using mammography, or may be used to guide fine-needle aspirations. Ultrasound is being studied as a screening tool in high-risk women, but at the current time is not recommended for screening in the general population.[72] Limitations for the use of ultrasound as a screening tool include a lack of standardized exam techniques and interpretation criteria and a higher

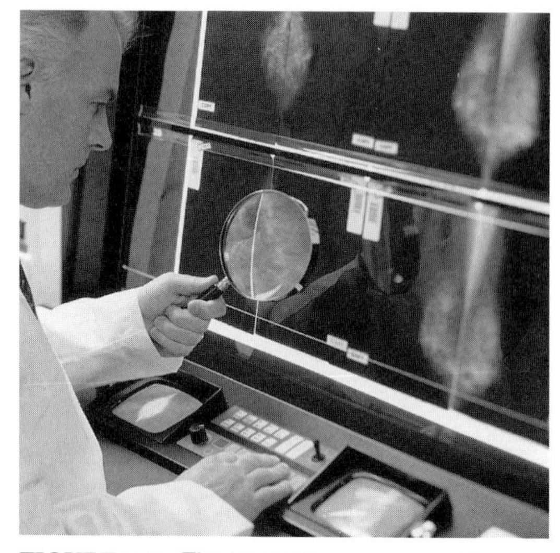

FIGURE 5-5 The ImageChecker computer-aided detection (CAD) system assists radiologists in reviewing mammograms by calling attention to regions of interest that may be associated with breast cancer. To interpret a case, the radiologist reviews the original mammograms at the viewer, then activates the R2 display button to review the marked images on the two video display monitors. (From ImageChecker by R2 Technology, Inc. Sunnyvale, California, 2005, R2 Technology. Web address: www.r2tech.com)

rate of false positive results when compared to mammography.[74] A recent study, for example, indicated that the false positive rate (based on solid lesion for ultrasound) ranged from 2.4% to 12.9% for ultrasound and between 0.7% and 6% for mammography.[75]

Magnetic Resonance Imaging

Magnetic resonance imaging (MRI) uses magnetic fields and radio waves to create images of the breast, a technology that allows the breast to be visualized in any plane and from any orientation. Gadolinium, an intravenous contrast medium, is often used to enhance the quality of MRI breast images. MRI is used to further evaluate abnormal mammographic or physical exam findings and can be particularly helpful in the following clinical situations: identifying abnormalities in augmented breasts that can sometimes be obscured by the implant on a mammogram; identifying contralateral tumors; evaluating close or positive surgical margins; identifying lobular cancers; identifying occult breast cancers; helping to determine whether breast cancer has spread to the chest wall; identifying multicentric or multifocal disease; improving the accuracy of tumor size classification, nodal status, or therapeutic response; and in the setting of high-risk screening.[72,76]

The FDA approved MRI in 1991 as a diagnostic (not screening) tool. MRI has been studied as a screening tool in women who are at high risk to develop breast cancer, but not in the general population. Although individual study results vary, in general the specificity of MRI tends to be lower than that of mammography. Screening MRI may be useful in specific populations such as young women with known BRCA1 or BRCA2 mutations.[72] In a study of 1,909 high-risk women (identified through family history or genetic mutation), breast MRI was effective in identifying more tumors than mammography. Researchers concluded that breast MRI was effective in detecting breast cancers at an early stage in high-risk women. Additional studies are warranted to more precisely define the population and settings where MRI would be most appropriately recommended.[77]

Positron Emission Tomography Scan

Positron emission tomography (PET) scanning can play an adjunctive role in the diagnosis and staging of breast cancer. PET scanning involves the administration of a radioactive form of glucose that is more rapidly metabolized by tumor than by normal cells. The increased uptake is translated into images by the scanner. PET scanning may be able to detect tumors that are not identified by other diagnostic means; however, PET scans are substantially more expensive than many other breast diagnostics. As such, they should be used in clearly defined circumstances. The American College of Radiology Imaging Network (ACRIN), a part of the National Cancer Institute's Clinical Trials Cooperative Group

Program, is currently sponsoring a clinical trial investigating the effectiveness of PET scans compared to other diagnostic modalities in the setting of breast cancer.[78] Results of this investigation will inform recommendations on the use of PET scans in this population in the future.

DIAGNOSIS AND STAGING

Surgical Techniques to Obtain Breast Tissue

Surgical techniques used in the diagnosis and treatment of breast cancer have evolved significantly over the past 30 years; the trend in all instances is to use minimally invasive techniques.[79,80] There are a variety of techniques for obtaining tissue for analysis from both palpable and nonpalpable lesions to establish a pathologic diagnosis (Table 5-3). The decision to use a particular technique depends on the patient's clinical status and preference, clinical and radiologic features of the mass, and expertise of the surgeon performing the procedure.[61] Figures 5-6 and 5-7 shows an example of a stereotactic table and the positioning of the patient on the stereotactic table.

Histopathologic Types of Breast Cancer

Distinct histopathologic features categorize breast cancers; a review of these features is briefly presented in Table 5-4.

Breast Cancer Staging

Clinical staging of breast cancer involves careful inspection of the skin, the mammary gland, and the axillary, supraclavicular, and cervical lymph nodes, and pathologic examination of tissue. Pathologic staging is based on all data obtained during clinical staging, findings obtained during any surgical procedures, and pathologic analysis of the primary tumor, the lymph nodes, and any metastatic sites. Breast cancers are classified using the Tumor, Node, Metastasis (TNM) classification schema. Essential characteristics of this schema include the size of the primary tumor, the level of invasion or microinvasion, the presence of regional lymph nodes, and metastasis. Staging for breast cancer is shown in Table 5-5.

In addition to determining disease stage, histologic grading of invasive breast cancer provides significant prognostic information. Histologic grading is accomplished by assessing specific morphologic characteristics including the mitotic count, nuclear pleomorphism, and tubule formation. Each of these features is assigned a score ranging from 1 to 3 based on whether they are favorable or unfavorable. Lower scores are associated with more favorable cellular characteristics. Tumors that are assigned a score of 3-5 points are histologic grade 1; those with 6-7 points are histologic grade 2; those with 8-9 points are a grade 3. The histologic grade of some tumors cannot be assessed; these tumors are classified as GX.[87] Additional information on prognostic indicators can be found in Table 5-6.

SURGICAL TREATMENT OF BREAST CANCER

The current surgical options for women with breast cancer are conservative resection followed by radiation therapy, or mastectomy. The trend towards increasingly conservative therapy is based on changes in the understanding of the biology of breast cancer. Conservative resections include those procedures designed to remove the tumor while retaining enough normal tissue to ensure a satisfactory cosmetic result. The advantage of this approach over more extensive procedures is purely cosmetic. Larger tumors or multicentric presentations are treated with mastectomy. A variety of reconstructive approaches have been used effectively to ameliorate the cosmetic alterations associated with mastectomy.

Lumpectomy

Lumpectomy (also called wide local resection or partial mastectomy) involves the removal of all tissue containing tumor to microscopically clean margins. Lumpectomy was shown to be as effective as total mastectomy in the NSABP-06 trial. This study evaluated the effectiveness of breast conservation therapy with or without irradiation. Women participating in the trial were randomized to receive total mastectomy,

Table 5-3 BIOPSY TECHNIQUES FOR PALPABLE AND NONPALPABLE BREAST MASSES

Biopsy Technique	Description	Indication	Reliability	Comments
Fine-needle aspiration (FNA)	Aspiration using 20- to 25-gauge needle and syringe to obtain fluid/ cells for cytologic analysis.	Palpable breast mass	• False-positive rate of 1% to 2%;[87] False-negative rate as high as 40%[81] • Negative results often require core-needles or excisional biopsy[61] • Atypia → open biopsy warranted	• Local anesthesia usually not required • Immunohistochemical analysis for hormone receptors available in most cytology labs • Requires both operator and cytologist expertise • Easily performed in office setting
Core-needle (cutting-needle biopsy)	Removal of narrow cylinder of tissue using 14-gauge needle pathologic analysis imaging breast analysis.	Palpable breast mass	• Highly accurate when successful targeting is confirmed by breast imaging • Benign or fibrocystic tissue should be considered suspiciously because it may represent sampling error. • Atypia → open biopsy warranted	• Local anesthesia required • May be technique of choice if not for cytopathologist available • Can be performed in office setting
Open biopsy	Open surgical procedure to obtain mass as a single specimen with small margin.	Palpable breast mass	• Provides complete pathologic diagnosis.	• Majority performed with local anesthesia or local anesthesia plus IV sedation (monitored anesthesia care). • Performed in operating room as same-day procedure.
Image-guided core-needle biopsy (ultrasound and stereotactic)	Biopsy of lesion using large core (11-14 gauge)-needle under direct visualization via ultrasound or stereotactic mammography.	Nonpalpable breast mass	• False negative rate 1% to 3%[88,85] • False positives are rare. • Equivocal findings necessitate open biopsy.	• Stereotactic approach used to biopsy microcalcifications or other subtle mammographic findings not seen on ultrasound.[81] • Stereotactic approach depends on location within breast; lesions close to chest wall or nipple may not be accessible.[61]

Continued

Table 5-3 Biopsy Techniques for Palpable and Nonpalpable Breast Masses—cont'd

Biopsy Technique	Description	Indication	Reliability	Comments
				• Stereotactic approach requires positioning of patient face-down on stereotactic table (see Figures 5-6 and 5-7) with the breast placed in compression through opening on table. • Ultrasound approach done with patient lying on back or side • Performed in breast imaging center • Low complication rate[83]
Open biopsy with needle (wire) localization	Using mammogram or ultrasound as a guide, the lesion or suspicious area is identified. A thin wire is inserted until the tip of the wire is at the location of the lesion. The wire is secured and the patient is transported to the operating suite. The breast surgeon removes a core of tissue around and along the wire. The specimen is immediately examined by radioimaging techniques to ensure that the suspicious area has been removed.	Nonpalpable breast masses	• Allows a complete pathologic analysis	• Local anesthetics are used for wire insertion. Local anesthesia or local anesthesia plus intravenous sedation are used for the open biopsy. • Performed in breast imaging center and operating room.

Continued

Table 5-3 BIOPSY TECHNIQUES FOR PALPABLE AND NONPALPABLE BREAST MASSES—CONT'D

Biopsy Technique	Description	Indication	Reliability	Comments
Directional vacuum-assisted biopsy (mammotomy)	Image-guided probe that vacuums, cuts, and removes cores of tissue for pathologic analysis. Following tissue sampling, inert metallic clips are inserted through the trochar for follow-up purposes.	Nonpalpable breast masses	• Allows complete pathologic analysis	• Target lesions • Local anesthesia is administered before procedure • Most technologically advanced core-needle biopsy technique • More successful at removing microcalcifications than core-needle biopsy • More sensitive in detecting ductal carcinoma in situ and atypical duct hyperplasia • Complications are uncommon

lumpectomy alone, or lumpectomy plus radiation therapy. Breast radiation following lumpectomy was found to significantly ($p < .000005$) decrease the likelihood of tumor recurrence in women who had margins that were histologically free of tumor.[26] In addition, there is conclusive evidence that adding radiation to the therapeutic plan decreases the occurrence of ipsilateral breast cancers. Lumpectomy is generally performed under local anesthesia as a same-day procedure and does not require surgical drain placement.

Axillary Node Dissection

Lymph node status is the single most important variable in determining breast cancer prognosis.

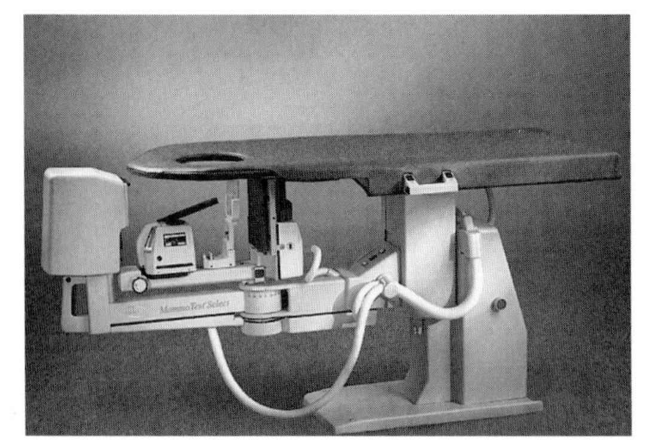

FIGURE 5-6 Stereotactic table. (From Fischer Imaging, Denver, Colorado, 2005, www.fisherimaging.com.)

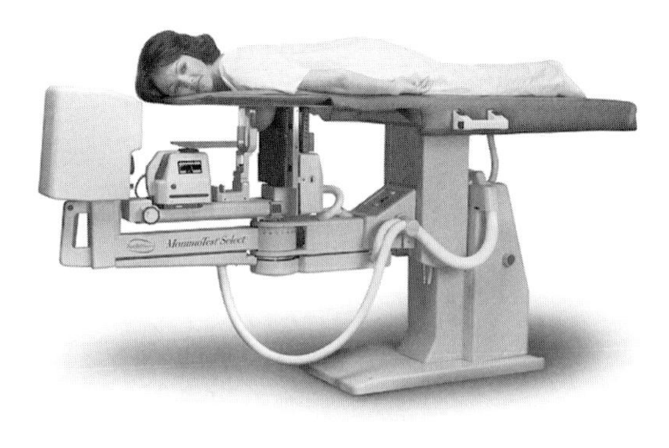

FIGURE 5-7 Stereotactic table with patient. (From Fischer Imaging, Denver, Colorado, 2005, www.fisherimaging.com.)

Table 5-4 Major Types of Breast Cancer

Type	% Occurence[84]	Clinico-Pathologic Description
Ductal carcinoma in situ (DCIS)		Proliferation of epithelial cells confined to the mammary ducts Identifiable through mammography Associated with a number of histological patterns that correlate to biologic behavior
Lobular carcinoma in situ (LCIS)		Precancerous growth that originates in the small end ducts of the breast and is confined to the lobules; often does not progress to infiltrating cancer.
Infiltrating ductal adenocarcinoma (IDC)	80%[29]	Develops from DCIS, spreads through the duct walls and invades fatty tissue of breast; characterized clinically by hardness to palpation, frequent metastases to the axillary lymph nodes, and poor prognosis
Invasive lobular carcinoma	10-15%	Originates in mammary glands and extends to the fatty tissue of the breast
Mucinous or colloid	3%[29]	Forms in mucin-producing cells which spread to surrounding breast cells; characterized on microscopy by nests and strands of epithelial cells floating in a mucinous matrix Small and usually slow-growing
Tubular	2%	An invasive carcinoma in which tubule formation is a prominent feature Typically well differentiated Presence of microcalcifications assists in early diagnosis Usually small and nonpalpable, tumor is formed by cells of high nuclear grade; it may exhibit extensive infiltration by small lymphocytes
Medullary	5%	May present bilaterally Usually large and well circumscribed
Inflammatory/dermal lymphatic carcinomatosis	1-3%	Characterized by diffuse erythema, tenderness, induration, warmth, a visible erysipeloid margin, enlargement of the breast, and diffuseness (or absence) of a tumor on palpation[85,86]

Historically, lymph node sampling has been accomplished through axillary node dissection. Axillary dissection for clinically node-negative breast cancers includes the resection of level I and II lymph nodes and the fibrofatty tissue around these nodes. Anatomically, the extent of this dissection includes the area from the latissimus dorsi muscle laterally, the axillary vein superiorly, and the medial border of the pectoralis minor muscle medially. There are a number of vessels, nerves, and venous and capillary channels that are located in the axillary region. It is important to identify and preserve these structures because damage to them during surgery may lead to a number of postoperative sequelae. Following the procedure, a surgical suction drain is placed to facilitate healing by removing excess blood and fluid from the surgical area.

Table 5-5 American Joint Committee on Cancer Staging for Breast Cancer Tumor-Node-Metastases (TNM) Classifications

Stage Grouping			
STAGE 0	Tis	N0	M0
STAGE I	T1*	N0	M0
STAGE IIA	T0	N1	M0
	T1*	N1	M0
	T2	N0	M0
STAGE IIB	T2	N1	M0
	T3	N0	M0
STAGE IIIA	T0	N2	M0
	T1*	N2	M0
	T2	N2	M0
	T3	N1	M0
	T3	N2	M0
STAGE IIIB	T4	N0	M0
	T4	N1	M0
	T4	N2	M0
STAGE IIIC	Any T	N3	M0
STAGE IV	Any T	Any N	M1

*T1 includes T1 microscopic.
Used with permission of the American Joint Committee on Cancer (AJCC), Chicago, Illinois. The original source for this material is the *AJCC cancer staging manual*, sixth edition (2002), published by Springer-Verlag New York, www.springer-ny.com.

Lymphatic Mapping and Sentinel Lymph Node Biopsy

Lymphatic node mapping and dissection is a less invasive approach to sampling axillary lymph nodes for pathologic analysis. The technique was developed for use in the melanoma population and adapted for use in breast cancer. Sentinel lymph node biopsy is based on the principle that the sentinel node is the first node where cancer cells will spread. Sentinel lymph node techniques involve the injection of a dye and a radionuclide. The dye is injected peritumorally, and gamma camera imaging is used to identify sites of drainage (Figure 5-8). The surgeon makes a small incision in the axilla and examines the area for the node containing dye and/or radionuclide (assessed using a hand held gamma probe). The sentinel lymph node is identified and undergoes pathologic analysis. If the sentinel node is free of tumor, an assumption is made that the axillary nodes are negative. If the sentinel node is positive, then an axillary node dissection will be performed. Contraindications to sentinel lymph node sampling include the presence of palpable axillary nodes, prior axillary surgery, or pregnancy.[61]

Mastectomy

In some clinical situations, mastectomy is the most appropriate surgical intervention. Simple mastectomy is indicated for ductal carcinoma in situ, in the case of prophylactic surgery, following lumpectomy and axillary node dissection when lumpectomy margins are positive, for the treatment of local recurrence following lumpectomy, radiation, and node dissection, and in elderly patients with comorbidities or other contraindications to axillary node dissection.[61] Mastectomy involves the removal of all breast tissue with conservation of well-perfused flaps to allow adequate skin approximation for primary closure or in preparation for reconstructive surgery.

Breast Reconstruction

The range and sophistication of breast reconstructive procedures has evolved substantially over the past few decades. Goals of breast reconstruction include restoring breast symmetry and recreating volume, shape, and contour using the opposite breast as the aesthetic reference. The timing of reconstructive surgery varies; reconstruction may be done immediately following mastectomy, or at a time after the initial surgery has been completed (delayed reconstruction). Placement of a submuscular inflatable prosthesis at the time of the surgical intervention allows skin flap approximation without tension. After healing takes place, sterile saline can be injected into the implant (usually over a period of weeks) until the desired size is achieved (Figure 5-9). After the expansion process is complete, the tissue expander is exchanged for a permanent saline prosthesis.

If inadequate skin is available to allow for expansion using an implant, autologous tissue may be used to reconstruct the breast. Autologous

Table 5-6 Prognostic Indicators of Breast Cancer

TUMOR SIZE	Survival rates vary by tumor size. Small tumors (<1 cm in diameter) have an overall survival rate of 99% at 5 years. Tumors between 1-3 cm and >3 cm have 91% and 85% 5-year survival rates respectively.[88,89]
HISTOLOGIC TYPE AND GRADE	Nuclear pattern, morphology, and mitotic activity are all important histopathologic characteristics of breast cancers. Tumors that are well differentiated and have characteristics more typical of normal breast cells and low mitotic counts are considered low-grade; these tumors have low metastatic potential. Tumors demonstrating abundant mitotic activity and cellular characteristics atypical of normal breast cells are considered high-grade and have high metastatic potential.[88]
HORMONE RECEPTOR STATUS	Breast tissue contains estrogen and progesterone receptors. Many breast tumors will retain hormone receptors; this allows estrogen to influence proliferation of the tumor. Well-differentiated, lower-grade tumors often retain receptors for both estrogen and progesterone. Determining hormonal receptor status enables the prediction of response to hormonal intervention. Estrogen receptor (ER) and progesterone receptor (PR) tumors have >75% likelihood of responding to hormonal therapy. Tumors lacking ER and PR receptors are generally of a higher histologic grade and do not respond to endocrine therapy.[88]
LYMPH NODE STATUS	Lymph node (LN) status is the single most important prognostic variable in breast cancer.[60,90] Prognosis worsens as the number of positive lymph nodes increases. The number of positive lymph nodes has been directly correlated to recurrence of disease at 5 years. Women with 1-3 positive LNs have a 40% chance of recurrence at 5 years; women with 10 or more positive nodes have a 78% chance of recurrence.[91]
MOLECULAR MARKERS	Several molecular markers have been investigated to determine their predictive ability in the setting of breast cancer.
HER2/NEU	HER2/neu is a protooncogene that is amplified in approximately 15% to 25% of women with breast cancer.[92,93] HER2/neu overexpression is associated with decreased survival rates, particularly in women with node-negative disease. HER2/neu–positive breast cancers have been shown to respond well to chemotherapy and to respond poorly to hormonal therapy. A subset of patients (25%) with HER2/neu overexpression respond favorably to trastuzumab therapy.
VEGF	Vascular endothelial growth factor (VEGF) is a proangiogenic factor that supports tumor growth through neovascularization. VEGF is overexpressed in many women with breast cancer. Overexpression of VEGF is associated with decreased survival in women with node-negative disease. Preliminary results from a very recent clinical trial have demonstrated a delay in time-to-progression in patients treated with an anti-VEGF agent (bevacizumab) given with chemotherapy, as compared to women who received chemotherapy alone.[94]
p53	p53 is a tumor-suppressor gene that may be an independent prognostic indicator of relapse. This may help in identifying node-negative women who could benefit from adjuvant therapy.

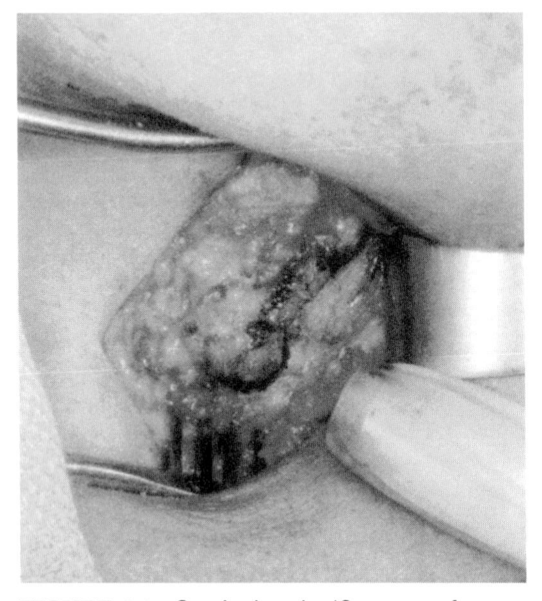

FIGURE 5-8 Sentinel node. (Courtesy of Thomas J. Kearney, MD, FACS, New Brunswick, New Jersey, 2005.)

reconstruction involves the transfer of flaps of tissue from donor sites to the anterior chest wall. These flaps can be transferred while they are still attached to their original blood supply (known as pedicled flaps) or as free flaps, in which tissue is isolated, transferred, and anastamosed to recipient blood vessels using microsurgical techniques. Myocutaneous flaps can be donated from a number of anatomic sites. The latissimus dorsi flap for example, (Figure 5-10) is accomplished by bringing skin, subcutaneous tissue, and muscle on its neurovascular pedicle from the region of the scapula to the breast area. The transverse rectus abdominus myocutaneous (TRAM) flap and its variants constitute what many consider to be the gold standard in breast reconstruction because superior cosmetic results are generally achievable using this technique (Figure 5-11). Disadvantages of the free TRAM flap include a lengthy operation (usually 4-6 hours) and risk of total flap failure (between 0.4% and 5.0%); also, because a portion

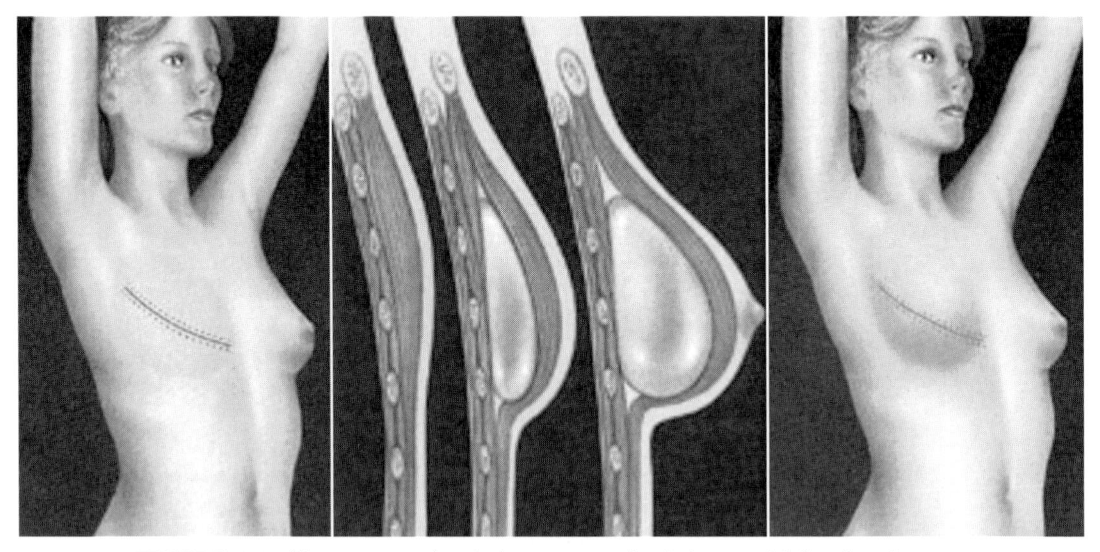

FIGURE 5-9 Tissue expander. A tissue expander is inserted following the mastectomy to prepare for reconstruction. The expander is gradually filled with saline through an integrated or separate tube to stretch the skin enough to accept an implant beneath the chest muscle. (From American Society of Plastic Surgeons: Arlington Heights, 2005, American Society of Plastic Surgeons. Retrieved from www.plasticsurgery.org/public_education/procedures/BreastReconstruction.cfm.

of rectus muscle and fascia is harvested, there is a risk of abdominal hernia following surgery.[95]

Nipple reconstruction can be accomplished using a variety of techniques; these include transplanting skin from the labia or the inner thigh or nipple sharing, a technique where a part of the nipple from the opposite breast is grafted to the reconstructed breast. Intradermal tattooing is frequently used to achieve desired cosmetic results.

Radiation therapy can be delivered to the chest wall and regional nodes either in the adjuvant setting or if local disease recurs after reconstructive surgery. Radiation can influence the cosmetic result of reconstructive surgery, can induce fibrosis, and may increase pain.[96]

Complications of surgical breast procedures include limitations in shoulder motion, arm edema, stiffness and pain, numbness, and infection. These issues may lead to decreased function and quality of life. As such, they must be proactively identified and managed. Nursing management of the patient undergoing breast surgery requires careful preoperative assessment that includes a thorough review of the history and the physical findings, comorbidities, medications, psychologic issues, self-care patterns, and financial support. Oncology nurses caring for patients preparing for surgery should be aware of specific institutional policies that guide perioperative care. The Joint Commission on Accreditation of Health Care Organizations has identified operative procedures as processes that have the potential to jeopardize patient safety.[97] Oncology nurses are in a pivotal position to ensure that patients receive high quality care in this setting.

Preoperative teaching should include information about the specific procedure and instructions for the preoperative and postoperative periods. Patients should be prepared for what to expect after the surgery, including symptoms to anticipate, wound care, complications such as infection or seroma formation, the follow-up plan, and contact numbers to call with questions or problems.[98] A subset of patients who undergo

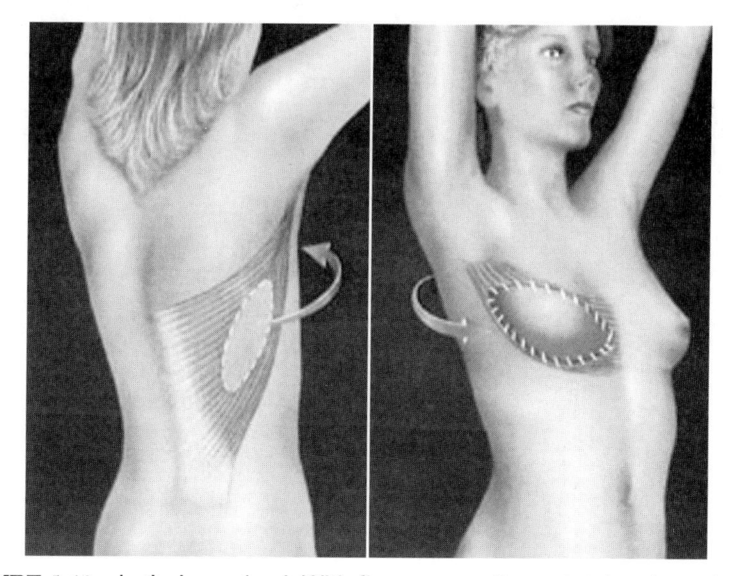

FIGURE 5-10 Latissimus dorsi. With flap surgery, tissue is taken from the back and tunneled to the front of the chest wall to support the reconstructed breast. The transported tissue forms a flap for a breast implant, or it may provide enough bulk to form the breast mound without an implant. (From American Society of Plastic Surgeons: Arlington Heights, 2005. Retrieved from www.plasticsurgery.org/public_education/procedures/BreastReconstruction.cfm.)

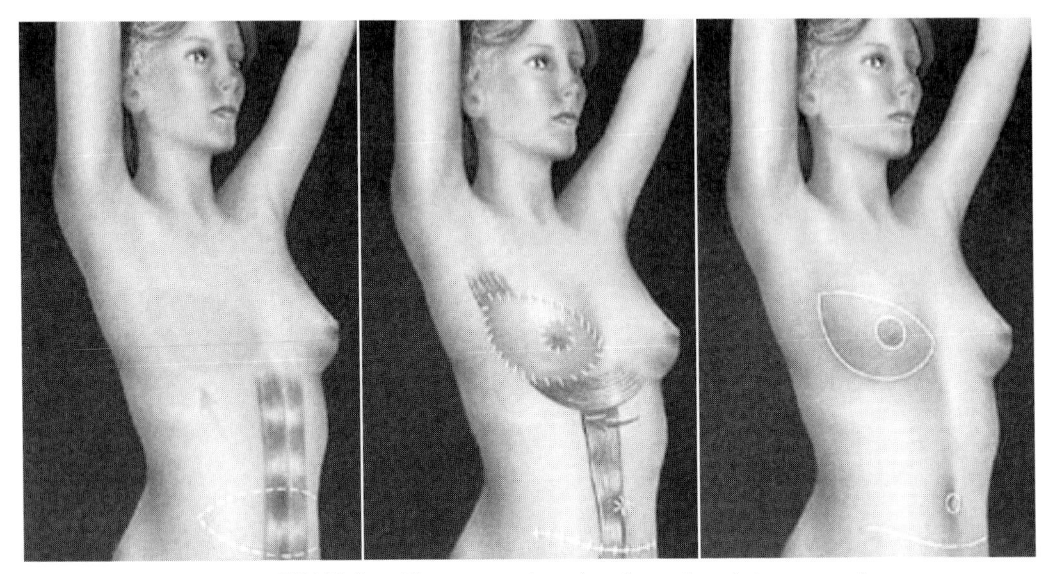

FIGURE 5-11 TRAM flap. Tissue may be taken from the abdomen and tunneled to the breast or surgically transplanted to form a new breast mound. After surgery, the breast mound, nipple, and areola are restored. (From American Society of Plastic Surgeons: Arlington Heights, 2005. Retrieved from www.plasticsurgery.org/public_education/procedures/BreastReconstruction.cfm.

breast surgery will be discharged from the hospital with drainage devices. Very specific drain care must be taught before the surgery. This should include information on milking and emptying the drainage tubes, and recording amounts and handling and disposal of any drainage material. Optimally, patients should receive written instructions for postoperative care. An example of postsurgical care instructions for patients undergoing surgical breast biopsy or lumpectomy is shown in Box 5-2.

RADIATION THERAPY

Radiation therapy plays a critical role in the management of breast cancer. The benefits of radiation therapy in early-stage breast cancer have been discussed previously. Radiation may also be used to treat local recurrence or more advanced disease. Radiation is typically administered as conventional external beam therapy. This requires 1 to 2 days of planning followed by a prescribed number of daily visits to complete the treatment. Current research is investigating alternative scheduling strategies for the administration of radiation to determine if the treatment times can be shortened, making this intervention more convenient to administer. Radiation therapy is generally well tolerated with low rates of long-term morbidity. Side effects include both acute and late effects. The most common acute effects, occurring during or immediately following treatment, include treatment-related fatigue and dermatitis. Skin changes are frequently seen in patients receiving breast radiation because of the tangential angle of the treatment beam. The skin in the treatment field may become erythematous or hyperpigmented. More severe reactions include moist or dry desquamation. Discomfort in the breast and axilla may also occur. This tends to be transient in nature and is often relieved by nonsteroidal antiinflammatory agents.[99] Other possible radiation-induced changes include breast atrophy and shrinkage, and an increase in breast

Box 5-2 INSTRUCTIONS FOLLOWING SURGICAL BREAST BIOPSY OR LUMPECTOMY

BIOPSY RESULTS

The final results of your biopsy or lumpectomy will be available in about 5 business days (not counting weekends and holidays). Your health care team will call you within 24 hours of receiving the written pathology report.

PAIN

For mild pain, most patients can take over-the-counter pain medications such as acetaminophen *(Tylenol)* or ibuprofen *(Motrin)*. Be sure to follow the instructions on the bottle or box of the medication. These medications may not be indicated for all patients, so please check with your health care team.

Your health care team may also give you a prescription for pain medication. This should be taken if the pain is not relieved with over-the-counter pain medication, or if the pain is severe. Remember to stop taking over-the-counter pain medications if you are using a prescription pain medication.

SHOWERING AND BANDAGES

You may remove the bandage in 2 to 3 days, and then take a shower. After you remove the bandage, leave the small paper strips *(Steri-Strips)* alone. They will start to peel off in about 1 to 2 weeks. Then you may peel them off the rest of the way. You may shower as long as you pat the area dry.

FOLLOW-UP

All of the stitches will dissolve in about a month. You may still feel a lump at the surgery site for 3 to 6 months, until healing is complete. There may be bruising that lasts for 2 to 4 weeks or more, along with some mild tenderness during the first few weeks. It may take up to 6 months for healing to be complete. The area usually heals very well. About 2% of patients will develop an infection. Signs of an infection include red skin around the scar, fever, increasing tenderness, increasing pain, or any drainage from the wound. If you have any of these symptoms, please call the Nursing Help Line at the number located in the box below. If you have any questions, please call.

If your results are benign, you will need a routine breast screening and a mammogram in 6 months. If your results show breast cancer or a precancerous condition, further surgery or care is needed. Your health care team will let you know and you can make an appointment for follow-up.

firmness. Rare complications of breast radiation include rib fractures, radiation pneumonitis, brachial plexus complications, secondary tumors, and cardiac complications. Key nursing responsibilities for patients undergoing radiation therapy include the following: ensuring that patients and families are knowledgeable about symptoms to anticipate during therapy; careful skin assessments to monitor for changes; teaching skin care; managing alterations in skin integrity; and monitoring for and managing fatigue. Self-care strategies should be addressed in detail with patients because the majority of breast radiation is administered on an outpatient basis, and many patients are able to work while receiving therapy.

SYSTEMIC TREATMENT OF BREAST CANCER

Hormonal Therapy

A variety of strategies have been used to alter the hormonal environment in the setting of breast cancer. The oldest form of endocrine therapy is ovarian ablation via surgical removal of the ovaries or, less frequently, by using radiation therapy. Side effects of this intervention include hot flashes, mood changes, and other signs and symptoms of estrogen deprivation. Long-term effects include accelerated bone demineralization and increased risk for cardiovascular disease.

SERMs are agents that cause regression in breast cancer cells by binding competitively to estrogen receptors, blocking estrogens binding ability. Tamoxifen was the first SERM to be used in clinical practice and it is the most frequently prescribed drug in the setting of breast cancer. In addition to its ability to block estrogen, tamoxifen has a number of other actions that are beneficial in the setting of breast cancer: these include lowering the production of TGF-α, blocking angiogenesis, and inducing natural killer cell activity and the production of TGF-β, protein kinase C, and calmodulin. Tamoxifen has both agonist and antagonist properties; as such, it increases the risk of the development of endometrial hyperplasia and dysplasia, and endometrial carcinoma as well as inducing a number of benign gynecologic changes. Tamoxifen's effect on endometrial tissue was investigated in over 2800 women with node-negative, ER-positive breast cancer who participated in the NSABP B-14 trial. In this study, two cases of endometrial cancer occurred in the placebo group and 23 were found in the group who received tamoxifen. Newer SERMS, such as toremefine, which has been approved for use in postmenopausal women with ER-positive metastatic breast cancer, and raloxifene, approved to minimize osteoporosis, lack the agonist activity on the uterus. Selective estrogen receptor down-regulators (SERDs) are pure estrogen antagonists. These agents block estrogen receptor transactivation and degradation, resulting in a decrease in receptor concentration on the cell. The only currently approved SERD is fulvestrant (Faslodex).[100]

Aromatase inhibition represents another strategy used to alter the hormonal environment. In premenopausal women, estrogen production mainly occurs in the ovaries. Following menopause, the ovaries no longer produce estrogen; it is primarily synthesized in the adrenal glands, muscle, and adipose tissues through the conversion of androgens by the enzyme aromatase. Aromatase is a cytochrome P450 enzyme required for the biosynthesis estrogen.[101] Aromatase is concentrated in adipose and hepatic tissue and is found in elevated concentrations in breast cancer. Agents that inhibit aromatase lower the serum and tumor levels of estrogen. The nonsteroidal aromatase inhibitors (AIs) anastrozole, letrozole, vorozole, and fadrozole bind reversibly to aromatase; steroidal AIs (exemestane and formestane) bind irreversibly, causing permanent inactivation.

The majority of studies of AIs have focused on their use in the adjuvant setting. As shown in these investigations, the use of adjuvant AIs has demonstrated efficacy in three instances: as an initial adjuvant hormonal therapy; in patients who had already received 2 to 3 years of therapy with adjuvant tamoxifen; and as extended adjuvant hormonal therapy after completion of 5 years of tamoxifen. In each of these settings, the use of AIs improved disease-free survival rates. Moreover, consistent reductions in the rates of contralateral breast cancers were reported in these investigations. Based on these data, AIs are increasingly prescribed in each of these clinical settings.[52,102,103] A number of studies have investigated the use of AIs in the setting of advanced breast cancer. Although these agents have demonstrated promise, additional studies are needed to more clearly define their role in this setting. AIs are generally well tolerated. Side effects include hot flashes, mild nausea, fatigue, mood disturbances, musculoskeletal problems, ischemic cardiovascular disease, thromboembolic events, and vaginal bleeding.

Chemotherapy

Chemotherapy plays a fundamental role in the medical management of breast cancer. Anthracycline-based regimens continue to play a pivotal role, but over the past several years the benefits of adding taxanes has been clearly established and novel chemotherapeutic and biological agents have been investigated and approved for use in breast cancer. Chemotherapy for breast cancer may be administered in a variety of settings; several of these will be briefly discussed.

Neoadjuvant Chemotherapy

Neoadjuvant therapy refers to chemotherapy administered before locoregional therapy. In the setting of breast cancer, this modality is often used to down-stage tumors and facilitate breast-conservation therapy. The first study to evaluate the effectiveness of neoadjuvant chemotherapy in breast cancer was initiated in 1973 at the Milan Cancer Insitiute.[104,105] Since that time, several clinical trials have demonstrated that larger breast cancers treated with neoadjuvant chemotherapy had higher rates of clinical response and greater likelihood of successful breast conservation. Stage of disease as well as type and duration of chemotherapy varied widely in these trials, making cross-comparisons difficult. The largest trial, conducted by the NSABP (B-18), reported a pCR of 13% using anthracycline-based chemotherapy regimens. More recent trials, employing taxanes, have shown even better results.[106,107] Although neoadjuvant therapy has been effective in down-grading tumors and improving surgical outcomes, recurrence rates are higher after neoadjuvant chemotherapy followed by breast-conserving surgery, as compared to mastectomy. Moreover, overall or disease-free survival rates have not been effectively improved using neoadjuvant chemotherapy. Although several early trials demonstrated a survival benefit, upon long-term follow-up of subjects, no substantial differences have been appreciated.[108,109]

Adjuvant Chemotherapy

Early clinical trials clearly established the role of adjuvant therapy in improving survival in women with early-stage breast cancer. These studies indicated that anthracycline-based regimens had higher rates of efficacy than other combination regimens and that adjuvant therapy administered for periods of greater than 6 months was no more effective than regimens administered over a 6-month period. Treatment approaches for early-stage breast cancer continue to evolve based on emerging evidence from clinical trials.[110] Recently, the use of taxanes, either combined with or following doxorubicin and cyclophosphamide administration, have demonstrated improvements in overall and disease-free survival rates. Newer schedules of adjuvant therapy administration are also being investigated. The administration of dose-dense therapy (a strategy that accelerates the drug administration schedule from 3 to 2 week cycles) for example, has shown greater efficacy than conventional schedules in several studies.[111-113] This approach requires more intensive supportive therapy, particularly with regard to the management of neutropenia.

Metastatic Chemotherapy

The goals of chemotherapy in the metastatic setting include controlling disease while ensuring quality of life. Selection of therapy in the setting of advanced disease is based on individual patient- and tumor-related factors and should be influenced by patient concerns and preferences. Although studies continue to define roles for chemotherapy and biotherapy, there is no standard of care in terms of a specific chemotherapeutic regimen for patients with metastatic breast cancer. A variety of antineoplastics have demonstrated efficacy when used as single agents or in combination: these agents include anthracyclines (doxorubicin and epirubicin), pegylated anthracyclines (liposomal doxorubicin), taxanes (paclitaxel and docetaxel), capecitabine (a prodrug of fluorouracil that is effective in paclitaxel-resistant patients), vinorelbine, and gemcitabine. However, no single agent therapy confers a survival advantage over any other agent.[114] The optimal sequencing and administration schedules of these agents have not been definitively established. Combination chemotherapy is also administered in the metastatic setting. Combinations of anthracycline plus a taxane, a taxane plus capecitabine, or a taxane plus gemcitabine have all demonstrated some benefit in this setting.[115]

Combinations of chemotherapy and trastuzumab (a monoclonal antibody discussed below) have resulted in increased overall survival as compared to chemotherapy alone in *human epidermal growth factor 2* (*HER2*) positive patients with breast cancer. When administered with anthracyclines, however, the toxicities of these agents, particularly cardiotoxicities, may be exacerbated. Newer anthracyclines, such as pegylated doxorubicin, are associated with less toxicity than conventional doxorubicin. The lower toxicity profile of this agent has led to increased use in the metastatic setting.

Targeted Therapies

Targeted therapies are being used and studied in the setting of breast cancer. Based on an increased understanding of the biology of breast cancer, newer treatments that target specific abnormalities known to occur in breast cancer are being developed. Epidermal growth factor receptors (EGFR) are overexpressed in a number of solid tumors including breast cancer. A member of the EGFR family, *HER2* is overexpressed in 20% to 30% of breast cancers. *HER-2* is a gene that is involved in the regulation of cell growth. Cellular proliferation is regulated by extracellular factors that trigger signaling cascades from surface receptors through cytoplasmic effectors.[116]

When *HER2* is overexpressed, it can lead to changes in the signaling process of cells. Breast cancers that overexpress *HER2* are associated with more aggressive biologic activity, including higher rates of relapse, earlier relapse, and increased mortality. Trastuzumab *(Herceptin)* is a monoclonal antibody that binds to the extracellular domain of the *HER2* protein on the surface of breast cancer cells. This binding prevents the initiation of the aberrant cell-signaling process. Trastuzumab is currently the only approved targeted therapy in the setting of breast cancer; however, many newer targeted therapies are under investigation. Historically, trastuzumab has been used (combined with chemotherapy) primarily in the metastatic setting;[91] however, new evidence from a recent interim analysis of two large, randomized clinical trials indicated that there was a significant decrease in breast cancer recurrence and improved survival[117] in patients who were treated with chemotherapy and trastuzumab for early-stage breast cancer as opposed to those who received chemotherapy alone.

Side effects of chemotherapy include myelosuppression, alopecia, acute and delayed nausea and vomiting, oral and gastrointestinal mucositis, diarrhea, constipation, and neuropathy. Neutropenia is the most serious and potentially life-threatening complication following the administration of chemotherapy. Long-term effects of chemotherapy include secondary malignancies. The oncology nurse's role in caring for breast cancer patients receiving chemotherapy includes being knowledgeable about the antineoplastic agents being administered, performing agent-specific targeted toxicity assessments, administering antineoplastics according to established standards, and providing anticipatory care, patient education regarding self-care, and psychologic support of the patient and family. Over the past several years, there has been an increased amount of attention to understanding the physiologic basis for the development of common chemotherapy symptoms and in identifying effective strategies to manage such events. Oncology nurses should be aware of changes in evidence about these issues and use this information to guide their clinical practice.

NURSING CONSIDERATIONS

The Role of Oncology Nursing Across the Breast Cancer Continuum

Breast and breast cancer care can be conceptualized on a continuum that ranges from prevention to terminal illness from advanced disease. Oncology nurses play a critical role at all points along this trajectory. Both generalist and advanced practice nurses are well positioned to provide public education on the risk factors associated with breast cancer and methods of screening and early detection. The Oncology Nursing Society's Position Statement on Prevention and Early Detection of Cancer in the United States[118] has indicated that oncology nurses must strive to provide educational and early detection services in a manner that is consistent with the cultural background and health care beliefs of the individuals and families to whom they provide care. There is very little evidence on breast health and breast cancer screening information needs among minority ethnic groups.[119] Oncology nurses need to work with cultural and ethnic groups in the areas where they practice to ensure that they develop strategies to provide appropriate and relevant information of screening activities for women.

Oncology nurses are instrumental during the diagnostic and treatment phases of care as well as in the setting of both advanced disease and survivorship phases of breast cancer care. The role of oncology nurses in managing several common clinical issues that occur in breast cancer will be discussed in the following material.

Managing Bone Health

Alterations in the hormonal milieu seen in breast cancer are associated with cumulative dysregulation of bone mineral homeostasis.[120] Women receiving treatment for early-stage breast cancer often experience rapid and progressive treatment-induced bone loss. Patients with more advanced disease are at risk for significant bone loss that occurs as a result of tumor-induced osteolysis (this occurs even in the absence of bone metastases). Changes in bone mineral density result in osteoporosis with an associated increased risk for fractures and other skeletal complications. Osteoporosis is defined using World Health Organization criteria as a bone mineral density (BMD) of ≥ 2.5 standard deviations below the mean for young adults of the same sex and race.[121]

It is estimated that 63% to 96% of women who are diagnosed with premenopausal breast cancer will experience ovarian failure during the first year of treatment with standard therapy. Several studies have demonstrated decreases in BMD in those women who experience ovarian failure as compared to those who do not. In addition, tamoxifen use in the premenopausal patient has been shown to decrease BMD as compared with placebo. The use of aromatase inhibitors is also associated with changes in BMD. Studies in this area have shown variable results depending on the specific agent studied. Additional investigations are currently in progress to more precisely define the relationship of these agents to alterations in bone density.

Proactive monitoring for bone loss and management of bone health during treatment for breast cancer are important responsibilities of the oncology nurse. Recommendations for the management of bone loss include performing baseline bone mineral analysis in postmenopausal women and in premenopausal women who experience ovarian failure as a result of cancer treatment. Dietary counseling to ensure adequate intake of calcium and vitamin D should also be provided. Antiresorptive therapy with bisphosphonates should be considered in patients who are osteopenic and at risk for continued bone loss, and should be initiated in patients who have documented osteoporosis. FDA-approved antiresorptive therapies for the prevention of osteoporosis include the bisphosphonates residronate and alendronate. Bisphosphonates are synthetic pyrophosphate analogs with strong affinity for bone mineral; as such, they are potent inhibitors of normal and abnormal bone resorption.[122] Clinical trials have clearly demonstrated that these agents are effective in maintaining BMD and preventing fractures. Moreover, in women with bony metastases, these agents promote bone healing, prevent or slow the development of new disease in the bone, decrease pain and the use of analgesic medications, and decrease the need for radiation therapy. After antiresorptive therapy, follow-up bone mineral density studies should be conducted. In addition, serum biomarkers of bone turnover (such as urinary deoxypirdinoline or collagen N-telopeptide) may be monitored.

Symptom Management

Women with breast cancer can experience a variety of symptoms related to both the disease and the treatments process. Symptoms may be present at the time the patient is first seen, may occur acutely as a result of therapeutic plan, or may first appear in the posttreatment phase. Changes in cognitive function, fatigue, anxiety, and the development of menopausal symptoms are commonly reported in women undergoing treatment for breast cancer. These symptoms are associated with increased distress and have been strongly correlated to quality of life.[134] Several reports have now indicated that symptoms experienced during treatment may linger for extended periods after the completion of therapy. Oncology nurses play a major role in the assessment and proactive management of symptoms. Key responsibilities of the oncology nurse include being knowledgeable about symptoms that are expected to occur, identifying risk factors, performing focused assessments, providing anticipatory care, using evidence-based interventions, and teaching patients self-care strategies to prevent, minimize, and effectively manage these events.

Survivorship Issues

There are over 2 million breast cancer survivors in the US today.[135] Breast cancer survivors are at risk for disease recurrence, second primary cancers, long-term effects of treatment, and a number of potential psychosocial issues. Recommendations for follow-up after primary treatment for breast cancer include performing monthly breast self-examination, having a mammogram annually, and undergoing a history and physical examination by a health care professional every 6 months for 5 years and then annually.[136] More intensive monitoring has not been shown to be more effective than routine follow-up testing on survival rates and health-related quality of life in breast cancer patients in a multicenter randomized controlled trial.[137,138] Most breast cancers recur within 5 years of the initial diagnosis; recurrence rates are lowest for small primary tumors (<1 cm) with no positive lymph nodes. Nonspecific symptoms, such as weight loss or weakness, or physical findings, such as changes in the chest wall or the development of adenopathy, may be indicators of recurrence and should be investigated thoroughly. Patients should also be monitored for second primary cancers known to occur in this population: these include cancers of the ipsilateral and contralateral breast and ovarian, colon, and rectal cancers. Women on long-term tamoxifen therapy also have an increased risk of developing endometrial cancer.[139]

As more people are surviving breast cancer, the long-term sequelae of treatment are now becoming a major area of research exploration. Treatment-induced cognitive alterations, fatigue, depression, sleep disturbances, vasomotor symptoms, lymphedema, osteopenia and osteoporosis, psychologic distress, premature menopause, and infertility have all been reported following completion of therapy.[140-142] Younger women may be at greater risk for distress associated with prolonged symptoms following treatment for breast cancer. Studies have demonstrated that younger women often experience more pronounced changes in mood and poorer emotional functioning than older women.[142] While chemotherapy has clearly improved survival rates in this group, the long-term effects on patients need to be effectively addressed. Optimal management of long-term symptoms requires an understanding of the underlying pathobiology and symptom patterns and the effects of symptoms on functional status and quality of life outcomes. It is essential that a more in-depth knowledge base regarding these issues be developed so that appropriate interventions and support can be provided. Issues confronting survivors are of great interest to oncology nurses. Historically, research on survivorship focused on survivors of childhood cancers.[143] As cancer treatments become more effective and survival rates improve, the research agenda is expanding to investigate many of the issues experienced after the acute phase of treatment. Oncology nurses need to stay abreast of emerging evidence on the issues of cancer survivorship and use this knowledge to inform their clinical practice.

IMPLICATIONS FOR NURSING PRACTICE, EDUCATION AND RESEARCH

Breast cancer represents a major health problem. Oncology nurses are involved in care at every point along the trajectory from prevention through survivorship or terminal illness from advanced disease.

Knowledge about breast cancer is evolving on a daily basis. Research on the topic spans a continuum that extends from the basic science work on molecular mechanisms to interventions designed to test strategies for breast cancer prevention, improve the ability to diagnose breast cancers at ever earlier time points, determine the most effective, minimally-invasive operative techniques, optimize clinical outcomes in patients receiving treatment for breast cancer, identify strategies to enhance quality of life in cancer survivors, and ensure optimal symptom control and relief of suffering in patients with advanced disease. The evolving research agenda requires oncology nurses to be committed to ongoing education so that they can keep abreast of new evidence that should be used in the practice setting. In addition, it is essential to advance the research agenda, particularly in areas that may be influenced by nursing practice, such as in the area of symptom control, improving coping, adaptation, or self-care.

REFERENCES

1. Jemal A and others: Cancer Statistics, 2005, *CA Cancer J Clin* 55(1):10-30, 2005.
2. Weiss JR, Moysich KB, Swede H: Epidemiology of male breast cancer, *Cancer Epidemiol Biomarkers Prevent* 14(1):20-26, 2005.
3. Fletcher SW, Elmore JG: Mammographic screening for breast cancer, *N Engl J Med* 348(17):1672-1680, 2003.
4. Domchek SM, Weber BL: Recent advances in breast cancer biology, *Curr Opin Oncol* 14(6):589-593, 2002.
5. U. S. National Cancer Institute, Surveillance, Epidemiology and End Results (SEER) Program with Emory University, Atlanta SEER Cancer Registry: *Quadrants of the Breast*, 2005. On the Web at http://training.seer.cancer.gov/ss_module01_breast/unit02_sec02_breast_quadrants.html.
6. Domchek SM and others: Application of breast cancer risk prediction models in clinical practice, *J Clin Oncol* 21(4):593-601, 2003.
7. Pharoah PDP and others: Family history and the risk of breast cancer: a systematic review and meta-analysis, *Int J Cancer* 71:800-809, 1997.
8. National Comprehensive Cancer Network Genetic/Familial High-Risk Assessment Panel—Mary B. Daly, MD, PhD/Chair and sole Writing Committee Member: Clinical Practice Guidelines in Oncology—v.1.2005, *Genetic/Familial High-Risk Assessment: Breast and Ovarian*, 2005. On the Web at www.nccn.org/ professionals/ physician_gls/pdf/genetics_screening.pdf.
9. National Cancer Institute, U.S. National Institutes of Health: *Breast cancer risk assessment tool*, 2000. Retrieved from http://brca.nci.nih.gov/brc/q1.htm.
10. Wooster R, Weber BL: Genomic medicine: breast and ovarian cancer, *N Engl J Med* 348(2):2339-2347, 2003.
11. Shattuck-Eidens D and others: BRCA1 Sequence analysis in women at high risk for susceptibility mutations: risk factor analysis and implications for genetic testing, *JAMA* 278(15):1242-1250, 1997.
12. Khoury-Collado F, Bombard AT: Hereditary breast and ovarian cancer: What the primary care physician should know, *Obstet Gynecol Surv* 59(7):537-542, 2004.
13. Easton DF, Ford D, Bishop DT, and the Breast Cancer Linkage Consortium: Breast and ovarian cancer incidence in BRCA1-mutation carriers, *Am J Hum Genet* 56:265-271, 1995.
14. Verhoog LC and others: Survival and tumour characteristics of breast-cancer patients with germline mutations of BRCA1, *Lancet* 351:316-321, 1998.
15. Verhoog LC and others: Survival in hereditary breast cancer associated with germline mutations of BRCA2, *J Clin Oncol* 17:3396-3402, 1999.
16. Levine DA and others: Fallopian tube and primary peritoneal carcinomas associated with BRCA mutations, *J Clin Oncol* 21:4222-4227, 2003.
17. Hilakivi-Clarke L: Estrogens, BRCA1, and breast cancer, *Cancer Res* 60:4993-5001, 2000.
18. Hedenfalk I and others: Gene-expression profiles in hereditary breast cancer, *N Engl J Med* 344(8):539-548, 2001.
19. Turner N, Tutt A, Ashworth A: Hallmarks of 'BRCAness' in sporadic cancers, *Nature Rev Cancer* 4:814-819, 2004.
20. Pavelic K, Gall-Troselj K: Recent advances in molecular genetics of breast cancer, *J Molec Med* 79:566-573, 2001.
21. BayesMendel Lab: BRCAPRO. Chavez OA and others, editors. On the Web at http://astor.som.jhmi.edu/BayesMendel/brcapro.html, 2005.
22. American Society of Clinical Oncology: *American Society of Clinical Oncology Policy Statement Update: Genetic Testing for Cancer Susceptibility*, *J Clin Oncol* 21(12):2397-2406, 2003.
23. Vadaparampil ST, Wey JP, Kinney AY: Psychosocial aspects of genetic counseling and testing, *Semin Oncol Nurs* 20(3):186-195, 2004.
24. Travis RC, Key TJ: Oestrogen exposure and breast cancer risk, *Breast Cancer Res* 5(5):239-247, 2003.
25. Pike MC and others: Oral contraceptive use and early abortion as risk factors for breast cancer in young women, *Br J Cancer* 43(1):72-76, 1981.
26. Margolese RG, Hortobagyi GN, Buchholz TA: Neoplasms of the breast. In Kufe DW and others, editors: *Cancer medicine*, Hamilton, Ontario, 2003, BC Decker.
27. de Carvalho M and others: The role of estrogens in BRCA1/2 mutation carriers: reflections on the past, issues for the future, *Cancer Nurs* 26(6):421-430, 2003.
28. Hamajima N and others as the Collaborative Group on Hormonal Factors in Breast Cancer: Alcohol, tobacco and breast cancer—collaborative reanalysis of individual data from 53 epidemiological studies, including 58,515 women with breast cancer and 95,067 women without the disease, *Br J Cancer* 87(11):1234-1245, 2002.
29. Shlipak MG and others: Estrogen and progestin, lipoprotein(a), and the risk of recurrent coronary heart disease events after menopause, *JAMA* 283(14):1845-1852, 2000.
30. Grady D and others for the HERS Research Group: Cardiovascular disease outcomes during 6.8 years of hormone therapy: heart and estrogen/progestin replacement study follow-up (HERS II), *JAMA* 288(1):49-57, 2002.

31. Hulley S and others for the HERS Research Group: Noncardiovascular disease outcomes during 6.8 years of hormone therapy: heart and estrogen/progestin replacement study follow-up (HERS II), *JAMA* 288(1):58-66, 2002.
32. Writing Group for the Women's Health Initiative Investigators: Risks and benefits of estrogen plus progestin in healthy postmenopausal women: principal results from the women's health initiative randomized controlled trial, *JAMA* 288(3):321-333, 2002.
33. McPherson K, Steel CM, Dixon JM: ABC of breast diseases: breast cancer—epidemiology, risk factors, and genetics, *BMJ* 321:624-628, 2000.
34. Dumitrescu RG, Cotarla I: Understanding breast cancer risk—where do we stand in 2005? *J Cell Molec Med* 9(1):208-221, 2005.
35. Sweeney C and others: Risk factors for breast cancer in elderly women, *Am J Epidemiol* 160(9):868-875, 2004.
36. Key TJ and others as the Endogenous Hormones and Breast Cancer Collaborative Group: Body mass index, serum sex hormones, and breast cancer risk in postmenopausal women, *J Natl Cancer Inst* 95(16):1218-1226, 2003.
37. Kuhl H: Breast cancer risk in the WHI study: The problem of obesity, *Maturitas Eur Menopause J* 51:83-97, 2005.
38. Carmichael AR, Bates T: Obesity and breast cancer: a review of the literature, *Breast* 13(2):85-92, 2004.
39. Kropp S and others: Low-to-moderate alcohol consumption and breast cancer risk by age 50 years among women in Germany, *Am J Epidemiol* 154(7):624-634, 2001.
40. Horn-Ross PL and others: Patterns of alcohol consumption and breast cancer risk in the California Teachers Study Cohort, *Cancer Epidemiol Biomarkers Prevent* 13:405-411, 2004.
41. Singletary KW, Gapstur SM: Alcohol and breast cancer review of epidemiologic and experimental evidence and potential mechanisms, *JAMA* 286(17):2143-2151, 2001.
42. Horn-Ross PL and others: Recent diet and breast cancer risk: the California Teachers Study (USA), *Cancer Causes Control* 13(5):407-415, 2002.
43. Tjonneland A and others: Alcohol intake, drinking patterns and risk of postmenopausal breast cancer in Denmark: a prospective cohort study, *Cancer Causes Control* 14(3):277-284, 2003.
44. Ellison RC and others: Exploring the relation of alcohol consumption to risk of breast cancer, *Am J Epidemiol* 154(8):740-747, 2001.
45. Kenney LB and others: Breast cancer after childhood cancer: a report from the childhood cancer survivor study, *Ann Intern Med* 141(8):590-597, 2004.
46. Dupont WD and others: Breast cancer risk associated with proliferative breast disease and atypical hyperplasia, *Cancer* 71(4):1258-1265, 1993.
47. McDivitt RW and others: Histologic types of benign breast disease and the risk for breast cancer. The Cancer and Steroid Hormone Study Group, *Cancer* 69(6): 1408-1414, 1992.
48. AstraZeneca Pharmaceuticals LP: *Nolvadex (tamoxifen citrate) tablets* (package insert). Wilmington, 2005, AstraZeneca Pharmaceuticals LP.
49. Kinsinger LS and others: Chemoprevention of breast cancer: a summary of the evidence for the U.S. Preventive Services Task Force, *Ann Intern Med* 137(1):E59-E69, 2002.
50. National Comprehensive Cancer Network Breast Cancer Risk Reduction Panel, Carlson RW and others: Clinical practice guidelines in oncology—v.1.2000, *Breast Cancer Risk Reduction*, 2004. On the Web at www.nccn.org/professionals/physician_gls/pdf/breast_risk.pdf.
51. Dunn BK, Wickerham DL, Ford LG: Prevention of hormone-related cancers: breast cancer, *J Clin Oncol* 23(2): 357-367, 2005.
52. Cuzick J: Aromatase inhibitors for breast cancer prevention, *J Clin Oncol* 23(8):1636-1643, 2005.
53. Lonning PE: Aromatase inhibitors in breast cancer, *Endocr-Related Cancer* 11(2):179-189, 2004.
54. Serrano D and others: Progress in chemoprevention of breast cancer, *Crit Rev Oncol/Hematol* 49:109-117, 2003.
55. Kong G and others: The retinoid X receptor-selective retinoid, LGD1069, down-regulates cyclooxygenase-2 expression in human breast cells through transcription factor crosstalk: implications for molecular-based chemoprevention, *Cancer Res* 65(8):3462-3469, 2005.
56. Decensi A and others: Breast cancer prevention trials using retinoids, *J Mammary Gland Biol Neoplasia* 8(1): 19-30, 2003.
57. Emens LA, Jaffee EM: Toward a breast cancer vaccine: work in progress, *Oncology (Huntingt)* 17(9):1200-1211, 2003.
58. Calderon-Margalit R, Paltiel O: Prevention of breast cancer in women who carry BRCA1 or BRCA2 mutations: a critical review of the literature, *Int J Cancer* 112:357-364, 2004.
59. Hartmann LC and others: Efficacy of bilateral prophylactic mastectomy in women with a family history of breast cancer, *N Engl J Med* 340(2):77-84. 1999.
60. Rebbeck TR and others et al for The Prevention and Observation of Surgical End Points Study Group: Prophylactic oophorectomy in carriers of BRCA1 or BRCA2 mutations, *N Engl J Med* 346(21):1616-1622, 2002.
61. Lind DS, Smith BL, Souba WW: Breast procedures. In *ACS surgery: principles and practice*, Section 3 Breast, skin and soft tissue, 2004. On the Web at www.acssurgery.com/sample/ch0305s.htm.
62. Love S: Ductal lavage. In SusanLoveMD.org, the website for women, 2004. On the Web at www.susanlovemd.org/lavage_frames.html.
63. Arun B: Ductal lavage and risk assessment of breast cancer, *Oncologist* 9(6):599-605, 2004.
64. Fabian CJ and others: Breast cancer chemoprevention phase I evaluation of biomarker modulation by arzoxifene, a third generation selective estrogen receptor modulator, *Clin Cancer Res* 10(16):5403-5417, 2004.
65. U.S. Preventive Services Task Force: Screening for breast cancer: recommendations and rationale, *Ann Intern Med* 137(5 Part 1):344-346, 2002.
66. Gotzsche PG, Olsen O: Is screening for breast cancer with mammography justifiable? *Lancet* 355:129-134, 2000.
67. Olsen O, Gotzsche PC: Screening for breast cancer with mammography, *Cochrane Database Systematic Reviews* 4(CD001877):1-63, 2001.
68. Health Council of the Netherlands: The benefit of population screening for breast cancer with mammography, *Health Council of the Netherlands; Reports 2002*. The Hague: Health Council of the Netherlands, 2003, 2002/2003 publication no. A03/05.

69. National Cancer Institute, U.S. National Institutes of Health: *NCI statement on mammography screening,* in News February 21, 2002. Retrieved from http://www.nci.nih.gov/ newscenter/mammstatement31jan02.
70. Astley SM, Gilbert FJ: Computer-aided detection in mammography, *Clin Radiol* 59(5):390-399, 2004.
71. American College of Radiology Imaging Network (ACRIN): ACRIN Protocol No. 6652: Digital vs. film-screen mammography. In Pisano E, principal investigator, Hendrick E, study co-chair, Masood S, pathology chair, Gatsonic C, study statistician: *Current Protocols,* activation date 10/29/2001, version date 10/27/2003. On the Web at www.acrin.org/current_protocols.htm.
72. Elmore JG, and others: Screening for breast cancer, *JAMA* 293(10):1245-1256, 2005.
73. Liberman M and others: Breast cancer diagnosis by scintimammography: a meta-analysis and review of the literature, *Breast Cancer Res Treatment* 80(1):115-126, 2003.
74. Gordon PB: Ultrasound for breast cancer screening and staging, *Radiol Clin North Am* 40(3):431-441, 2002.
75. Irwig L, Houssami N, van Vliet C: New technologies in screening for breast cancer: a systematic review of their accuracy, *Br J Cancer* 90:2118-2122, 2004.
76. Porter BA: Current best clinical indications for breast MR. In *American Society of Breast Disease Symposium—April 14-16, 2005,* Las Vegas, Nev., American Society of Breast Disease.
77. Kriege M and others: Efficacy of MRI and mammography for breast-cancer screening in women with a familial or genetic predisposition, *N Engl J Med* 351(5): 427-437, 2004.
78. National Cancer Institute, U.S. National Institutes of Health: *Cancer facts: improving methods for breast cancer detection and diagnosis.* Bethesda, 2001. On the Web at http://cis.nci.nih.gov/fact/5_14.htm.
79. Cody HS: Current surgical management of breast cancer, *Curr Opin Obstet Gynecol* 14(1):45-52, 2002.
80. Cotlar AM, Dubose JJ, Rose M: History of surgery for breast cancer: radical to the sublime, *Curr Surg* 60(3): 329-337, 2003.
81. Stanley MW and others: Current issues in breast cytopathology, *Am J Clin Pathol* 113(5 Suppl 1):S49-S75, 2000.
82. Klimberg VS: Advances in the diagnosis and excision of breast cancer, *Am Surg* 69(1):11-14, 2003.
83. Bold RJ: Surgical management of breast cancer: today and tomorrow, *Cancer Biother Radiopharmaceut* 17(1): 1-9, 2002.
84. National Comprehensive Cancer Network Breast Cancer Panel Members, Carlson RW and others: Clinical practice guidelines in oncology—v.1.2005, *Breast Cancer,* 2005. Retrieved from http://www.nccn.org/professionals/physician_gls/PDF/breast.pdf.
85. Anderson WF, Chu KC, Chang S: Inflammatory breast cancer noninflammatory locally advanced breast cancer carcinoma: distinct clinicopathologic entities? *J Clin Oncol* 21(12):2254-2259, 2003.
86. Cristofanilli M: Inflammatory breast carcinoma: time to define new standards for diagnosis and treatment, *Am J Oncol Rev* 2(11):638-639, 2003.
87. Singletary S and others: Breast. In Greene FL and others, editors: *AJCC cancer staging manual,* ed 6, Chicago, 2002, Springer.
88. Clark GM: Prognostic and predictive factors. In Harris JR and others, editors: *Diseases of the breast,* Philadelphia, 2000, Lippincott Williams & Wilkins.
89. Carter CL, Allen C, Henson DE: Relation of tumor size, lymph node status, and survival in 24,740 breast cancer cases, *Cancer* 63(1):181-187, 1989.
90. Schnitt SJ: Traditional and newer pathologic factors, *J Natl Cancer Inst Monogr* 20:22-26, 2001.
91. Nemoto T and others: Management and survival of female breast cancer: results of a national survey by the American College of Surgeons, *Cancer* 45(12):2917-2924, 1980.
92. Vogel CL, Franco, SX: Clinical experience with trastuzumab (herceptin), *Breast J* 9(6):452-462, 2003.
93. Simon R and others: Patterns of her-2/neu amplification and overexpression in primary and metastatic breast cancer, *J Natl Cancer Inst* 93(15):1141-1146, 2001.
94. National Cancer Institute, U.S. National Institutes of Health: *Bevacizumab combined with chemotherapy improves progression free survival for patients with advanced breast cancer,* in *News,* 2005. On the Web at www.nci.nih.gov/newscenter/pressreleases/AvastinBreast.
95. Ahmed S and others: Breast reconstruction, *BMJ* 330: 943-948, 2005.
96. Kuske RR and others: Radiotherapy and breast reconstruction: clinical results and dosimetry, *Int J Radiat Oncol Biol Phys* 21(2):339-346, 1991.
97. Joint Commission on Accreditation of Healthcare Organizations (JCAHO): *National patient safety goals & FAQs.* Washington, D.C., 2005, JCAHO. On the Web at www.jcaho.org/index.htm.
98. Gillespie TW: Surgical therapy. In Yarbro CH, Frogge MH, Goodman M, editors, *Cancer nursing: principles and practice,* Sudbury, Mass, 2005, Jones and Bartlett.
99. Maher KE: Radiation therapy: toxicities and management. In Yarbro CH, Frogge MH, Goodman M, editors, *Cancer nursing: principles and practice,* Sudbury, Mass, 2005, Jones and Bartlett.
100. AstraZeneca Pharmaceuticals LP: *Faslodex fulvestrant injection (package insert).* Wilmington, 2002, AstraZeneca Pharmaceuticals LP.
101. Janicke F: Are all aromatase inhibitors the same? A review of the current evidence, *Breast* 13(1 Suppl 1): 10-18, 2004.
102. Strasser-Weippl K, Goss PE: Advances in adjuvant hormonal therapy for postmenopausal women, *J Clin Oncol* 23(8):1751-1759, 2005.
103. Winer EP and others: American Society of Clinical Oncology technology assessment on the use of aromatase inhibitors as adjuvant therapy for postmenopausal women with hormone receptor-positive breast cancer: status report 2004, *J Clin Oncol* 23(3):619-629, 2005.
104. Chen AM and others: Neoadjuvant chemotherapy to permit breast conservation for patients with locally advanced breast cancer, *Am J Oncol Rev* 3(12):692-696, 2004.
105. Charfare HL, Limongelli S, Purushotham AD: Neoadjuvant chemotherapy in breast cancer, *Br J Surg* 92(1):14-23, 2005.
106. Heys SD and others, Aberdeen Breast Group: Neoadjuvant docetaxel in breast cancer: 3-year survival results from the Aberdeen trial, *Clin Breast Cancer* 3(Suppl 2):S69-74, 2002.

107. Bear HD and others: The effect on tumor response of adding sequential preoperative docetaxel to preoperative doxorubicin and cyclophosphamide: preliminary results from National Surgical Adjuvant Breast and Bowel Project protocol B-27, *J Clin Oncol* 21(22):4165-4174, 2003.
108. Van der Hage JA and others and cooperating Investigators: Preoperative chemotherapy in primary operable breast cancer: Results from the European Organization for Research and Treatment of Cancer Trial 10902, *J Clin Oncol* 19(22):4224-4237, 2001.
109. Mauriac L and others: Neoadjuvant chemotherapy for operable breast carcinoma larger than 3cm: a unicentre randomized trial with a 124-month median follow-up, Institut Bergonie Bordeax Groupe Sein (IBBGS), *Ann Oncol* 10(1):47-52, 1999.
110. Adjuvant therapy for breast cancer. NIH consensus statement 2000, November 1-3, *Cancer Control* 17(4):1-35.
111. Campos SM: Evolving treatment approaches for early breast cancer, *Breast Cancer Res Treatment* 89(Suppl 1): S1-7, 2005.
112. Ellis GK and others: Dose-dense anthracycline-based chemotherapy for node-positive breast cancer, *J Clin Oncol* 20(17):3637-3643, 2002.
113. Hudis C: Dose-dense chemotherapy for breast cancer: the story so far, *Br J Cancer* 82(12):1897-1899, 2000.
114. Hamilton A, Hortobagyi G: Chemotherapy: What progress in the last 5 years? *J Clin Oncol* 23(8):1760-1775, 2005.
115. Gralow JR: Optimizing the treatment of metastatic breast cancer, *Breast Cancer Res Treatment* 89(Suppl 1): S9-S15, 2005.
116. Fornier M and others: HER2 testing and correlation with efficacy of trastuzumab therapy, *Oncology (Huntingt)* 16(10):1340-1348, 2002.
117. National Cancer Institute, U.S. National Institutes of Health: *Herceptin combined with chemotherapy improves disease-free survival for patients with early-stage breast cancer, News,* 2005. On the Web at www.nci.nih.gov/newscenter.
118. Oncology Nursing Society: Prevention and early detection of cancer in the United States. In *ONS Positions,* approved April 2001; revised August 2002. On the Web at www.ons.org/publications/positions/Prevention Detection.shtml.
119. Watts T, Merrell J, Murphy F, Williams A: Breast health information needs of women from minority ethnic groups, *J Adv Nurs* 47(5):526-535, 2004.
120. Aapro MS: Long-term implications of bone loss in breast cancer, *Breast* 13(1 Suppl 1):29-37, 2004.
121. Nissl J: Bone mineral density. In Van Houten S, editor: *WebMDHealth: health guide A-Z,* Boise, last update, December 7, 2004, Healthwise. On the Web at http://my.webmd.com/hw/osteoporosis/hw3738.asp.
122. Rosen LS and others: Zoledronic acid versus pamidronate in the treatment of skeletal metastases in patients with breast cancer or osteolytic lesions of multiple myeloma: a phase III, double-blind, comparative trial, *Cancer J* 7(5):377-387, 2001.
123. Tchen N and others: Cognitive function, fatigue, and menopausal symptoms in women receiving adjuvant chemotherapy for breast cancer, *J Clin Oncol* 21(22): 4175-4183, 2003.
124. Reuben S for The President's Cancer Panel: *Living beyond cancer: finding a new balance*; President's Cancer Panel 2003-2004 Annual Report, Bethesda, 2004, National Cancer Institute, National Institutes of Health, U.S. Department of Health and Human Services.
125. Rojas MP and others: Follow-up strategies for women treated for early breast cancer, *The Cochrane Database of Systematic Reviews 2 (Cochrane Library)* 2:1-28, 2005.
126. GIVIO Investigators, Interdisciplinary Group for Cancer Care Evaluation, Milan, Italy: Impact of follow-up testing on survival and health-related quality of life in breast cancer patients: a multicenter randomized controlled trial, *JAMA* 271(20):1587-1592, 1994.
127. Del Truco MR and others for the National Research Council on Breast Cancer Follow-up: Intensive diagnostic follow-up after treatment of primary breast cancer: a randomized trial, *JAMA* 271(20):1593-1597, 1994.
128. Sunga AY and others: Care of cancer survivors, *Am Fam Phys* 71(4):699-706, 2005.
129. Gelinas C, Fillion L: Factors related to persistent fatigue following completion of breast cancer treatment, *Oncol Nurs Forum* 31(2):269-278, 2004.
130. Carpenter JS and others: Sleep, fatigue, and depressive symptoms in breast cancer survivors and matched healthy women experiencing hot flashes, *Oncol Nurs Forum* 31(3): 591-598, 2004.
131. Ganz PA and others: Breast cancer in younger women: reproductive and late health effects of treatment, *J Clin Oncol* 21(22):4184-4193, 2003.
132. Duffy CM, Allen SM, Clark MA: Discussions regarding reproductive health for young women with breast cancer undergoing chemotherapy, *J Clin Oncol* 23(4):766-773, 2005.

CHAPTER

6 Cervical Cancer

Alice Spinelli

INTRODUCTION

This chapter focuses on cervical intraepithelial neoplasia and invasive cervical cancer. The incidence, risk factors, screening, and treatment of cervical cancer will be discussed. In addition, nursing care including education and counseling are explored.

CERVICAL INTRAEPITHELIAL NEOPLASIA

Incidence and Mortality

Cancer of the cervix is the second most common cancer among women worldwide; about 490,000 new cases will be diagnosed in 2005. About 80% of cervical cancer cases occur in developing countries where, in many regions, it is the most common cancer among women.[1] In the US, cervical cancer is the fourteenth most common type of cancer in women with 10,370 new cases and 3,710 deaths projected for 2005. Incidence and mortality for cervical cancer have decreased dramatically in the US, largely because of Pap test screening. Over the past 5 decades, Pap tests have reduced cancer incidence by detecting precancerous lesions that can be successfully treated before they progress to cancer.[2] The 5-year survival rate for precancerous lesions is 100%, and 92% for early stage cancers.[3] Approximately half of the cervical cancers diagnosed in the US are in women who have never been screened, and an additional 10% of cancers occur in women who have not been screened within the past 5 years.[4] Significant disparities exist between races, ethnicities, and geographic regions. In the US, the highest incidence is observed among Hispanic/Latino women and the highest mortality rates are among African American women. This disproportionate burden of cervical cancer in medically underserved populations is mainly due to lack of screening.[5]

Risk Factors and HPV

A strong causal relationship between human papilloma virus (HPV) and cervical cancer (and its precursors) has been established, given that HPV is present in virtually all of invasive cervical cancers.[4,6] HPV is also detected in approximately 50% to 80% of vaginal, 50% of vulvar, and nearly all penile and anal cancers.[7] Genital infection with HPV is the most common sexually transmitted viral infection in the US; approximately 6.2 million new infections occur each year. Overall about 75% of the US adult population have been exposed to HPV.[8] Genital infection with HPV is especially common among sexually active young women (less than 25 years of age), with prevalence decreasing with older age. The higher rates in younger women appear to be related to transmission of new infection during the years of early sexual activity, with infection clearing over time in most women.[6]

Despite the high prevalence of HPV, exposure most often results in latent infection. Latent infection implies the presence of HPV DNA without evidence of disease and may never result in

Table 6-1 Cervical Neoplasia Risk Factors[32]

Risk Factors	Risk-Reducing Behaviors
Intercourse at an early age	Routine PAP test
Multiple sexual partners	Limit sexual activity in teen years
Male partner risk factors	Barrier contraceptive use
Human papilloma virus infection	Health education:
Cigarette smoking	• Risks of sexual contact
Oral contraceptive use	• Safe sexual practices and disease prevention methods and purpose
Immunosuppression	
Low socioeconomic status	• Need and frequency of PAP testing and pelvic exams
	Avoid smoking
	Increase vitamin A intake
	Seek prompt treatment of cervical epithelial neoplasia when recommended

neoplasia. Once women become infected with HPV, there are two potential outcomes: a transient or self-limited infection and a persistently expressed infection. Most commonly, HPV infections are self-limited or transient. Less than half of HPV infections persist for 24 months or more.[9] Whether or not HPV infection remains latent or progresses to neoplasia is dependent primarily on the presence or absence of "high-risk" types of HPV, and other cofactors.[5] (Table 6-1).

To date, over 120 distinctive types of HPV have been identified, of which over 30 are considered genital types. The various subtypes of HPV hold different levels of oncogenic potential. "High-risk" HPV types are associated with a high relative risk of cervical cancer, "low-risk" viruses are associated with low risk of invasive cervical cancer, and "intermediate-risk" viruses are occasionally associated with cervical cancer[9] (Table 6-2).

The most common of the "high-risk" viruses is HPV-16, and the second most common is HPV-18. HPV-16 is found in almost half of all women with cervical cancer and is also the most common type found in women with high-grade cervical intraepithelial neoplasia (CIN) types 2 and 3. HPV-6 and HPV-11 are the most common types found in genital warts and are uncommonly found in association with invasive cervical cancer.[10,11] HPV DNA testing for high-risk types of HPV has been approved by the FDA for primary screening in combination with the Pap test for women aged 30 years and older and as triage for women of all ages who have an equivocal cytology (Pap) result.[12,13]

Screening

The purpose of screening, in addition to detecting cervical cancer at an early stage, is to detect and remove high-grade lesions and thus prevent potential progression to cervical carcinoma. Pap test sensitivity for high-grade CIN is 70% to 80%.[14] The majority of false-negative results can be

Table 6-2 Anogenital HPV Types

	HPV Type
"LOW-RISK" TYPES	6, 11, 40, 42, 43, 44, 53, 54, 61, 72, 73, 81
"HIGH-RISK" TYPES	16, 18, 31, 33, 35, 39, 45, 51, 52, 56, 58, 59, 68, 82
POSSIBLE "HIGH-RISK" TYPES	26, 66, 73

Adapted with permission from Munoz N and others: Epidemiologic classification of human papillomavirus types associated with cervical cancer, *New Eng J Med* 348:518-527, 2003.

Table **6-3** AMERICAN CANCER SOCIETY GUIDELINES FOR CERVICAL CANCER SCREENING[32]

BEGIN SCREENING	3 years after beginning vaginal intercourse, but no later than at 21 years of age
ANNUAL SCREENING WITH CONVENTIONAL PAP OR EVERY 2 YEARS WITH LIQUID-BASED	>30 years old: If 3 consecutive PAP tests are negative, may be performed every 2-3 years unless immunocompromised or DES-exposed
MAY STOP SCREENING	>70 years old who have had 3 or more consecutive, normal PAP tests and no abnormal tests in 10 years Women with a history of hysterectomy: PAP testing not necessary unless hysterectomy performed for cervical neoplasia Women with severe comorbid or life-threatening illnesses may forego screening.

attributed to sampling error. Liquid-based, thin-layer preparations have been developed in an attempt to improve the sensitivity of Pap tests in detecting abnormalities and thereby reduce false-negative rates associated with conventional Pap tests.[15] While liquid-based cytology methods are more expensive, the data demonstrate improved diagnostic sensitivity.[16-18] HPV DNA testing can be performed using the same liquid-based cervical samples that are obtained for Pap testing. This means DNA testing can be performed at the time of initial screening, when applicable, or as "reflex testing" should the Pap test result be equivocal, obviating the need for a return visit for DNA sampling.

Screening Guidelines

The American Cancer Society has developed updated guidelines for the early detection of cervical neoplasia and cancer (Table 6-3). Screening should begin approximately 3 years after a girl or woman begins having vaginal intercourse. Screening should begin no later than at 21 years of age. Screening should then be performed annually with the conventional cervical cytology smears or every 2 years using liquid-based cytology; or after age 30, women who have had three consecutive tests with satisfactory normal/negative results may be screened every 2 to 3 years (unless they have a history of *in utero* diethylstilbestrol [DES] exposure or are immunocompromised). Women who are infected with human immunodeficiency virus (HIV) and/or are immunocompromised should have a Pap test twice in the first year after diagnosis of HIV infection and, if the results are normal, annually thereafter. Women aged 70 and older who have had three or more documented, satisfactory normal/negative Pap test results within the 10-year period before age 70 may elect to cease cervical cancer screening. Women with severe comorbid or life-threatening illnesses may forego cervical cancer screening. Screening with vaginal cytology tests following total hysterectomy (with removal of the cervix) for benign gynecologic disease is not indicated. Screening should continue annually if the hysterectomy was performed for cervical neoplasia, as well as in women with a history *of in utero* DES exposure.[19]

THE BETHESDA REPORTING SYSTEM

The Bethesda System was developed in 1988 as a uniform system of terminology that would provide clear guidance for clinical management. It was revised in 1991 and again in 2001 to reflect evolving knowledge and technology.[20-22] Table 6-4 provides a comparison of Pap test

Table 6-4 Comparison of Pap Smear Classifications[20,24,28]

Numerical System	Dysplasia, Cytologic Classification	Cervical Intraepithelial Neoplasia (CIN)	Bethesda System
Class I	Negative: squamous metaplasia	No designation	Negative for intraepithelial lesion or malignancy
Class II	Atypical squamous cells	No designation	Atypical squamous cells • ASC-US • ASC-H
Class III	Mild dysplasia	CIN 1	LSIL
	Moderate dysplasia	CIN 2	HSIL
Class IV	Severe dysplasia Carcinoma in situ	CIN 3	HSIL
Class V	Invasive cancer	Invasive cancer	Invasive cancer

SIL, Squamous intraepithelial lesion.

classifications and cervical pathology. The term "squamous intraepithelial lesion (SIL) may refer to a low-grade (LSIL) or high-grade (HSIL) lesion. With regard to equivocal results, the reporting of "atypical squamous cells" is qualified either as "of undetermined significance (ASC-US)" or "cannot exclude HSIL (ASC-H)." Glandular cell abnormalities are classified as "atypical endocervical, endometrial, or glandular cells."[22] The presence of endometrial glandular cells will be mentioned if the woman is age 40 or older. Atypical glandular cells are detected on cervical Pap tests in 17% of cases and indicate significant cervical pathology such as endometrial hyperplasia, or adenocarcinoma of the endocervix or endometrium in all combined cases. Although it is rare for atypical glandular cells to appear in Pap results, they necessitate immediate work-up with colposcopy and biopsy.[23]

COLPOSCOPY

The colposcope is a magnifying instrument used to identify an abnormal area of the cervix and to perform directed biopsies. Colposcopy is also used to evaluate the vulva and vagina in a similar manner. Recognition of a colposcopic abnormality is followed with a biopsy of the suspicious area, because histologic support is necessary to confirm a diagnosis. Treatment is then based on the continuity of findings from the Pap, the colposcopic exam, and the histologic diagnosis.[24]

Studies of women's reactions to colposcopy have demonstrated that women experience uncertainty about the experience, fear of pain, anxiety about diagnosis, and fear of cancer; these feelings create barriers to recommended follow-up treatment.[25,26] Therefore it is important to let women know that the colposcope will not touch them, but that they will likely experience mild to moderate cramping for a few minutes as a result of the cervical biopsy.[24]

PATHOLOGY OF CERVICAL NEOPLASIA

Although the Pap test is an effective screening tool, the diagnosis of neoplasia requires tissue for diagnostic study obtained by colposcopy with directed biopsy. Intraepithelial neoplasia, also referred to as dysplasia, describes premalignant changes of the epithelial tissue. CIN defines the spectrum of changes that precede invasive cancer. These changes are classified into three grades:

CIN 1 (mild dysplasia), representing involvement of up to one third of the thickness of the epithelium, CIN 2 (moderate dysplasia), representing involvement of one third to two thirds, and CIN 3 (severe dysplasia or carcinoma-in-situ), representing two-thirds to full-thickness involvement without involvement of the underlying stroma. Stromal involvement represents invasive cancer.[27,28] (Figure 6-1).

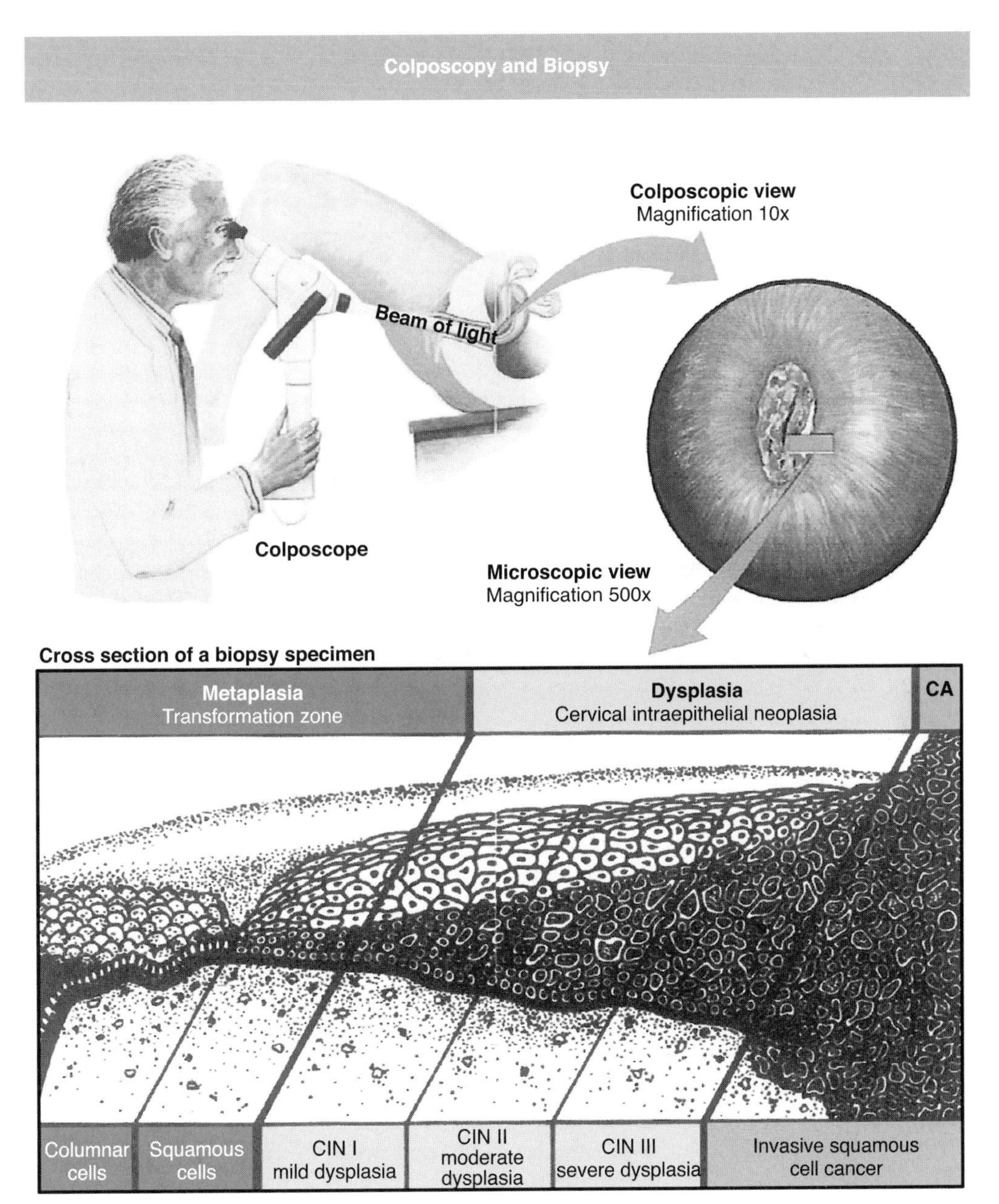

FIGURE 6-1 Cross section of a biopsy specimen. From Wayne, RD: *The Pap smear and your cervix,* 1990, Chicago MedFax Sentinel, Inc.

ABNORMAL PAP RESULTS

Management of women with ASC depends on whether the Pap test is subcategorized as ASC-US or ASC-H. Women with ASC-US should be managed using a program of two repeat Pap tests (one at 4 and one at 6 months), immediate colposcopy, or DNA testing for high-risk HPV. When liquid-based cytology is used or when collection for HPV DNA can be done, reflex HPV DNA testing is the preferred approach. Women who test negative for high-risk HPV DNA can be followed with a repeat Pap test in 12 months. Those who test positive should be referred for colposcopy. With consideration to special circumstances, pregnant women with ASC-US should be managed the same as nonpregnant women. Immunosuppressed women should be referred for colposcopy. This includes all HIV-infected women, irrespective of the degree of immunosuppression. Postmenopausal women may be provided a trial of vaginal estrogen for 3 months followed by repeat Pap testing a week after completion, barring any contraindications to intravaginal estrogen. If ASC-US persists, the woman should be referred for colposcopy. The recommended management of women with ASC-H obtained using either liquid-based or conventional cervical cytology is referral for colposcopic examination.[28]

Women with LSIL should be referred for colposcopy. The exception is for adolescent girls and postmenopausal women. Cytologic abnormalities secondary to transient HPV infections are quite common among adolescents, but clinically significant CIN 3 is distinctly uncommon, and cervical cancer is almost nonexistent. The 2001 Consensus Guidelines found that an acceptable management option for adolescent girls with LSIL is follow-up *without* initial colposcopy using a protocol of HPV DNA testing at 12 months with referral to colposcopy if testing is positive for high-risk DNA. Postmenopausal women with adequate prior screening and no previous history of CIN 2, CIN 3, or glandular abnormality may be managed with HPV DNA testing at 12 months or immediate reflex testing, rather than being referred for immediate colposcopy.[10,29]

A cytologic result of HSIL identifies a woman at significant risk for having CIN 2 or CIN 3 (70% to 75%) or invasive cancer (1% to 2%).[22,30,31] Therefore, colposcopy with endocervical assessment is the recommended management of women with HSIL.[28] Pregnant women with HSIL should be referred for colposcopy. Biopsy of lesions suspicious for high-grade disease or cancer is preferred; biopsy of other lesions is acceptable. Endocervical curettage is unacceptable in pregnant women. In the absence of invasive disease, follow-up with colposcopy and cytologic testing are recommended, with repeat biopsy limited to worsening of the lesion. Unless invasive disease is identified, treatment is unacceptable during pregnancy. Reevaluation with colposcopy and Pap test is recommended no sooner than 6 weeks postpartum.[28]

TREATMENT OF CIN

The treatment of CIN includes observation and ablative or excisional procedures. The choice of treatment depends on several factors including site, the grade of the lesion, desire for childbearing, and cost. Both ablative and excisional procedures, which involve destroying or removing the abnormal tissue of the cervix, are performed on an outpatient basis and have success rates of 90% to 98%.[32] CIN 1 may be managed with repeat cytologic investigation every 6 months, because an estimated 50% to 70% of these lesions will resolve spontaneously. Persistent CIN for up to 2 years, or progressive lesions, should be treated. CIN types 2 and 3 should be treated, except during pregnancy.[33,34]

Ablative therapies include cryotherapy and laser vaporization. Cryotherapy is performed in the office or clinic setting. It is reliable and inexpensive and has a low complication rate. The procedure is well tolerated, with mild cramping during the procedure. After treatment, women experience a watery vaginal discharge for approximately 2 weeks.[24,32] Laser vaporization is effective, yet costly. CIN is more commonly treated with loop electrosurgical excisional procedure (LEEP), or conization.

LEEP conization of the cervix uses a thin wire loop through which an electric current is passed that turns the loop into a very effective cutting tool. It is also a clinic or office procedure that is well tolerated; mild cramping is usually experienced during the procedure.[33] The advantage of the LEEP is that excising the lesion serves as both a diagnostic and treatment procedure. Cold knife conization uses the scalpel to remove the abnormal portion of the cervix. The procedure requires general anesthesia and is used when the lesion is higher in the endocervix for LEEP, or if glandular disease is present.[33]

Hysterectomy may be an acceptable method of management in women who have completed childbearing, provided they are made aware of other more conservative options.[33] If hysterectomy is planned, it should always be preceded by a cone biopsy (LEEP or cold knife) to rule out invasive disease.

EDUCATION AND COUNSELING

An HPV infection has many implications for a woman's health, yet many women are unaware of HPV and its role in cervical and other genital cancers. Ideally, providers should teach patients about HPV at the beginning of the cervical screening experience. Primary prevention strategies include educating women, especially adolescents, regarding the risk factors including early sexual activity and number of sexual partners. Sexual abstinence is ideal, but often unrealistic; therefore, the use of barrier contraceptives should be encouraged. Condoms can reduce but not eliminate the risk of HPV transmission. Women should also be educated about other risk factors including smoking, and empowered with smoking cessation interventions (see Table 6-4).[34,36]

Once HPV is diagnosed or Pap test results are abnormal, the nurse's role is to assess the woman's understanding of the diagnosis and options for treatment. Because most women are unfamiliar with HPV, the diagnosis of an STD and its relationship to cancer often results in feelings of fear, anxiety, uncertainty, and shame. There may also be feelings of anger, confusion, and blame. It is most important that patients understand that the majority of sexually active individuals will be infected with HPV at some point in their lifetimes and that HPV is generally transient and cleared by the immune system. It should be emphasized that the risk of invasive cancer is very low.[34,35]

HPV VACCINE DEVELOPMENT

HPV types 16 and 18 cause about 70% of invasive cervical cancer and high-grade CIN.[36] HPV types 6 and 11 cause 90% of anogenital warts. Genital warts (condyloma) affect approximately 1% of, or 2 million, young adults in the United States annually.[37] A prophylactic vaccine that targets these four types should thus substantially reduce the burden of HPV-associated clinical diseases.[38]

In a placebo-controlled study of 2,392 young women (16 to 23 years of age), administration of an HPV-16 vaccine reduced the incidence of both HPV-16 infection and HPV 16–related CIN. The women were followed for a median of 17.4 months after completing the vaccine regime. The incidence of persistent HPV infection was 3.8 per 100 woman-years at risk in the placebo group and 0 per 100 woman-years at risk in the vaccine group. All nine HPV-related cases of CIN occurred in the placebo recipients.[39]

A study of a bivalent vaccine targeting HPV-16 and HPV-18 also demonstrated efficacy. At 27 months of follow-up the vaccine was 100% effective against persistent HPV-16 and HPV-18 infections.[40]

In a phase II, randomized, multicenter, double-blind trial, Villa and others investigated the efficacy of a prophylactic quadrivalent vaccine targeting HPV types 6, 11, 16, and 18. The study included 277 young women with a mean age of 20.2 years. After 35 months of follow-up, incidence of persistent infection associated with HPV types 6, 11, 16, and 18 decreased by 89% in women allocated active vaccine who had at least one dose as compared with the placebo group. In addition to prophylactic vaccines, therapeutic HPV vaccine research is also quite promising. Various forms of HPV vaccines have been described in experimental systems targeting HPV-16 E6 and E7 viral proteins.[41]

These proteins have been found to stimulate a significant immune response. Development of a therapeutic vaccine is less evolved than the development of a prophylactic vaccine. Given the prevalence of existing HPV infection and cervical cancer worldwide, it is critical to continue in parallel the development of both prophylactic and therapeutic vaccines.[41]

A prophylactic vaccine will most likely be available within the next few years. Questions remain regarding the duration of protection. In addition, the economic, ethical, and social impact has yet to be articulated. At what age should one be vaccinated? Should both sexes be vaccinated or just females? Should developing nations receive priority? Will a conservative political climate in the US influence approval of a vaccine for a sexually transmitted disease? Nurses must remain informed and must advocate for the health of the women.

INVASIVE CERVICAL CANCER

HISTOLOGY

The ectocervix and vagina are lined with squamous epithelial cells. The endocervix is lined with columnar epithelial cells. Where these two types of tissue meet is the squamocolumnar junction, or transformation zone, which is the usual site of neoplasia.[42] Squamous cell carcinoma accounts for approximately 85% of all invasive cervical cancer. Adenocarcinomas and mixed adenosquamous carcinomas accounts for approximately 10%. The remaining 5% consists of more rare cancers including clear cell adenocarcinomas, endometrioid adenocarcinomas, small cell cancers, and undifferentiated carcinomas. Squamous cell carcinomas arise from the ectocervix. Adenocarcinomas arise from the endocervical mucus-producing glandular cells. For this reason, adenocarcinomas may be less clinically evident.[43]

CLINICAL PRESENTATION

Cervical carcinoma grows locally and may extend in continuity to the paracervical tissues and to the pelvic organs, spread to regional lymph nodes, and only later metastasize to distant structures.[44] The symptoms of early cervical cancer often go unrecognized by the patient. She may experience a thin, watery, blood-tinged vaginal discharge. It is painless, and may be noticeable after douching or intercourse. As the tumor progresses, the discharge may be foul-smelling, and more bleeding episodes may occur with subsequent anemia. Indications of advanced disease include pelvic or sciatic pain, dysuria, hematuria, constipation, or rectal bleeding.[33,45] Lower extremity edema may occur as a result of lymphatic and venous blockage by extensive pelvic disease. Ureteral obstruction may also occur.[46]

STAGING AND TREATMENT

Cervical cancer is the only gynecologic cancer that is staged clinically (Table 6-5). A staging workup includes the following: history and physical examination, complete blood count (CBC), platelet count, cervical biopsy, cone biopsy as indicated, chest x-ray, and intravenous pyelogram (IVP). Computed tomography (CT) or magnetic resonance imaging (MRI) is optional for stage IB1 or below. Optional for stage IB2 or above are the following: exam under anesthesia (EUA) with cystoscopy/proctoscopy, positron emission tomography scan (PET), lymphangiography, and liver and renal function studies.[47]

Because cervical cancer is clinically staged, lymph node involvement does not influence staging; however, it significantly affects survival and treatment planning (Table 6-6). Women with stage IB disease and negative pelvic lymph nodes have an 85% 5-year survival rate as opposed to 60% for those with positive lymph nodes.[33] The prevalence of lymph node disease correlates with stage and grade of the malignancy. Lymph node involvement in stage I is 15% to 20% and in stage II 25% to 40%, and in stage III it is assumed at least 50% have positive pelvic nodes.[33] Treatment is based on stage of disease and lymph node involvement, age, and general medical condition or comorbidities (Table 6-7).

Table 6-5 CARCINOMA OF THE CERVIX UTERI STAGING[44]

Figo Stages		TNM Categories
	Primary tumor cannot be assessed	TX
	No evidence of primary tumor	T0
0	Carcinoma in situ (preinvasive carcinoma)	Tis
I	Cervical carcinoma confined to uterus (extension to corpus should be disregarded)	T1
IA	Invasive carcinoma diagnosed only by microscopy. All macroscopically visible lesions—even with superficial invasion—are stage 1B/T1b	T1a
IA1	Stromal invasion no greater than 3 mm and not more than 5 mm with a horizontal spread ≤7 mm	T1a1
IA2	Stromal invasion >3 mm in depth and ≤7 mm in horizontal spread	T1a2
IB1	Clinically visible lesion confined to the cervix or microscopic lesions >Ia2/T1a2	T1b
IB1	Clinically visible lesion ≤4 cm in greatest dimension	T1b1
II	Tumor invades beyond the uterus but not pelvic wall or to lower third of the vagina	T2
IIA	Without parametrial invasion	T2a
IIB	With parametrial invasion	T2b
III	Tumor extends to pelvic wall and/or involves lower third of vagina and/or causes hydronephrosis or nonfunctioning kidney.	T3
IIIA	Tumor involves lower third of vagina, no extension to pelvic wall	T3a
IIIB	Tumor extends to pelvic wall and/or causes hydronephrosis or nonfunctioning kidney	T3b
IVA	Tumor invades mucosa of bladder or rectum and/or extends beyond true pelvis	T4
	Distant metastasis	M1

Fertility Considerations

In women of reproductive age, consideration must be given to the woman's desire for future childbearing. Opening this conversation may appear insensitive when the priority concern at the time of diagnosis is cancer treatment. However, this may also be the only time that interventions to preserve fertility are an option.[48] In very early cervical cancer (stage IA1), a cone biopsy with Pap test follow-up at 4 months, 10 months, and then annually (if both Pap tests are negative), is appropriate in women who desire fertility.[44] If a hysterectomy or radical hysterectomy is indicated, the ovaries may remain intact, leaving surrogacy as an option. In women who are to receive pelvic radiation therapy, the ovaries may be surgically suspended outside the pelvic field.[44] Finally, recent studies have demonstrated vaginal radical trachelectomy (amputation of the cervix below the isthmus of the uterus) with laparoscopic pelvic lymphadenectomy can offer a select population of women with early cervix cancer the opportunity to conceive and carry a pregnancy to term.[49]

Treatment by Stage

- Stage IA1: Total abdominal hysterectomy or vaginal hysterectomy. If fertility is desired, observation after cone biopsy is appropriate as described above.

Table **6-6** Five-year Survival by Stage[33]

Preinvasive disease	100%
Stage Ia	90%
Stage Ib with negative nodes	85%
Stage Ib with positive nodes	60%
Stage II	60-80%
Stage III	45%
Stage IV	14%
Recurrent disease	10%

- Stage IA2: Modified radical hysterectomy and pelvic lymphadenectomy. If there is no lymph or vascular space invasion, consideration may be given to extrafascial hysterectomy and pelvic lymphadenectomy. If fertility is desired, options include a large cone biopsy and pelvic lymphadenectomy or radical trachelectomy with pelvic lymphadenectomy.[44,50]
- Stage IB1-IIA (<4 cm): Radical hysterectomy with pelvic lymphadenectomy or external pelvic irradiation plus intracavitary brachytherapy. As there is no survival advantage to either method, the treatment decision is based on available resources and the age and general health of the patient. The patient should be informed of the therapeutic alternatives, including toxicity and potential outcomes.[44]

Adjuvant Therapy after Surgery

The risk of recurrence after radical surgery is increased with the presence of positive nodes, positive parametria, or positive surgical margins. Adjuvant concurrent chemoradiation (using 5-fluorouracil (5FU) + cisplatin or cisplatin alone) improves survival compared with pelvic irradiation alone in such patients.[51]

- Stages IB2-IIA (>4cm): Options for primary therapy include (1) primary chemoradiation; (2) primary radical hysterectomy and pelvic lymphadenectomy, which usually has to be followed with adjuvant radiation; (3) neo-adjuvant chemotherapy (three rapidly delivered courses of platinum based chemotherapy) followed by radical hysterectomy and pelvic lymphadenectomy with or without adjuvant postoperative radiation or chemoradiation.[52]
- Stages IIB-IVA: Standard primary treatment is irradiation given as a combination of external radiation and intracavitary brachytherapy with concurrent chemotherapy.[53,54] Primary pelvic exenteration may be considered for stage IVA disease not extending to the pelvic sidewall, particularly if vesicovaginal or rectovaginal fistula is present.[44]
- Stage IVB or recurrent disease: Treatment of recurrent and stage IVB cervical cancer is palliative and radiation therapy to control bleeding and pain, and systemic chemotherapy.[55] Cisplatin is the single most active drug to treat cervical cancer. Response rates to chemotherapy

Table **6-7** Treatment of Invasive Disease[44]

Disease Type	Treatment
Ia1	Cervical conization or simple hysterectomy
Ia2	Modified radical hysterectomy and pelvic lymphadenectomy
Ib-IIa	Radical hysterectomy, pelvic lymphadenectomy, and/or radiation therapy and chemotherapy
IIb-IVa	Radiation therapy and chemotherapy
IVb and recurrent disease	Pelvic exenteration for central recurrence, or palliative chemotherapy and/or radiation treatment and palliative care

are 10% to 40%.[45] Almost 80% of recurrences occur within 2 years, and 1-year survival averages 6 to 10 months.[56] The triad of symptoms consisting of leg edema, pain, and weight loss is ominous. Leg edema is usually secondary to progressive lymphatic obstruction; however, thrombophlebitis should be ruled out. Pain is often sciatic; patients describe it as radiating to the buttock and/or thigh. Others describe deep pelvic pain or pain in the groin.[45] The coordinated effort of a team of professionals is optimal; this may include gynecologic oncologists, radiation and medical oncologists, pain specialists, oncology nurses, oncology social workers, and hospice professionals. Relief of pain and other symptoms, along with psychosocial support for the patient and her family, are paramount.[44]

Pelvic Exenteration

The only potentially curative treatment after primary irradiation is pelvic exenteration. Because the goal is cure, and the procedure highly morbid, patients should be selected carefully: those with resectable central recurrences that involve the bladder and/or rectum without evidence of intraperitoneal or extrapelvic spread and who have a disectable tumor-free space along the pelvic sidewall are potentially suitable. The triad of unilateral leg edema, sciatic pain, and ureteral obstruction almost always indicates unresectable disease on the pelvic sidewall, and palliative measures are indicated.[44]

In addition to physical criteria, psychosocial adjustment must also be assessed. Preoperative teaching must ensure that the patient comprehends the extensiveness of surgery, associated potential complications, and recovery and rehabilitative needs. She should convey understanding of permanent changes that will influence her quality of life, including living with ostomies and alterations to sexual function.

Total pelvic exenteration includes radical hysterectomy, pelvic lymph node dissection, and removal of the bladder and rectosigmoid colon. It often also includes vaginectomy with neovaginal reconstruction. Occasionally, a posterior exenteration (with preservation of the bladder), or anterior exenteration (with preservation of the rectum) can be performed. Fibrotic tissue changes secondary to prior radiation therapy usually prohibits these approaches.[56]

Postoperative care includes assessing for acute complications of extensive pelvic surgery such as pulmonary emboli, pulmonary edema, cerebrovascular accident, hemorrhage, myocardial infarction, deep vein thrombosis, sepsis, and small bowel obstruction. Long-term complications include urinary obstruction and infection, sepsis, and fistula formation.[33,56,57] Care should be multidisciplinary and address the physical, psychosocial, and psychosexual implications of disease recurrence and surgery.

The prognosis is better for patients with a disease-free interval of greater than 6 months, a recurrence 3 cm or less in diameter, and no sidewall fixation.[58] The 5-year survival for patients following pelvic exenteration is in the order of 30% to 60%, and the operative mortality should be less than 10%.[44]

RADICAL HYSTERECTOMY

Radical hysterectomy involves the removal of the uterus, the upper third of the vagina, and the entirety of the parametrium on each side, along with pelvic node dissection encompassing the four major pelvic node chains: urethral, obturator, hypogastric, and iliac.[33] The ovaries are left intact in young women since metastasis to the ovaries is rare.[46]

Acute complications, which occur in less than 5% of patients, include infection, ureteral fistula (0% to 3%), pulmonary embolism, and small bowel obstruction, which is rare unless the patient received preoperative radiation therapy.[59] Subacute complications include postoperative bladder atony, formation of lymphocysts, and lymphedema. Temporary bladder atony during the immediate postoperative period (1 to several weeks) is expected. During a radical hysterectomy the ureters are dissected out of the parametrial tissue, and there is subsequent trauma resulting in temporary injury to the sensory and motor nerve supply to the detrusor muscle.[60] The patient most often will experience a reduced sensitivity to bladder filling, and an inability to initiate voiding or empty the bladder. Maintaining bladder drainage with a Foley or suprapubic catheter for at least several days after surgery promotes the return to normal bladder function. Once the catheter is removed, adequate bladder emptying must be assessed either with ultrasound or intermittent catheterization. Postvoid residual urine should be less than 100 cc.[45] It is not uncommon for bladder dysfunction to persist for several weeks. Patient education should include catheter care or intermittent self-catheterization every 4 hours after attempts to void. Patients often require considerable reassurance that their bladder function will improve, and encouragement to be patient with bladder training.

The formation of pelvic lymphocysts is reduced with the provision of adequate drainage of the retroperitoneal space after surgery via continuous suction catheters,[33] (e.g., Jackson-Pratt drains). Lower-extremity lymphedema rarely occurs following radical hysterectomy alone, yet the incidence increases with the addition of radiation therapy.[61]

RADIATION THERAPY

Radiation therapy for cervical cancer consists of a combination of high-energy megavoltage pelvic irradiation to treat regional lymph nodes and the central cervical disease, and intracavitary brachytherapy to treat the rest of the central tumor (one cGy = 1 rad of absorbed dose).[33] External beam radiation therapy uses a linear accelerator to deliver radiation from a specific distance to a defined target volume.[62] Treatment for cervical cancer involves delivering daily fractions (single dose of ionized radiation) over 4 to 6 weeks, followed by brachytherapy. Brachytherapy is the temporary or permanent placement of a radioactive source into a body cavity, into tissue (interstitial), or on the surface of the body. Brachytherapy delivers a high radiation treatment dose to a specified tumor volume with a rapid fall-off rate in radiation dose to normal tissue. It can be either LDR (low dose rate) or HDR (high dose rate). LDR for cervix cancer is an in-patient procedure involving the placement of intracavitary applicators including tandem and ovoids, and may also include placement of transperineal interstitial vaginal template and needles.[62] This is performed under general anesthesia. The implant remains for 2 to 3 days while the patient is hospitalized with radiation isolation precautions. This process is repeated based on the total dose to be delivered. The patient must remain on strict bed rest with log roll for care to prevent possible dislodgement of the applicators. A Foley catheter is placed, and bowel management with antidiarrheal medication is given, as well as a low-residue diet to prevent bowel movements. The head of the bed cannot be elevated more than 30 degrees. Radiation precautions are necessary to prevent exposure to others, and this can result in the patient feeling socially isolated.[62] Nursing care priorities include providing comfort measures and adequate nutrition, preventing complications of immobility, and providing emotional support. The patient is considered radioactive only when the source is in the applicator. The staff wears a radiation badge to monitor radiation exposure. The time spent in the room is minimized to limit exposure. Patients may bring items from home to occupy their time. The items in the room do not become radioactive because the source used is sealed.

HDR brachytherapy involves the use of an automated remote afterloading device for the placement of the radioactive source into the applicators, which have been placed in the tumor cavity. The source is delivered via source guide tubes that are in the afterloader, which is then attached to the patient's treatment device (tandem and ovoids).[63] Like LDR, the procedure is performed under general anesthesia. HDR allows patients to be treated on an out-patient basis. It is an all-day procedure. The actual treatment lasts approximately 10 to 20 minutes and is given on an average of twice a week for a total of 3 to 5 times. The number of treatments depends on whether or not the patient will undergo surgery following completion of radiation therapy.

Complications of pelvic radiation therapy can be categorized as acute or delayed. Acute complications are related to the ionized effects on the bowel and bladder. Symptoms include cystitis, cramping, diarrhea, tenesmus, dysuria, skin irritation, and hair loss. A low-fiber diet and antidiarrheal or antispasmodic agents may be helpful. Pain related to cystitis or bowel or perineal irritation requires analgesic intervention. A week of rest from radiation therapy may be indicated for severe symptoms. Most patients also experience fatigue, which may worsen as treatment progresses.[64] Late complications related to radiotherapy may include vaginal stenosis, proctitis, fistula formation, intestinal obstruction, ureteral stricture, and severe cystitis. The risk of vaginal stenosis can be minimized by the patient using vaginal dilators with a water-soluble lubricant or by having sexual intercourse.[62] Most women experience dyspareunia during treatment, prohibiting intercourse until vaginal irritation subsides. Patients should initiate use of the vaginal dilator once they are able to insert it comfortably. This might be 4 to 6 weeks after the completion of radiation therapy.

Nurses need to initiate discussion regarding the importance of preventing vaginal stenosis and educate patients on the use of dilators. This will also provide the patient the opportunity to discuss sexuality concerns related to her diagnosis and treatment.

CONCLUSION

Although the incidence and mortality of cervical cancer has decreased dramatically in developed countries since the development of the Pap test, worldwide and here in the United States, it remains predominantly a disease of the poor and underserved. For a disease that is essentially preventable with recommended screening, this is unconscionable. As technologic advances and evolving knowledge provide the opportunities to improve our management of women with HPV and cervical neoplasia, remember that at this time, there is no better tool than education and screening. In caring for women with invasive disease, provide knowledge-based care with compassion, empathy, intellect, and advocacy.

REFERENCES

1. Cancers of the female reproductive tract. In Stewart BW, Kleihues P, editors: *World cancer report*, Lyon, France, 1995, IARC Press.
2. American Cancer Society Cancer Facts and Figures 2005: *Cancer: Basic Facts,* Atlanta, 2005, American Cancer Society.
3. American Cancer Society Cancer Facts and Figures 2002, Atlanta, 2002, American Cancer Society.
4. U.S. National Institutes of Health: *Consensus Statement on Cervical Cancer,* National Institutes of Health, Bethesda, Md., Apr 1-3, 1996. On the Web at http://consensus.nih.gov/1996/1996CervicalCancer102html.htm, accessed October, 2005.
5. Nolte S, Walczak J: Screening and prevention of gynecologic malignancies. In Moore-Higgs GJ, editor: *Women and cancer: a gynecologic oncology nursing perspective,* Boston, Mass., 2000, Jones and Bartlett.
6. Association of Reproductive Health Professionals: Cervical cancer prevention and HPV DNA testing, 10:1, 2005, on the Web at www.arhp.org, accessed 4/25/2005.
7. Sisk E, Robertson E: CJON writing mentorship program paper, *Clin J Oncol Nurs* 7(3):271-274, 2003.
8. Koutsky LA for the Atypical Squamous Cells of Undetermined Significance/Low-Grade Squamous Intraepithelial Lesions Triage Study ALTS Group: HPV triage as a management strategy for women with low-grade squamous intraepithelial lesions, *J Natl Cancer Inst,* 92:397-402, 2000.
9. Wright TC, Schiffman M: Adding a test for human papilloma virus DNA to cervical-cancer screening, *New Eng J Med* 348:489-490, 2003.
10. American Society for Colposcopy and Cervical Pathology: Human papilloma viruses HPV-different types and natural history of infection, *Clin Uses of HPV DNA Testing* 1:7, 2004.
11. Munoz N and others: Epidemiologic classification of human papillomavirus types associated with cervical cancer, *New Eng J Med* 348:518-527, 2003.
12. Sherman ME and others: Baseline cytology, human papillomavirus testing and risk for cervical neoplasia: a ten-year cohort analysis, *J Natl Cancer Inst* 95(1):46-52, 2003.
13. ALTS Group: Results of a randomized trial on the management of cytology interpretations of atypical squamous cells of undetermined significance, *Am J Obstet Gynecol* 188:1383-1392, 2003.
14. Sherman ME and others: Performance of a semi-automated Papanicolaou smear screening system, results of a population-based study conducted in Guanacasta, Costa Rica, *Cancer* 84:273-280, 1998.
15. Ball C, Madden JE: Update on cervical cancer screening, current diagnostic and evidence-based management protocols, *Postgrad Med* 113(2):59-70, 2003.
16. Austin RM, Ramzy I: Increased detection of epithelial cell abnormalities by liquid-based gynecologic cytology preparations, a review of accumulated data, *Acta Cytol* 42(1):178-184, 1998.
17. Lee KR and others: Comparison of conventional Papanicolaou smears and a fluid-based thin layer system for cervical cancer screening, *Obstet Gynecol* 43:65-68, 1999.

18. Vassilaskos P, Samuel J, Rondez R: Direct-to-vial use of the AutoCyte PREP liquid-based preparation for cervical-vaginal specimens in three European laboratories, *Acta Cytol* 43:65-68, 1999.
19. Saslow D and others: ACS guideline for the early detection of cervical neoplasia and cancer, *CA Cancer J Clin* 52(6): 342-362, 2002.
20. National Cancer Institute Workshop: The 1988 Bethesda System for reporting cervical/vaginal cytologic diagnosis, *JAMA* 262:931-934, 1989.
21. National Cancer Institute Workshop: The revised Bethesda System for reporting cervical/vaginal cytologic diagnosis, report of the 1991 Bethesda workshop, *JAMA* 267:1892, 1992.
22. Solomon D and others: The 2001 Bethesda System terminology for reporting results of cervical cytology, consensus statement, *JAMA* 287(16):2114-2119, 2002.
23. Kennedy AW and others: Results of the clinical evaluation of atypical glandular cells of undetermined significance detected on cervical cytology screening, *Obstet Gynecol Survey* 52:177-178, 1997.
24. Spinelli A: Preinvasive diseases of the cervix vulva and vagina, *Semin Oncol Nurs* 18(3):184-191, 2002.
25. Barsevick AM, Johnson JE: Preference for information and involvement information seeking and emotional responses of women undergoing colposcopy, *Res Nurs Health* 13:1-7, 1990.
26. Lerman C and others: Telephone counseling improves adherence to colposcopy among lower-income minority women, *J Clin Oncol* 10:330-333, 1992.
27. Wayne RD: The Pap smear and your cervix, 1990, MedFax Sentinel.
28. Yoder L, Rubin M: The epidemiology of cervical cancer and its precursors, *Oncol Nurs Forum* 19:485-493, 1992.
29. Wright TC: 2001 Consensus guidelines for management of women with cervical cytologic abnormalities, consensus statement, *JAMA,* 287(16):2120-2129, 2002.
30. Kinney WK and others: Where's the high-grade cervical neoplasia? *Obstet Gynecol* 91:973-976, 1998.
31. Massad LS, Collins YC, Meyer PM: Biopsy correlates of abnormal cervical cytology classified using the Bethesda System, *Gynecol Oncol* 82:516-522, 2001.
32. Nolte S, Hanjani PO: Intraepithelial neoplasia of the lower genital tract, *Semin Oncol Nurs* 6:181-189, 1990.
33. Disaia PJ, Creasman WT: *Clinical Gynecologic Oncology,* ed 5, St Louis, Mosby, 1997.
34. Likes WM, Itano J: HPV and cervical cancer: not just a sexually transmitted disease, *CJON,* 7(3):271-276, 2003.
35. Association of Reproductive Health Professionals: Advances in cervical cancer prevention, *ARHP Clin Proc* 1:22, 2003.
36. Bosch FX, de Sanjose S: Chapter 1: Human papilloma virus and cervical cancer-burden and assessment of causality, *J Natl Cancer Inst Monogr* 31:3-13, 2003.
37. Von Krogh G: Management of anogenital warts condylomata acuminata, *Eur J Dermatol* 11:598-604, 2001.
38. Villa LL, Costa RL, Petta CA and others: Prophylactic quadrivalent human papilloma virus (types 6 11 16 and 18) L1 virus-like particle vaccine in young women: a random double blind placebo controlled multicentre phase II efficacy trial, April 7, 2005: Retrieved from www://oncology.thelancet.com.
39. Koutsky LA and others: A controlled trial of a human papilloma virus type 16 vaccine, *N Eng J Med,* 347(21): 1645-1651, 2002.
40. Harper DM and others: Efficiency of a bivalent L1 virus-like particle vaccine in prevention of infection with human papilloma virus types 16 and 18 in young women: a randomized controlled trial, *Lancet* 13:364(9447):1757-1765, 2004.
41. Richard BS and others: Perspectives in pathology: vaccination to prevent and treat cervical cancer, *Hum Pathol* 35(8):971-982, 2004.
42. McChance KL, Huether SE: *Pathophysiology: the biological basis for disease in adults and children,* ed 3, St Louis, 1998, Mosby.
43. Hording U, Duagaard S, Visfeldt J: Adenocarcinoma of the cervix and adenocarcinoma of the endometrium: distinction with PCR-mediated detection of HPV DNA. *APMIS* 105(4):313-316, 1997.
44. Federation International Gynaecology and Obstetrics: Staging classifications and clinical practice guidelines of gynaecologic cancers, *Int J Gynecol Obstet* 70,207:312, 2000. Online reprint retrieved from www.FIGO.org/content/pdf/staging-booklet.pdf, 2005.
45. Lamb MA: Invasive cervical cancer. In Moore-Higgs GJ, editor: *Women and cancer: a gynecologic oncology nursing perspective,* Boston, MA. Jones and Bartlett, 2nd ed. 1:49, 2000.
46. Hopkins MP, Morley GW: Prognostic factors in advanced stage squamous cell cancer of the cervix, *Cancer* 72(8): 2389-2393, 1993.
47. National Comprehensive Cancer Network: Clinical practice guidelines in oncology—v.1, *Cervical Cancer* 1:1-6, 2004.
48. Gossfield LM, Cullen ML: Sexuality and fertility issues. In Moore-Higgs GJ, editor: *Women and cancer: a gynecologic oncology nursing perspective,* ed 2, Boston, 2000, Jones and Bartlett.
49. Plante M and others: Vaginal radical trachelectomy: an oncologically safe fertility-preserving surgery. An updated series of 72 cases and review of the literature, *Womens Oncol Rev* 4(4):275-276, 2004.
50. Plante RM: Pregnancies after radical vaginal trachelectomy for early stage cervical cancer. *Am J Obstet Gynecol* 179: 1491-1496, 1998.
51. Peters III WA and others: Concurrent chemotherapy and pelvic radiation therapy compared with pelvic radiation therapy alone as adjuvant therapy after radical surgery in high risk early stage cancer of the cervix, *J Clin Oncol* 18(8):1606-1613, 2000.
52. Sardi J and others: Results of a prospective randomized trial with neoadjuvant chemotherapy in stage Ib, bulky, squamous carcinoma of the cervix, *Gynecol Oncol* 49:156-165, 1993.
53. Rose PG and others: Concurrent cisplatin-based radiotherapy and chemotherapy for locally advanced cervical cancer, *N Eng J Med* 340:1144-1153, 1999.
54. Whitney CW and others: Randomized comparison of fluorouracil plus cisplatin vs. hydroxyurea as an adjunct to radiation therapy in stage IIb-Iva carcinoma of the cervix with negative paraaortic lymph nodes: a Gynecologic Oncology Group and Southwest Oncology Group study, *J Clin Oncol* 17:1339-1348, 1999.

55. Coleman RL, Monk, BJ: Challenging *cases in the treatment of gynecologic malignancies*, New York, 2004, Global Edge.
56. Shingleton HM, Orr JW: *Cancer of the Cervix*, Philadelphia, 1995 Lippincott.
57. Hatch KD, Fu YS: Cervical and vaginal cancer. In Berek JS, Adashi EY, Hillard P editors: *Novak's gynecology*, Baltimore, 1996, Williams and Wilkins.
58. Shingelton H and others: Clinical and histopathologic factors predicting recurrence and survival after pelvic exenteration for cancer of the cervix, *Obstet Gynecol* 73: 1027-1034, 1989.
59. Hatch KD: Cervical cancer. In Berek JS, Hacker NF, editors: *Practical gynecologic oncology*, Baltimore, 1989, Williams and Wilkins.
60. Carenza L, Nobili E, 7 Glacobini S: Voiding disorders after radical hysterectomy, *Gynecol Oncol* 13(2):213-219, 1982.
61. Werngren-Elgstrom M, Lidman D: Lymphedema of the lower extremities after surgery and radiotherapy for cancer of the cervix, *Scand J Plast Reconst Surg Hand Surg* 28(4):289-293, 1994.
62. Watkins-Bruner D, Haas ML, Gosselin-Acomb TK: *Manual for radiation oncology nursing practice and education*, ed. 3, Pittsburgh, 2005, Oncology Nursing Society.
63. Bruner DW and others, editors: *Manual for radiation oncology nursing practice and education*, Pittsburgh, 1998, Oncology Nursing Society.
64. Ogino I and others: Late rectal complication following high dose rate intracavitary brachytherapy in cancer of the cervix, *Int J Radiat Oncol Biol Phys*, 31(4):725-734, 1995.

CHAPTER

7 Ovarian Cancer

Virginia R. Martin and Carol Cherry

INTRODUCTION

When compared to other cancers that affect women, ovarian cancer has a relatively low incidence. However, the incidence is disproportional to the high morbidity and mortality the disease affords. Of the 22,210 American women predicted to be affected in 2005, likely 75% will be diagnosed in advanced stages and mortality will exceed 16,000.[1] Increased research funding has led to advances in understanding the molecular basis of disease and improvement in chemotherapeutic options. There has been an increase in 5-year survival from 30% in the 1960s to over 50% in the past several years.[2] Committed survivors have raised the general level of awareness of symptoms. Once thought not to exist, symptoms are now known to be present in even early-stage disease. A reliable screening test for ovarian cancer remains elusive. Women identified at increased risk due to family history or genetic predisposition face the choice between early detection tests of limited efficacy or risk-reducing surgery with physical and psychologic implications. Nurses are challenged to promote awareness and manage the physical and emotional sequelae of the disease.

Epidemiology

Ovarian cancer is the seventh most common cancer affecting women in the US, accounting for 3% of cases. Cancer of the ovary is the most common cause of gynecologic cancer death and the fourth cause of cancer deaths overall.[1] General population lifetime risk is less than 2%. This risk rises significantly according to family history or hereditary cancer syndromes, although such cases account for only 5% to 10% of the total incidence. In the US, non-Hispanic white women and black women have the highest incidence, compared to American Indian and Asian women, although it should be noted that very little is published about racial variations. Worldwide, the incidence is 192.4 per 100,000.[3] Ovarian cancer occurs more commonly among women in North America, Eastern Europe, and Scandinavia, as contrasted to Asia and Africa.[4]

Most ovarian cancers arise from the surface epithelium and present primarily as a disease of aging, with a median occurrence age of 60.[5] When the disease presents in a woman's 30s and 40s, a concern for a hereditary syndrome should prompt family history evaluation. There are ovarian tumors that typically occur in adolescence. These are much less common and are derived from the primitive female reproductive cells (ova or germ cells). Survival varies significantly with tumor histology and stage of presentation. If diagnosed when disease is confined to the ovaries, survival is greater than 90%, but in advanced stages the 5-year survival rate is a discouraging 25% to 30%.[6] It is notable that improved treatment options and side effects management afford better quality of life during the course of chronic, recurrent disease.

Etiology

There is no definitive understanding of ovarian cancer causation, but various risk factors and hypotheses of carcinogenesis have been identified.

Hormonal, reproductive, genetic, and lifestyle factors all play a role, and most likely a complex interaction of many factors leads to tumor development (Table 7-1). Three major hypotheses attempt to explain the physiologic basis of ovarian cancer.

Incessant Ovulation

Much research has been focused on changes the ovarian surface epithelium undergoes during malignant transformation. Ovulation causes a repetitive trauma-and-repair cycle that may lead to malignancy. According to the incessant ovulation hypothesis, risk of ovarian cancer is directly related to the number of ovulatory cycles a woman experiences. This theory is supported by the epidemiologic data indicating that risk of ovarian cancer is inverse to use of oral contraceptives, number of pregnancies, and long-term breastfeeding, all of which suppress ovulation.[7]

Gonadotropin Hormone Effect

The phenomenon of inclusion cysts and their role in ovarian tumor formation has been studied. Inclusion cysts are thought to occur when surface cells find their way into the connecting tissue (or stroma) of the ovary and become trapped. Here the gonadotropin hormone hypothesis postulates that excessive levels of follicle-stimulating hormone (FSH) and luteinizing hormone (LH) stimulate overgrowth of the trapped cells, and eventually malignancy occurs.[8] Factors that reduce a woman's exposure to gonadotropins, such as pregnancy and oral contraceptive use, would be protective and data to this effect lends support to this theory.

Inflammation

A more recent hypothesis involves the role of inflammation and is supported by its association with the risk factors of endometriosis and talc use. Endometriosis is linked to the endometrioid and clear cell types of ovarian cancer.[9] Talc, an asbestos-like powder, has been found in diseased ovaries. A possible association of women's talcum powder use with ovarian cancer has been studied, but the connection is modest at best. These hypotheses offer insight but are less than conclusive for a clear cause of disease.

OTHER RISK FACTORS

Diet may play a role in up to 30% of human cancers,[4] but there is no definitive association between specific foods and ovarian cancer. Overweight and obesity have been linked to many cancers, including ovarian cancer, in animal and epidemiologic studies.[10] In response to the high proportion of overweight and obese Americans, the American Cancer Society, the American Diabetes Association, and the American Heart Association have established collaborative guidelines

Table 7-1 FACTORS RELATED TO OVARIAN CANCER RISK

Risk Factors	Risk-reducing Factors
Advanced age	Parity
Family history of ovarian cancer	Breastfeeding
Genetic predisposition	Oral contraceptives
• Hereditary breast and ovarian cancer syndrome	
• Hereditary nonpolyposis colorectal cancer syndrome	
Nulliparity	Risk-reducing surgery
	• Tubal ligation
	• Oophorectomy
Infertility	
Endometriosis	
Industrialized Western environment	
Talc exposure	

Table 7-2 Diet and Physical Activity Guidelines for Preventing Cancer, Cardiovascular Disease, and Diabetes[10]

Diet	Physical Activity
Choose: at least 5 servings of fruits and vegetables daily Choose: whole-grain carbohydrates Limit: saturated fat, alcohol, refined carbohydrates	Moderate exercise at least 30 minutes on 5 or more days per week

for diet and physical activity (Table 7-2). Obesity has been linked with increased mortality from all cancers, including ovarian.[11]

The relationship between infertility, fertility drug use, and ovarian cancer has been studied. A large, pooled analysis suggests that disease is linked to the condition of infertility, rather than effects of the fertility drugs.[12]

GENETICS

After increasing age, family history is the most significant risk factor. Lifetime risk in the general population is 1.4%.[13] Assigning risk based on family history is not an exact science, but it is estimated that a woman with one or more first-degree relatives with ovarian cancer has a risk of 5% to 9%.[14] Families with multiple members affected by ovarian and/or breast cancer may exhibit a hereditary cancer syndrome related to mutations in the *BRCA1* or *BRCA2* genes.

The majority of ovarian cancers occur sporadically; the minority (5% to 10%) is due to inherited predisposition of an altered gene. Alterations in two tumor-suppressor genes—*BRCA1*, located on chromosome 17, and *BRCA2*, on chromosome 13—are responsible for the hereditary breast/ovarian cancer syndrome (HBOC). Numerous alterations have been discovered within these genes; three in particular are highly prevalent in the Ashkenazi Jewish population. Characteristics of the syndrome are found in Box 7-1. Families exhibiting these characteristics should be referred for cancer risk assessment by professionals with specialized training in cancer genetics. A national directory of trained genetics professionals may be found at www.cancer.gov/search/genetics_services. Commercial genetic testing, now often covered by insurance, is available. Women found to be carriers of mutations in the *BRCA1* gene have up to a 44% lifetime risk of developing ovarian cancer. The risk approaches 27% in *BRCA2*-mutation carriers.[15] *BRCA1*-related cancers typically present 7 years earlier than sporadic cases. *BRCA2* cancers typically present at a later stage; but interestingly, survival is better than in sporadic disease.[13]

The HBOC syndrome accounts for approximately 85% of hereditary ovarian cancers.[15] Another 10% are attributed to alterations in DNA mismatch repair genes (*hMLH1, hMSH2, hMSH6,* and *PMS2*). Mutations in these genes are responsible for the hereditary nonpolyposis colorectal cancer syndrome (HNPCC). The HNPCC syndrome is diagnosed clinically using a

Box 7-1 Characteristics of Hereditary Breast and Ovarian Cancer Syndrome

- Multiple family members in the same lineage affected with breast and/or ovarian cancer
- Younger-than-typical age of onset (≤ 50 years)
- More than one primary cancer in an individual
- Autosomal dominant pattern of inheritance
- Male breast cancer

Box 7-2 Criteria for Hereditary Nonpolyposis Colorectal Cancer

Colon cancer in ≥ 3 relatives, one of whom is a first-degree relative of the other two
Colon cancer in at least two generations
One or more colon cancers diagnosed <50 years of age
Extracolonic cancers may be associated: ovary, uterine, stomach, kidney, biliary tract

specific criteria system known as the Amsterdam criteria and/or by genetic testing. These criteria are found in Box 7-2. After careful genetic counseling, commercial genetic testing for the *MLH1* and *MSH2* genes, which account for the majority of HNPCC cases, is available. Carriers of an HNPCC-related gene alteration have a 9% to 12% lifetime risk of ovarian cancer.[14] The average age for development of ovarian cancer in carriers is the mid-40s.[16]

Pathogenesis

Ovarian cancers are very complex solid tumors with a high number of genetic mutations in both sporadic and hereditary disease. In addition to the genes associated with the HBOC and HNPCC syndromes, numerous other genes such as *AKT, TP53, RAS, MYC, PI3-K, AR, HER2, EGFR, DAB2,* and *PTEN* are implicated, but their role in tumor development remains under investigation.[2]

Current research is focused on the association of certain gene changes; the various pathologic subtypes and their origins are illustrated in Figure 7-1. The majority of ovarian tumors (60%) are surface epithelial, meaning they arise from the cells covering the outer surface of the ovary. They may be benign, borderline (also known as low malignant potential), or malignant. Four main subtypes of epithelial cancers include serous (most common), mucinous, endometrioid, and clear cell. There is data to suggest that most tumors in the HBOC syndrome are serous, and that borderline and mucinous subtypes are not a part of the syndrome.[17] The major focus of the information presented in this chapter corresponds to the epithelial ovarian cancer type.

Sex-cord stromal tumors are those that originate in various cells such as theca and granulosa cells that surround ovarian follicles. They represent 8% of ovarian tumors. They are typically rare, often are benign, or present in stage I.[18] Subtypes include granulosa cell, thecoma, fibroma, Sertoli cell, Sertoli-Leydig cell, and steroid cell tumors.

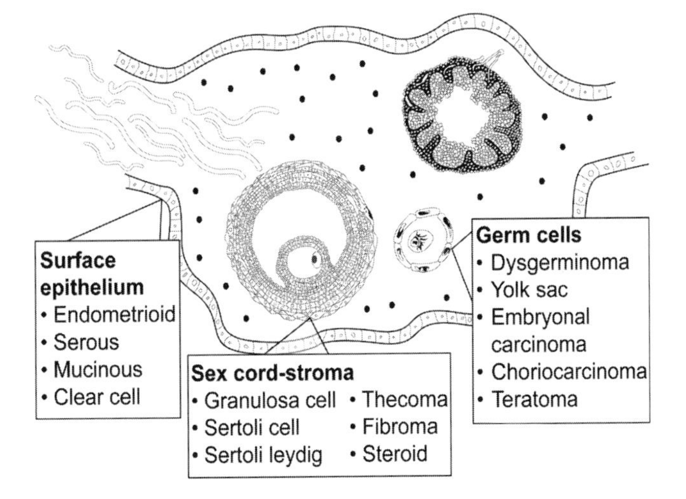

FIGURE 7-1 Ovarian tumor types and their origins. Adapted from Chen VW and others: Pathology and classification of ovarian tumors, *Cancer* 97:2631-2642, 2003.

Germ cell tumors account for 25% of ovarian tumors; up to 7% of these are malignant. The majority present during adolescence. Dysgerminomas and teratomas are the most common subtypes and have a good prognosis. Ovarian teratomas are also known as dermoid cysts. These are nonmalignant and can contain teeth, skin, or hair. Yolk sac tumors, embryonal carcinomas, and choriocarcinomas are highly malignant.[18]

It is hoped that further discovery in the genetic pathways related to ovarian tumor development will offer not only increased understanding of pathogenesis, but yield new markers for detection and prognosis and identification of targets for treatment. A major advance that will assist in this research is the recent generation of a genetically engineered mouse in which ovarian cancer can be studied.[19]

Primary Prevention

Women have no control over the major ovarian cancer risk factors of age and family history. Decisions regarding number of pregnancies, breastfeeding, and healthy lifestyle may have an impact on risk, but it is difficult to quantify that impact and a preventive effect is not guaranteed. There are two proven primary prevention options: use of oral contraceptives and risk-reducing surgery. These options are typically discussed with women whose risk exceeds that of the general population.

ORAL CONTRACEPTIVES

The effect of taking oral contraceptive pills (OCPs) on reducing risk of ovarian cancer has been well studied in the general population. When averaged together, these studies show about a 40% reduction in risk.[2] Fewer studies have looked at this issue in African American women, but those that have show similar results. There is not one clear recommendation on how long to take the pill or which particular pill to take. However, it does appear that the protective effect lasts for many years after the pills are discontinued. It is not fully understood how OCPs provide protection. There is evidence that progestins are the most protective component of oral contraceptives.[13] They may work by suppressing ovulation or by increasing cell death of abnormal ovarian cells. Data on the effect of OCPs in carriers of *BRCA1/BRCA2* mutations is less conclusive, but a 38% risk reduction in long-term users was found in a recent international pooled analysis.[20]

RISK-REDUCING SURGERY

Surgical options for reduction of ovarian cancer risk include tubal ligation and bilateral salpingo-oophorectomy (BSO) with or without removal of the uterus. Prospective data from the Nurses' Health Study shows a large reduction of risk (relative risk 0.33) from tubal ligation.[21] In *BRCA1*-mutation carriers (but not *BRCA2*), risk may be reduced by as much as 60%.[22] The mechanism is not fully understood, but tubal ligation may reduce blood supply or restrict the passage of inflammatory agents into the ovary.

Elective surgical removal of the ovaries is an option chosen with increasing frequency by women at high risk. Given the lack of a reliable screening test and the high mortality rate of ovarian cancer, consensus and expert opinion guidelines recommend that hereditary cancer syndrome patients consider prophylactic oophorectomy when childbearing is complete or by age 35.[14] This is best done in the context of risk assessment counseling, where the benefits and risks are fully explored. Women with a family history of ovarian cancer often have a high perceived risk of vulnerability to cancer, even when the status of genetic predisposition is unknown. In known carriers of *BRCAl* mutations, BSO affords a risk reduction of 85% to 96%.[23] Women should be counseled that surgery does not reduce risk by 100%. A less than 5% risk remains for primary peritoneal carcinomatosis, a lethal malignancy that behaves like ovarian cancer. Breast cancer risk is also reduced by BSO in *BRCA1/BRCA2* carriers by 50%.[23]

It should be noted that the fallopian tubes should be removed along with the ovaries, given the finding of occult cancers found incidentally during preventive surgery for carriers of *BRCA1/BRCA2* mutations. Given this finding, careful sectioning of the ovaries and tubes by a pathologist familiar with gynecologic malignancies is also recommended.[24] Women may choose hysterectomy in addition to BSO, particularly if there are benign reasons to do so, as with painful fibroids. Surgery may be performed via abdominal incision or laparoscopic technique. For women with HNPCC- syndrome risk, hysterectomy should be included, given the elevated risk for uterine cancer in these families. As with any surgery, complications are possible. Infection, bladder perforation, and small bowel obstruction have been observed in *BRCA1/BRCA2* carriers following BSO.[25]

Premenopausal women who choose ovary removal will experience an abrupt surgical menopause with quality of life implications. Hot flashes, vaginal dryness, urinary tract infections, loss of libido, joint pains, and osteoporosis can occur from estrogen deprivation. Use of hormone replacement therapy (HRT) may be considered, but given the link between long-term use of HRT and breast cancer, some clinicians prefer nonhormonal management. Drugs such as venlafaxine and fluoxetine, in the antidepressant class of selective serotonin reuptake inhibitors (SSRIs), have proven useful in hot flash control.[26] Vaginal dryness may be managed with vaginal lubricants or vaginal preparations of estrogen that do not cause systemic absorption. Women report the benefits of oophorectomy outweigh the side effects, but they need more comprehensive preparation when considering this option of risk reduction.[27] Nurses can assist in education, decision making, and side effects management of primary prevention strategies.

Secondary Prevention

The only recommended ovarian cancer screening for the general population is an annual rectovaginal pelvic exam. Palpation of the ovaries should be attempted but may not be possible because of small size or body habitus.

Available screening tests are limited in sensitivity and specificity. Women at high risk are offered the CA125 blood test and transvaginal ultrasound on an annual basis, but need to know the limitations of these studies. CA125 is a protein in the blood, the levels of which are used to track status of disease in affected women. It is a reliable test in the disease setting but as a screening test detects only 50% of stage I cancers. Measuring CA125 levels at short intervals over time is an approach currently under study, and may provide a more informative use of the test. False-positive CA125 results are caused by numerous benign conditions including ovulation, endometriosis, ovarian cysts, uterine fibroids, hepatitis, diverticulitis, autoimmune diseases, and pancreatitis.

The study of protein patterns in the blood—proteomics—offers hope for identifying early-stage disease. A protein pattern for ovarian cancer and numerous other biomarkers are the focus of ongoing research.[28]

Aside from CA125 the only other available screening test is transvaginal ultrasonography (TVUS). Pelvic ultrasound via the vagina affords the best image of the ovaries, although the transabdominal view can also prove useful. Cysts are a common finding on ultrasound and are classified as simple or complex. A complex cyst may have solid features and septations, and is considered more suspicious.[5] TVUS is limited in detecting primary peritoneal carcinoma and cancer in normal-sized ovaries. Both CA125 and TVUS should be scheduled with the first 10 days of the menstrual cycle, to avoid equivocal findings related to ovulation.

SYMPTOM AWARENESS

With limited ability to detect ovarian cancer and no clear-cut presentation of early-stage disease, raising the general level of awareness of symptoms becomes important. A growing number of advocacy groups are countering the prevailing notion that ovarian cancer has no symptoms. Rather than lack of symptoms, both women and health care providers have failed to attribute nonspecific symptoms to this disease. An increasing number of studies describe women's experience of numerous symptoms before diagnosis in all stages of disease (Box 7-3). When women were surveyed retrospectively about their symptoms before diagnosis, only 5% reported no symptoms and over 70%

BOX 7-3 SYMPTOMS ATTRIBUTED TO OVARIAN CANCER BY WOMEN WITH THE DISEASE

Bloating
Pain (pelvic, abdominal, back)
Urinary frequency/urgency
Gastrointestinal distress (heartburn, early satiety, loss of appetite, nausea, vomiting)
Change in bowel habits (constipation, diarrhea, gas)
Fatigue
Painful intercourse
Weight loss/gain
Abnormal vaginal bleeding
Shortness of breath

reported symptoms present for 3 months or more.[29] Nurses who are aware of the symptoms and the disease are uniquely positioned to increase the awareness in the community.

Clinical Factors

The presence of an ovarian mass should be investigated if found during a physician assessment. Most palpable masses found on exam in a premenopausal woman are not indicative of a malignancy. The general guideline for a premenopausal woman with a mass smaller than 8 cm is that the physician will observe it and do a repeat pelvic exam in 1 to 3 months because many masses regress during subsequent menstrual cycles.[30] Any mass in a postmenopausal woman should be fully investigated without delay. In addition, a full investigation is warranted if the mass is 10 cm or larger, enlarges to beyond 5 cm while under observation, or persists even though the woman is on oral contraceptives; if the mass is immobile, painless, or irregular, or has solid or mixed solid and cystic components; if there is bilateral ovarian involvement; and/or if on pelvic exam any other mass is present.[30]

An ultrasound—either transvaginal and/or abdominal, a chest x-ray, a computed tomography (CT) scan, and a full panel of laboratory studies including a CA125 level are usually ordered as part of the diagnostic workup. A barium enema or colonoscopy may also be ordered if symptoms are present or for preoperative full assessment.

Diagnosis and Staging

A diagnosis is made by a comprehensive surgical staging procedure. The surgery is called an exploratory laparotomy; its goal is to leave no tumor behind greater than 1 cm, because it has been established that minimal residual disease is associated with improved survival.[31]

The surgical procedure approach is abdominal with a vertical midline incision from the symphysis pubis to above the umbilicus to allow for maximum exposure of the upper abdomen and pelvis. A gynecologic surgical oncologist is the optimal trained specialist to perform the procedure. A total abdominal hysterectomy and bilateral salpingo-oopherectomy is performed as well as an omentectomy, careful examination of all peritoneal surfaces, biopsy of paraaortic lymph nodes, random biopsies of clinically uninvolved areas, and peritoneal washings. Ovarian cancer is staged based on the International Federation of Obstetrics and Gynecology (FIGO) staging system (Table 7-3).[32] Surgical staging provides important information that will guide postoperative treatment decision making. Patients are usually classified as optimally debulked or suboptimally debulked after surgery, based on the goal of leaving behind no tumor >1 cm. Histologic types include papillary serous (the most common), endometrioid, mucinous, or clear cell. A universally accepted grading system incorporating molecular markers or DNA cytometry is in development. At this time grade 1 tumors are well differentiated, grade 2 tumors are moderately differentiated, and grade 3 tumors are poorly differentiated.

Ovarian cancer spreads intraperitoneally, via the lymphatic channels, or by hematogenous dissemination. The most common method of spread is via the exfoliation of the cells that become implanted along the surfaces of the peritoneal cavity. These cells give rise to metastatic foci throughout the abdomen; the process is referred as peritoneal seeding.

Table 7-3 STAGING SYSTEM FOR EPITHELIAL OVARIAN CANCER

Stage	Characteristics
I	Tumor limited to ovary or ovaries[1]
A	One ovary involved; without ascites, positive peritoneal washings, surface involvement, or rupture
B	Both ovaries involved; without ascites, positive peritoneal washings, surface involvement, or rupture
C	Ascites, positive peritoneal washings, surface involvement, or rupture present
II	Ovarian tumor with pelvic extension1
A	Involvement of the uterus or fallopian tubes
B	Involvement of other pelvic organs (e.g., bladder, rectum, or pelvic sidewall)
C	Pelvic extension, plus findings indicated for stage IC
III	Tumor involving the upper abdomen or lymph nodes
A	Microscopic disease outside the pelvis, typically involving the omentum
B	Gross deposits ≤ 2 cm in diameter[2]
C	Gross deposits ≥ 2 cm in diameter or nodal involvement[2]
IV	Distant organ involvement, including pleural space or hepatic or splenic parenchyma[3]

These guidelines are from the International Federation of Gynecology and Obstetrics.
1. Patients with disease that appears to be confined to the ovaries or pelvis require nodal biopsy for compete staging to rule out the possibility of occult stage IIIC disease
2. Disease measurements for staging purposes are made before debulking has been attempted
3. Pleural effusion must be cytologically proven to be malignant if used to define stage IV disease

Surgery plays other important roles in managing ovarian cancer besides diagnosis and staging. Procedures can include a secondary surgical cytoreductive surgery, second-look surgery, laparoscopic surgery, and palliative surgery. In some cases, initial surgery may not be successful, and clinical trials designed to study interval debulking surgery found a benefit to this surgery.[33] Exploratory surgery at the end of primary treatment, or second-look surgery, remains a controversial approach because a negative second look does not mean the patient is cured, and the current available treatment for patients with positive results is not effective in obtaining a cure. Second-look surgery continues to be recommended only in the context of a clinical trial. Laparoscopic surgery is a less invasive approach and may be useful to inspect a certain area of concern on an imaging study or to document a recurrence. Palliative surgery is performed to relieve a symptom or a medical diagnosis such as a bowel obstruction.

TREATMENT

A curative treatment approach in ovarian cancer is challenging because most tumors are discovered at a late stage, and even though primary treatment leads to a complete remission, the majority of women with advanced disease relapse after primary therapy. The current standard approach after surgery for most ovarian cancers is combination chemotherapy (www.nccn.org).[34,35]

EARLY-STAGE DISEASE

There is a small subset of women with early-stage disease who require no further treatment after surgery. The low-risk group of women with early-stage disease have tumors that are stage IA–grade 1 disease, or stage IA–grade 2 and stage IB–grades 1 or 2 disease. Systemic therapy is required after surgery once early-stage disease develops any of the following: tumor on the external surface of the ovary, a ruptured capsule, ascites, positive peritoneal washings, or poorly differentiated disease; these women are classified as at high risk. The recurrence rate for patients at high risk is 25% to 40%.[36] Platinum-based adjuvant therapy can reduce the risk of relapse in this group, resulting in a disease-free survival of approximately 80%.[37,38] An overall survival advantage in high-risk patients with early-stage disease who had immediate postoperative chemotherapy was found in two randomized trials in Europe comparing immediate postoperative chemotherapy to chemotherapy at the time of relapse.[39,40] The chemotherapy regimen recommended is paclitaxel (175 mg/m^2 administered over 3 hours) combined with carboplatin (area under the curve [AUC] of 5 to 7.5).[35] (A description is also available at www.nccn.org)

The Gynecologic Oncology Group (GOG) recently compared three cycles with six cycles to determine the number of cycles necessary to achieve optimal benefit; so far, results have not shown a difference in overall survival and have indicated a slightly higher relapse rate in patients receiving the three-cycle regimen.[41] However the conclusion of this study's initial results is that the three cycles administered in addition to the standard three cycles of therapy did not significantly alter the rate of recurrence and that standard therapy for early-stage ovarian cancer patients consists of three cycles of paclitaxel plus carboplatin.[41,42] The current GOG trial for high-risk early-stage disease is three cycles of paclitaxel and carboplatin as the standard treatment arm; in the experimental arm the patients are treated with an additional 24 weeks of low-dose paclitaxel (40mg/m^2). This study is investigating the theory that this dose of paclitaxel may have antiangiogenic properties, and markers of angiogenesis are being collected.

ADVANCED DISEASE

Ovarian cancer has always been a chemotherapy-sensitive disease. Initially, regimens contained alkylating agents and were used as single agents. Anthracycline agents were also part of the early regimens. It became apparent that combinations of agents compared to single agents were superior, and the addition of the platinum agents to the armamentarium brought dramatic results, as summarized in Box 7-4. The GOG has led the way in identifying the standard of care for advanced ovarian cancer. Two groups of patients have been studied in many clinical trials, those patients with optimal disease (FIGO stage III with no tumor nodule >1 cm after surgery) and those with sub-optimal disease (FIGO stage IV and stage III with any residual tumor >1 cm).

The major milestone in research studies in the 1990s was the comparison of what had been

Box 7-4 Historical Summary of Chemotherapy in Ovarian Cancer

1970s	Most common drugs used as monotherapy Melphalan, cyclophosphamide, chlorambucil, and thiotepa
1980s	Cisplatin: first established as an active single agent Cisplatin and cyclophosphamide combined: results showed improved response rates and almost doubled survival rates Anthracyclines added to the cisplatin-alkylating agent regimen in many trials: modest gains in survival, but concern of cardiotoxicity outweighed clinical gain
1990s	Carboplatin: considerably less toxic; in the 1990s was compared to cisplatin and found equally effective
Mid-1990s	Paclitaxel: improved response rate, progression-free survival, and overall survival when compared to older regimens Platinum compound and paclitaxel combination: improved median survival, progression-free survival, and overall survival by substituting cyclophosphamide with paclitaxel
2005	Carboplatin and paclitaxel

the standard combination of therapy up to that time, cisplatin and cyclophosphamide, to the combination of cisplatin and paclitaxel. The latter was found to be superior with an improved response rate, an increased complete response rate, an increase in progression-free survival, and an increased overall median survival.[43] A Canadian and European trial confirmed the GOG results with the only difference being that this group administered paclitaxel over a 3-hour infusion, compared to the GOG's regimen, where it was given over 24 hours.[44] Carboplatin was introduced next as a substitute for cisplatin because of its ease of administration in the outpatient setting and its better profile of toxicity. It was compared in a series of randomized trials, where no significant difference was demonstrated when compared to cisplatin except in patients with optimal stage III disease.[45] The international consensus conference in 1993 recommended that carboplatin should not replace cisplatin in stage III optimally debulked patients.[46] As a result, a new GOG trial was designed to investigate this issue along with several other research questions. GOG 158 compared the efficacy and toxicity of carboplatin plus paclitaxel, as opposed to cisplatin plus paclitaxel, in optimally debulked stage III patients. The results showed no difference in the progression-free survival or overall survival, and the carboplatin and paclitaxel arm was less toxic.[47]

Three other trials studied paclitaxel and platinum therapy in various combinations and comparisons. GOG 132 (a three-arm trial) compared standard doses of cisplatin and paclitaxel in combination versus high-dose paclitaxel (200 mg/m^2) versus high-dose cisplatin (100 mg/m^2). There was no difference in the median overall survival between the treatment arms, but the platinum-containing regimens had a superior response rate and progression-free survival.[48]

The second and third International Collaborative Ovarian Neoplasm Groups' (ICON-2, ICON-3) studies provided more insight into ovarian cancer treatment. ICON-2 compared carboplatin administered as a monotherapy to cyclophosphamide, doxorubicin, and cisplatin (CAP). There was no significant difference in survival between the two groups, and the CAP arm was more toxic.[49] ICON-3 compared single-agent carboplatin versus carboplatin and paclitaxel versus carboplatin and paclitaxel and CAP. The follow-up showed no significant difference in overall survival at 51 months between the three arms.[50] There was a wide range of patient types recruited to this study; one third of the patients in the control arm went on to receive a taxane at some point. Therefore one conclusion may be that the efficacy of taxane and platinum agents, together or as a monotherapy, may depend at least in part on the manner in which they are sequenced.[51] All of the clinical trial information compiled to this point has led to written guidelines supporting the use of paclitaxel and carboplatin for first-line therapy in cases of advanced disease.[35] In the United Kingdom the NICE guidelines support the use of paclitaxel/platinum combination therapy or platinum therapy alone for first-line advanced ovarian cancer treatment.[52]

A second taxane agent, docetaxel, began to be investigated, and phase II trials indicated a level of efficacy comparable to paclitaxel and in addition, docetaxel had clinical activity in paclitaxel-resistant patients.[53,54] In light of this activity and after testing the feasibility of the docetaxel and carboplatin combination, a trial was initiated to compare combinations. Docetaxel plus carboplatin was compared to the standard combination of paclitaxel and carboplatin in a randomized trial. After a follow-up of 23 months, both groups had similar progression-free survival rates and response rates.[55] The docetaxel/carboplatin arm was associated with more myelosuppression and the paclitaxel/carboplatin arm had more neurotoxicity.[55] These authors conclude that this combination may represent an alternative first-line regimen, but a longer follow-up is needed to provide a definitive statement on survival.[55]

The most recent GOG trial for first-line therapy was closed in the US in the summer of 2004 and in Europe a short time afterward, and analysis is underway. It is a multiarmed phase III trial of the Gynecologic Cancer Inter Group (GCIG) and accrued 4000 patients.[56] This trial included three newer drugs with activity in recurrent ovarian cancer: gemcitabine, topotecan, and liposomal doxorubicin. The schema included five arms and examined whether the new combinations should include triplets or sequential doublets. The results of this trial are anxiously anticipated. The next proposed GOG trial for first-line treatment for suboptimal patients compares carboplatin plus paclitaxel to carboplatin, plus paclitaxel, plus bevacizumab.

CONSOLIDATION AND MAINTENANCE THERAPY

Despite very high response rates and clinical complete response rates, about 75% of patients eventually relapse. Many investigators have been interested in studying ways to consolidate or maintain these initial responses. Until recently, none of these studies has shown a benefit for consolidation or maintenance therapy.[57] A recently reported phase III trial of extended duration paclitaxel as maintenance therapy was originally designed to randomize 450 patients with a clinical complete response to either 12 or 3 additional monthly cycles of paclitaxel.[58] The study was closed early because of differences in progression-free survival favoring the 12 additional cycles. Survival will not be able to be assessed because patients were allowed to cross over to the 12-cycle regimen after study closure. The GOG is planning further trials to confirm the value of prolonged paclitaxel by doing a study that will randomize patients who achieve a clinical complete response to standard paclitaxel/carboplatin–based therapy to either no further treatment, 12 monthly cycles of paclitaxel, or 12 months of a polyglutamated paclitaxel.[59]

INTRAPERITONEAL THERAPY

Intraperitoneal therapy (IP) can provide a pharmacologic advantage, namely a higher ratio of peak peritoneal drug levels to plasma levels. The drugs administered via the IP route will also enter the systemic circulation and achieve a 50% to 75% uptake of intravenous (IV) administration exposure via the lymphatic channels or by passive diffusion. There has continued to be a great deal of interest in pursuing the IP method of drug administration in ovarian cancer because the disease even in its advanced stages is predominantly confined to the abdomen. Cisplatin is the drug most frequently used in IP therapy for ovarian cancer. IP therapy has been evaluated in three large, randomized trials of patients with small-volume residual disease.[60-63] In the Southwest Oncology Group (SWOG)/GOG trial for optimal stage III patients, IP cisplatin and IV cyclophosphamide were compared to IV cisplatin and cyclophosphamide. The complete response rate and the overall median survival was superior in the IP arm.[60] The next GOG trial compared IV cisplatin and paclitaxel to two doses of IV carboplatin followed by six cycles of IP cisplatin and IP paclitaxel. Progression-free survival and overall survival were statistically significantly better in IP arm.[62] The third trial compared IV paclitaxel (day 1) plus IP cisplatin (day 2), and IP paclitaxel (day 8) to IV paclitaxel and cisplatin.[61,63]

This phase III study resulted in an improvement in progression-free and overall survival for the arm with intraperitoneal treatment (GOG proceedings July 2005). These results spurred much discussion regarding the possible inclusion of IP therapy in future GOG trials of optimally debulked patients. However, IP therapy has produced significantly more toxicity than the IV regimens. In addition, the logistics of administration, including challenges with catheter placement and continued patency, have not made this regimen widely accepted outside a clinical trial. Current research efforts are following up on the use of more tolerable IP regimens, such as the substitution of cisplatin with carboplatin, that will maintain the efficacy advantage of the IP regimens.

DOSE INTENSITY

Dose intensity has been widely studied in this disease with both cisplatin and carboplatin. Results from trials show no advantage over standard doses, just increased toxicity.[33] Paclitaxel has also been studied for a dose intensity benefit, and there has been no evidence to support doses greater than 175 mg/m^2. Weekly paclitaxel has been associated with an antiangiogenic effect.[64] This schedule has shown encouraging activity and an improved therapeutic index in relapsed ovarian cancer, so investigation continues in upfront therapy.[33,64-69] High-dose chemotherapy has also been studied, and at present this approach is not recommended outside the context of a clinical trial. A phase III European study of high-dose sequential chemotherapy compared to standard chemotherapy in patients with optimal stage III and IV disease may help clarify the role.[33]

Radiation Therapy

Initially, before chemotherapy, radiation therapy was the postoperative treatment of choice. After the arrival of active chemotherapy, radiation and single-agent chemotherapy were compared and produced similar outcomes. Since radiation therapy produced much greater morbidity, chemotherapy quickly became the standard treatment. Radiation therapy of the whole abdominal area is a toxic treatment. With the new techniques of intensity-modulated radiotherapy and new fractionation schedules, toxicity appears to be reduced. Possible roles for radiation therapy may include consolidation treatment after postoperative chemotherapy, as palliative or salvage therapy in persistent or recurrent disease, and as consolidation in patients with no or minimal residual disease at second-look laparotomy after postoperative chemotherapy.

Debby and others evaluated 32 patients who had no pathologic evidence of disease; they received 800 cGY single-dose whole abdominal radiotherapy by an 8 MeV linear accelerator in a single fraction.[70] The results indicate a favorable long-term survival in patients and suggests that a prospective randomized study may be worthwhile.[70] Palliative radiotherapy in platinum-resistant patients provided 39% with relief of their symptoms for longer than 12 months; 30% obtained relief of their symptoms for 6-12 months, and the authors concluded that radiation could provide effective and durable palliation of symptoms.[71]

Recurrent Disease Treatment

Although primary or first-line therapy has continued to yield improved results, the majority of women relapse and are then incurable. An elevated CA125 is a sensitive indicator of relapse with a preclinical lead time of 3 to 9 months.[72,73] This indicator makes it especially challenging for clinicians, since the marker becomes elevated before the symptoms or definitive disease progression become apparent. The information contributes to anxiety on the part of the patient who monitors her tumor markers closely and understands the meaning of a rise in value. In Europe, two trials are underway to address the rising CA125 treatment issue. Serial CA125 results are monitored on registered women and not made routinely available to the clinician.[73] Upon elevation of the level to twice the upper limit of normal, women are randomized to either receive immediate treatment or no treatment until relapse is clinically indicated.[73]

In the US, treatment decisions are based on an increased CA125 alone, on recurrent disease found on the CT scan, or on a change in the physical exam. Decisions are made on individual basis following discussion with the patient. An alternative approach to an elevated tumor marker may be to use the drug tamoxifen or an aromatase inhibitor until clinical evidence of disease recurrence exists.[74-77] Some patients may have a prolonged period of stable disease, an occasional patient may have a dramatic reduction in her CA125 level, and less than 20% overall have a response to hormonal therapy; in addition to these potential benefits, it is an alternative that avoids the side effects of toxic treatment.[5]

Most clinicians use the platinum-free interval guideline as a basis for decisions regarding recurrent disease therapy. In a woman whose disease relapses less than 6 months after first-line chemotherapy, there is about a 10% chance of further response.[73,78] This increases to 31% after a platinum-free interval of 5 to 12 months, and to 59% with intervals of more than 24 months.[73,79] Hence, platinum-sensitive patients are defined as patients with a disease-free interval of more than 6 months, platinum-resistant patients are those who had a disease-free interval shorter than 6 months, and refractory patients had no response to first-line therapy.

There is no evidence at this time that rechallenging a patient by using original primary treatment drugs is any better than using new agents. For the platinum-sensitive patient, second-line therapy has consisted of single-agent therapy with either paclitaxel or carboplatin. Two more recent trials suggest combination therapy (paclitaxel plus platinum) in the platinum-sensitive group improves both survival and progression-free survival when compared to single-agent therapy.[68,80,81] There was more toxicity in the combination therapy arm, leading other experts to conclude single-agent therapy was superior.[73]

Phase II studies have investigated combining platinum with various other active cytotoxic agents including etoposide, epirubicin, and gemcitabine, and results have been reported.[73,82-86] Peglylated liposomal doxorubicin, an active agent in ovarian cancer, was compared with topotecan in patients with refractory and recurrent ovarian cancer. The results demonstrated the group who received liposomal doxorubicin had a prolonged survival and that survival benefit was more pronounced in patients with platinum sensitive disease.[87] The oxaliplatin, fluorouracil, and leucovorin combination was active in two recently reported studies with relapsed ovarian cancer for both platinum-sensitive and platinum-resistant and taxane-pretreated ovarian cancer patients and had a good toxicity profile.[88,89] Additional chemotherapy agents to be considered for the platinum-resistant patient include oral etoposide, gemcitabine, liposomal doxorubicin, epirubicin, paclitaxel, docetaxel, topotecan, altretamine, ifosfamide, and vinorelbine. All patients should be considered candidates for clinical trials. The drug-refractory patients should be offered investigational therapy.

The response in second-line therapy is not durable. The likelihood of benefit must be weighed against the toxicity of treatment. The patients most likely to benefit from second-line treatment include those with small-volume disease, a good performance status, a long treatment-free interval, serous histology, and a low number of disease sites. The clinicians should consider the following parameters when choosing a treatment for recurrent disease: prior response; toxicity of prior treatment and toxicity profile; quality of life; age, comorbid illness, and extent of disease; cost; and patient goals and preferences. Overall the standard approach is to treat for two to three cycles, evaluate the response, and make a decision as to whether to continue based on results and patient symptoms.

FUTURE DIRECTIONS OF THERAPY

A combination of new agents and the identification of molecular targets are leading the next phase of treatment for ovarian cancer in a new exciting direction. Several of the molecular targets for drug development have been identified including the pathway mediated by p53, lysophosphatidic acid, the *BCL2* family, the epidermal growth factor receptor (EGFR) and the vascular endothelial growth factor receptor (VEGFR).[5]

Angiogenesis is emerging as a most interesting target for ovarian cancer treatment, and the anti-vascular endothelial factor antibody bevacizumab and thalidomide are currently being investigated.[90] HER2 protein is known to be expressed in approximately 10% to 15% of ovarian cancer; however, the anti-HER2 monoclonal antibody trastuzumab showed low activity in the GOG trial.[91] OSI-774 (Erlotinib), an oral EGFR-tyrosine kinase inhibitor, showed modest activity, and ZD 1839 (gefitinib, Iressa) showed growth inhibition and acted synergistically with chemotherapy in ovarian cancer.[92-94] Iressa as a single agent had a low response rate in a phase II GOG trial.[95] B43.13 (OvaRex), a monoclonal antibody developed to target CA125-expressing ovarian cancer cells, was studied in a phase II trial that followed 345 patients who received either B43.14 or placebo after surgery and standard chemotherapy. An interim analysis showed a correlation between the immune response and better progression-free survival.[96] A phase III trial is planned to confirm these results.[33]

Bryostatin, a protein kinase C inhibitor, was used in a phase II GOG trial as a single agent, and those results are not yet available. ET-743, a new cytotoxic agent, showed a response rate of 28% in previously treated platinum-sensitive ovarian cancer patients.[97] A novel anticancer agent with angiogenesis target MSI-1256F (Squalamine) was administered in combination with carboplatin and yielded a response rate as high as 36% in platinum-resistant/refractory ovarian cancer patients.[98] CT-2103 (Xyotax), a novel conjugate of paclitaxel and poly-L-glutamic acid, is active in patients with ovarian cancer.[99] It is conjugated, so there was no need for Cremophor as a solubilizing agent, and there was enhanced permeability and retention on the tumor tissue.[90]

In these two phase I trials with CT-2103, eight ovarian cancer patients were treated; six of those had a partial response, and two had stable disease.[100,101] These results propelled the GOG to begin a phase II trial and explore the development of a phase III trial.[90] TLK 286, a glutathione analog, was administered to about 70 patients with platinum-resistant disease and produced a response rate of 15%. It is being combined with conventional chemotherapy in phase I and phase II trials.[102,103] Novel classes of microtubule-stabilizing agents with activity similar to that of paclitaxel, the epothilones, are in clinical trials.

Table 7-4 lists a summary of these investigational agents and the potential targets. Another new direction is the use of microarray gene-expression profiling, which holds promise as a prognostic tool. It may provide insight into the mechanisms of drug resistance, which develops frequently in this tumor.

At this time the clinical impact of all these new therapies remains unknown, but they do point to an exciting time of research in ovarian cancer treatment. Most of these agents are in the early stages of clinical trials and have been mostly evaluated as single agents; the next phase will bring even more interest, since those that have activity will be combined with some of the known active chemotherapy agents in this disease, to yield what are hoped to be improved results.

Symptom Management

Ovarian cancer treatment is aggressive and at times unrelenting for the patient, especially during the recurrent stage. Nurses have many opportunities to partner with the patient and family to offer support and education. Nurses are best positioned

Table 7-4 Summary of Investigational Agents in Ovarian Cancer

Agent	Target or Action
	Angiogenesis
Thalidomide	Angiogenesis
MSI-1256F (Squalamine)	Angiogenesis
	Signal transduction
Bevacizumab	VEGFR
Cetuximab	EGFR
Trastuzumab	Anti-HER2
Gefitinib (Iressa)	EGFR
Erlotinib	(OSI-774) EGFR
	Novel cytotoxic or other action
MAbB43.13 (OvaRex)	Monoclonal antibody to CA125
CT-2103	Tubulin
ET 742	Cytotoxic
Bryostatin	Protein kinase inhibitor
TLK 286	Glutathione analog

to help the patient manage the toxicity profile of treatment, the advanced disease problems that occur, and the psychosocial issues surrounding living with a chronic and often terminal disease.

Nursing intervention revolves around three different periods in the management of the ovarian cancer patient. Before surgery the nurse will prepare the patient and family for surgery and its potential complications, and he or she will monitor the patient during the acute postoperative phase for infection, circulatory complications, fluid and electrolyte imbalances, and pain. Coordinating home care support at discharge will help provide continuous support.

Chemotherapy starts early after surgery, and the office or ambulatory nurse will provide the detailed information on the side effects of the regimen chosen for the patient. Some of the many side effects the patient may experience include alopecia, nausea, vomiting, fatigue, diarrhea, constipation, mucositis, neuropathy, arthralgias and myalgias, and myelosuppression. A treatment nurse must prepare the patient and family for the potential problems and provide them with strategies to tackle any of these problems if they occur. Having patients keep a diary of their problems and carry it with them from office visit to office visit allows the practitioner to provide more customized care and will prevent patients from having repetitive problems. Keeping in close contact by phone between visits allows the patient and family to use the nursing support and cements the relationship of a partnership.

As the disease recurs the patient may encounter a different set of problems, and the nurse in the community is the potential source of support. Ascites, intermittent bowel obstruction, lymphedema, and malnutrition are the most frequently occurring management challenges of the advanced ovarian cancer patient and are due to the disease in the abdomen. A chronic problem with pleural effusions may also occur because of the cancer cells leaking into the pleural cavity at the diaphragm. Some of these side effects are covered in depth in other chapters of this book; here an effort will be made to concentrate on the problems that are not covered elsewhere.

Ascites can occur in up to two thirds of women with ovarian cancer. The peritoneal fluid is normally present in a small volume, and it provides lubrication in the abdominal cavity. When tumor obstructs the diaphragmatic or abdominal lymphatic channels or the tumor itself produces excess amounts of fluid, ascites occurs because the fluid produced exceeds the amount fluid cleared.[104,105] With a fluid increase of about 500 cc the patient begins to develop symptoms. A patient may experience weight gain, abdominal bloating, shortness of breath, indigestion, or altered bowel habits; may feel quickly full after small meals or lack an appetite; or be unable to bend or sit upright. If there is no intervention, the symptoms progress and the patient will not be able to perform normal activities. Nursing assessment reveals shiny and tense abdominal skin, an everted umbilicus, diminished bowel sounds, shifting dullness, a bulging flank, increased venous distention, increased abdominal girth, weight gain, a fluid wave, or midabdomen tympany.[106,107] An abdominal ultrasound will confirm the presence of ascites, and a therapeutic paracentesis may be ordered for symptomatic relief. Systemic treatment of the primary tumor will usually be attempted, since all measures to deal with the fluid are temporary unless the underlying problem is addressed.

Diuretic therapy is usually not effective in malignant ascites. A peritoneovenous shunt may be used for the patient who is refractory to medical interventions and has disabling symptoms. This is a continuous shunt to rechannel ascites fluid from the peritoneal cavity to the superior vena cava and eventually into the venous circulation. The shunt is placed with one end in the peritoneal cavity and the other end in the superior vena cava, and the ascites flows upward via a one-way valve.[105,106,108,109] Unfortunately, shunts often fail early after placement from malfunctions such as kinking or occlusion, so the decision to use one is often only made after much discussion.

Patient education is the key to successfully managing ascites. Nurses teach the patient about keeping track of her weight and abdominal girth weekly. Trying to intervene at a stage that is less acute is helpful to the patient. Instructions about a bowel regimen are necessary to relieve any symptoms such as constipation. Adjustments will need to be made in meals and intake to maintain nutrition and promote comfort. Small, frequent meals or snacks are suggested, with adequate protein intake. Since many women with ovarian cancer present with advanced disease, ascites is often a presenting symptom at diagnosis. The recurrence of this symptom produces anxiety as well as physical discomfort, since the disease is again at a stage where it is out of control. Helping patients become aware of the symptom and the need to report its manifestations, and helping prepare the patient for interventions and the accompanying side effects, helps the patient in maintaining control.

Another gastrointestinal problem in the advanced stages of disease is the medical diagnosis of a bowel obstruction. Several retrospective reviews estimate that it occurs in 25% to 50% of patients with ovarian cancer.[110] An obstruction may be acute, chronic, or recurrent, and 90% of bowel obstructions in general involve the small bowel, although in ovarian cancer either small or large bowel can be involved.[111] In ovarian cancer the tumor or adhesions cause extrinsic compression of the bowel, and the obstruction can be partial or complete. When obstruction occurs, the bowel responds at first by increasing the force of peristalsis and attempting to move the bowel contents beyond the obstructions; thus the first sounds heard are hyperactive bowel sounds. After a time the bowel tires, peristalsis slows, and hypoactive bowel sounds are noted.[112] The signs and symptoms are abdominal pain that is spasmodic, colicky, crampy in the mid-to-upper abdominal region and either diffuse or localized; abdominal distention; reduced amount and caliber, or absence, of stool; fever; chills; retching and vomiting; and no flatus if the obstruction is complete.[111]

The nursing assessment reveals abdominal tenderness and distention and hyperactive bowel sounds and, as the bowel tires, absent bowel sounds. Assess the patient for dehydration and for orthostatic hypotension, tachycardia, and tachypnea. Laboratory tests are assessed, especially electrolytes and blood urea nitrogen and creatinine levels. A plain abdominal x-ray film or an obstruction series is ordered. Medical intervention consists of relieving the distention, correcting the fluid imbalances, and removing the source of obstruction. A complete obstruction of the bowel indicates emergency surgical intervention. Partial obstructions can be managed conservatively. Initial treatment may involve simple bowel rest for 24 to 48 hours with no oral intake. After that time, decompression of the bowel with a nasogastic tube, a long intestinal tube, or a venting gastrostomy tube may be indicated. A retrospective chart review of 24 patient records was done to examine the effectiveness of managing a bowel obstruction with a percutaneous gastrostomy tube (PEG). No nausea or vomiting was noted by 75% of the patients at discharge, 92% resumed a clear liquid diet, 83% were discharged from the acute care setting, and 70% did not require readmission.[113] Pharmacologic management may include narcotics, anticholinergic agents, and antiemetics. If indicated, systemic treatment of the disease have an impact on the underlying cause of the bowel obstruction problem.

Decisions about surgical intervention for advanced cancer are always difficult; sometimes in an acute episode there is no other alternative, but often, in the more chronic setting, the physician will carefully weigh options with the patient and family. Quality of life issues must be considered against the possible complications of surgery, since the nature of this disease may well lead to another bowel obstruction episode and the surgical procedure itself entails its owns challenges and possible complications. The goal of treatment at this stage of disease is often palliative. Nurses caring for patients can educate the patient and support her to make the best decision. Having medication in the home for acute pain and vomiting may be part of a plan. Since a partial or complete bowel obstruction produces symptoms of a dramatic nature, patients must learn to recognize when a potential problem is developing and call to alert the caregiver of the onset of symptoms. It is critical in preventing progression of the problem.

OPPORTUNITIES FOR NURSING RESEARCH

Women with advanced disease seem the most vulnerable for physical problems and psychologic distress.[114] Certain types of cancer are associated with uncertainty, anxiety, and depression as a result of a late stage at diagnosis.[114-116] The majority of ovarian cancer patients are diagnosed at this stage of the disease and are immediately faced with aggressive combinations of therapy. There is a growing body of literature documenting a woman's response to living with ovarian cancer; however, many nursing research opportunities remains.

A review of the literature about the distress associated with some of the physical symptoms revealed that women reported problems with pain, appetite, fatigue, and finances, all of which had a significant impact on their quality of life and the worsening of symptoms as the disease progressed.[117,118] Women who experienced pain and fatigue lost the ability to enjoy life, engage in normal relationship activities, and maintain employment status.[119]

The psychosocial distress in the literature reveals high rates of anxiety and depression during chemotherapy treatment, and high distress scores continue for one third of the long-term survivors.[116,117,120,121] Emotional distress in ovarian cancer patients worsened with disease progression over a 2-year period, as did psychologic distress that impaired function.[114,121] For these women, relief came from psychologic counseling and support and also from improvement in their physical symptoms. An increase in family stress was also noted that resulted from the patient's increased anxiety about the diagnosis, treatment, and prognosis. One qualitative study describing the concerns of women with ovarian cancer found increased distress because of the compressed time frame to confront life-threatening issues.[122] This group expressed overwhelming feelings of helplessness and uncertainty while facing mortality and the need to redefine goals and expectations.

A review of over 21,000 letters, cards, and e-mails from ovarian cancer survivors to the editor of the ovarian cancer newsletter called "Conversations!" provided insight into the psychologic concerns of women throughout all stages of the disease. There were some unique findings: women experienced isolation from being diagnosed with a lesser known cancer; there was anxiety over the genetic association with the disease and a fear for their daughters; and there was stress and uncertainty because of the disease trajectory.[123] The investigators hope to use the coping strategies identified in this study to build an intervention that health care providers would be able to use to assist women with ovarian cancer.[123]

In another study, 263 women returned surveys on important issues associated with ovarian cancer. These women included 93 who had experienced recurrent disease and 170 who had not. A greater proportion of the women with recurrent disease reported bowel problems, fear of dying, pain, and difficulty getting around, and feelings of self-blame.[124] On average, women with recurrent disease reported experiencing more problems since diagnosis than those without recurrent disease.[124] A particular concern raised in this study was that a significant proportion of women felt they had not received adequate help for the problems they experienced. Two specific areas of inadequate assistance were difficulties with bowel and sexual function.[125] These women perceived nurses as being helpful to them, thereby indicating opportunities for nurses to provide more support.

In another, more recent study, 18 women with ovarian cancer were interviewed who identified the following major challenges: living with uncertainty, lack of control, fear of the unknown, the stigma of cancer, and facing death.[126] These authors outline the implications of their findings for nursing practice, which involve family-centered care to help deal with the adjustments in roles and relationships, a sensitivity to financial issues, facilitating the expression of fears and anxieties about death, and giving assistance in planning for the future.[126] As these women faced recurrent disease, four primary themes surfaced: waiting for recurrence, facing the diagnosis of recurrence, managing treatment-related concerns, and attempting to regain control.[119] More importantly, these women described changed communication with their health care providers when recurrent disease was found. They felt increased hopelessness as a result of their perception that the provider was not listening to their symptoms and had no treatment options to present.[119] The message these patients received was that symptom management had become the goal, rather than prolongation of life, and this caused them distress.

Patient support groups are another way of providing emotional support to patients. A support group for patients with ovarian cancer over a 2-year period was described.[127] The group of 30 women discussed two consistent themes. "Fate vs. freedom" (the struggle to face the real possibility of dying as opposed to the freedom to enjoy life) and "despair vs. hope" (the struggle to give in to loss, pain, and dejection as opposed to maintaining optimism).[127] Struggling with these existential issues stood out as the most important therapeutic factor in this support group.

Positive changes have also been reported about the way women's lives changed after the diagnosis.[117] A new appreciation of life and an adoption of a live for-the-moment philosophy were reported.

Since ovarian cancer is a disease that frequently recurs, research looking at the period after primary therapy and during disease recurrence has added to the knowledge base for nurses. The continual monitoring of CA125 is a reminder of the potential for recurrence. Hamilton noted that women identify their CA125 levels as evidence of disease status, and their emotions are governed by the value of the marker.[128]

Finally, following women without active disease yielded additional information. Responses were collected to a survey from 200 women who had ovarian cancer, were without evidence of active disease, and not on treatment for at least 2 years. Most respondents reported good physical, psychologic, social, and spiritual health. The cancer experience did have a detrimental effect (reported by 57% of respondents) on the women's sex lives.[129] Nurses therefore should take the opportunity to get education to these women during office visits about their sexual health and questions.

Information gained from ovarian cancer patient surveys and interviews provides nurses with valuable insight into the experience of living with ovarian cancer over the course of the disease and its treatment. Nurses can help patients understand information about and meaning of monitoring for disease recurrence and provide more sensitive communication about their treatment options. Nurses are key to helping women with ovarian cancer by providing both physical and emotional care during the disease trajectory and improving quality of life. A nurse can support the patient best by understanding the individual's unique personality and circumstances and then lending support to her most effective coping strategies. Weisman suggests the following to facilitate patient coping: nurses should clarify problems; help maintain control by encouraging patients to explore options; offer a willing and noncritical ear to help relieve pent-up emotions; direct patients to constructive channels to reduce anxiety; discourage hasty actions; and be comfortable sharing periods of silence.[114,130,131]

Nursing research can build on the information gathered to this point and craft interventions that address the identified stressors and symptom management issues. The nursing assessment must be broadened to include both the physical and the psychosocial domains. Women must be screened routinely for psychologic distress using a standard tool such as a distress scale.[114] Patients should be surveyed regularly, and the most distressing symptoms should be identified and interventions planned. It is important to enlist the support of multiple providers including mental health providers, community agencies and support services, and formal home care services to provide the most comprehensive care.[114] There are many opportunities for nurses to design interventions to facilitate better coping at different transition points in the process, such as at diagnosis, recurrence, and end of life. Continuing to gather information from the woman's perspective about recurrent ovarian cancer and what strategies are supportive to her will provide nurses with valuable data.

OVARIAN CANCER RESOURCES

Ovarian cancer has followed the successful path of other cancer advocacy groups and in the late 1990s two large organizations were established. One is the Ovarian Cancer National Alliance (OCNA), on the Web at www.OvarianCancer.org, whose mission is to unite organizations and individuals in addressing ovarian cancer. The group's primary goal was to establish a coordinated national effort to place ovarian cancer education, policy, and research issues prominently on the agendas of national policy makers and women's health care leaders. The other is the National Ovarian Cancer Coalition (NOCC), whose Web site is at www.ovarian.org; the group's mission is to raise awareness about ovarian cancer and to promote education about the disease. By dispelling myths and misunderstandings, the coalition is committed to improve the overall survival rate and quality of life for women with ovarian cancer. Additional ovarian cancer awareness resources are listed in Box 7-5. At Fox Chase Cancer Center the Family Risk Assessment Program coordinated a project to increase awareness about ovarian cancer. Figure 7-2 shows a photo of the quilt that was made by patients, staff, and family and friends whose lives were affected by cancer. This quilt is moved around to different sites and functions to increase community awareness.

Box 7-5 Ovarian Cancer Resource Information

Conversations! The International Newsletter for Those Fighting Ovarian Cancer
806-355-2565
www.Ovarian-News.org

Gilda Radner Familial Ovarian Cancer Registry
800-OVARIAN
www.OvarianCancer.com

Gilda's Club Worldwide
888-GILDA-4-U
www.GildasClub.org

Gynecologic Cancer Foundation
800-444-4441
www.WCN.org/GCF

National Ovarian Cancer Association (NOCA)
877-413-7970
www.OvarianCanada.org

National Ovarian Cancer Coaltion (NOCC)
888-OVARIAN
www.Ovarian.org

Ovarian Cancer National Alliance (OCNA)
202-331-1332
www.OvarianCancer.org

Ovarian Cancer Research Fund, Inc. (OCRF)
800-873-9569
www.ocrf.org

SHARE: Self-help for Women with Breast or Ovarian Cancer
866-891-2392
www.sharecancersupport.org

Society of Gynecologic Oncologists (SGO)
312-321-4099
www.SGO.org

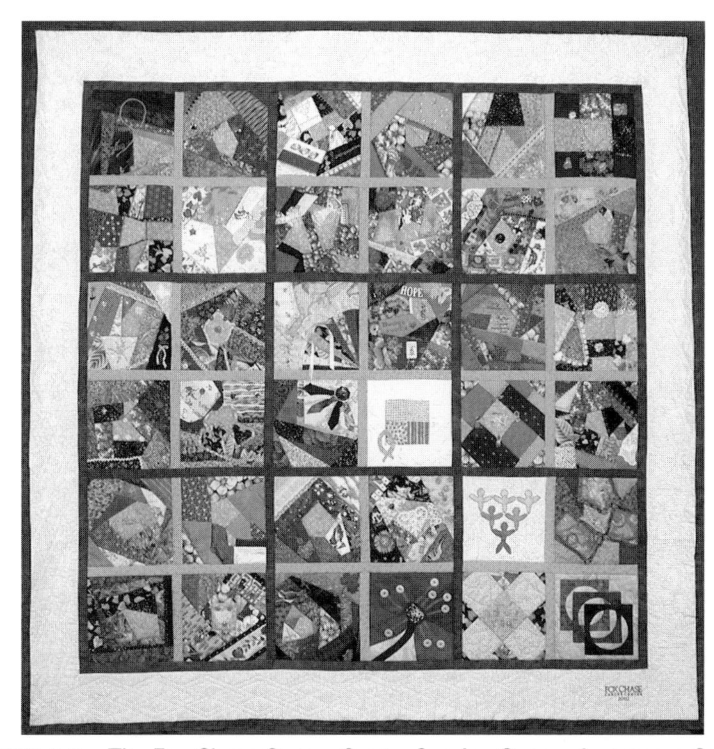

FIGURE 7-2 The Fox Chase Cancer Center Ovarian Cancer Awareness Quilt is composed of quilt squares designed by Fox Chase Cancer Center of Philadelphia staff, patients, family members, and friends whose lives were affected by cancer. It is displayed to raise awareness of ovarian cancer symptoms, screening and prevention options, the benefits of risk assessment, and the commitment to state-of-the-art ovarian cancer care and research. © Fox Chase Cancer Center. Photo courtesy of James Borders.

SUMMARY

The outlook for ovarian cancer patients has made definite strides over the last several decades. Awareness of the disease and its symptoms by committed survivors has made the disease "silent no more." Familial syndromes are recognized, and risk-reduction strategies are being implemented. Proteomics, or protein identification strategies, holds promise for future screening. First-line therapy has improved survival and there are more options for recurrent disease treatment. The future holds promise as new drugs are under investigation, molecular targets identified, and pathways targeted, and research leads to new understanding of the disease and its treatment.

REFERENCES

1. Jemal A and others: Cancer statistics, 2005, *CA Cancer J Clin* 55:10-30, 2005.
2. Ozols RF and others: Focus on epithelial ovarian cancer, *Cancer Cell* 5:19-24, 2004.
3. Parkin D and others: Estimating the world cancer burden: Globocan 2000, *Int J Cancer* 94:153-156, 2001.
4. Stewart BW, Kleihues P, International Agency for Research on Cancer: World cancer report, Lyon, France, 2003, IARC Press.
5. Cannistra SA: Cancer of the ovary, *N Engl J Med* 351: 2519-2529, 2004.
6. Hogg R, Friedlander M: Biology of epithelial ovarian cancer: implications for screening women at high genetic risk, *J Clin Oncol* 22:1315-1327, 2004.
7. Goodman M, Howe H: Descriptive epidemiology of ovarian cancer in the United States, 1992-1997, *Cancer* 97(Suppl):2615-2630, 2003.

8. Modugno F: Ovarian cancer and high-risk women-implications for prevention, screening, and early detection, *Gynecol Oncol* 91:15-31, 2003.
9. Seidman JD, Kurman RJ: Pathology of ovarian carcinoma, *Hematol Oncol Clin North Am* 17:909-925, vii, 2003.
10. Eyre H, Kahn R, Robertson RM: Preventing cancer, cardiovascular disease, and diabetes: a common agenda for the American Cancer Society, the American Diabetes Association, and the American Heart Association, *CA Cancer J Clin* 54:190-207, 2004.
11. Calle EE and others: Overweight, obesity, and mortality from cancer in a prospectively studied cohort of U.S. adults, *N Engl J Med* 348:1625-1638, 2003.
12. Ness RB and others: Infertility, fertility drugs, and ovarian cancer: a pooled analysis of case-control studies, *Am J Epidemiol* 155:217-224, 2002.
13. Modugno F: Ovarian cancer and polymorphisms in the androgen and progesterone receptor genes: a HuGE review, *Am J Epidemiol* 159:319-135, 2004.
14. Cherry C, Vacchiano SA: Ovarian cancer screening and prevention, *Semin Oncol Nurs* 18:167-173, 2002.
15. Shahin M, Sorosky J: Prevention and early diagnosis of ovarian cancer. In Manetta A, editor: Cancer prevention and early diagnosis in women, Philadelphia, 2004, Mosby.
16. ACOG practice bulletin: Prophylactic oophorectomy. Number 7, September 1999 (replaces Technical Bulletin Number 111, December 1987). Clinical management guidelines for obstetrician-gynecologists. American College of Obstetricians and Gynecologists, *Int J Gynaecol Obstet* 67:193-199, 1999.
17. Piver S: Hereditary ovarian cancer lessons from the first twenty years of the Gilda Radner familial ovarian cancer registry, *Gynecol Oncol* 85:9-17, 2002.
18. Chen VW and others: Pathology and classification of ovarian tumors, *Cancer* 97:2631-2642, 2003.
19. Connolly DC and others: Female mice chimeric for expression of the simian virus 40 TAg under control of the MISIIR promoter develop epithelial ovarian cancer, *Cancer Res* 63:1389-1397, 2003.
20. Whittemore AS and others: Oral contraceptive use and ovarian cancer risk among carriers of *BRCA1* or *BRCA2* mutations, *Br J Cancer* 91:1911-1915, 2004.
21. Hankinson SE: *Healthy women, healthy lives: a guide to preventing disease from the landmark Nurses' Health Study,* New York, 2001, Simon & Schuster Source.
22. Narod SA and others: Tubal ligation and risk of ovarian cancer in carriers of *BRCA1* or *BRCA2* mutations: a case-control study, *Lancet* 357:1467-1470, 2001.
23. Schwartz MD and others: Bilateral prophylactic oophorectomy and ovarian cancer screening following *BRCA1/BRCA2* mutation testing, *J Clin Oncol* 21: 4034-4041, 2003.
24. Leeper K and others: Pathologic findings in prophylactic oophorectomy specimens in high-risk women, *Gynecol Oncol* 87:52-56, 2002.
25. Kauff ND and others: Risk-reducing salpingo-oophorectomy in women with a *BRCA1* or *BRCA2* mutation, *N Engl J Med* 346:1609-1615, 2002.
26. Shanafelt TD and others: Pathophysiology and treatment of hot flashes, *Mayo Clin Proc* 77:1207-1218, 2002.
27. Hallowell N and others: High-risk premenopausal women's experiences of undergoing prophylactic oophorectomy: a descriptive study, *Genet Test* 8:148-156, 2004.
28. Bast RC, Jr: Status of tumor markers in ovarian cancer screening, *J Clin Oncol* 21:200-205, 2003.
29. Goff BA and others: Ovarian carcinoma diagnosis, *Cancer* 89:2068-2075, 2000.
30. Eriksson JA, Frazier SR: Epithelial cancers of the ovary and fallopian tube. In Moore-Higgs GJ, editor: *Women and cancer: a gynecologic oncology nursing perspective,* Boston, 2000, Jones and Bartlett.
31. Bristow RE and others: Survival effect of maximal cytoreductive surgery for advanced ovarian carcinoma during the platinum era: a meta-analysis, *J Clin Oncol* 20: 1248-1259, 2002.
32. Gynecologic sites—Part VIII. In Greene FL, American Joint Committee on Cancer, and American Cancer Society, editor: *AJCC cancer staging manual,* New York, 2002, Springer-Verlag.
33. Mano MS and others: Remaining controversies in the upfront management of advanced ovarian cancer, *Int J Gynecol Cancer* 14:707-720, 2004.
34. Ozols RF: Update of the NCCN ovarian cancer practice guidelines, *Oncology (Huntingt)* 11:95-105, 1997.
35. Morgan RJ and others: Ovarian cancer. In: Clinical practice guidelines in oncology, v.1.2005, pages 1-35, National Comprehensive Cancer Network.
36. Vergote I and others: Prognostic importance of degree of differentiation and cyst rupture in stage I invasive epithelial ovarian carcinoma, *Lancet* 357:176-182, 2001.
37. Young RC: Early-stage ovarian cancer: to treat or not to treat, *J Natl Cancer Inst* 95:94-95, 2003.
38. Young RC and others: Adjuvant treatment for early ovarian cancer: a randomized phase III trial of intraperitoneal 32P or intravenous cyclophosphamide and cisplatin—a gynecologic oncology group study, *J Clin Oncol* 21:4350-4355, 2003.
39. Colombo N and others: International Collaborative Ovarian Neoplasm trial 1: a randomized trial of adjuvant chemotherapy in women with early-stage ovarian cancer, *J Natl Cancer Inst* 95:125-132, 2003.
40. Trimbos JB and others: International Collaborative Ovarian Neoplasm trial 1 and adjuvant chemotherapy in Ovarian Neoplasm trial: two parallel randomized phase III trials of adjuvant chemotherapy in patients with early-stage ovarian carcinoma, *J Natl Cancer Inst* 95:105-112, 2003.
41. Ozols RF: Update on Gynecologic Oncology Group (GOG) trials in ovarian cancer, *Cancer Invest* 22(Suppl 2):11-20, 2004.
42. Bell J and others: A randomized phase III trial of three vs. six cycles of carboplatin and paclitaxel as adjuvant treatment in early stage ovarian epithelial carcinoma: a Gynecologic Oncology Group Study, *Ann Meet Soc Gynecol Oncol* 34:125-132, 2003.
43. McGuire WP and others: Cyclophosphamide and cisplatin compared with paclitaxel and cisplatin in patients with stage III and stage IV ovarian cancer, *N Engl J Med* 334:1-6, 1996.
44. Piccart MJ and others: Randomized intergroup trial of cisplatin-paclitaxel versus cisplatin-cyclophosphamide in women with advanced epithelial ovarian cancer: three-year results, *J Natl Cancer Inst* 92:699-708, 2000.

45. Aabo K and others: Chemotherapy in advanced ovarian cancer: four systematic meta-analyses of individual patient data from 37 randomized trials. Advanced Ovarian Cancer Trialists' Group, *Br J Cancer* 78:1479-1487, 1998.
46. Allen DG and others: Advanced epithelial ovarian cancer: 1993 consensus statements, *Ann Oncol* 4:S83-S88, 1993.
47. Ozols RF and others: Phase III trial of carboplatin and paclitaxel compared with cisplatin and paclitaxel in patients with optimally resected stage III ovarian cancer: a Gynecologic Oncology Group study, *J Clin Oncol* 21: 3194-3200, 2003.
48. Muggia FM and others: Phase III randomized study of cisplatin versus paclitaxel versus cisplatin and paclitaxel in patients with suboptimal stage III or IV ovarian cancer: a gynecologic oncology group study, *J Clin Oncol* 18:106-115, 2000.
49. Collaborators I: ICON2: randomised trial of single-agent carboplatin against three-drug combination of CAP (cyclophosphamide, doxorubicin, and cisplatin) in women with ovarian cancer, *Lancet* 352:1571-1576, 1998.
50. ICON: Paclitaxel plus carboplatin versus standard chemotherapy with either single-agent carboplatin or cyclophosphamide, doxorubicin, and cisplatin in women with ovarian cancer. The ICON 3 randomized trial, *Lancet* 360:505-515, 2002.
51. McGuire WP 3rd, Markman M: Primary ovarian cancer chemotherapy: current standards of care, *Br J Cancer* 89 (Suppl 3):S3-S8, 2003.
52. Ozols RF: NICE guidelines for ovarian cancer: recommendations versus standard care, *Cancer Invest* 22: 815-817, 2004.
53. Rose PG and others: A phase II study of docetaxel in paclitaxel-resistant ovarian and peritoneal carcinoma: a Gynecologic Oncology Group study, *Gynecol Oncol* 88:130-135, 2003.
54. Kaye SB and others: Phase II trials of docetaxel (Taxotere) in advanced ovarian cancer—an updated overview, *Eur J Cancer* 33:2167-2170, 1997.
55. Vasey PA and others: Phase III randomized trial of docetaxel-carboplatin versus paclitaxel-carboplatin as first-line chemotherapy for ovarian carcinoma, *J Natl Cancer Inst* 96:1682-1691, 2004.
56. Bookman MA, Greer BE, Ozols RF: Optimal therapy of advanced ovarian cancer: carboplatin and paclitaxel vs. cisplatin and paclitaxel (GOG 158) and an update on GOG0 182-ICON5, *Int J Gynecol Cancer* 13:735-740, 2003.
57. Ozols RF: Maintenance therapy in advanced ovarian cancer: progression-free survival and clinical benefit, *J Clin Oncol* 21:2451-2453, 2003.
58. Markman M, and others: Phase III randomized trial of 12 versus 3 months of maintenance paclitaxel in patients with advanced ovarian cancer after complete response to platinum and paclitaxel-based chemotherapy: a Southwest Oncology Group and Gynecologic Oncology Group trial, *J Clin Oncol* 21:2460-2465, 2003.
59. Thigpen T: First-line therapy for ovarian carcinoma: what's next? *Cancer Invest* 22(Suppl 2):21-28, 2004.
60. Alberts DS and others: Intraperitoneal cisplatin plus intravenous cyclophosphamide versus intravenous cisplatin plus intravenous cyclophosphamide for stage III ovarian cancer, *N Engl J Med* 335:1950-1955, 1996.
61. Armstrong DK: Relapsed ovarian cancer: challenges and management strategies for a chronic disease, *Oncologist* 7(Suppl 5):20-28, 2002.
62. Markman M and others: Phase III trial of standard-dose intravenous cisplatin plus paclitaxel versus moderately high-dose carboplatin followed by intravenous paclitaxel and intraperitoneal cisplatin in small-volume stage III ovarian carcinoma: an intergroup study of the Gynecologic Oncology Group, Southwestern Oncology Group, and Eastern Cooperative Oncology Group, *J Clin Oncol* 19:1001-1007, 2001.
63. Armstrong DK and others: Randomized phase III study of intravenous (IV) paclitaxel and cisplatin vs. IV paclitaxel, intraperitoneal (IP) cisplatin, and IP paclitaxel in optimal stage III epithelial ovarian cancer (OC): a Gynecologic Oncology Group trial (GOG 172), *Proc Am Soc Clin Oncol* 21:803, 2002.
64. Belotti D and others: The microtubule-affecting drug paclitaxel has antiangiogenic activity, *Clin Cancer Res* 2: 1843-1849, 1996.
65. Fennelly D and others: Phase I and pharmacologic study of paclitaxel administered weekly in patients with relapsed ovarian cancer, *J Clin Oncol* 15:187-192, 1997.
66. Kaern J, Baekelandt M, Trope CG: A phase II study of weekly paclitaxel in platinum and paclitaxel-resistant ovarian cancer patients, *Eur J Gynaecol Oncol* 23:383-389, 2002.
67. Markman M and others: Phase II trial of weekly single-agent paclitaxel in platinum/paclitaxel-refractory ovarian cancer, *J Clin Oncol* 20:2365-2369, 2002.
68. Dizon DS and others: Retrospective analysis of carboplatin and paclitaxel as initial second-line therapy for recurrent epithelial ovarian carcinoma: application toward a dynamic disease state model of ovarian cancer, *J Clin Oncol* 20:1238-1247, 2002.
69. Thomas H, Rosenberg P: Role of weekly paclitaxel in the treatment of advanced ovarian cancer, *Crit Rev Oncol Hematol* 244:S43-S51, 2002.
70. Debby A and others: Whole-abdomen, single-dose consolidation radiotherapy in patients with pathologically confirmed complete remission of advanced ovarian epithelial carcinoma: a long-term survival analysis, *Int J Gynecol Cancer* 14:794-798, 2004.
71. Gelblum D and others: Palliative benefit of external-beam radiation in the management of platinum refractory epithelial ovarian carcinoma, *Gynecol Oncol* 69:36-41, 1998.
72. Rustin GJ and others: Defining response of ovarian carcinoma to initial chemotherapy according to serum CA125, *J Clin Oncol* 14:1545-1551, 1996.
73. Ledermann JA, Wheeler S: How should we manage patients with "platinum-sensitive" recurrent ovarian cancer? *Cancer Invest* 22(Suppl 2):2-10, 2004.
74. Ozols RF: Chemotherapy of ovarian cancer, *Cancer Treat Res* 95:219-234, 1998.
75. Markman M and others: Tamoxifen in platinum-refractory ovarian cancer: a Gynecologic Oncology Group Ancillary Report, *Gynecol Oncol* 62:4-6, 1996.
76. Van Der Velden J and others: Tamoxifen in patients with advanced epithelial ovarian cancer, *Int J Gynecol Cancer* 5:301-305, 1995.

77. Bowman A and others: CA125 response is associated with estrogen receptor expression in a phase II trial of letrozole in ovarian cancer: identification of an endocrine-sensitive subgroup, *Clin Cancer Res* 8:2233-2239, 2002.
78. Blackledge G and others: Response of patients in phase II studies of chemotherapy in ovarian cancer: implications for patient treatment and the design of phase II trials, *Br J Cancer* 59:650-653, 1989.
79. Markman M and others: Second-line platinum therapy in patients with ovarian cancer previously treated with cisplatin, *J Clin Oncol* 9:389-393, 1991.
80. Parmar MK and others: Paclitaxel plus platinum-based chemotherapy versus conventional platinum-based chemotherapy in women with relapsed ovarian cancer: the ICON4/AGO-OVAR-2.2 trial, *Lancet* 361:2099-2106, 2003.
81. Gonzalez Martin A and others: Randomised phase II study of carboplatin vs. paclitaxel-carboplatin in platinum-sensitive recurrent advanced ovarian carcinoma with assessment of quality of life: a GEICO study (Spanish Group for Investigation on Ovarian Carcinoma), *Proc Am Soc Clin Oncol* 22:1812, 2003.
82. Van der Burg ME and others: Weekly cisplatin and daily oral etoposide is highly effective in platinum pretreated ovarian cancer, *Br J Cancer* 86:19-25, 2002.
83. Bolis G and others: Carboplatin alone vs carboplatin plus epidoxorubicin as second-line therapy for cisplatin- or carboplatin-sensitive ovarian cancer, *Gynecol Oncol* 81: 3-9, 2001.
84. Lund B and others: Phase II study of gemcitabine (2',2'-difluorodeoxycytidine) in previously treated ovarian cancer patients, *J Natl Cancer Inst* 86:1530-1533, 1994.
85. Du Bois A and others: Second-line carboplatin and gemcitabine in platinum sensitive ovarian cancer—a dose-finding study by the Arbeitsgemeinschaft Gynakologische Onkologie (AGO) Ovarian Cancer Study Group, *Ann Oncol* 12:1115-1120, 2001.
86. Pfisterer J and others: Gemcitabine/carboplatin (GC) vs. carboplatin (C) in platinum sensitive recurrent ovarian cancer (OVCA). Results of a Gynaecologic Cancer Intergroup randomised phase III trial of the AGO, OVAR, the NCIC CTG and the EORTC GCG, *Proc Am Soc Clin Oncol* 22:450s, 2001.
87. Gordon, AN and others: Long-term survival advantage for women treated with pegylated liposomal doxorubicin compared with topotecan in a phase 3 randomized study of recurrent and refractory epithelial ovarian cancer. Gynecol Oncol 95:1-8, 2004.
88. Sundar S and others: Phase II trial of oxaliplatin and 5-fluorouracil/leucovorin combination in epithelial ovarian carcinoma relapsing within 2 years of platinum-based therapy, *Gynecol Oncol* 94:502-508, 2004.
89. Pectasides D and others: Oxaliplatin plus high-dose leucovorin and 5-fluorouracil (FOLFOX 4) in platinum-resistant and taxane-pretreated ovarian cancer: a phase II study, *Gynecol Oncol* 95:165-172, 2004.
90. See H, Kavanagh JJ: Novel agents in epithelial ovarian cancer, *Cancer Invest* 22(2):29-44, 2004.
91. Bookman MA and others: Evaluation of monoclonal humanized anti-HER2 antibody, trastuzumab, in patients with recurrent or refractory ovarian or primary peritoneal carcinoma with overexpression of HER2: a phase II trial of the Gynecologic Oncology Group, *J Clin Oncol* 21: 283-290, 2003.
92. Finkler N and others: Phase 2 evaluation of OSI-774, a potent oral antagonist of the EGFR-TK in patients with advanced ovarian carcinoma, *Proc Am Soc Clin Oncol* 20:208a, 2001.
93. Sewell JM and others: Targeting the EGF receptor in ovarian cancer with the tyrosine kinase inhibitor ZD 1839 ("Iressa"), *Br J Cancer* 86:456-462, 2002.
94. Finn RS and others: ZD1839 ("Iressa") acts synergistically with chemotherapy in ovarian cancer cells expressing high levels of the epidermal growth factor receptor, *Proc Am Soc Clin Oncol* 21:29b, 2002.
95. Schilder RJ and others: Phase II trial of gefitinib in patients with recurrent ovarian or primary peritoneal cancer. Gynecologic Oncology Group 170C, *Proc Am Soc Clin Oncol* 22:451, 2003.
96. Ehlen TG and others: Adjuvant treatment with monoclonal antibody, OvaRex MAb-B43.13 (OV) targeting CA125, induces robust immune responses associated with prolonged time to relapse (TTR) in a randomized, placebo-controlled study in patients (pts) with advanced epithelial ovarian cancer, *Proc Am Soc Clin Oncol* 21:Abstract 31, 2002.
97. Colombo N and others: Phase II and pharmacokinetics study of 3-hr infusion ET-743 in ovarian cancer patients failing platinum-taxanes, *Proc Am Soc Clin Oncol* 21:221a, 2002.
98. Davidson SA and others: A phase IIA trial of continuous 5-day infusions of MSI-1256F (squalamine lactate) plus carboplatin for therapy of persistent or recurrent advanced ovarian cancer, *Proc Am Soc Clin Oncol* 21: 220a, 2002.
99. Sabbatini P and others: Phase II study of CT-2103 in patients with recurrent epithelial ovarian, fallopian tube, or primary peritoneal carcinoma, *J Clin Oncol* 22: 4523-4531, 2004.
100. Kudelka A and others: Phase I study of CT-2103/cisplatin in patients with solid tumors, *Proc Am Soc Clin Oncol* 22: 457, 2003.
101. Nemunaitis J, Bolton MG: Phase I study of CT-2103 (Xyotax) with carboplatin in patients with solid tumors, Proc 12th Eur Cancer Conf, *Eur J Cancer* 1:S171, 2003.
102. Kavanagh JJ and others: Phase 2 study of TLK286 (GST P1-1 activated glutathione analog) administered weekly in patients with platinum refractory or resistant third-line advanced ovarian cancer, *Proc Am Soc Clin Oncol* 22: 452, 2003.
103. Kavanagh JJ and others: Phase II study of TLK 286 in patients with platinum resistance ovarian cancer, *Proc Am Soc Clin Oncol* 21:208a, 2002.
104. Puls LE and others: The prognostic implication of ascites in advanced-stage ovarian cancer, *Gynecol Oncol* 61:109-112, 1996.
105. Collins CA: Ascites, *Clin J Oncol Nurs* 5:43-45, 2001.
106. Kraemer K, Luynch MP: Ascites. In Preston FA, editor: *Clinical guidelines for symptom management in oncology*, New York, 1998, Clinical Insights Press.
107. Sansivero GE: Ascites. In Camp-Sorrell D, Hawkins RA, editors: *Clinical manual for the oncology advanced practice nurse*, Pittsburgh, 2000, Oncology Nursing Press.
108. Iyengar TD, Herzog TJ: Management of symptomatic ascites in recurrent ovarian cancer patients using an intra-abdominal semi-permanent catheter, *Am J Hosp Palliat Care* 19:7-8, 2002.

109. Kelvin JF, Scagiola J: Metastases involving the gastrointestinal system, *Semin Oncol Nurs* 14:187-198, 1999.
110. Pothuri B and others: Reoperation for palliation of recurrent malignant bowel obstruction in ovarian carcinoma, *Gynecol Oncol* 95:193-195, 2004.
111. Held-Warmkessel J: Bowel obstruction and ileus. In Camp-Sorrell D, Hawkins RA, editors: *Clinical manual for the oncology advanced practice nurse*, Pittsburgh, 2000, Oncology Nursing Press.
112. Waldman AR: Bowel obstruction, *Clin J Oncol Nurs* 5:281-286, 2001.
113. Jolicoeur L, Faught W: Managing bowel obstruction in ovarian cancer using a percutaneous endoscopic gastrostomy (PEG) tube, *Can Oncol Nurs J* 13:212-219, 2003.
114. McCorkle R, Pasacreta J, Tang ST: The silent killer: psychological issues in ovarian cancer, *Holistic Nurs Pract* 17:300-308, 2003.
115. Zabora J and others: The prevalence of psychological distress by cancer site, *Psycho-Oncol* 10:19-28, 2001.
116. Bodurka-Bevers D and others: Depression, anxiety, and quality of life in patients with epithelial ovarian cancer, *Gynecol Oncol* 78:302-308, 2000.
117. Ersek M and others: Quality of life in women with ovarian cancer, *Western J Nurs Res* 19:334-350, 1997.
118. Lakusta CM and others: Quality of life in ovarian cancer patients receiving chemotherapy, *Gynecol Oncol* 81: 490-495, 2001.
119. Howell D, Fitch MI, Deane KA: Impact of ovarian cancer perceived by women, *Cancer Nurs* 26:1-9, 2003.
120. Kornblith AB and others: Quality of life of women with ovarian cancer, *Gynecol Oncol* 59:231-242, 1995.
121. Guidozzi F: Living with ovarian cancer, *Gynecol Oncol* 50:202-207, 1993.
122. Burnett CB, Midler A, Steiner A: Concerns of women with ovarian cancer: a qualitative investigation, *Qual Life: A Nursing Challenge* 6:92-101, 1998.
123. Ferrell B and others: Psychological well being and quality of life in ovarian cancer survivors, *Cancer* 98:1061-1071, 2003.
124. Fitch MI, Gray RE, Franssen E: Women's perspectives regarding the impact of ovarian cancer, *Cancer Nurs* 23: 359-366, 2000.
125. Fitch M and others: Women's experiences with ovarian cancer: reflections on being diagnosed, *Can Oncol Nurs J* 12:152-159, 2002.
126. Howell D, Fitch MI, Deane KA: Women's experiences with recurrent ovarian cancer, *Cancer Nurs* 26:10-17, 2003.
127. Sivesind DM, Baile WF: An ovarian cancer support group, *Cancer Pract* 5:247-251, 1997.
128. Hamilton AB: Psychological aspects of ovarian cancer, *Cancer Invest* 17:335-413, 1999.
129. Stewart DE and others: "What doesn't kill you makes you stronger": an ovarian cancer survivor survey, *Gynecol Oncol* 83:537-542, 2001.
130. Weisman A: *Coping with Cancer*, New York, 1979, McGraw-Hill.
131. Weisman A: A model for psychosocial phasing in cancer. In Moos RH, editor: *Coping with physical illness*, New York, 1984, Plenum.

CHAPTER

8 Endometrial, Vulvar, and Vaginal Cancers

Lynn Cloutier

ENDOMETRIAL CANCER

INTRODUCTION AND OVERVIEW

Endometrial cancer is the most common gynecologic cancer and the fourth most common cancer in women in the US. Worldwide, it is the fifth most common cancer in women. In 2005, it is estimated that 40,800 cases of endometrial cancer will be diagnosed and 7,310 women will die of the disease. The death rate from endometrial cancer has been increasing. Between 1987 and 2003, deaths from endometrial cancer rose 134%.[1-3] Though the incidence of endometrial cancer rose rapidly for a while in the 1970s, presumably as a result of an increased use of unopposed menopausal estrogen therapy, it has since stabilized. However, its incidence is increasing in many economically underdeveloped countries. Five-year survival rates have not changed in 30 years.[2,4] For those patients with advanced disease, prognosis is poor, with a 5-year survival rate of approximately 27%.[5]

Endometrial cancer is a disease of postmenopausal women, and occurs infrequently (5%) in women under 40 years of age. Only 20% to 25% of women are diagnosed before menopause.[6] Most cases are diagnosed at an early stage. The probability of developing invasive cancer is small in women up to age 39. That probability doubles in women aged 60 to 79, in comparison with those aged 40 to 59.[2]

Approximately half of cases occur in women older than 65 years. In the US, the incidence rates of endometrial cancer are much higher for Caucasian women than for African American women. Although the incidence rate in Caucasian women has been declining over the past 30 years, it has remained steady for African American women. Importantly, however, the incidence-to-mortality ratio (the number of women who have endometrial cancer and die from the disease) is much lower—2:1, for African American women and 7:1 for Caucasian women. Thus even though a greater percentage of Caucasian women are diagnosed with endometrial cancer, a smaller percentage of them die from the disease. The ratio of incidence to mortality for Hawaiian women is 3:1. The smaller incidence-to-mortality ratios among African American and Hawaiian women suggest that access to health care may be an issue. It is likely that endometrial cancer in Caucasian women is diagnosed at an earlier stage and thus easier to treat.[7]

EPIDEMIOLOGY

Endometrial cancer is considered an estrogen-dependent disease. Chronic exposure to estrogen, either endogenous or exogenous, without the accompanying balancing effects of progesterone, is considered the major risk factor for endometrial cancer and may play a causal role in the development of the disease. Any factor that leads to increased relative exposure to estrogen over time also leads to an increased risk of endometrial cancer. A precancerous condition called endometrial hyperplasia, or adenomatous hyperplasia, may cause irregular uterine bleeding. This condition can be mild, moderate, or severe. Severe hyperplasia with atypia is considered carcinoma in situ, the earliest detectable stage of endometrial cancer.

ETIOLOGY AND RISK FACTORS

Endometrial cancer refers specifically to tumors that originate in the glandular mucosa of the innermost lining of the uterus. The mucosa is dependent on cyclical changes in estrogen and progesterone, and any condition that leads to an abnormal imbalance in these hormones is the most causative factor.

- **Chronic Estrogen Exposure:** the best-recognized risk factor is chronic estrogen exposure, either endogenous or exogenous.
- **Age:** 65% of women with endometrial cancer are 60 to 70 years old. Only 5% are less than 40.[2,6,7]
- **Obesity:** Studies have estimated that women with excess body weight have a 2 to 5 times greater risk of developing endometrial cancer than women with no excess body weight. This correlation is likely due to the face that fat cells (adipocytes) convert androstenedione to estrone, creating chronic estrogen exposure. Obesity has a particularly strong association with endometrial cancer, with morbidly obese women having a 9 times increased risk for the disease as compared to ideal body weight counterparts. Of women with uterine cancer, 78.6% have comorbidities; the most common is an increased body mass index (BMI), usually greater than 40. Obese women develop endometrial cancer through a hormone-dependent pathway (type I end CA), in comparison to thin women who may develop the disease through autonomous oncogenesis (type II).[8]
- **Diabetes Mellitus and Hypertension:** The relationship between these risk factors and endometrial cancer is unclear, although obesity may play a role. An interaction between obesity and diabetes significantly increases the risk of endometrial cancer.[9] Women with a history of diabetes mellitus are twice as likely to develop endometrial cancer. Type I diabetes carries a greater risk than type 2 diabetes. Hypertension may increase risk among obese women.[10]
- **Few or No Children:** Pregnancy is a period of intense progesterone stimulation by the placenta. Because progesterone counterbalances the growth-stimulating effects of estrogen, women who have experienced pregnancy are at a lower risk for developing endometrial cancer. Nulliparity is often associated with infertility, which is an independent risk factor for endometrial cancer. Conditions associated with infertility are Stein-Leventhal syndrome (polycystic ovary syndrome) and granulose-thecal cell ovarian tumors.[8]
- **Early Menarche and Late Menopause:** Late menopause (and possibly early age at menarche) is both associated with more estrogen exposure. Women who started menstruating at an early age or stopped at a late age might have a higher risk for developing endometrial cancer. Women with a menstrual span longer than 39 years have 4.2 times the risk of women with menstrual history of a 25 years or less.[9]
- **Unopposed Estrogen Replacement Therapy:** Estrogen replacement therapy that is used to relieve the symptoms of menopause puts women at high risk for endometrial cancer. It is believed that the increase in endometrial cancer that occurred in the United States in the 1970s was due to the introduction and widespread use of unopposed estrogen as postmenopausal hormone therapy. The risk is reduced when the estrogen is combined with progesterone.[8]
- **Tamoxifen:** Tamoxifen is an antiestrogenic drug and is the most widely prescribed hormonal treatment for women with breast cancer. One of the side effects of tamoxifen is that it induces growth of noncancerous uterine tumors, some of which develop into endometrial cancer. Only 1 in 500 women who are taking tamoxifen develop endometrial cancer, and the small risk is more than justified by the enormous benefits that tamoxifen can have for women with breast cancer.[8]

- **Genetic Predisposition/Family History:** Some women appear to have a genetic predisposition to endometrial cancer. The risk may approach 50% in some families. But these account for few cases of endometrial cancer overall. Women with a family history or hereditary nonpolyposis colon cancer (HNPCC) are predisposed to develop endometrial cancer before the age of 50.[8]
- **Previous Cancer:** Women who have had cancer of the breast, colon, or ovary are at an increased risk for developing endometrial cancer. The time interval between diagnosis of the two different cancers can be as long as ten years.[7]

SCREENING

Routine screening of women for endometrial cancer has not proven to be beneficial. Screening for endometrial cancer is beneficial in those women who are identified as an "at risk" population. Those women include premenopausal women with anovulatory cycles (polycystic ovarian syndrome/Stein-Leventhal syndrome), and women with a family history. About 50% to 70% of hereditary uterine cancers are linked to the HNPCC syndrome, also known as Lynch syndrome. This syndrome is due to mutations in DNA mismatch repair genes. At least five of these genes are known. In addition to an increased uterine cancer risk, there are increased risks for colon, ovarian, stomach, bile duct, and urinary tract cancers. In women with a genetic predisposition, cancers occur at an earlier age than in the general population. All women should be informed about the risks and symptoms of endometrial cancer, and counseled to report any unexpected bleeding or spotting to their doctors. For women with or at high risk for HNPCC, annual screening should be offered for endometrial cancer with endometrial biopsy beginning at age 35.[2] The American Cancer Society recommends that all women at high risk for endometrial cancer (e.g., women with a history of infertility or obesity) should undergo an endometrial biopsy at menopause.[7]

CLINICAL FACTORS

More than 90% of women with endometrial cancer complain of postmenopausal bleeding or irregular vaginal bleeding,[11] and one of three women who develop vaginal bleeding after menopause is found to have endometrial cancer. Other symptoms associated with endometrial cancer may be difficult or painful urination or pain during intercourse. In later stages of the disease, women may feel pelvic pain and experience unexplained weight loss. Symptoms that occur may include the following:

- Unusual bleeding, spotting, or vaginal discharge
- Abdominal cramps, which are caused when the tumor blocks the cervical canal and keeps the blood from being expelled
- Postmenopausal bleeding
- Irregular bleeding in younger women. Profuse bleeding that does not stop in a few days like a normal menstrual cycle should be screened.
- In advanced stages, symptoms include intense lumbosacral pain, weight loss, and anemia.

PREVENTION

Prevention is aimed at decreasing exposure to unopposed estrogen, either exogenous or endogenous. Early detection is the best prevention from developing invasive endometrial cancer. As the disease progresses, the chances of survival decrease markedly. Average 5-year survival rates for endometrial cancer are 90% for stage I, 60% for stage II, 40% for stage III, and 5% for stage IV. Treating precancerous hyperplasia with hormones (progestins), a hysterectomy, or a D & C (dilatation and curettage) can prevent abnormal, precancerous cells from developing into cancer. Progesterone may be used to treat endometrial hyperplasia and subsequently stop the transition to a cancerous condition. About 10% to 30% of all hyperplasia cases eventually develop into cancer, if left untreated.[7] Any woman with abnormal vaginal bleeding should visit her physician immediately.

DIAGNOSIS

A thorough history and physical examination is required for those women with a suspicion of endometrial cancer. The most important symptom used to diagnose endometrial cancer is abnormal vaginal bleeding. Postmenopausal bleeding is the classic symptom for 90% of all endometrial cancer cases. Perimenopausal women relate a history of intermenstrual bleeding, excessive bleeding lasting longer than 7 days, or an interval of less than 21 days between menses. Heavy, prolonged bleeding in patients known to be at risk for anovulatory cycles should be followed up by histologic evaluation of the endometrium. Eighty percent of postmenopausal women will have a complaint of abnormal purulent or blood-tinged vaginal discharge. Physical examination of the abdomen may reveal ascites; further evaluation may show omental and liver metastases. Some women will first be seen with pelvic pain and may have retained blood in the uterine cavity (hematometra) related to cervical stenosis.

Hematometra may present as a large, midline mass arising from the pelvis. These patients require surgical intervention to obtain a specimen of the endometrium. A careful pelvic exam should be performed with inspection and palpation of the vulva, vagina, and cervix to exclude metastatic spread or other causes of abnormal vaginal bleeding. The uterus may or may not be enlarged. A rectovaginal exam should be performed to evaluate the fallopian tubes, ovaries and cul-de-sac.[12] Women with endometrial cells on a Pap smear should be evaluated, particularly if atypical cells are present. Fifteen percent of women in the general population with postmenopausal bleeding will develop endometrial cancer.[13] Presenting symptoms of advanced disease include pelvic pressure, ascites, and hemorrhage; these are related to uterine enlargement and extrauterine spread of tumor.[6,14] All patients suspected of having endometrial cancer should have endocervical curettage and an endometrial biopsy. If the biopsy in a symptomatic patient is negative, then further examination by D & C under anesthesia is warranted.[15] Because abnormal uterine bleeding is an important symptom of endometrial cancer, a woman who has unexplained uterine bleeding should have her endometrial tissue sampled. This can be done by aspiration, biopsy, or curettage of the endometrium. Transvaginal ultrasound may be effective in evaluating symptomatic patients whose tissue specimen is nondiagnostic. If either a biopsy or D & C reveals hyperplasia or endometrial cancer, the extent of the disease must be determined with other tests. The tissue that is sampled from either procedure is sent to a laboratory, where the cells can be examined under a microscope and evaluated for any abnormalities. If cancerous cells are found, the type of cancer and tumor grade is evaluated.

Pretreatment Medical Evaluation

When a woman is diagnosed with endometrial cancer, the extent of the disease and an optimal treatment plan must be determined. The treatment of endometrial cancer requires surgery, unless for some reason a woman cannot or chooses not to have surgery; therefore the pretreatment evaluation usually focuses on determining whether the disease has spread to other parts of the body and is inoperable. Metastasis to other parts of the body is uncommon for endometrial cancer. Metastases occur via local extension to adjacent structures such as the cervix and vagina. Metastasis to local lymph nodes occurs via lymphangitic spread. Distant metastasis is rare. Tumors in the lung, for example, occur in only 2% to 3% of all endometrial cancer patients. Hematologic involvement by endometrial cancer is very rare.

Imaging Studies

Imaging can assist in two main respects: (1) determining the local extent of the tumor; and (2) determining evidence of extrauterine spread, particularly lymph node metastases and, less often, direct spread to the tissues surrounding the uterus.

In all cases, a chest radiograph (CXR) is mandatory to look for metastases and evaluate the cardiopulmonary status of the patient. Magnetic resonance imaging (MRI) may be the most accurate technique for assessing the local extent of disease in terms of myometrial invasion and cervical involvement. MRI and computerized tomography (CT) cannot replace surgical evaluation of nodes.[16] Transvaginal sonography (TVS) is considered useful for identifying endometrial malignancies; it is a very sensitive study but not very specific, since it has a low positive value and a high false-positive rate. TVS is useful for identification of patients who require further diagnostic evaluation including endometrial biopsy. TVS may also be helpful in determining which patients should have a biopsy and useful for surveillance in women on tamoxifen therapy.[17] TVS has been studied as an alternative to hysteroscopy, which is an invasive procedure.[18] More extensive preoperative assessment such as MRI, CT scan, or barium enema may be indicated for patients whose disease has features that put them at high risk for metastases (e.g., poorly differentiated, papillary serous, clear cell, or sarcomatous histologic study results). Evaluation for metastases is indicated in patients with abnormal liver function tests, clinical evidence of metastases, and parametrial or vaginal tumor extension. For locally advanced disease, cystoscopy, proctoscopy, and/or barium enema should be obtained.

HISTOLOGY

Type I, or adenocarcinoma, is the most common pathology and comprises the majority of cases. Of all endometrial cancers, 97% are adenocarcinomas with endometrioid the most common histologic subtype.[19] Atypical hyperplasia is the malignant precursor of the more common endometrioid adenocarcinomas. Endometrial hyperplasia is an overgrowth of the endometrial lining of the uterus that results from prolific stimulation of the endometrium. This presents clinically as abnormal bleeding. It can occur in progesterone-deficient young women who are infertile because of anovulation.[20] Hyperplasia with atypia is a complex pattern with crowding of the glands. The presence of atypical cells indicates high risk for the progression to cancer. Hyperplasia and endometrial cancers are two different entities, and the distinguishing feature is the presence or absence of cytologic atypia. These two cytologic variants can exist simultaneously. Seventy-five percent of women with a typical hyperplasia have a history of exposure to unopposed estrogen, either exogenous or endogenous. There are three grades of adenocarcinomas based on the percentage of tumor growth: grade 1, grade 2, and grade 3. Grade 1 tumors are the least solid. They have at least 95% normal endometrial tissue, and the glands that are so prominent in the endometrium are distinct from the cancer cells. Grade 3 tumors are characterized by solid tumor growth, and the endometrial glands are not well differentiated.[13]

Type II endometrial cancers are less common and can appear simultaneously with hyperplasia, but are not clearly related to a transition from atypical hyperplasia. They arise in a background of inert or atrophic endometrium and are associated with more undifferentiated cell types, lower overall survival rates, and a higher risk of metastatic disease at the time of surgical staging. Patients with serous (also known as papillary serous) and clear cell carcinomas tend to be older than those with other types and are more likely to have abnormal cervical cytologic features. A minority of women develop these types of endometrial cancer, and these neoplasms tend to be associated with a more undifferentiated cell type and a poorer prognosis.[13]

STAGING

Originally, endometrial cancer was staged by physical exam, radiologic exam, and sounding of the uterus. Surgical staging replaced clinical staging in 1988, when it was found that clinical staging alone was inadequate and inconsistent, leading to either undertreatment or overtreatment. Surgical staging allowed for the identification of patients at risk for treatment failure. Uterine findings and presence or absence of lymph node metastases was recommended to guide adjuvant therapy options. In a recent retrospective analysis of 153 cases,[21] preoperative tumor grade did not accurately predict histologic study results. Thus all patients with endometrial cancer should undergo lymph node staging.

Surgical staging has become the standard of care for the treatment of women with endometrial cancer. Although the extent of staging has not yet been defined, growing evidence suggests that preoperative studies and intraoperative clinical opinion cannot be consistently counted on to be predictive of postoperative histologic status.[22] The main goal of staging a cancer is to determine the extent of the disease before treatment begins and to evaluate an appropriate treatment protocol. Endometrial tumors are also graded to aid in the evaluation. Most endometrial cancers are staged according to the surgical system approved in 1988 by the International Federation of Gynecology and Obstetrics (Table 8-1). Factors used to stage the disease include the depth of the tumor, whether the tumor has spread to the cervix and other nearby organs, the cytologic features of the cancer (the cellular make-up and activity), whether it has metastasized to the lymph nodes, and the extent to which it has spread to other parts of the body. If a patient does not undergo surgical evaluation, because of her age or other conditions that make surgery prohibitive, then the older, a clinical staging system is used.

TREATMENT

The extent of treatment and prognosis are strongly dependent on stage and grade. Prognosis is dependent on the following:[9,15]

- Histologic cell type
- Tumor grade
- Depth of myometrial involvement
- Extension into cervix
- Vascular space invasion
- Patient age

About two thirds of newly diagnosed women with endometrial cancer have early-stage tumor confined to the uterus with favorable prognostic factors, and are typically cured with surgery with or without adjuvant radiation therapy. The remaining one third of women newly diagnosed with endometrial cancer have more advanced disease (e.g., FIGO stages III and IV) and have poor prognostic features. The depth of myometrial invasion—especially invasion of the outer third of the myometrium, cervical involvement, high-grade histologic variants (e.g., serous-papillary and clear cell), and aortic node involvement all appear to be important signs of more aggressive

Table **8-1** FIGO® SURGICAL STAGES FOR ENDOMETRIAL CANCER

Stage	Description
0	Carcinoma in situ
Stage I	The tumour is confined to the corpus uteri
Stage IA	The tumour is limited to the endometrium
Stage IB	The tumour invades up to less than one half of the myometrium
Stage IC	The tumour invades to more than one half of the myometrium
Stage II	The tumour invades the cervix but does not extend beyond uterus
Stage IIA	Endocervical glandular involvement only
Stage IIB	Cervical stromal invasion
Stage III	There is local and regional spread as specified in IIIA, IIIB, or IIIC
Stage IIIA	The tumour involves the serosa and/or adnexa and/or cancer cells in ascites or peritoneal washings
Stage IIIB	Vaginal involvement (direct extension or metastasis)
Stage IIIC	Metastasis to pelvic and/or paraaortic lymph nodes
Stage IVA	Tumour invades bladder mucosa and/or bowel mucosa
Stage IVB	Distant metastasis (excluding metastasis to vagina, pelvic serosa, or adnexa, including metastasis to intraabdominal lymph nodes other than the paraaortic and or inguinal nodes)

From International Federation of Gynecology and Obstetrics: Staging classifications and clinical practice guidelines of gynaecologic cancers, 2003: www.figo.org. Reprinted with permission.

disease that is prone to metastasize to distant sites.[11,23-25] Vascular space invasion is associated with both lymphatic and hematogenous dissemination.[26,27] The presence of deep myometrial invasion is the strongest predictor of hematogenous dissemination in endometrial cancer and, together with stage IV disease, independently predicts lung recurrence.[26]

Age has been found to be a predictor of survival for endometrial cancer unrelated to surgical stage or grade of adenocarcinoma. As the age of the woman increases, factors such as advanced disease at time of diagnosis and deep myometrial invasion cause survival rates to decline.[13] Standard therapies include surgery, radiation therapy (RT), chemotherapy, and hormonal therapy. The best outcomes are associated with surgery, or surgery in combination with RT.[28] Women who have endometrial cancer with high-risk features or documented extrauterine disease require adjuvant therapy.

Surgery

Gynecologic oncologists are more likely to offer comprehensive surgical care for all women with endometrial cancer.[22] However, only one third of all women with endometrial cancer are seen preoperatively by a gynecologic oncologist.[29-31] The majority of patients are medically able to undergo surgery. The treatment generally recommended for patients with endometrial cancer is total abdominal hysterectomy with staging.[15] A hysterectomy can be either abdominal or vaginal. In an abdominal hysterectomy, the surgeon makes an incision in the front of the abdomen and removes the uterus. In a vaginal hysterectomy, the uterus is removed through the vagina. Because endometrial cancer originates in the uterine body, a hysterectomy should be sufficient, but the ovaries are removed because they are the most common sites of undetected metastasis. Also, most women who undergo the surgery are postmenopausal, and their ovaries are no longer providing the hormonal function that is so important before menopause. During an abdominal hysterectomy, the lymph nodes are also almost always sampled (a pelvic lymph node dissection) to detect any spread of cancer to the lymph nodes.

Operative laparoscopy, combined with vaginal hysterectomy, is an alternative to laparotomy for patients with early-stage endometrial cancer. Laparoscopy is also used in patients who were incompletely staged initially. Thus women can opt for a vaginal hysterectomy and still have their lymph nodes examined. This method involves inserting a tube through a very small opening in the abdomen. The vaginal hysterectomy, combined with the laparoscope, is much less invasive and requires less recovery time than an abdominal hysterectomy. In a survey of members of the Society of Gynecologic Oncologists, 56% of respondents were proponents of laparoscopic-assisted vaginal hysterectomy. Laparoscopic lymph node dissection is appropriate first-line treatment for uterine cancer, showing no difference in survival when compared to those patients treated with traditional abdominal hysterectomy.[22]

Vaginal hysterectomy has a high rate of cure for elderly patients and also for those women with multiple medical comorbidities with endometrial cancer. The long-term survival following vaginal operations was comparable to that after standard abdominal approach, with better operative outcomes.[32]

Radiation Therapy

Primary radiation therapy with curative intent is reserved for those women who are medically inoperable and have been clinically staged. This includes patients with advanced age and severe cardiopulmonary disease or compromise and those with extreme morbid obesity. Disease-specific survival rates may be 10% to 20% lower than for patients of similar clinical stage who undergo surgery. In patients at high risk for relapse after surgery, radiation therapy is used, most often with concurrent chemotherapy as a sensitizing agent to improve loco-regional control. Radiation procedures include external beam radiation therapy, brachytherapy, and whole pelvic and whole abdomen radiation therapy; P-32 (radioactive phosphorus-32) may be used as intraperitoneal radioactive treatment. These procedures are shown to have an impact on the local control of disease, but not on survival. For some women with high-grade lesions and/or cervical involvement, brachytherapy may be performed before surgery. Vaginal vault brachytherapy used postoperatively has been shown to increase survival and disease-free interval.[33]

High-risk histologic tumor types, such as papillary serous and clear cell, and presence of lymphvascular space invasion (LVSI), deep invasion, or grade 3 lesions may warrant adjuvant radiation therapy. Patients with paraaortic and pelvic lymph node involvement should receive radiation therapy to the involved field.[34]

Vaginal radiation can be delivered with high-dose-rate (HDR) or low-dose-rate (LDR) radiation equipment. Both techniques have resulted in excellent local control rates and low morbidity. Each technique has its advantages. HDR treatments require multiple insertions, generally with one insertion done every week for 3 to 6 weeks. However, hospitalization is not required, and each insertion takes only a brief amount of time, approximately 10 minutes. LDR treatments are delivered once but do require hospitalization for 2 to 3 days.[13] HDR vaginal brachytherapy in thoroughly staged patients with intermediate-risk endometrial cancer provides excellent overall and disease-free survival with less toxicity and less cost compared with whole pelvic radiation.[35,36]

Adjuvant whole pelvic radiation therapy is an effective treatment for stage I to stage III endometrial cancer with high-risk pathologic factors for intraabdominal recurrence, including serous papillary and clear cell variants.[25] Intraoperative radiation therapy (IORT) is used as a boost technique in patients who would otherwise require high doses of external radiation therapy. IORT treatment can deliver a single high dose of radiation to a tumor or tumor bed after surgical resection. A linear accelerator that produces high-energy electron beams is used to deliver precise, highly concentrated doses of radiation directly to the tumor site while avoiding adjacent normal tissues. A single dose delivered in one treatment during a surgical procedure is equivalent to several weeks of daily radiation treatments.[37] The rationale for this treatment is to increase the therapeutic ratio of local tumor control without significantly increasing the risk of complication. IORT has been used at various medical centers as a component of aggressive treatment approaches for locally advanced primary or recurrent gynecologic cancers.

The use of intraoperative radiation therapy in the treatment of endometrial cancer continues to be studied. Palliative radiation therapy may be used in women with isolated advanced or recurrent disease located in areas not previously irradiated. When palliation is the goal of therapy, it is important to fully evaluate the patient's medical status.[28] In advanced disease, namely stages III and IV, radiation therapy, chemotherapy, and hormonal therapy are employed.

Hormonal Therapy

Endocrine or hormonal therapy is used in treating endometrial cancer with the aim of prolonging the progression-free interval and time to recurrence in Stage I and Stage II lesions after initial surgery and RT. Conservative management with progestational agents has an effect on patients with well-differentiated adenocarcinoma and who are at high risk for surgical morbidity.[38] It has been shown that the increasing of the dose of the medication does not offer a greater response; therefore higher doses leading to a higher side effect profile are not advocated. The best responders to hormonal therapy are those with well-differentiated lesions and positive estrogen receptors (ER) and progesterone receptors (PR) disease.[39,40]

Depo-Provera, Provera, Delalutin, and Megace are the most common progestational agents currently used for women who are ER- and PR-positive.[41] Although regarded as an antiestrogen in breast tissue, tamoxifen is known to have estrogenic or agonist activity at other sites.[42] Tamoxifen blocks the binding of estradiol to the ER of endometrial carcinomas. The benefit of treatment with the drug should outweigh the risk of thromboembolic events and weight gain in women who may already be obese.[43]

Advances in hormonal and chemotherapy have emerged from studies using mifepristone, aromatase inhibitors, and selected estrogen receptor modulators, also known as SERMs. Mifepristone is an antiprogesterone and noncompeting antiestrogen. It blocks the capacity of the endometrial tissue to grow in response to estrogen. It fights tumors that have progesterone receptors by binding those receptors and also by blocking the growth of new blood vessels that the cancer needs to grow.

Aromatase expression is hormonally controlled in adipose cells. Aromatase activity has been reported in endometrial cancer cell lines and endometrial cancer tissues. Disease-free endometrium does not express aromatase. Treatment with aromatase inhibitors decreases cell proliferation in endometrial cancer cells.

SERMs mimic the effect of estrogens in some tissues, but act as estrogen antagonists in others. All SERMs act by binding with high affinity to the estrogen receptor, and yet produce tissue- and drug-specific responses.[42] SERMs are ER-antagonists in the uterus. SERM studies show that the new SERMs are better antagonists in the endometrium, the basic mechanism of action again binding both ER sites. Each SERM has a specific affinity for the organ-specific ER alpha and/or ER beta that leads to the unique conformation of the ER-SERM complex. This structure allows coregulatory proteins to induce or stop gene activation.[44] SERMs have low toxicity and are easily administered. Progestins, tamoxifen, SERMs and gonadotropin releasing hormone agonists have shown to affect patients with advanced or recurrent endometrial cancer.[45] While less toxic than chemotherapy, hormonal agents are associated with and increased risk for DVT and cardiovascular side effects, which can be problematic when used in an elderly population.

Chemotherapy

Studies have not yet produced clear results on the effectiveness of chemotherapy to treat endometrial cancer. Chemotherapy is potentially most useful for cancers that have spread to distant parts of the body. Systemic therapy is required in cases of initial advanced disease and at the time of relapse. The number of effective chemotherapeutic agents has been found to be limited.[46] Although several agents have been shown to induce clinical responses, most of these responses were partial and of short duration.

Chemotherapy has a role in endometrial cancer in patients with a high risk of relapse, those with stage IIIB or high-grade disease, and those with stage III or stage IV papillary serous histologic features. Also, those women with recurrent disease may benefit from chemotherapy.[46]

The chemotherapy modality may be a single agent, multiple agents, or a combination therapy with radiation. Active agents include doxorubicin, cisplatin, carboplatin, and paclitaxel. In clinical trials enrolling women with advanced or recurrent disease, it has been shown that multiagent therapy with a taxane, anthracycline, and platinum regimen is most effective and may increase survival rates from 50% to 59%. Studies have also shown that the combination of platinum, doxorubicin, and cyclophosphamide has improved the 5-year survival rate in women with stage I and stage II disease;[47] however, the outcome for stage III patients is still unfavorable depending on the degree of LVSI and deep myometrial invasion.[48] Carboplatin has a low toxicity and is active in chemotherapy-naïve advanced endometrial cancer patients. The choice of the initial dose can be determined according to whether the patient has received prior radiotherapy.[49]

Paclitaxel is an active agent in the treatment of endometrial cancer in patients who have had previous chemotherapy or advanced disease.[50] The Gynecologic Oncology Group (GOG) has reported a 35% response rate in previously untreated women.[9]

Combination Therapy

Most studies examining the use of chemotherapy with radiation therapy in the treatment of endometrial cancer show efficacy; however, they are of small numbers. Studies combining cyclophosphamide, doxorubicin, and cisplatin with radiation have shown 5-year survival up to 84%.[51] Paclitaxel, doxorubicin, and carboplatin with radiation in patients with high-risk endometrial cancer provides both local control and systemic control in advanced endometrial or endometrial cancer of any stage with high-risk histologic features.[52] In patients with advanced, recurrent, or refractory disease, the use of paclitaxel, carboplatin and amifostine has been shown to be of benefit to those women in this clinically difficult situation.[53]

RECURRENT DISEASE

Recurrence is more likely in women with advanced disease and in those whose tumor had certain high-risk features such as deep myometrial invasion, moderately or poorly differentiated tumors, or cervical involvement. Usually recurrence happens within 3 years of the original diagnosis.[7] Recurrent endometrial cancer is initially confined to the pelvis in 50% of patients. The major sites of distant metastases are the abdominal cavity, the liver, and the lungs.[13] The treatment of recurrent disease is dependent upon the location, extent, and nature of recurrence.

Isolated recurrences, most often seen in the vagina, are still highly curable, especially if confined to the pelvis and are treated definitively with surgery or RT. Patients with recurrent endometrial cancer confined to the pelvis should be treated with external pelvic irradiation and intracavitary or interstitial brachytherapy.[28]

Selected patients with isolated central pelvic recurrence may benefit from pelvic exenteration. The procedure consists of hysterectomy with bilateral salpingo-oophorectomy, removal of the vagina, rectum, bladder, urethra, and supporting structures. The procedure carries with it a potential for both physiologic and psychosexual morbidity. Although the long-term survival rate after this procedure is only 20%, it remains the only potentially curative option for the few patients with central recurrence of endometrial cancer who have not responded to standard surgery and radiation therapy.[13] Systemic recurrences may be treated with chemotherapy.[13,19] Chemotherapy for recurrent disease is palliative. Agents in GOG studies include doxorubicin, cisplatin, ifosfamide, and paclitaxel.[41] Topotecan has been shown to have activity in women with advanced or recurrent endometrial cancer who have not received prior cytotoxic therapy; however, more studies are needed to determine the maximum tolerated dose (MTD) and the most efficacious dose, in light of the intolerable side effects of hematologic and gastrointestinal toxicities and neurotoxicities. Support with hematopoietic growth factors is also necessary.[54-56] Burke and others[57] reported a response rate of 45% in 87 evaluable patients with advanced or recurrent disease when using the combination of doxorubicin, cisplatin, and cyclophosphamide. Progression-free survival was limited to 4.8 months.

Patients with recurrent endometrial carcinoma often receive hormonal therapy with progestins. These agents most often offer only palliation, but with minimal toxicity. Response rates to progestins range from 15% to 30%, and therapy can be continued indefinitely.[13,58] Tamoxifen has been used in the treatment of endometrial cancer both in the salvage setting and as a first-line systemic therapy, although it has not been found as active as progestins and is of little value as second-line therapy in patients who do not respond to progestins.[13] Hormone therapy can be used to treat recurrent disease. If an objective response is obtained, the progestin should be continued indefinitely.[15]

IMPLICATIONS FOR PRACTICE, EDUCATION, AND RESEARCH

One in ten women with uterine cancer may have a genetic predisposition for the disease. Genetic cancer risk assessment should be considered if a woman has any of the following:

- Uterine cancer before age 50
- Uterine cancer and another cancer such as colon, ovarian, stomach, or bile duct
- A history of colon polyps before age 40
- Family member with any of the above

Obese women should consider weight reduction with the assistance of a health care professional. Women should be encouraged to eat a diet low in fat and with the majority of food items coming from the vegetable, fruit, and whole grains categories. Data support the conclusion that many survivors exercise less often and have a higher rate of obesity. A study[59] found that exercise and BMI were meaningfully and independently associated with quality of life (QOL). Too little exercise and high BMI have an additive effect on poor QOL. These findings were not altered after controlling for important demographic and medical variables. Like many other cancer survivor populations, the majority of endometrial cancer survivors do not obtain adequate exercise for health benefits.[59] This increased rate of obesity places these survivors at greater risk than the general population for hypertension, diabetes, cardiovascular disease, and cancers.[60]

FOLLOW-UP CARE

Follow-up for women who have endometrial cancer and subsequent therapy is every 2 to 4 months for 2 to 3 years depending on the risk recurrence, then a revisit 6-month schedule is recommended.[20] Several goals for follow-up for women with endometrial cancer are identified: (1) early detection and treatment of recurrent disease, (2) psychologic support of the patient, (3) provision of health maintenance and other screening services, and (4) diagnosis and management of treatment side effects.

Premature Menopause

Women who undergo removal of their ovaries during treatment for endometrial cancer will become menopausal. Because of the lack of estrogen, the patient may report hot flashes and/or night sweats. Patients need to be apprised of interventions that may assist in decreasing frequency of hot flashes and night sweats. Relief can be achieved by (1) general measures such as reduction of caffeine and nicotine, avoidance of warmth, exercise in fresh air, breathing and relaxation exercises, and a balanced diet; (2) treatment with phytopreparations; (3) treatment trial with medroxyprogesterone or megestrol acetate; (4) low-dose estrogen therapy with vaginal gel/cream, offering nonsystemic relief of urogenital symptoms; and (5) administration of opipramol or an SSRI such as venlafaxine if the patient declines hormonal treatment.[61]

Hormone therapy can be given after endometrial cancer surgery in women with stage I disease. Prospective randomized studies are needed to ensure safety in those women with higher stage diseases. A review of estrogen replacement in patients with stages I and II endometrial cancer found no difference in progression-free or overall survival associated with estrogen use. Of note, 53% of patients treated with estrogen received progestin therapy. In addition, patients with estrogen replacement had a lower-stage and lower-grade cancer, and also less depth of invasion, as compared to patients who did not receive estrogen. There are studies in progress that may possibly resolve the issue of HRT in the endometrial cancer patient. The patient may also report decreased vaginal lubrication, vaginal burning and pruritus, and dyspareunia. Nurses can advise on the use of a vaginal moisturizer to restore moisture to vaginal mucosa, and water-based lubricants to facilitate sexual relations. Patients may also report joint pain and backache as a result of osteoporosis. A calcium supplement and physical exercise are essential in protecting against bone loss.[20]

Early and Late Effects of Treatment

Lower extremity lymphedema is a potential acute and chronic complication of lymph node dissection.[62] Treatment consists of elevation of the lower extremities; compression therapy, with elastic stockings, ace wrapping, or compression devices; manual massage; exercise; and effective skin care. Obvious avoidance of injuries and activities that impede lymphatic flow are stressed. Early and late side effects of radiation therapy include diarrhea, dysuria, and urinary frequency and can extend to fistulas, bladder irritation, and vaginal stenosis. Symptom management with appropriate medications should be employed to prevent or stop acute symptoms. Chronic use of a vaginal dilator may be necessary to prevent problems with vaginal shortening and stenosis following brachytherapy and teletherapy. Management of fistulas ranges from conservative management with total parenteral nutrition (TPN), somatostatin, and bowel rest to use of aggressive surgical procedures. Patients may also have neurotoxicity issues from the use of cisplatin and taxanes. Peripheral foot and hand care is important, and the possible deep tendon effect must be addressed to keep patients mobile and safe.

VULVAR INTRAEPITHELIAL NEOPLASIA

INCIDENCE

Vulvar intraepithelial neoplasia (VIN) is dysplasia involving the epidermis. The condition is uncommon, approximately 1.8 new cases per 100,000 women, with a greater tendency for occurrence in younger women.

EPIDEMIOLOGY

VIN-1 corresponds to the basal third of cells exhibiting dysplasia, VIN-2 includes the basal two thirds, and VIN-3 includes the full thickness.[63] The three levels of dysplasia are divided into two clinically meaningful categories. Low-grade VIN includes subclinical human papillomavirus (HPV) infection and VIN-1 or mild dysplasia. High-grade VIN includes VIN-2 moderate dysplasia and VIN-3 dysplasia/carcinoma in situ.[64]

ETIOLOGY AND RISK FACTORS

HPV is associated with VIN in 86% of cases.[63,65] High-risk HPV types, mainly HPV-16, is associated with undifferentiated VIN in women 30 to 40 years of age.[66] Other risk factors include infection, smoking, poor personal hygiene, pregnancy, and immunosuppression.

CLINICAL FEATURES

There is a division of clinical features into two distinct types. Type 1 is VIN that is directly related to HPV infection, particularly HPV-16, and most often includes premenopausal women with multifocal disease that may coalesce to develop a large field of disease. The second type occurs most often in postmenopausal, HPV-negative women and is unifocal, localized disease associated with lichen sclerosis that most often presents as invasive disease.

The most common presenting symptom is pruritis; however, VIN may be asymptomatic and found coincidentally on annual exam. Women also display symptoms of burning in the area, pain, or difficult/painful urination. Delay in diagnosis is common in patients, even in those with symptoms, because of embarrassment or because treatment is attempted first for another condition that does not resolve.

Lesions are found on hair-bearing and non–hair-bearing areas of the vulva, and on the perineum and perianal area. Lesions appear pigmented, and white, brown, or red and are often visible to the naked eye. There may be raised, reddened areas with demarcation. Some areas may be ulcerated. Mosaicism, the presence of a defined vascular pattern, alerts the clinician that the lesion has developed a vessel mechanism. In dark-skinned women, areas may be hypopigmented and appear pink. Because of the variable appearance of VIN, the practitioner should perform diagnostic biopsies liberally, particularly for recurrent lesions or lesions that change color, ulcerate, or are hyperpigmented.

DIAGNOSIS

All suspicious lesions should be examined under colposcopic guidance. A 3% to 5% acetic acid solution is applied for 5 minutes before obtaining biopsies. The areas will turn white when acetic acid is applied. The goal is to distinguish benign from malignant disease.

TREATMENT

The treatment goal is to prevent progression of dysplasia, and subsequently malignant disease. Treatment for undifferentiated VIN consists of physical destruction of lesions by partial vulvectomy, cryotherapy, laser vaporization, or electrocautery.[66] CO_2 laser ablation may be used in VIN-1 and VIN-2. Wide local excision with disease-free margin of at least 5 mm should be used in VIN-3. Extensive confluent lesions require more extensive excisional procedures.[63] Imiquimod 5% cream is effective in treating VIN-2 and VIN-3; however, invasive disease must be excluded before use. Studies on using the cream 1 to 3 times a week at night are promising, this treatment preserving anatomy and function of the vulva. Efficacy was measured clinically, with the use of serial photography and histologic confirmation.[64,66] In women older than 45 years of age, VIN should be treated with an excisional procedure, since the incidence of progression to invasive cancer increases at this age.[67]

FOLLOW-UP CARE

Long-term follow-up is required. Many pre-invasive lesions are associated with HPV infection and will recur. Close colposcopic observation is necessary to detect new and recurrent lesions when they are small. This will minimize the need for multiple episodes of treatment.[68] Patients should be counseled to quit smoking, since smoking is directly correlated with recurrence of VIN.

VULVAR CANCER

INCIDENCE

Vulvar carcinoma affects the external female genitalia. Primary cancer of the vulva is uncommon and represents less than 4% of all gynecologic cancers. In 2005, 3,870 women in the US were diagnosed with vulvar cancer and 870 women were projected to die of the disease.[2] The peak incidence is seen in the sixth and seventh decades of life. Approximately 15% of all vulvar cancers occur in women younger than age 40.[69]

EPIDEMIOLOGY

Current opinion focuses on vulvar cancer as two distinct types of disease. The first type occurs in younger patients as multifocal disease. It is related to HPV and smoking and is commonly associated with basaloid or warty VIN. The second type is more common and is seen mainly in elderly patients. It is unrelated to smoking or HPV infection and is associated with a high incidence of dystrophic lesions including lichen sclerosis adjacent to the tumor.[68] Lichen sclerosis is thought to be a predisposing factor in the development of HPV-negative vulvar cancer.[68]

RISK FACTORS

Factors that increase a woman's risk for vulvar cancer include VIN, smoking, and chronic vulvar dystrophy and inflammation. Smoking also increases the risk of recurrence of the disease after initial treatment is completed.

SCREENING

There is no screening procedure for vulvar cancer. However, routine annual visual inspection should be performed by a health care provider. Female patients should be instructed on vulvar self-examination as part of preventive health care measure.[66] Those patients with VIN or lichen sclerosis should be kept under surveillance.[29]

CLINICAL FEATURES

Pruritis is the predominate presenting sign. The patient may also have raised fleshy lesions or ulcerated, leukoplakic, or warty lesions. Pain and bleeding may occur if ulceration is present. Other symptoms include swelling, discharge, and a painful or nonpainful lump. Careful examination must be performed because most squamous cell carcinomas are unifocal and occur on the labia majora. Approximately 5% of cases are multifocal, and the labia minora, clitoris, or perineum may be involved as primary sites. Occasionally women will present with a large mass in the groin, signaling a suspicion for disease outside the vulva.[69]

PREVENTION

An active approach is needed to diagnose and manage precursor lesions that often lead to the development of vulvar cancer. Studies indicate there is a delay in treatment on the part of both the physician and patient. In some cases, women went undiagnosed for up to 6 months and had visited a health care professional 3 or more times prior to diagnosis. Women should be instructed to perform vulvar self-examination on a monthly basis.

DIAGNOSIS

Diagnosis is based on biopsy alone. Biopsy must be performed on any suspicious lesions, symptomatic or asymptomatic. All grossly suspicious lesions must be biopsied including confluent areas, any wartlike mass, persistent ulceration, or itchy area; or those areas with change in color, elevation, or appearance of a surface of lesion.[69] Colposcopic exam is required with 3% acetic acid and subsequent biopsy. Serial sectioning of small lesions must be performed to assess depth of invasion[29] if the lesion is less than 2 cm in diameter and depth on invasion.

A careful history and physical exam are necessary. An important aspect of vulvar cancer is the generally delayed presentation. Factors affecting this late presentation include fear, embarrassment, and lack of access to medical care. Physicians may lack experience with vulvar lesions and may provide prolonged treatment of lesions presumed benign.[63] Patients often fail to seek treatment for 2 to 16 months for symptomatic lesions or chronic pruritis, and physicians often provide medical care of vulvar lesions for up to 12 months before obtaining a biopsy or considering referral to a gynecologic oncologist.[6,68] If a primary care physician or gynecologist is unable to or uncomfortable in performing a biopsy, the patient should be referred to a gynecologic oncologist for treatment.

HISTOLOGY

Since vulvar cancer is in close association with the skin, 85% are found to be squamous cell carcinomas. The second most common histologic type is melanoma, accounting for 5% to 10% of cases. Other rare lesions include adenocarcinoma, Paget's disease, Bartholin's gland, or sarcoma.[68,70] Squamous cell occurs often in elderly women.[63] Staging (Table 8-2) reflects the characteristics of vulvar cancer growth, first by direct extension, then onto distant sites via the lymphatic system.[66]

Table **8-2** VULVAR CANCER FIGO® STAGING

Stage	Description
0	Carcinoma in situ (preinvasive disease)
I	Tumour confined to vulva or vulva and perineum, 2 cm or less in greatest dimension
IA	Tumour confined to vulva or vulva and perineum, 2 cm or less in greatest dimension and with stromal invasion no greater than 1 mm*
IB	Tumour confined to vulva or vulva and perineum, 2 cm or less in greatest dimension and with stromal invasion greater than 1 mm*
II	Tumour confined to vulva or vulva and perineum, more than 2 cm in greatest dimension
III	Tumour invades any of the following: lower urethra, vagina, anus, and/or unilateral regional node metastasis
IVA	Tumor invades any of the following: bladder mucosa, rectal mucosa; or is fixed to bone and/or bilateral regional node metastases
IVB	Any distant metastasis including pelvic lymph nodes

**The depth of invasion is defined as the measurement of the tumour from the epithelial-stromal junction of the adjacent most superficial dermal papilla, to the deepest point of invasion*

From International Federation of Gynecology and Obstetrics: Staging classifications and clinical practice guidelines of gynaecologic cancers, 2003: www.figo.org. Reprinted with permission.

The incidence of lymph node metastases is 30% overall. The risk increases as the size and depth of invasion increases. Pelvic node metastases are uncommon and are not usually found in absence of suspicious groin nodes. Positive pelvic nodes are found in 20% of patients with inguinal node metastases.[71]

TREATMENT

Definitive treatment aims at eradicating tumor on the vulva and also assessment and treatment of regional lymph nodes. Survival is generally good when timely treatment is attained. The treatment of choice for vulvar cancer remains individualized surgery. Advances in management of vulvar cancer since the 1980s include the following:[71]

- Individualization of treatment for patients with invasive disease
- Vulvar conservation for patients with unifocal disease and normal vulva
- Omission of groin dissection in women with T1 tumors and less than 1 mm invasion
- Elimination of routine pelvic lymphadenectomy
- Use of separate groin incisions for groin dissection
- Avoidance of contralateral groin dissection in women with T1 tumors and negative ipsilateral nodes
- Use of preoperative radiation in advanced disease to avoid pelvic exenteration
- Use of postoperative radiation in those patients with multiple positive groin nodes

Microinvasive disease is resected with a 1-cm margin of normal tissue. T1 and T2 tumors with invasion can be excised using wide radical excision with 2-cm margin, or by radical vulvectomy. Large T3 and T4 lesions require an abdominal-perineal approach.[68] Lymphatic mapping is considered experimental in the treatment of vulvar cancer. The most common postoperative side effects include numbness of anterior thigh secondary to femoral nerve injury, deep vein thrombosis, wound breakdown, and seroma.[69]

Radiation therapy with or without the addition of concurrent chemotherapy has an increasingly important role in the management of vulvar cancer. Radiation therapy alone is indicated in women before surgery with advanced disease or in women with small tumors in the clitoral or periclitoral area, and after surgery to treat pelvic lymph nodes and groins to prevent recurrence.[71]

RECURRENT DISEASE

Margin status, depth of invasion, and lymph node involvement are independent risk factors for local recurrence of disease. Repeat wide radical excision for local recurrences is often successful salvage treatment. Local recurrent disease may also be treated with radiation therapy, either external beam or with interstitial needles. Regional and distant recurrence and metastases are difficult to treat, chemotherapy responses are low, and long-term survival is very uncommon. Multifocal disease and those with nodal metastases are at high risk for recurrence. Recurrence in the groin is difficult to treat due to close proximity to vessels, and inability to irradiate again. The majority of patients with recurrent disease will die of it.[71]

LATE EFFECTS

Lymphedema may be a late-occurring effect and is related to the extent of surgery and radiation therapy. There is a high incidence of psychosexual morbidity (e.g., dyspareunia), and urinary dysfunction (stress incontinence). Hernia may also form in the femoral area.[69]

FOLLOW-UP CARE

Women who have been treated for vulvar cancer are recommended to have follow-up every 6 months for 2 to 3 years, then annually. Prognosis correlates with stage of disease and lymph node status. Lymph node metastasis is the single most important prognostic factor in vulvar cancer.[68] Patients need long-term follow-up and surveillance because of the ability of this cancer to recur many years after the initial diagnosis. Smoking cessation should be a routine part of care because of the prevalence of recurrent disease and its correlation to smoking.

VAGINAL INTRAEPITHELIAL NEOPLASIA

INTRODUCTION

Vaginal intraepithelial neoplasia (VAIN) is classified as three progressive levels of dysplasia. VAIN-1 indicates mild dysplasia and is a human papillomavirus (HPV)-induced change. VAIN-2 is moderate dysplasia. VAIN-3 is severe dysplasia/carcinoma in situ and is considered a premalignant lesion. VAIN-2 and VAIN-3 involve the upper third of the vagina in more than 70% of cases. Mean age at diagnosis of VAIN has decreased to 30 years, probably from increased awareness, improved screening, and an absolute increase in incidence.[63] Risk factors include a prior history of cervical intraepithelial neoplasia (CIN), HPV infection, prior irradiation for pelvic malignancy, smoking, and immunosuppresion.[67]

CLINICAL FEATURES

Most patients with VAIN are asymptomatic and are identified during an annual clinical vaginal exam and Pap smear. Women affected may complain of postcoital bleeding or vaginal discharge. Most often, lesions present as multifocal, flat, and inconspicuous; however, they may also be pink, red, or white in color.

DIAGNOSIS

Diagnosis is made under colposcopic examination using 3% to 5% acetic acid applied for 5 minutes. Rotation of the speculum is required to survey the entire vaginal vault. Biopsy of all suspicious lesions is undertaken to establish diagnosis and to rule out malignancy.

TREATMENT

Treatment for VAIN should be individualized and based on extent and location of disease. CO_2 laser ablation is the treatment of choice for most VAIN cases.[63] For patients with noninvasive disease that is multifocal and would require extensive surgical intervention to remove lesions, an effective treatment is 5-FU (5-fluorouracil) cream. Upper vaginectomy is used in the treatment of high-grade VAIN when suspicion of invasive disease is present.

VAGINAL CANCER

INCIDENCE

Vaginal cancer is rare, accounting for less than 1% of all gynecologic cancers. Up to 30% of patients with primary vaginal carcinoma may have a history of previously treated in situ or invasive cervical cancer.[29] New cases in 2005 will number 2,140, and up to 810 women will die of the disease.[2] Vaginal cancer generally occurs in older women, and most is located in the upper, posterior wall of the vagina. Mean age of diagnosis is 60 years of age.

EPIDEMIOLOGY

Of women with primary vaginal cancer, 59% have previously undergone hysterectomy. Exposure to diethylstilbestrol (DES) in utero during the first 12 weeks of pregnancy increases the incidence of clear cell carcinoma of the vagina.[72]

RISK FACTORS

Risk factors include low socioeconomic status, history of HPV infection, chronic vaginal irritation, and prior treatment for cervical cancer.

SCREENING

Routine screening for vaginal cancer is not cost-effective. Women with a history of CIN or invasive cervical cancer should be followed with regular exams and PAP smears.[29,71]

CLINICAL FACTORS

Most women are first seen with symptoms similar to those of cervical cancer. These include painless vaginal discharge that is frequently bloody, postcoital bleeding, and irregular or postmenopausal bleeding. Urinary problems may cause women to seek medical assistance who are then found to have disease compressing or involving the bladder. Pelvic pain signifies advanced disease.[72]

DIAGNOSIS

Clinicians must acquire a comprehensive history and physical and perform inspection of the vagina with a colposcope, bimanual exam, and rectal exam. Lesions vary in size and may be indurated, ulcerated, or fungating. Small lesions may be missed on first exam if located in the lower vagina and obscured by the speculum.[70] Definitive diagnosis requires biopsy.

HISTOLOGY

Squamous cell neoplasms account for 80% to 85% of vaginal cancers, 9% are adenocarcinomas, and fewer than 5% are melanomatous. Verrucous carcinomas are very rare and often have multiple episodes of indolence and local recurrence. Other rare types include sarcoma and smooth muscle tumors. Staging (see Table 8-3) for vaginal cancer is clinical and is based on the findings of general physical and pelvic examination, cystoscopy, proctoscopy, and chest x-ray.[73]

TREATMENT

The rarity of this disease requires the expertise of a gynecologic oncologist. Treatment is based on site of vaginal involvement, stage, and extent of disease. Surgery is difficult because of the close proximity of the tissues to the bladder and rectum. The majority of primary vaginal cancers are treated with irradiation. Stage I is usually treated with radiation. Surgical intervention is an option for patients with stage I lesions involving the upper vagina, in patients with stage I clear cell carcinoma, those with nonepithelial lesions, and those with tumors that recur after irradiation. Surgery also has a role in patients who develop a rectovaginal or colovaginal fistula. Radiation therapy is standard treatment for stages II through IV and comprises a combination of external beam therapy with intracavitary/interstitial treatment.[73] Chemotherapy is limited to use in salvage therapy.

LATE EFFECTS

Anatomical closeness of the vagina with other anatomical structures may cause effects such as radiation cystitis and proctitis, fistula formation, and vaginal necrosis and stenosis.

Table **8-3** Vaginal Cancer FIGO® Staging

Staging	Description
0	Carcinoma in situ, intraepithelial neoplasia grade 3
I	The carcinoma is limited to the vaginal wall.
II	The carcinoma has involved the subvaginal tissue but has not extended to the pelvic wall.
III	The carcinoma has extended to the pelvic wall.
IV	The carcinoma has extended beyond the true pelvis or has involved the mucosa of the bladder or rectum; bullous oedema as such does not permit a case to be allotted to Stage IV.
IVA	Tumour invades bladder and/or rectal mucosa and/or direct extension beyond the true pelvis.
IVB	Spread to distant organs

From International Federation of Gynecology and Obstetrics: Staging classifications and clinical practice guidelines of gynaecologic cancers, 2003: www.figo.org. Reprinted with permission.

FOLLOW-UP CARE

The reported overall survival for vaginal cancer is 44%.[73] Prognosis depends on the stage of the disease. The majority of recurrences appear within 2 years of primary therapy and occur in the pelvis. If previous radiation therapy has been given, recurrent disease is generally managed surgically. Patients who have undergone radiation therapy should be encouraged to use a vaginal dilator and estrogen cream to maintain vaginal function.

REFERENCES

1. Dowdy SC and others: Overexpression of the TGF-beta antagonist Smad7 in endometrial cancer, *Gynecol Oncol* 96:368, 2005.
2. Jemal A and others: Cancer statistics, *CA: Cancer J Clin* 55:10, 2005.
3. Silverberg E, Lubera J: Cancer statistics, *CA Cancer J Clin* 37:2, 1987.
4. Elit L, Hirte H: Current status and future innovations of hormonal agents, chemotherapy, and investigation agents in endometrial cancer, *Curr Opin Obstet Gynecol* 14:67, 2002.
5. Ries LAG and others, editors: *SEER cancer statistics review, 1975-2000*, Bethesda, 2003, National Cancer Institute.
6. Disaia PJ, Creasman WT: Adenocarcinoma of the uterus. In Disaia PJ, Creasman WT, editors: *Clinical gynecologic oncology*, ed 4, St Louis, 2002, Mosby.
7. Endometrial cancer. On the Web at OncologyChannel online, www.oncologychannel.com/endometrialcancer, 2005.
8. Pavelka JC and others: Morbid obesity and endometrial cancer: surgical, clinical, and pathologic outcomes in surgically managed patients, *Gynecol Oncol* 95:588, 2004.
9. Salazar-Martinez E and others: Case control study of diabetes, obesity, physical activity and risk of endometrial cancer among Mexican women, *Cancer Causes Control* 11(8):707, 2000.
10. Weiderpass E and others: Body size in different periods of life, diabetes mellitus, hypertension, and risk of postmenopausal endometrial cancer, *Cancer Causes Control* 11(2):185, 2000.
11. Purdie DM, Green AC: Epidemiology of endometrial cancer, *Best Pract Res Clin Obstet Gynaecol* 15:341, 2001.
12. Hacker NF: Uterine cancer. In Berek JS, Hacker NF, editors: *Practical gynecologic oncology*, ed. 4, Philadelphia, 2005, Lippincott.
13. Barakat RR and others: Endometrial cancer. In Pazdur R, Coia LR, Hoskins WJ, and Wagman LD, eds: Cancer management: a multidisciplinary approach, ed. 5, 2001, CMP Media.
14. RR and others: Corpus epithelial tumors. In Hoskins WJ, Perez CA, Young RC, editors: *Principles and practice of gynecologic oncology*, ed. 3, Philadelphia, 2000, Lippincott Williams and Wilkins.
15. Hacker NF: Uterine cancer. In Berek JS, Hacker NF, editors: *Practical gynecologic oncology*, ed 4, Philadelphia, 2005, Lippincott Williams and Wilkins.
16. Kitchener HC: Surgery for endometrial cancer: what type and by whom? *Best Pract Res Clin Obstet Gynaecol* 15:407, 2001.
17. Canavan TP, Doshi NR: Epidemiology of endometrial cancer, *Am Fam Phys* 59:3069, 1999.
18. Symonds I: Ultrasound, hysteroscopy, and endometrial biopsy in the investigation of endometrial cancer, *Best Pract Res Clin Obstet Gynecol* 15:381, 2001.
19. Society of Gynecologic Oncologist. Management of endometrial cancer. On the Web at: www.sgo.org/policy/state_of_state_2005.pdf.
20. Paniscotti BM: Cancer of the endometrium. In Moore-Higgs GJ, editor: *Women and cancer: a gynecologic oncology nursing perspective*, ed 2, Sudbury, Mass., 2000, Jones and Bartlett.
21. Frumovitz M and others: Predictors of final histology in patients with endometrial cancer, *Gynecol Cancer* 95:463, 2004.
22. Orr JW and others: Endometrial cancer: is surgical staging necessary? *Curr Opin Oncol* 13:408, 2001.
23. Mariani A and others: Surgical stage I endometrial cancer: Predictors of distant failure and death, *Gynecol Oncol* 87:272, 2002.
24. Mariani A and others: Assessment of prognostic factors in stage IIIA endometrial cancer, *Gynecol Oncol* 86:38, 2002.
25. Stewart KD and others: Ten-year outcome including patterns of failure and toxicity for adjuvant whole abdominopelvic irradiation in high-risk and poor histologic feature patients with endometrial carcinoma, *Int J Radiat Oncol Biol Phys* 54:527, 2002.
26. Mariani A and others: Hematogenous dissemination in corpus cancer, *Gynecol Oncol* 80:233, 2001.
27. Mariani A and others: Role of wide/radical hysterectomy and pelvic lymph node dissection in endometrial carcinoma with cervical involvement, *Gynecol Oncol* 83:72, 2002.
28. Grigsby PW: Update on radiation therapy for endometrial cancer, *Oncology* 16:777, 2002.
29. International Federation of Gynecology and Obstetrics: Staging classifications and clinical practice guidelines of gynaecologic cancers, 2003: retrieved from www.figo.org.
30. Roland PY: The benefits of a gynecologic oncologist: a pattern of care study for endometrial cancer treatment, *Gynecol Oncol* 93:125 2004.
31. Carney M, Wiggins C: A population-based study on patterns of care for endometrial cancer: who is seen by a gynecologic oncologist and who is not? *Gynecol Oncol* 84: 529, 2002.
32. Susini T and others: Vaginal hysterectomy and abdominal hysterectomy for treatment of endometrial cancer in the elderly, *Gynecol Oncol* 96:362, 2005.
33. Ng TY and others: Local recurrence in high-risk node negative stage I endometrial carcinoma treated with postoperative vaginal vault brachytherapy, *Gynecol Oncol* 79:490, 2000.
34. Look K: Stage I-II endometrial adenocarcinoma evolution of therapeutic paradigms: the role of surgery and radiation, *Int J Gynecol Cancer* 12:237, 2002.

35. Alektiar KM and others: Intravaginal high-dose rate brachytherapy for stage IB (FIGO grade 1, 2) endometrial cancer, *Int J Radiat Oncol Biol Phys* 53:707, 2002.
36. Horowitz NS and others: Adjuvant high-dose rate vaginal brachytherapy as treatment of stage I and II endometrial cancer, *Obstet Gynecol* 99:235, 2002.
37. Domanovic M and others: Using intraoperative radiation therapy—a case study, *AORN* 77:412, 2003.
38. Ramirez PT, Frumovitz M, Bodurka DC et al: Hormonal therapy for the management of grade 1 endometrial adenocarcinoma: a literature review, *Gynecol Oncol* 95:133, 2004.
39. Loibl S, von Minckwitz G, Kaufmann M: Adjuvant therapy following primary therapy for endometrial cancer, *Eur J Cancer* 38:S41, 2002.
40. Von Minckwitz G and others: Adjuvant endocrine treatment with medroxyprogesterone acetate or tamoxifen in stage I and stage II endometrial cancer—a multicentre, open, controlled, prospectively randomized trial, *Eur J Cancer* 38:2265, 2001.
41. Otto, SE: Endometrial cancer. In *Oncology Nursing*, ed 4, St Louis, 2001, Mosby.
42. Podczaski E, Mortel R: Hormonal treatment of endometrial cancer: past, present, and future, *Best Pract Res Clin Obstet Gynaecol* 15:469, 2001.
43. Jain MG and others: A cohort study of nutritional factors and endometrial cancer, *Eur J Epidemiol* 16:899, 2000.
44. Neven P: New SERMs in development, *Eur J Cancer* 38:S26, 2002.
45. Ferguson GG, Herzog TJ: Current research on the use of hormonal therapy in the treatment of advanced or recurrent endometrial cancer, *Women's Oncol Rev* 4:175, 2004.
46. Hoskins PJ and others: Paclitaxel and carboplatin, alone or with irradiation, in advanced or recurrent endometrial cancer: a phase II study, *J Clin Oncol* 19:4048, 2001.
47. Fleming GF, Muggia FM: Doxorubicin/cisplatin/paclitaxel regimen improves survival in endometrial cancer, *Oncol News* 11, 2002.
48. Aoki Y and others: Stage III endometrial cancer: analysis of prognostic factors and failure patterns after adjuvant chemotherapy, *Gynecol Oncol* 83:1, 2001.
49. van Wijk FH and others: Phase II study of carboplatin in patients with advanced or recurrent endometrial cancer. A trial of the EORTC Gynaecologic Cancer Group, *Eur J Cancer* 39:78, 2003.
50. Ramondetta L and others: Treatment of uterine papillary serous carcinoma with paclitaxel, *Gynecol Oncol* 82:156, 2001.
51. Onda T and others: Treatment of node-positive endometrial cancer with complete node dissection, chemotherapy and radiation therapy, *Br J Cancer* 75:1836, 1997.
52. Duska LR and others: A pilot trial of TAC (paclitaxel, doxorubicin, and carboplatin) chemotherapy with filgastrim (r-metHuG-CSF) support followed by radiotherapy in patients with "high-risk" endometrial cancer, *Gynecol Oncol* 96:198, 2005.
53. Scudder SS and others: Paclitaxel and carboplatin with amifostine in advanced, recurrent, or refractory endometrial adenocarcinoma: a phase II study of the Southwest Oncology Group, *Gynecol Oncol* 96:610, 2005.
54. Traina TA and others: Weekly topotecan for recurrent endometrial cancer: a case series and review of the literature, *Gynecol Oncol* 2004.
55. Wadler S and others: Topotecan is an active agent in the first-line treatment of metastatic or recurrent endometrial carcinoma: Eastern Cooperative Group study E3E93, *J Clin Oncol* 21:2110, 2003.
56. Miller DS and others: A Phase II trial of topotecan in patients with advanced, persistent, or recurrent endometrial carcinoma: a Gynecologic Oncology Group study, *Gynecol Oncol* 87:247, 2002.
57. Burke TW and others: Prospective treatment of advanced or recurrent endometrial carcinoma with cisplatin, doxorubicin, and cyclophosphamide, *Gynecol Oncol* 40:264, 1991.
58. Mirashemi R, Nieves-Nera W, Averette HE: Gynecologic malignancies in older women, *Oncology* 15:580, 2001.
59. Corneya KS and others: Associations among exercise, body weight, and quality of life in a population-based sample of endometrial cancer survivors, *Gynecol Oncol* 97:422, 2005.
60. World Health Organization: Diet, nutrition, and the prevention of chronic diseases, Technical report series 916, Geneva, 2003, World Health Organization.
61. Mueck AO, Seeger H: Hormone therapy after endometrial cancer, *Hormone Res* 62:40, 2004.
62. Nunns D and others: The morbidity of surgery and adjuvant radiotherapy in the management of endometrial carcinoma, *Int J Gynecol Cancer* 10:233, 2000.
63. Hall KL: Clinical considerations in vulvar cancer, *J Women's Imaging* 4:114, 2002.
64. Campion MJ: Preinvasive disease. In Berek JS, Hacker NF, editors: *Practical gynecologic oncology*, ed. 4, Philadelphia, 2005, Lippincott Williams and Wilkins.
65. Joura EA: Epidemiology and precursors of vulvar cancer: review article, *J Women's Imaging* 4:126, 2002.
66. Wendling J and others: Treatment of undifferentiated vulvar intraepithelial neoplasia with 5% imiquimod cream: a prospective study of 12 cases, *Arch Dermatol* 140:1220, 2002.
67. Bodurka DC, Bevers MW: Preinvasive disease of the lower female genital tract. In Barakat RR and others, editors: *Handbook of gynecologic oncology*, ed. 2, London, 2002, Martin Dunitz.
68. Burke TW: Vulvar cancer. In Barakat RR and others, editors: *Handbook of gynecologic oncology*, ed 2, London, 2002, Martin Dunitz.
69. Canavan TP, Cohen D: Vulvar cancer, *Am Fam Phys* 66(7):1269-1274, 2002.
70. de Hullu JA, Oonk M, van der Zee A: Modern management of vulvar cancer, *Curr Opin Obstet Gynecol* 16:65, 2002.
71. Hacker NF: Vulvar cancer. In Berek JS, Hacker NF, editors: *Practical gynecologic oncology*, ed 4, Philadelphia, 2005, Lippincott Williams and Wilkins.
72. Bodurka DC, Wharton JT: Vaginal cancer. In Barakat RR and others, editors: *Handbook of gynecologic oncology*, ed 2, London, 2002, Martin Dunitz.
73. Hacker NF: Vaginal cancer. In Berek JS, Hacker NF, editors: *Practical gynecologic oncology*, ed 4, Philadelphia, 2005, Lippincott Williams and Wilkins.

CHAPTER

9 Colorectal Cancer

Tracy K. Gosselin-Acomb

INTRODUCTION AND OVERVIEW

Colorectal cancer (CRC) is one of the most studied and talked about cancers today. Many popular people in society have been diagnosed with the disease including past president Ronald Reagan, cartoonist Charles Schultz, Katie Couric's late husband, Jay Monahan, and recently, the CEO for McDonald's, Charlie Bell. Unfortunately, many of these people succumbed to the disease, leaving us with many questions that still need to be examined. Despite increased education and awareness regarding the disease, CRC still remains the third most common cancer diagnosed in women. Treatment for CRC includes a variety of different options based upon individual patient staging. Newer treatment agents such as antiepidermal growth factors (EGFRs) and ongoing clinical trials exploring the role of chemoprevention agents are providing new information about the prevention and management of this disease.

EPIDEMIOLOGY

Colorectal cancer is the most common gastrointestinal cancer (GI) and the third most common cancer diagnosed in the US.[1] The American Cancer Society (ACS) estimates that approximately 73,470 women will be diagnosed in 2005 with CRC: of these, 56,660 will be colon and 16,810 will be rectal.[1] 25,750 women are expected to succumb in 2005 to the disease, representing 10% of all cancer deaths in women. The incidence rates for CRC are similar in men and women.

Colorectal cancer incidence rates have stabilized since the mid-1990s after experiencing a decline in the mid-1980s to mid-1990s.[1] As a woman ages, her chances of being diagnosed with CRC also increase. It is currently estimated that 1 in 17 women in the US will be diagnosed with CRC. Incidence rates for colorectal cancer vary by a factor of 20 around the world.[2] The incidence pattern for females differs based upon race and ethnic background (Figure 9-1). African Americans have the highest incidence rates followed by Caucasians, while American Indian/Alaskan Natives have the lowest incidence rates. A woman's lifetime risk of developing CRC in the US is about 6%.[3]

ETIOLOGY AND RISK FACTORS

There are a variety of risk factors that put a woman at risk for the development of CRC, the two most common being age and family history. As many as 15% of patients with CRC have a strong family history of the disease; if at least one first-degree relative has had colorectal cancer, the relative risk for developing the disease is 1.7.[4] In addition, the relative risk of developing CRC is associated with preexisting adenomatous polyps or adenomas, genetic predisposition, preexisting diseases of the bowel, and environmental factors such as nutrition, alcohol, sedentary lifestyle, and cigarette smoking.[5]

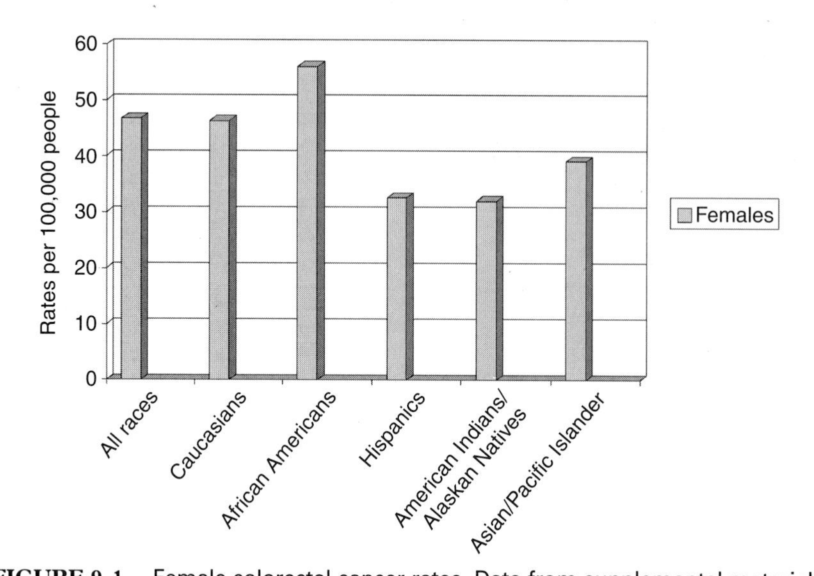

FIGURE 9-1 Female colorectal cancer rates. Data from supplemental materials #1: rates and trends for the top 15 cancer sites by sex and race/ethnicity for 1992-2000. (Retrieved 1/4/05 from http://seer.cancer.gov/report_to_nation/1975_2000/other/top15sites.incd.females.pdf.)

Polyps/Adenomatous Polyps

It is thought that CRC arises from normal epithelial cells that grow into adenomatous colonic polyps and then into adenocarcinoma based on a series of genetic events. Polyps are typically described as an outpouching of the bowel wall (Figure 9-2). As people age, the chance of developing polyps increases, and therefore the role of cancer screening is critical to early diagnosis and intervention. Polyps themselves are not considered cancerous unless they undergo a series of changes and enlarge: the larger the polyp, the greater the chance of it being cancerous. In fact, it can take up to 5 to 10 years for a polyp to become malignant.[5] Adenomatous polyps (adenomas) can be classified as villous, tubular, or tubulovillous. Tubulovillous polyps are a combination of villous and tubular, and typically the villous or flat adenomas are more likely to be cancerous. The overall risk of a adenomatous polyps progressing to malignancy is

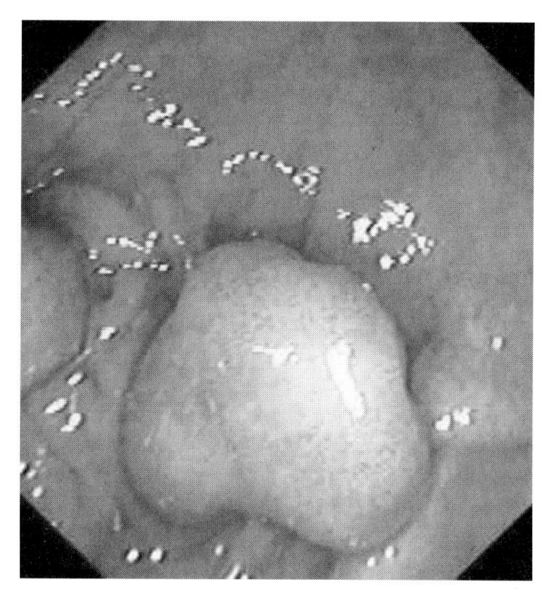

FIGURE 9-2 Polyp. (Courtesy Robert Beebe, Gastroenterology Division, Duke University Health System.)

approximately 2% to 5%, with polyp size being a major determinant of risk.[6] Early identification and removal decreases the risk of CRC developing.

Preexisting Bowel Disease

Women who have a history of inflammatory bowel disease such as Crohn's disease or ulcerative colitis are at risk of developing CRC that is increased by thirtyfold.[5] It is theorized that inflammatory bowel disease causes mucosal wall destruction with a high cell turnover rate and enhances genetic mutations that can lead to proliferation of a cell line containing malignant clones.[6] It is these malignant clone cells that develop into CRC. One of the difficulties in caring for patients with ulcerative colitis is that they can develop an endophytic growth pattern, and therefore visual endoscopic surveillance may fail to detect a cancer until it has become advanced and blind biopsies of normal mucosal tissue may be warranted.[7,8] Women who have more severe cases of inflammatory bowel disease, dysplastic cellular changes, and a greater time period with active disease are more at risk for developing CRC.

Genetics

The majority of CRC cases are sporadic, although a few familial syndromes have been discovered. Familial adenomatosis polyposis (FAP) and hereditary nonpolyposis colorectal cancer (HNPCC) are the two most common hereditary syndromes associated with CRC. In the US, 1 in 5,000 to 10,000 people are affected by FAP, but because of the routine use of prophylactic colectomy when it is found it accounts for 1% of treated colorectal cancers.[9] The colectomy is then followed by an ileoanal anastomosis. Women may also then undergo a prophylactic bilateral salpingo-oophorectomy after they have children.

FAP is an autosomal dominant condition associated with mutation in the adenomatous polyposis coli (APC) tumor suppressor gene on chromosome 5q. This mutation can sometimes be found in Jews of Eastern European ancestry. FAP is characterized by hundreds to thousands of polyps (Figure 9-3) that spread throughout the colon. Families that have a history of FAP may often have their children undergo early screening for this condition. Colorectal adenomas appear at puberty and colorectal cancer appears in the 30s.[10] If FAP is left untreated, the risk of cancer is almost 100%. There are two syndromes associated with FAP, Gardner's and Turcot's. Gardner's syndrome is associated with desmoid tumors, sebaceous cysts, and osteomas, whereas Turcot's syndrome is associated with brain tumors.

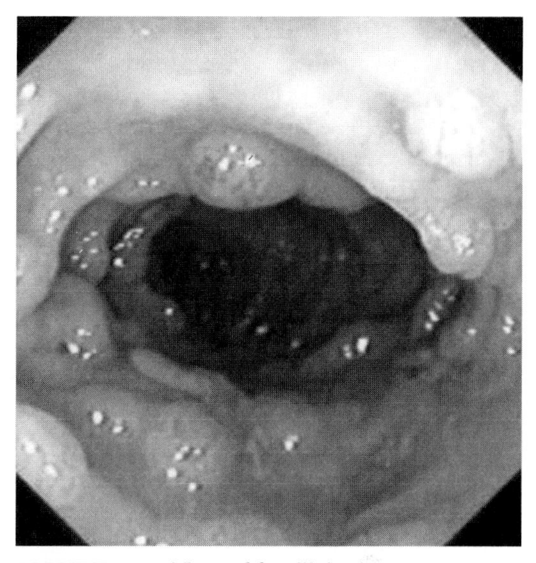

FIGURE 9-3 View of familial adenomatous polyposis (FAP). (Courtesy Robert Beebe, Gastroenterology Division, Duke University Health System.)

Attenuated FAP is characterized by a paucity of colonic adenomas, and the ones that do occur are primarily in the proximal colon.[11] CRC in these patients is typically diagnosed later in life (in the 50s) and is often harder to diagnose. These patients do not experience congenital hypertrophy of the retinal pigment epithelium (CHRPE), which looks like small freckles in the retina of the eye.

HNPCC, also referred to as Lynch syndrome, is the most common familial syndrome associated with CRC and places women at risk for extracolonic cancers of the uterus and ovary. HNPCC is believed to account for 5% to 15% of colorectal cancers.[12] In this syndrome, multiple generations are affected with colorectal cancer at an early age (a mean of approximately 45 years), with a predominance of right-sided colorectal cancer (approximately 70% proximal to the splenic flexure).[11] HNPCC is an autosomal dominant condition that is caused by defective mismatched repair genes. Most patients with HNPCC show widespread alterations in the DNA-base sequences, or microsatellite sequences distributed throughout the genome.[13]

Before genetic testing was available for HNPCC, the Amsterdam criteria were used to classify the disease; today, with genetic testing, most often *MLH1* and *MLH2* are the genes that account for HNPCC.[11] If someone should test positive, it is important to pursue the family history because, in many cases, it is recommended that relatives begin CRC screening earlier than at age 50 and have more frequent follow-up testing.[14] The *RAS* oncogene is commonly mutated in patients with cancer, and mutation to the K-*ras* may be associated with poorer prognosis.

Advancement in the field of molecular genetics has assisted clinicians with prevention, management, and treatment strategies. Patients face difficult questions when they decide whether or not to choose genetic testing. In a study of patients with colorectal cancer, Kinney and others[15] identified the most frequently cited reasons for wanting genetic testing: to inform family members and thereby help them make decisions about lifestyle changes and to prompt appropriate colorectal screening behaviors to reduce their risk (46%); to determine the patient's own risk of recurrence or overall prognosis (23%); and curiosity (6%). The most common reasons for not wanting genetic testing were confidentiality issues that might influence insurability or employability (4%) and adverse psychologic effects (4%). Other reasons for not wanting genetic testing were cost, old age, belief that the cancer was not due to hereditary causes, and that the personal physician discouraged testing.[15]

Lifestyle Risk Factors

There have been a variety of case control, cohort, prospective, and retrospective studies looking at dietary factors and their influence on CRC development. Dietary fiber, red meat, and fruit and vegetable consumption have been the most widely studied variables. Before considering the influence of any specific dietary component, it is important to understand how overall food consumption – specifically total energy intake relative to energy requirement – is related to the occurrence of colon cancer.[16] The impact of physical activity, body size, and body mass index (BMI) also play a role in the development of CRC, and although the mechanisms are not clearly understood, both obesity and physical inactivity should be considered risk factors.[16] Wei and others[17] found that physical inactivity is more strongly correlated with colon cancer, and Slattery and others[18] found that vigorous activity performed at leisure or around the home was associated with reduced risk of rectal cancer. The Nurses' Health Study reported that women with a higher level of leisure-time activity had a significant reduction in the risk of colon cancer.[18]

Dietary fiber including fruit and vegetables has been thought to increase intestinal transit time, thus decreasing exposure time in the bowel to carcinogens. It was thought until recently a high-fiber diet with fruit and vegetables decreased the risk of CRC. Recent studies have shown this not to be the case.[16,19-22] In a prospective study of 88,757 women, no association between dietary fiber and the risk of CRC or adenoma was found.[20] Studies with wheat bran fiber also do not show a reduction in bile acid, which is thought to contribute to CRC.[23]

Red meat contributes more to the development of colon cancer than other protein sources.[16] It is thought that the fatty acid, high stearic acid content, and nonlipid components of red meat contribute to colon cancer.[16] A large body of data supports the suggestion that substituting fish, poultry, and low-fat dairy products for red meat will lower one's risk of colon cancer.[16]

In an analysis of 10 cohort studies, researchers found high intakes of dietary and total calcium were associated with a lower risk of colorectal cancer. They also assumed that if the association between calcium and colorectal cancer is causal, 15% of CRC cases could be avoided if women who consume less than 1000 mg/day of calcium could increase their calcium intake to 1000 mg/day or more.[24] Calcium has also shown a decrease in the recurrence rates of CRC adenomas.[25]

Alcohol and tobacco have both been shown to be risk factors for adenomas and CRC.[16,17,21] Alcohol is thought to have an antagonist role with folate, thus affecting its ability to metabolize products in the methyl group. Smoking may increase the prevalence of tubular adenomas that may grow slowly into large adenomas, explaining the long induction period between smoking initiation and colorectal cancer development.[26]

A risk factor unique to women is prior diagnosis and treatment of a gynecologic cancer. Women with a history of ovarian cancer have a CRC rate of average-risk women who are 4 to 8 years older. The relative risk (RR) for all CRCs is greater for patients who received radiation therapy (RT).[27] In addition, relatives of women with ovarian cancer have a higher risk of developing CRC and elevated rates of death from CRC.[28] Endometrial cancer has a similar risk, and the increased risk of rectal cancer was significant in those patients who received RT; these cancers appeared in the period consistent with the delayed carcinogenic effects of RT.[27] African American women with endometrial cancer seem to have a higher-than-expected risk for CRC.[27] There is currently no reported risk for those diagnosed with cervical cancer.[28]

An association also exists between colorectal cancer and certain occupational circumstances such as exposure to solvents, abrasives, fuel oils, formaldehyde, and particulate compounds.[29]

PREVENTION, SCREENING, AND DETECTION

Prevention of CRC looks at how women can modify/minimize their risk factors for developing CRC. Both age and family history of the disease increase a woman's risk of developing CRC (Figure 9-4). Body composition, level of activity, and BMI can also put a woman at risk. There is currently a high level of awareness in the US regarding weight and obesity. It is important for women to eat a well-balanced, low-fat diet that includes fiber, fruit, and vegetables and to exercise regularly. Women should also avoid alcohol and tobacco-related products. Ongoing education and support of women who are attempting to change their lifestyle is critical to their success.

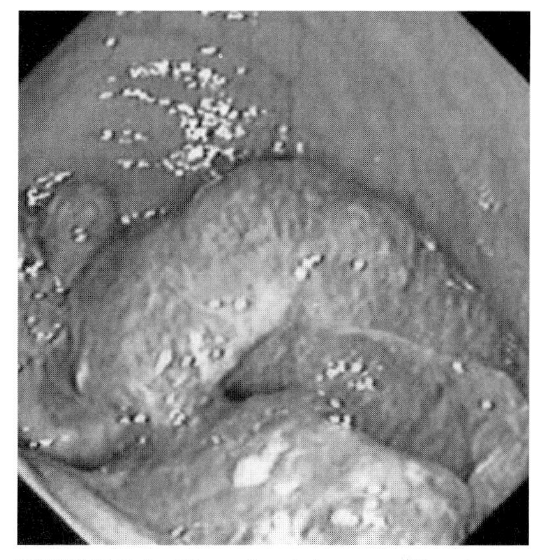

FIGURE 9-4 View of rectal cancer. (Courtesy Robert Beebe, Gastroenterology Division, Duke University Health System.)

Hormone replacement therapy (HRT) in postmenopausal women is another strategy that researchers are investigating that has shown to have a protective effect. A metaanalysis of 18 epidemiologic studies of hormone replacement therapy in postmenopausal women showed a 20% reduction in the risk of colorectal cancer.[30] It is thought that exogenous estrogens also decrease bile acid synthesis by up to 15%; this is important because bile acids, which are absorbed in the proximal colon, are thought to promote malignant changes in the colonic epithelium.[31]

Chemoprevention

Current studies are looking at chemoprevention agents including folic acid; bile acid modifiers such as calcium, wheat bran fiber, low fat, high fruit and vegetables and fiber, ursodeoxycholic acid; and nonsteroidal antiinflammatory drugs (NSAIDs) such as piroxicam, sulindac, sulindac sulfone, and celecoxib [Celebrex]).[32] NSAIDs, including aspirin, are the most widely investigated chemopreventive agents in colorectal neoplasia.[33] Most people are familiar with NSAIDs; they inhibit the cyclooxygenase-2 *(COX-2)* gene, which is sometimes found to be overexpressed in CRC patients. Results of epidemiologic studies are consistent with an approximate 50% reduction in colorectal cancer risk associated with the use of aspirin or other NSAIDs.[34] NSAIDs are also known to cause irritation to the GI tract, and patients who use them may have bleeding, diarrhea, and/or pain.

Ongoing chemoprevention studies continue to look at the role of NSAIDs, folic acid, and other antioxidants.

Screening

Healthy People 2010 goals for CRC screening are that 50% of the population can report having fecal occult blood testing (FOBT) within the past 2 years and that 50% can report previous sigmoidoscopy.[35] The proportion of adults aged 50 and older reporting recent CRC screening with an endoscopic procedure (either sigmoidoscopy or colonoscopy) was nearly twice that of adults reporting recent screening with FOBT.[36] In 2002, 40.4% of adults in this age group reported having received either a sigmoidoscopy or colonoscopy procedure within the past 5 years, whereas the prevalence of having an FOBT within the past year was 21.8%.[36] Because the disease progresses gradually, the conversion of normal mucosa to carcinoma typically takes up to 10 years.[37] CRC is a highly preventable disease: precancerous polyps and adenomas that are typically precursors to the disease can be endoscopically or surgically removed, thus decreasing the risk of CRC. Researchers determined that 67% of colon cancer deaths could be prevented if women were universally screened for colon cancer.[38]

A variety of health care groups have developed CRC screening guidelines including the Agency for Healthcare Research and Quality, ACS, the American Gastroenterological Association, the National Comprehensive Cancer Network (NCCN), the National Cancer Institute (NCI), and the U.S. Preventive Services Task Force (USPSTF). Each of these guidelines incorporates the use of FOBT, a noninvasive screening method, and other, invasive studies such as flexible sigmoidoscopy, double-contrast barium enema (DCBE), and colonoscopy. Both the ACS and the NCCN guidelines provide information for average-risk, intermediate-risk and high-risk persons. The most up-to-date guidelines can be accessed via their websites at www.acs.org or www.nccn.org.

The ACS guidelines (Table 9-1) for asymptomatic, average-risk individuals over the age of 50 provide clinicians with different options depending upon the patient.[36] It is estimated that between 70% and 80% of all CRCs occur among patients at average risk, and that by adopting these principles the mortality from CRC could decrease by 50%.[31,37] FOBT is an easy, noninvasive test that women can perform yearly in their home.

Table 9-1 Colorectal Cancer Screening for Average-Risk, Increased-Risk, and High-Risk Patients[36]

Type of Test	Average Risk
Fecal occult blood test (FOBT) or fecal immunochemical test (FIT)	Every year
OR	
Flexible sigmoidoscopy	Every 5 years
OR	
FOBT and flexible sigmoidoscopy	Every 5 years
OR	
Double-contrast barium enema (DCBE)	Every 5 years
OR	
Colonoscopy	Every 10 years

Certain foods and medications may cause false-positive results, so patient education and instruction is important. Patients are given six testing cards on which they smear a sample of stool. Two samples are taken from three consecutive stools. Samples should come from different ends of the stool. Patients then mail or deliver the cards back to their provider. Once returned the reagent is applied, and if a positive test is found, further evaluation is warranted. The need to rule out the positive results from the false-positives is one of the disadvantages of this test.

A digital rectal exam (DRE) is often performed at the time of a yearly physical or when a patients comes in for follow-up care. A recent study from 13 Veterans Affairs Medical Centers found that single digital FOBT during an exam is a poor screening method for colorectal neoplasia and cannot be recommended as the only test.[39] When repeated annually, FOBT alone, with no other screening modality, has been shown to reduce the risk of CRC death by about one third.[40]

Flexible sigmoidoscopy is an invasive procedure that usually requires the patient to be on a clear liquid diet for 24 hours and to use Fleet's enemas prior to the exam. The benefit of the exam is that it allows the clinician to visualize the rectum and part of the colon (sigmoid colon, descending colon up to the splenic flexure). Biopsies and polypectomies can be performed with this procedure. The downside of this procedure is that the transverse colon, hepatic flexure, and ascending colon cannot be visualized. A colonoscopy may be recommended after biopsy or polypectomy to check for disease that could not be visualized with this procedure.

A DCBE (double contrast barium enema) requires the patient to perform a bowel prep before the procedure but requires no sedation. In this procedure a patient is given a barium enema followed by air into the colon. It is important that the patient be told that her next few stools may be white from the barium.

Colonoscopy requires the patient to have nothing by mouth (NPO) and to undergo bowel prep before the procedure. The bowel prep is essential to good visualization. Patients also receive conscious sedation during the procedure to assist with air insufflation during the procedure. This procedure allows visualization of the entire colon and is the best method to detect CRC. Virtual colonoscopy (VC), also known as computed tomography (CT) colonography, is another type of procedure that is being evaluated. This noninvasive procedure has an easier prep and is better accepted by patients. One of the issues that still has to be resolved is the type of software that should be used so the sensitivity of the test is consistent with traditional colonoscopy.[41]

The ACS recommends more intensive surveillance for (1) persons at increased risk because of a history of adenomatous polyps; (2) persons with a history of curative-intent resection of colorectal cancer; (3) persons with a family history of either colorectal cancer or colorectal adenomas diagnosed in a first-degree relative before age 60; (4) persons at significantly higher risk because of a history of inflammatory bowel disease of significant duration; or (5) persons at significantly higher risk because of a family history of or genetic testing indicating the presence of one of two hereditary syndromes.[36] In patients with HNPCC, annual full colonoscopy, initiated between the ages of 20 and 25, is recommended for those with strong clinical evidence or documented germ-line mutations in *MLH1*, *MSH2*, or *MSH6* (or a combination).

Patients with a family history of HNPCC are not only at risk for adenomas and cancers at a young age but also have an accelerated adenoma-carcinoma sequence, which means that they will have to be screened directly with colonoscopy every year.[10] Women diagnosed with HNPCC need yearly follow-up with a gynecologist. With respect to the endometrium, annual transvaginal ultrasonography and endometrial aspiration for pathologic assessment should be begun at the age of 30 and repeated annually.[11] In the case of the ovary, this evaluation should include transvaginal ovarian ultrasonography and CA125 screening, also beginning at the age of 30.[11] Children and young adults who test positive for the APC gene may receive yearly colonoscopies for surveillance until they may undergo a colectomy, and then they will receive ongoing evaluation for extracolonic and rectal tumors.

Screening strategies have also been adapted for surveillance of patients who have undergone treatment for CRC. Patients should undergo standard follow-up with a physician that includes a regular history, physical examination, and diagnostic studies (complete blood count, liver function studies, carcinoembryonic antigen [CEA] levels, and fecal occult blood test).[31] The American Society of Clinical Oncologists (ASCO) have evidenced-based guidelines for colorectal surveillance.[42] These guidelines recommend a history and physical every 3 to 6 months for the first 3 years after treatment, colonoscopy every 3 to 5 years, and serial CEAs every 2 to 3 months for the first few years to monitor for recurrence.

Screening Barriers

CRC screening rates are lower than breast, cervical, and prostate cancer screening rates. It is important to understand the barriers that affect screening in women from both a patient and provider standpoint. Research has identified the following patient barriers: (1) lack of knowledge, (2) no recommendation from health care provider, (3) not part of general care, (4) embarrassing/painful, (5) sexual orientation of patient, and (6) cost/insurance coverage.[43-49] Research has also identified provider barriers: these include (1) lack of knowledge, (2) attitudes and discouragement by patients, (3) need for better screening tools, (4) need for better processes, and (5) cost.[44-46] Women also tend to think that CRC is a man's disease.[43]

A variety of methods have been proposed to improve screening rates: these include patient education, reminders, and phone calls.[43,44] From a cost perspective: in 2000 Congress passed Medicare reimbursement for FOBT and flexible sigmoidoscopy; then in 2001 it provided Medicare reimbursement for screening colonoscopy. A recent article in the North Carolina Medical Journal provided an example of a quality improvement project related to improving CRC screening in a general internist practice. This article provided an overview of the process as well as the necessary steps that any office can implement.[50]

CLINICAL FACTORS

Women may experience a variety of symptoms related to CRC. Some may be more general, like fatigue and weakness, whereas others are more specific, like blood in the stool (dark or bright red) or a change in bowel habits (diarrhea or constipation). The signs and symptoms of the disease typically correspond to the area of the bowel where the disease is located. Approximately 75% of tumors develop in the left side of the colon (i.e., descending, rectosigmoid, and rectal areas), 15% develop in the right colon (i.e., cecum and ascending colon), and 10% develop in the transverse colon.[51] By knowing the signs/symptoms of the disease, clinicians can determine the approximate location of the tumor as well as potential metastases. Other symptoms may include bloating, tenesmus, pain, flatulence, and weight loss. If a patient reports bleeding, it is important to find out whether they have hemorrhoids, because these are also known to bleed. Patients who are first seen with complaints of obstruction typically have advanced disease at the time of diagnosis.

Younger patients may experience a delay in diagnosis. This may be due to a delay in the patient's seeking care, lack of access, or misdiagnosis by the physician.[52] It is important for young women who have a family history of the disease or who have had positive genetic testing to be evaluated promptly when they experience signs or symptoms of the disease.

DIAGNOSIS AND STAGING

A diagnosis of CRC can often be overlooked as a result of the symptoms of the disease being vague. For women who complain of fatigue and are found to be anemic based on complete blood count (CBC) results, further workup is warranted. A complete history and physical should be performed as well as a DRE for lower-lying lesions. DRE is often of limited benefit because of the inexperience of the examiner and the short area that can be palpated. The history and physical may be performed by a primary care physician, gynecologist, and/or midlevel provider. Further laboratory and radiology tests may include a chemistry panel, GI panel, carcinoembryonic assay (CEA), chest x-ray, CT of the abdomen and pelvis, colonoscopy, proctoscopy, and/or barium enema. In patients who may potentially have advanced disease, fluorodeoxyglucose positron emission tomography (FDG-PET), magnetic resonance imaging (MRI), and endorectal sonography may be used to determine the extent of tumor spread.

The diagnosis and treatment of CRC cancers by endoscopic polypectomy may become commonplace.[53] These cancers are not usually expected at the time of screening and are found after the endoscopy procedure is over and the pathology department is reviewing the polyp. Patients undergoing this procedure need follow-up care if the polyp is found to be malignant; otherwise they should continue with routine screening. Other tumors that may resemble colorectal carcinoma include colorectal lymphomas, carcinoid tumors, gastrointestinal stromal tumors (mural sarcomas), metastatic tumors that exhibit tropism for the GI tract (e.g., malignant melanoma), malignancies of adjacent organs that directly invade the colorectum (e.g., cancers of the ovary, endometrium, bladder or prostate), or appendiceal tumors that extend into the cecum.[53]

Each diagnostic test has its own strengths and weaknesses based on design. Women who undergo a barium enema cannot have a suspicious area biopsied. Colonoscopy requires the use of conscious sedation. Although CT and MRI are more than 90% accurate for identifying metastatic spread before treatment, both are limited with respect to their ability to reveal the spread of local disease.[31]

To determine a patient's prognosis, staging and pathology are important elements to be considered. A biopsy is needed to confirm diagnosis before the initiation of treatment. The majority of CRCs are adenocarcinomas; other types include squamous cell carcinoma, small cell carcinoma, and undifferentiated carcinoma. Patients diagnosed with signet ring adenocarcinoma typically have a poorer prognosis.[7] Tumor grade is also an important feature; high-grade tumors are poorly differentiated, and low-grade tumors are well or moderately differentiated.

Staging for CRC takes into account the depth of tumor invasion into the tissues and the extent of disease in the body. In colorectal cancer, the label of pM1 indicates that disease encompasses pathologically documented metastasis to any nonregional lymph node, the parenchyma of any distant organ or tissue, and/or the peritoneum of any abdominal structure.[53] The most common site of metastatic disease in CRC is the liver. Currently, there are three different staging systems used to classify CRC (Table 9-2). The Duke's system was the first system developed and has undergone modification to account for lymph node involvement and tumor depth; the Modified Astler-Coller (MAC) is another. Then, the American Joint Committee on Cancer (AJCC) and the International Union Against Cancer (UICC) developed tumor, nodes, metastasis (TNM) staging. The TNM staging system provides clinicians with a single system to use in caring for patients with CRC. This system is used nationally and internationally, is multidisciplinary in design, and is pertinent to all modern techniques of stage evaluation.[53]

Appropriate diagnosis and staging are critical to determining available treatment options to patients that may include clinical trials. Approximately 77% of patients are diagnosed with localized/regional disease, and 19% have evidence of distant metastasis at the time of diagnosis.[1] The overall 5-year survival rate for CRC is 63%, which is a 13% increase from the 1974 to the 1976 figures.[1] Patients diagnosed with distant metastasis have a 5-year survival of approximately 10%.[1]

TREATMENT

Treatment of CRC can range from simple to complex, depending upon the extent of the disease. Patients with stage I disease may only require surgery, whereas those with advanced T stage or the presence of lymph node metastases may require neoadjuvant or adjuvant chemotherapy and/or RT to improve their overall survival.

Table **9-2** AJCC Colon and Rectum Staging

	Category	Definition
PRIMARY TUMOR (T)	TX	Primary tumor cannot be assessed
	T0	No evidence of primary tumor
	Tis	Carcinoma *in situ: intraepithelial or invasion of lamina propria*[*]
	T1	Tumor invades submucosa
	T2	Tumor invades muscularis propria
	T3	Tumor invades through the muscularis propria into the subserosa, or into nonperitonealized pericolic or perirectal tissues
	T4	Tumor directly invades other organs or structures, and/or perforates visceral peritoneum
REGIONAL LYMPH NODES (N)	NX	Regional lymph nodes cannot be assessed
	N0	No regional lymph node metastasis
	N1	Metastasis in 1 to 3 lymph nodes
	N2	Metastasis in 4 or more regional lymph nodes
DISTANT METASTASIS (M)	MX	Distant metastasis cannot be assessed
	M0	No distant metastasis
	M1	Distant metastasis

Stage Grouping

Stage	T	N	M	Dukes[*]	MAC[*]
0	Tis	N0	M0	–	–
I	T1	N0	M0	A	A
	T2	N0	M0	A	B1
IIA	T3	N0	M0	B	B2
IIB	T4	N0	M0	B	B3
IIIA	T1-T2	N1	M0	C	C1
IIIB	T3-T4	N1	M0	C	C2/C3
IIIC	Any T	N2	M0	C	C1/C2/C3
IV	Any T	Any N	M1	–	D

[*]Dukes B is a composite of better (T3 N0 M0) and worse (T4 N0 M0) prognostic groups, as is Duke C (Any TN1 M0 and Any T N2 M0). MAC is the modified Astler-Coller classification.

Surgery and RT were the standard treatment for CRC for many decades. Until the mid-1980s, when newer drugs were developed that showed efficacy in treating CRC, 5-fluorouracil (5-FU) was used as a single agent. Today 5-FU is used in combination chemotherapy regimens. In the combined modality setting, RT is used to treat local disease while chemotherapy is used to treat both local and distant disease.

Surgery

Surgery is considered to be the primary treatment of CRC. Resection with curative intent is possible in about 75% of patients. Surgery for CRC has 4 goals: (1) cure, defined as the prevention of systematic spread; (2) local control; (3) preservation of the anal sphincter or anorectal function; and (4) preservation of sexual and urinary functions by preserving the integrity of the autonomic nervous system.[54] Depending upon the size, rectal tumors may be excised in one of three ways: 1) a low anterior resection for lesions in the upper rectum, 2) an abdominal-perineal resection for low rectal cancers, and 3) a transanal resection if adequate margins can be obtained.[55]

The type of surgical procedure for CRC depends upon the anatomic location of the tumor and the draining lymphatics of that particular area. The gold standard for removal of a rectal cancer is via transabdominal low anterior resection (LAR) or a combined abdominal-perineal resection (APR).[56] In both of these surgeries, the affected bowel is removed as well as the mesenteric lymph nodes. APR patients, who have the lower third of the rectum removed along with the bowel that has the anal sphincter, are then left with a colostomy. Patients undergoing an LAR have tumor in the middle to upper rectum and often do not require a permanent colostomy. The distal margin of the rectum is an important consideration when thinking about sphincter preservation as well as recurrence. The National Surgical Adjuvant Breast and Bowel Study (NSABP) [R-01] found that there was no difference in recurrence between resections with distal margins greater than 3 cm compared to those at 2 cm.[57]

In patients with curative colon cancer, surgery is the treatment of choice. There are a variety of different colectomy procedures that a patient can undergo depending upon the tumor location; these include right colectomy, left colectomy, transverse colectomy, splenic flexure colectomy, and sigmoid colectomy. In addition, sentinel lymph node mapping, dissection of the lymph nodes, and/or possible exploration of the abdominal cavity may also be done. When metastasis occurs in the liver, patients whose lesions are less than 5 cm may undergo surgical resection or ablative techniques such as cryoablation, radiofrequency ablation (RFA), ethanol injection, transarterial chemoembolization, hepatic artery transfusion, and systemic chemotherapy.[58] In a study of patients who underwent RFA for metastatic colon cancer, survival at 1, 2, and 3 years was found to be 87%, 77%, and 50%.[59]

Patients with obstructing tumors may have a temporary or permanent ostomy performed at the time of surgery. A temporary ostomy involves bringing the proximal bowel through the abdominal wall and suturing the distal bowel closed. Anastomosis of the proximal and distal bowel occurs several months later. Patients with a permanent ostomy need to be educated on how to care for their ostomy, as well as the impact that it will have on their lifestyle.

Care of the surgical patient focuses on many areas including minimizing infection, bowel changes, managing fluid and electrolytes, pain control, ileus, urinary retention, and wound care. Complications from the surgery can often affect a patient's recovery and quality of life (QOL). When looking at QOL in patients undergoing surgery for CRC, researchers found that lower pretreatment health-related quality of life scores correlated with surgical complications.[60] Ongoing research in this area will assist in developing appropriate interventions for patients both before and after surgery.

Radiation Therapy

Radiation therapy may be used as a neoadjuvant or adjuvant treatment. In the neoadjuvant setting the goal is to reduce the tumor burden, making the tumor more resectable and thus sparing healthy tissue at the time of resection, and to down-stage the tumor so that the chance of the patient requiring a permanent colostomy is decreased.[61] Adjuvant RT is used to eradicate any remaining disease as well as to reduce the risk of local recurrence.

In the neoadjuvant/preoperative setting, patients receive 45 Gy to 50.4 Gy of RT in 180 cGy fractions on a daily basis Monday through Friday for a total of 25 to 28 treatments over 5 to 6 weeks (Figure 9-5, Figure 9-6, Figure 9-7). RT is delivered as a three- or four-field arrangement to the pelvis that typically includes the presacral nodes and internal iliac nodes. There are a variety of techniques used to minimize the amount of radiation to the small bowel, which is the dose-limiting organ. Boost treatments may be given at the end of treatment to a smaller treatment field (Figure 9-7). 5-FU regimens may also be used in conjunction with RT as a sensitizing agent. 5-FU

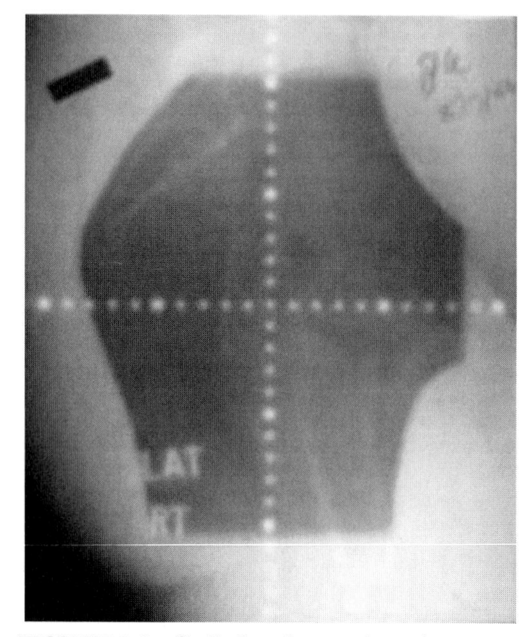

FIGURE 9-5 Radiation therapy lateral treatment field. (Courtesy Tracy K. Gosselin-Acomb, Department of Radiation Oncology, Duke University Health System.)

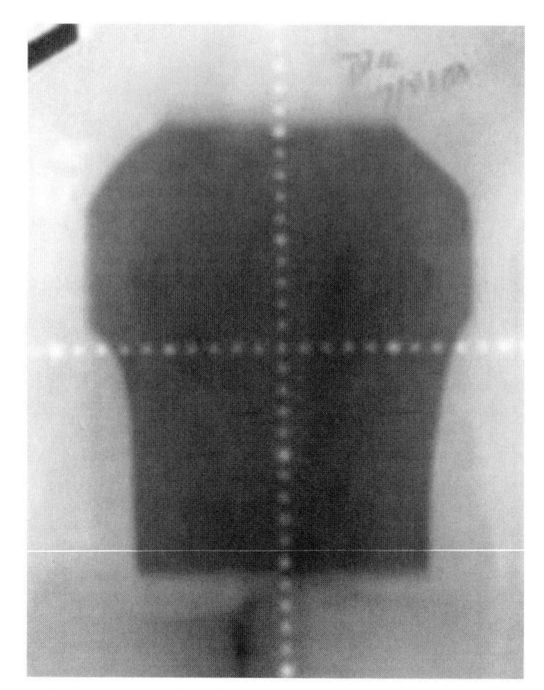

FIGURE 9-6 Radiation therapy posterior treatment fields: anterior, posterior and lateral. (Courtesy Tracy K. Gosselin-Acomb, Department of Radiation Oncology, Duke University Health System.)

may be given as an intravenous (IV) bolus, as a continuous IV infusion through a portable pump, or orally. Other agents that may be used in the preoperative setting include leucovorin, levamisole, and mitomycin-C. Decreased toxicity has been noted when chemotherapy and RT are delivered preoperatively.[62,63]

Postoperative chemotherapy and RT has been the standard of care for patients with locally advanced disease. Postoperative doses of RT are similar to those used in the neoadjuvant setting. Advantages of postoperative RT include that the stage is known (allowing the 10% to 15% of patients with T1-2 N0 M0 disease to be spared treatment) and that a more accurate definition of the tumor bed for radiation planning is obtained by the placement of surgical clips at the time of surgery.[64] Many studies have evaluated the roles of preoperative versus postoperative RT. A small study found that patients who had postoperative RT after anterior resection had markedly inferior anorectal function based upon laboratory and clinical findings.[65]

The NCCN recommends preoperative 5-FU/RT followed by resection and adjuvant chemotherapy, or surgery followed by observation or chemotherapy, for patients with T3 N0 or T any, N1-2 rectal cancer. Patients with T4 and/or locally unresectable disease receive preoperative chemotherapy/RT followed by resection and adjuvant chemotherapy. Patients with resectable M1 disease can receive chemotherapy and RT followed by resection with adjuvant chemotherapy, or combination chemotherapy with bevacizumab followed by resection and chemotherapy/RT, or resection and combination chemotherapy with or without RT.[66] The NCCN also has clinical practice guidelines for colon cancer.[67] RT is not used as commonly in colon cancer because most recurrences occur within the abdomen.

Intraoperative radiation therapy (IORT) is typically used in treating locally advanced disease or recurrent disease in patients who may have

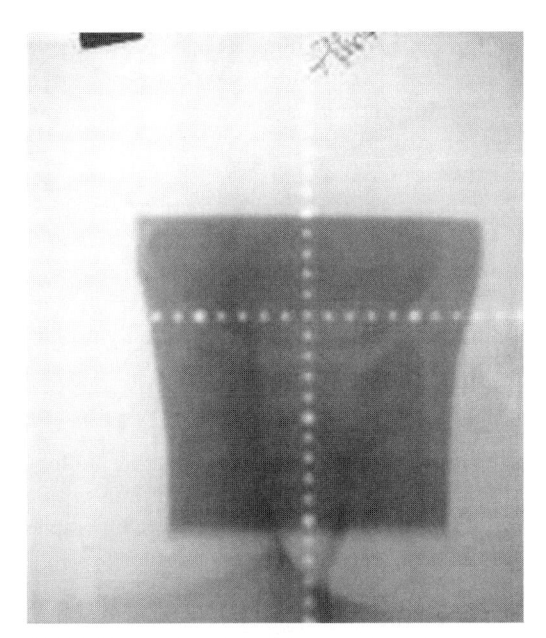

FIGURE 9-7 Radiation therapy boost treatment field. (Courtesy of Tracy K. Gosselin-Acomb, Department of Radiation Oncology, Duke University Health System.)

received RT with or without chemotherapy. The primary advantage of IORT is that radiation can be delivered at the time of surgery to the site with the highest risk of local failure (the tumor bed) while decreasing the dose to the surrounding normal tissues.[68] IORT can be delivered with high-energy electrons (IOERT), an orthovoltage unit, or a high-dose-rate (HDR) gamma-emitting isotope (HDR-IORT).[69] Centers have a dedicated operating room (OR) with a linear accelerator; or for HDR brachytherapy they transport a remote afterloader to the OR that holds the radioactive sources.

Clinical trials show promise for the use of hyperthermia (HT), or the application of heat, in addition to RT and chemotherapy; it can also be delivered to patients preoperatively or postoperatively. The goal is to heat the tumor to 40° to 43° C. In a study of patients with recurrent CRC, those who received chemotherapy, RT, and HT were found to have better responses to treatment than those in other studies who did not receive HT.[70] These results are similar to another study that used 5-FU, RT, and HT in locally advanced, unresectable, or recurrent rectal cancer.[71]

Chemotherapy

Chemotherapy for CRC has seen many advances over the past 10 to 15 years. Chemotherapy, like RT, may be given in the preoperative, the postoperative, or the palliative setting. It is most commonly used in stages III and IV disease and sometimes in stage II disease. As newer chemotherapy agents have been developed and incorporated into treatment, combinations of different agents are being used. When using chemotherapy for the treatment of CRC it is important to know the dose, timing, and route of the drug/s that are being used.

5-FU is the most common drug used to treat CRC in the adjuvant and metastatic setting. It is used today as a single agent or in combination regimens. An antimetabolite that interferes with cancer cell growth, it was initially used as a single agent in combination with surgery and RT. 5-FU may be given as a bolus, by continuous infusion, or as a bolus with continuous infusion. In most North American trials, bolus 5-FU is given over a 1- to 2-minute period, a practice that produces severe mucositis or diarrhea in about 30% of patients treated.[31] Many studies have examined the method of administration, and it has been found that continuous infusion has greater response and survival rates.[72] The folic acid derivative leucovorin (LV) was found to enhance 5-FU cytotoxicity and improve response rates. A recent metaanalysis demonstrated that 5-FU/LV improved both response rate and overall survival compared to 5-FU alone.[73] This regimen is commonly known as the "Mayo Clinic Protocol." Common side effects include diarrhea, myelosuppression, mucositis, and hand-foot syndrome, especially in patients receiving a protracted continuous infusion.

Irinotecan is a topoisomerase I enzyme inhibitor that inhibits DNA replication. Irinotecan has been studied as both a single agent and in combination with 5-FU/LV. In a phase III study of irinotecan, 5-FU/LV, and irinotecan in combination with 5-FU/LV (IFL), it was shown that in untreated patients with metastatic CRC, the IFL group had a greater response rate, greater time-to-disease-progression, and improved overall survival.[74] This regimen has commonly become known as the "Saltz" regimen and is used as first-line therapy in patients with advanced CRC. Common side effects include diarrhea, myelosuppression, mucositis, nausea and vomiting, and cholinergic syndrome, which is characterized by cramping, excessive sweating, and increased salivation.

Capecitabine is an oral fluoropyrimidine that was developed as an oral alternative to 5-FU. With capecitabine, response and survival rates are comparable with intravenous fluorouracil, but lead to significantly fewer treatment-related adverse events including decreased mucositis, neutropenia, febrile neutropenia, and alopecia (hair loss).[37] Capecitabine is first-line therapy in patients with metastatic CRC. Patients who are to receive oral chemotherapy need specific information regarding handling, storage, and dosing of the drug. Issues with patient compliance and drug safety are critical components to be considered in this home-based therapy.

Oxaliplatin is a third-generation platinum compound that is used in the treatment of advanced CRC and stage III colon cancer after resection of the primary tumor. Oxaliplatin inhibits DNA replication and transcription. In a study of 5-FU/LV and 5-FU/LV plus oxaliplatin in patients with stages II to III colon cancer, a higher rate of disease-free survival was found in patients who received the oxaliplatin.[75] Common side effects include diarrhea, nausea and vomiting, neutropenia, and acute sensory neuropathy. The most important toxicity of oxaliplatin, however, is a rather unique neurotoxicity that occurs in two distinct forms: a very common acute syndrome that is transient and appears during or shortly after the first exposure to oxaliplatin; and a dose-limiting chronic sensory neurotoxicity that is cumulative in nature and resembles characteristics of cisplatin neurotoxicity, but is more readily reversible.[76] Cold-induced dysesthesias are common, although the precise incidence is difficult to ascertain because this uncomfortable side effect is so easy to prevent through patient education.[77] Patients are taught to avoid cold exposure the first week after treatment including eating certain food items, going from inside to outside, and even handling cold/frozen items.

Hepatic artery infusion therapy (HAI) is done to treat liver metastasis. Chemotherapy is delivered to the liver via an implanted pump in the abdomen. Floxuridine (FUDR) a fluoropyrimidine, is one of the agents commonly used in this treatment along with LV.

Targeted Agents

In the last 5 years the advancement of technology and drug delivery has provided clinicians with a new type of treatment for CRC. Targeted therapies are treatments that (1) preferentially target specific tumor cells, (2) cause damage to those cells while sparing healthy cells, and (3) are targeted towards a specific signaling pathway. These agents may be monoclonal antibodies (mAbs), tyrosine kinase inhibitors (TKIs), ligand conjugates, immunoconjugates, and antisense oligonucleotides. Each of these agents works in its own way to block epidermal growth factor (EGFR) and promote apoptosis. Aberrant EGFR expression results in abnormal growth, tumor promotion, inhibition of apoptosis, and metastatsis.[78] Many epithelial tumors, including the majority of colorectal tumors, express EGFR, and such expression has important prognostic significance.[78]

Vascular endothelial growth factor (VEGF) is one type of growth factor known to activate endothelial cell growth. It is responsible for preventing apoptosis of vascular cells. As a tumor develops, signals are sent out and endothelial cells respond. Vascular endothelial growth factor rapidly stimulates endothelial cell functions, increases permeability and the survival of immature vasculature, promotes lymphangiogenesis, and may inhibit the tumoral immune response.[79] EGFR and VEGF are each responsible for the growth and development of new cells in different ways, but both also contribute to the development of tumors.

Bevacizumab is a first-line therapy for patients with metastatic CRC who are also receiving infusional 5-FU–based therapy. This agent is a recombinant humanized mAb that binds to and inhibits the interaction of VEGF with the receptors. This neutralizes human VEGF biologic properties, including endothelial mitosis, vascular permeability–enhancing activities, and angiogenesis.[80] A phase III study of first-line bolus IFL and bevacizumab showed statistically significant increases in median survival, progression-free survival, response rates, and duration of response as compared to IFL alone.[81] Side effects include fever, proteinuria, and vascular effects (bleeding, hypertension, and thrombolytic events).[82,83]

Cetuximab is indicated as a single agent for EGFR-expressing CRC patients who are intolerant of irinotecan, or in combination with irinotecan as second-line therapy in patients with EGFR-expressing metastatic CRC who are refractory to irinotecan. This agent is a recombinant chimeric mAb that binds extracellularly to EGFR and thus blocks the ability of EGF to initiate receptor activation and signaling to the tumor. This blockade results in an inhibition of tumor growth by interfering with downstream signaling, which inhibits tumor invasion and metastases, cell repair, and the stimulation of VEGF production leading to angiogenesis.[84] Side effects include allergic reactions and rashes that can be severe.

There is a variety of treatment regimens that incorporate the use of two or more of the drugs discussed above (Table 9-3). The regimens of FOLFIRI (Irinotecan, Leucovorin, Fluorouracil) and FOLFOX (Oxaliplatin, Fluorouracil, Leucovorin) differ on their use of irinotecan and oxaliplatin, and there are different regimens of FOLFOX. COX-2 inhibitors are not as active as EGFR and VEGF pathway inhibitors in the advanced disease, but are useful in preventing polyp formation in patients with FAP.[85] The majority of patients diagnosed with CRC receive treatment, although some patients are not referred for further treatment. Reasons patients are not referred for treatment include patient refusal, comorbidities, and death, and when a physician does not recommend chemotherapy.[86] As expected, older patient age reduced the likelihood of an oncology referral, whereas higher pathologic stage was associated with increased likelihood of referral.[86]

The role of palliative treatment is important in patients who are diagnosed with advanced disease or who experience recurrence. Palliative chemotherapy offers the ability to relieve symptoms and promote QOL, as well as prolonging survival for patients diagnosed at an advanced stage or who develop metastatic disease despite curative therapy.[87] Palliative resection is probably one of the most common palliative procedures for locally advanced disease; patients may suffer less from the potential sequelae including the severe pain of obstruction or even perforation.[88] RT may be used to shrink the tumor and assist with pain control.

In treating patients with CRC it is important to recognize if the chemotherapy agents have overlapping toxicities and if dose reduction of one

Table 9-3 Common Combination Chemotherapy Regimens[66,67,108]

Regimen Name	Chemotherapy Agents Used
Mayo	Fluorouracil Leucovorin
Roswell Park	Fluorouracil Leucovorin
Saltz	Irinotecan Leucovorin Fluorouracil
IFL/BV	Irinotecan Leucovorin Fluorouracil Bevacizumab
FOLFOX4	Oxaliplatin Fluorouracil Leucovorin
FOLFIRI	Irinotecan Leucovorin Fluorouracil
Cetuximab/Irinotecan	Cetuximab Irinotecan
IROX	Irinotecan Oxaliplatin

or more agents is needed. The same chemotherapy agents are often used for both adjuvant therapy and for metastatic disease. Intensity modulated radiation therapy (IMRT) is known to minimize toxicity in head and neck and prostate cancer patients; however, its usefulness in treating CRC has yet to be determined. The landscape of treating CRC is changing and will continue to evolve as new agents are developed and current agents are investigated further. New therapies do come with a significant cost, and this fact has not been lost on health care practitioners.

SYMPTOM MANAGEMENT

Acute and late toxicities of CRC therapy often affect patients' QOL (Table 9-4). The acute side effects arise while patients are undergoing treatment and typically resolve within a month after treatment has been completed. Late effects arise months to years after the treatment has been completed. The side effects of chemotherapy can often overlap and exacerbate the toxicities. RT side effects are localized to the area (organs/tissues) that are encompassed in the treatment field. These side effects may also be exacerbated by the use of chemotherapy. Prompt, accurate assessment and intervention is critical to keeping patients on track for their planned treatment and prevent the need for dose reduction and/or treatment breaks. The NCI has established common toxicity criteria that can be used to grade the severity of side effects. There are also a variety of different medications available to treat many of the side effects that patients experience (Table 9-5).

Table **9-4** COMMON ACUTE AND LATE TOXICITIES OF COLORECTAL TREATMENT

Symptom	Acute	Late
Allergic reaction	X	
Alopecia	X	
Anorexia	X	X
Cholinergic syndrome	X	
Diarrhea	X	X
Cystitis, dysuria, hematuria	X	
Enteritis		X
Fever	X	
Hand-foot syndrome	X	
Mucositis	X	
Myelosuppression	X	
Nausea, vomiting	X	
Peripheral neuropathy	X	X
Proteinuria	X	
Skin erythema, desquamation	X	
Skin fibrosis		X
Sterility		X
Tenesmus		X
Urgency, incontinence	X	
Vaginal dryness, dyspareunia, stenosis	X	X
Vascular effects	X	

Acute Effects

Nausea and vomiting in the CRC patient is typically related to the chemotherapy, although depending on the size of the RT treatment field, RT may also contribute to this. Patients in the postoperative setting may experience nausea and vomiting related to the anesthetic agents and ileus. Nausea arises in patients when neurotransmitters in the gut, such as serotonin and dopamine, are released by chemotherapy and/or RT. There are specific medications that are used to block the message they send from the gut to the vomiting center. The introduction of 5-HT_3 therapy has dramatically affected the care of patients with nausea and vomiting. The NCCN guidelines on the management of nausea and vomiting take into account the emetogenic potential of the treatment. In addition to the emetogenic qualities of individual agents, the use of combination chemotherapy, dosage, time of day, and length of administration may influence the incidence of nausea and vomiting.[89] Patients may also benefit from intravenous fluids (IVFs) and nonpharmacologic therapies to relieve nausea and vomiting. The American Society for Clinical Oncology (ASCO) has guidelines related to radiation-induced nausea and vomiting.

Diarrhea is the dose-limiting toxicity of 5-FU and also is a side effect of irinotecan. RT can also

Table 9-5 COMMON SYMPTOM MANAGEMENT MEDICATIONS

Symptom	Medication	Dosing
Myelosuppression	Darbepoetin alfa	2.25 mcg/kg SQ every week*
	Epoetin alfa	40,000 units SQ once a week*
	Filgrastim	5 mcg/kg/day SQ
	Oprelvekin	50 mcg/kg/day SQ**
Nausea/Vomiting	Prochlorperazine	5-25 mg PO every 4-6 hours
	Promethazine hydrochloride	12.5-25 mg every 4 hours
	Ondansetron hydrochloride	8-24 mg PO**
	Granisetron hydrochloride	1 mg PO
Diarrhea	Loperamide hydrochloride	OTC 4 mg PO followed by 2 mg after each unformed stool (maximum of 8 g a day or up to 16 g if prescribed by provider)
	Diphenyoxylate hydrochloride and atropine	
	Octreotide acetate	5 mg PO, 4 times a day; then titrate to response for 2 days
		Chemotherapy-induced: 300 mcg/day by continuous infusion radiotherapy-induced: 50 mcg SQ every 8 hours
Proctitis	Hydrocortisone (Protocort)	1 applicator (90 mg) 1-2 times/day for 2-3 weeks; then every second day

SQ, Subcutaneous; *PO*, by mouth; *OTC*, over-the-counter.
* Check titrating guidelines based on laboratory values.
** Check emetogenic potential of chemotherapy agent to determine dose.
Data from Wilkes GM, Barton-Burke M, editors: *2004 Oncology Nursing Drug Handbook.* Boston, 2004, Jones and Bartlett.

induce diarrhea. For patients who have diarrhea that is uncontrolled by medications, their chemotherapy and/or RT may be delayed. Patients who have an ostomy need to be educated about how to care for themselves when this challenging side effect arises. Dietary modification, the use of pharmacologic agents, and IVFs may be administered. In a study of 100 patients receiving chemotherapy for CRC, 37 patients used more than oral antidiarrheals to control diarrhea, 14 patients received emergency outpatient treatment, 23 were hospitalized, and 21 received intravenous fluids.[90]

Skin reactions typically arise in the perianal area of patients undergoing RT. Skin reactions initially appear in the second or third week of treatment and present as erythema in the area; this can then progress to dry desquamation and on to moist desquamation. For patients who are also experiencing diarrhea, this can be a challenging side effect to manage, and some type of barrier cream is typically recommended. Use of such a cream can ease the irritation and discomfort arising from dry desquamation of the perianal skin; it can also help prevent moist desquamation and the attendant risk of secondary infections from fecal bacteria, a particular concern when chemotherapy is given with radiation.[31] Sitz baths and Domeboro soaks may also be used to help alleviate the discomfort. A perineal-rectal skin care protocol may be helpful to both health care provider and patient (Box 9-1).

Late Effects

Enteritis is a late effect of RT that is characterized by dysmotility and malabsorption and may lead to complications requiring surgical intervention or long-term parenteral nutrition.[91] Late radiation-induced bowel changes may take years to develop and are typically characterized by small-bowel obstruction, fibrosis, adhesions, and fistulas.[61] The small and the large bowel are dose-limiting structures in abdominal and pelvic RT. Since RT planning and treatment delivery have become

Box 9-1 Perineal-Rectal Skin Care Protocol

ROUTINE CARE

During morning care and after each episode of urination or defecation, the patient will receive the following care:

- Gently cleanse skin with tepid water or a mild cleaning agent followed by gently patting areas dry or cleanse with tepid to cool sitz baths.
- If open lesions are present, cleanse with a wound cleanser or normal saline solution and treat.
- Apply a moisturizing cream.
- Recommend cotton undergarments; avoid restrictive clothing.
- Perform a full assessment of the perineal-rectal skin.
- Perform a nutrition assessment followed by nutrition consult, if needed.
- Consult an enterostomal therapy or wound-care nurse as needed.

ASSESSMENT	RECOMMENDATIONS FOR CARE
Erythema signs and symptoms	Gently cleanse using a mild cleansing agent (perineal skin cleansers).
Pinkness	Apply a moisturizing, protective cream.
Tenderness	If cleanser is not accessible and soap must be used, use a soap without perfumes and thoroughly rinse all soap residues from the skin. Avoid lotions or creams containing perfume and talc (if receiving radiation therapy to the area, avoid products containing metals or ointments or cleanse area prior to receiving radiation therapy). Frequency of skin care: daily and after toileting.

DRY DESQUAMATION SIGNS AND SYMPTOMS	RECOMMENDATIONS FOR CARE
Scaling	Cleanse with tepid water or a wound cleanser.
Flaking	Apply a protective cream.
Pruritis	
Pain	Assess for pruritis, if present. • Apply topical antihistamine creams. • Take a cool shower or bath. • Consider analgesics or antihistamines. Assess for fungal infection, if present. • Treat with topical antifungal or systemic antifungal agent. • Frequency of skin care: twice a day/as needed after toileting.

MOIST DESQUAMATION SIGNS AND SYMPTOMS	RECOMMENDATIONS FOR CARE
Pain	Recommend sitz bath, shower, whirlpool as needed.
Weeping	Cleanse with a wound cleanser as needed.
Sloughing	Apply a protective cream that will adhere to the skin.
Abscess	Apply an adhesive peripad or a pantyliner without deodorant to the undergarments. Assess need for analgesics, pain medications. If desquamation worsens, apply a wound hydrogel. Frequency of skin care: twice a day/as needed after toileting.

Continued

Box 9-1 Perineal-Rectal Skin Care Protocol—cont'd

POSSIBLE COMPLICATIONS OF MOIST DESQUAMATION	RECOMMENDATIONS FOR CARE
Vesicles Furuncle Carbuncles Abscess formation	Consult with physician or advanced practice nurse for treatment and systematic antibiotics. If vesicles are present, rule out herpes and treat appropriately.
REPORT TO PHYSICIAN	**DOCUMENTATION**
Worsening of skin alteration	Anatomical area involved Size of involvement
Increase in inflammation	Area may be difficult to measure because of the perineal-rectal anatomy.
Appearance of furuncle, carbuncles, abscess	Attempt to record in centimeters.
Appearance of vesicles	Measure from where the normal skin stops to where it begins again (use a disposable ruler). If open areas develop, measure width, length, and depth.
Pain or increase in pain, change in character of pain	Record daily in acute care or weekly in home or long-term care: • Changes in skin or wound conditions • Color(s) of skin • Drainage (i.e., amount, odor, color, consistency) • Presence of sloughing or necrosis • Presence and intensity of pain or pruritis • Patient outcomes

Haisfield-Wolfe ME, Rund C: Nursing protocol for the management of perineal-rectal skin alterations, Clin J Oncol Nurs *4, 2000. Copyright 2000 by Oncology Nursing Press.*

more sophisticated, the likelihood of severe complications is low (about 5% or less).[92]

Patients who experience this may complain of abdominal cramping, pain, and frequent and urgent stools. Mild cases of enteritis typically require a low-residue diet, stool softeners, and the occasional use of an antidiarrheal agent. Patients may use additional fiber in their diet to assist in forming and shaping their stool if they are having problems with rectal compliance. Anusol HC suppositories may be used for patients who complain of proctitis.

Sexuality issues face many survivors of CRC. For many women, sexuality is more than the ability to have intercourse: it encompasses their body image, their femininity, and their ability to bear children.[93] Each treatment for CRC has its own impact upon sexuality. In a retrospective study of patients undergoing multimodality treatment for CRC, 71% of patients had no documentation of sexuality issues in their consent form and women receiving RT were found to have no documentation in the consent.[94] Another study found that women with stomas had to learn to manage the devices, and even those with supportive partners described the stomas as a threat to their sexual identity.[95]

Women who undergo treatment experience both physiologic as well as psychosocial issues. The ovaries and/or vagina may become fibrotic from RT, which leads to premature menopause and vaginal stenosis. Women may experience dyspareunia related to sexual intercourse because of the vaginal stenosis. One of the challenges health care providers face is awareness of patients' pretreatment sexual practices. When this concern is not addressed early on, patients typically attempt to return to their usual sexual practices, only to find out that they cannot. Education should occur before, during, and after treatment. Appropriate educational materials such as the American Cancer Society's *Sexuality and Cancer* booklet can serve as a starting point between the patient and the health care team. This book provides women with practical suggestions and if needed, the patient can be referred to a counselor. If the patient is at risk for vaginal stenosis, a vaginal dilator may be given to her to use 3 times a week if she is not engaging in sexual intercourse.

Other acute and late side effects include myelosuppression, mucositis, peripheral neuropathy, hand-foot syndrome, and a variety of others that may arise. Each side effect should be thoroughly assessed by the health care provider and managed based on the best evidence to date. Clinical guidelines have been published by a variety of organizations to assist clinicians in making appropriate treatment recommendations.

PATIENT AND FAMILY EDUCATION

Treatment for colorectal cancer and the disease process itself may result in numerous events (i.e., symptoms, problems, and concerns) that affect patients, their families, and ultimately patient outcomes.[96] When a woman is diagnosed with CRC it is important to understand that the family system and her multiple roles within it are often disrupted, ultimately affecting QOL. In a study of 121 patients, researchers found that CRC imposed significant psychosocial and existential concerns, especially in those people under the age of 45.[96] When CRC appears in this younger population it is found to be more aggressive, diagnosed at a later stage, and has poorer pathologic findings.[52] Women who fall into this younger age group, therefore, face additional concerns regarding the disease and treatment than their older counterparts. This must be taken into consideration as individual treatment and surveillance plans are developed.

A diagnosis of CRC places a strain upon both the patient and the family. Relationships with spouse, significant other, and/or children all are affected by a cancer diagnosis. Early and ongoing education regarding procedures, treatment, and side effects management are initial components of how the health care team can assist in demystifying the cancer experience. Health care providers must be sure patients understand how to care for themselves in both the short- and the long-term. Open dialogue is an important component of establishing trust in the patient-provider relationship. If the patient should discuss the need for genetic testing of self and/or other family members, referral to a genetic counselor should be made to further discuss the process.

Appropriate referrals to counselors and cancer patient support groups can assist in facilitating dialogue about the disease, treatment, and their impact upon self and family. Support groups may be in place for both patients and caregivers and this often helps them in realizing they are not alone. Barriers to attendance include perceptions of adequate support at home, living too far away, no perceived need of support, and not feeling well.[97] Individual counseling appointments may be arranged in conjunction with other appointments for patients who cannot attend support groups. There are also online support groups that can be recommended if the patient wants to participate, but is unable to because of distance. The incorporation of the NCCN Distress Management Guidelines and assessment tool can also assist in referring patients to appropriate resources. Patients seeking complementary and/or alternative care should be referred to reputable clinicians who provide this service. Patients may also use a cancer patient education library or resource center to gather further information.

Depending upon the practice setting, patients may also seek assistance from social workers. Social workers may assist them with psychologic and monetary issues. There are many hidden costs associated with care that may include travel, parking costs, food, loss of work time due to treatment, medical equipment and supplies, and so on. Depending upon the distance from the patient's home to the treatment facility, some patients may apply for discounted housing or a host home, or there may be a facility that provides housing for patients.

Nutritional needs become an issue when the side effects of treatment affect oral intake and/or the absorption of nutrients. Early identification, assessment, and intervention with high-risk patients is critical in meeting the nutritional needs that the patient will have while undergoing therapy. In a study of 88 patients undergoing RT or chemotherapy/RT, 12 of the 13 GI patients surveyed needed to see a dietitian.[98] Education regarding dietary changes for ostomy patients is important as they learn how to care for the ostomy and manage bowel changes. Calorie count, sample diets to manage side effects, and the use of nutritional supplements as well as nutraceuticals should also be discussed.

A patient with a temporary or permanent ostomy may also see the wound care or ostomy nurse, who can provide her with education about the care and management of her ostomy. These nurses also assist patients with determining the appropriate supplies needed for care as well as adjusting to it.

There are a variety of websites that patients and their families may visit. It is important to guide patients to accurate websites that have up-to-date information (Box 9-2).

SPECIAL CONSIDERATIONS

Women who are diagnosed with CRC during pregnancy face a myriad of decisions. The treatment of the pregnant patient is the same as that of the nonpregnant patient, and a decision will have to be made regarding the pregnancy. Both chemotherapy and radiation can have detrimental affects upon the fetus, and most chemotherapy agents are considered teratogenic. Women who are of childbearing potential should be counseled not to become pregnant during treatment and immediately after treatment. Appropriate birth control methods should be recommended and selected based upon individual patient preference. If a woman is diagnosed with CRC and is breast-feeding, this should be discontinued.

CRC is the third most common cancer in females 60 to 79 years old and the second most common cancer in women in their 80s.[1] Cancer is the leading cause of death in 60- to 79-year-olds and in women in their 80s is the second leading cause of death next to heart disease.[1] Treatment of CRC, like many other cancers, has often not been thoroughly studied in the older/elderly population. Clinical trials have specific eligibility criteria that may omit this population based on criteria or may not have included similar numbers of older adults.

The Comprehensive Geriatric Assessment (CGA) tool provides health care providers with information about patients that might otherwise be overlooked. The CGA tool looks at eight specific elements including function, comorbidities, socioeconomic factors, cognition, emotional conditions, nutritional status, polypharmacy, and geriatric

Box 9-2 SELECTED INTERNET RESOURCES ON COLORECTAL CANCER

Cancer Care
www.cancercare.org

Coalition of National Cancer Cooperative Groups, Inc.
www.healthfinder.gov/orgs/HR3487.htm

Colorectal Cancer Network
www.colorectal-cancer.net

National Cancer Institute
www.cancer.gov

National Comprehensive Cancer Network
www.nccn.org

OncoLink
www.oncolink.upenn.edu

The American Cancer Society
www.cancer.org

syndromes.[99] Elderly patients undergoing treatment for CRC often receive the same treatment as and experience similar toxicities to their younger counterparts. While elderly patients with advanced colorectal cancer should not be denied chemotherapy on the sole basis of chronologic age, it is important to notice that the incidence of severe comorbidities increases from 35% in those less than 70 years to 60% in patients aged 70 or more.[100] One of the challenges in this population is the issue of polypharmacy, affecting chemotherapy agents as well as symptom management. A study of 158 patients with CRC who were 65 years of age or older found that patients who reported more limitations in their social activities with family and friends tended to be more depressed. This study also found that more attention should be paid to women, as they need more assistance.[101]

It is estimated that there are approximately 9.8 million cancer survivors in the US[102] of whom 1 million are CRC survivors.[103] Female survivors of CRC face many issues that have an impact on QOL. Younger women especially face issues of fertility, motherhood, and parenthood and, if they have a hereditary form of CRC, the possibility of passing the trait on to their children. Body image and altered sexuality may also cause distress that results from the treatment, the side effects, and/or having an ostomy. Short-term, younger survivors, compared to long-term survivors of CRC, experience greater distress, have higher risk perception, and more intrusive thoughts about recurrence.[104] Survivors in this study also reported that they had made behavior changes, (e.g., diet, weight loss, increased exercise) after treatment to improve their overall health and to reduce the likelihood of cancer recurrence.[104]

Female CRC survivors who have an ostomy or experience a recurrence within 5 years may experience a decline in the physical domain of QOL.[105] Newly-diagnosed women with CRC need to know that long-term CRC survivors have rated their health-related QOL as comparable to that of similarly aged women in the general population.[105] Social networks have also been found in long-term CRC survivors to contribute to mental health in female survivors.[106] The one factor most strongly associated with QOL in female, long-term CRC survivors is not the original diagnosis of CRC, but other medical conditions that exist along with CRC.[105]

IMPLICATIONS FOR PRACTICE, EDUCATION, AND RESEARCH

Health care providers are uniquely positioned to have a great impact in the areas of practice, education, and research by advocating for better programs, enhanced screening, and increased funding for research. Clinicians must look at the development of practice guidelines that incorporate the best evidence, as well as take into account cultural and geographic diversity. The care provided often encompasses the disease trajectory from diagnosis to end of life care. Practitioners have to ensure that patients are aware not only of the acute effects of treatment, but also the late effects that arise months to years later.

It is estimated that each year in the US, 4,200 to 6,300 people die because of a failure to receive the recommended colorectal cancer screening.[107] It is important to understand not only the barriers that patients have to screening, but also one's own biases and knowledge. Education has to happen in a variety of ways and must be tailored to the intended audience. Involvement of local agencies as well as community and faith-based centers allows for dissemination of information in a nonthreatening setting and can often stimulate discussion among participants. As therapies become more advanced, health care providers need to remain up to date on the treatments, as well as patients' comorbid conditions that could exacerbate the side of effects of treatment. Lastly, ongoing education to survivors who need long-term follow-up is critical for ongoing screening, as well as to determine the late effects of treatment.

The need for ongoing research in a variety of areas is critical as we continue to learn more about the human genome and the role that pharmacogenomics will play in the future. Researchers have identified many genes that are linked to the development of CRC. Ongoing work in molecular biology will continue to change the way care is delivered. The role of oncogenes (e.g., K-*ras*), tumor suppressor genes (e.g., p53), and DNA mismatch repair genes (e.g., *hMSH2*) and how they affect the development of CRC will have to be considered as future chemoprevention studies are developed. There is still mixed opinion about dietary influences upon CRC development, and it is important that both clinicians and researchers determine recommended lifestyle guidelines for the general public as well as survivors.

Much research has been done on the barriers to screening, and it is now time to focus on the interventions and factors that enhance screening compliance and ongoing surveillance. As new treatments are developed to improve overall survival rates, nursing research must look at appropriate interventions for both monotherapy and combined therapy. QOL, symptom clusters, late effects, and survivorship studies are long overdue in this population. The impact of pharmacogenomics on treatment decision making has yet to be determined, but how it impacts patient decision making will be of future interest.

REFERENCES

1. Jemal A and others: Cancer statistics, *CA Cancer J Clin* 55:10-30, 2005.
2. Potter JD: Colorectal cancer: molecules and populations, *J Natl Cancer Inst* 91:916-932, 1999.
3. Osias GL, Osias KB, Srinivasan R: Colorectal cancer in women: an equal opportunity disease, *JAOA* 101:S7-S12, 2001.
4. Fuchs CS and others: A prospective study of family history and the risk of colorectal cancer, *N Engl J Med* 331:1669-1674, 1994.
5. Berg DT: Epidemiology and risk of cancer of the colon and rectum. In Berg DT, editor: *Contemporary issues in colorectal cancer*, Boston, 2001, Jones and Bartlett.
6. Wong NA, Harrison DL: Colorectal neoplasia in ulcerative colitis-recent advances, *Histopathology* 39:221-234, 2001.
7. Myerson RJ: Colon and rectum. In Perez CA and others, editors: *Principles and practice of radiation oncology*, ed 4, Philadelphia, 2004, Lippincott Williams & Wilkins.
8. Itzkowitz SH: Inflammatory bowel disease and cancer, *Gastroenterol Clin North Am* 26:129-139, 1997.
9. Ryan DP, Willett CG: Colon and rectal carcinoma: an overview. In Willett CG, editor: *Cancer of the lower gastrointestinal tract*, Hamilton, 2001, B.C. Decker.
10. Winawar SJ: A quarter century of colorectal cancer screening: progress and prospects, *J Clin Oncol* 19:6s-12s, 2001.
11. Lynch HT, Chapelle A: Hereditary colorectal cancer, *N Engl J Med* 348:919-932, 2003.
12. Aaltonen LA and others: Incidence of hereditary nonpolyposis colorectal cancer and the feasibility of molecular screening for the disease, *N Engl J Med* 338:1481-1487, 1998.
13. Loescher LJ, Whitesell L: The biology of cancer. In Tranin AS, Masny A, Jenkins J, editors: *Genetics in oncology practice*, Pittsburgh, 2003, Oncology Nursing Society.
14. Sifri R, Gangadharappa S, Acheson LS: Identifying and testing for hereditary susceptibility to common cancers, *CA Cancer J Clin* 54:309-326, 2004.
15. Kinney AY and others: Attitudes toward genetic testing in patients with colorectal cancer, *Cancer Practice* 8:178-186, 2000.
16. Giovannucci E, Willett WC: Dietary factors and risk of colon cancer, *Ann Med* 26:443-452, 1994.
17. Wei EK and others: Comparison of risk factors for colon and rectal cancer, *Int J Cancer* 108:433-442, 2004.
18. Slattery ML and others: Physical activity and cancer, *Am J Epidemiol* 158:214-224, 2003.
19. Martinez ME and others: Leisure-time physical activity, body size, and colon cancer in women, *J Natl Cancer Inst* 89:948-955, 1997.
20. Fuchs CS and others: Dietary fiber and the risk of colorectal cancer and adenoma in women, *N Engl J Med* 340: 169-176, 1999.
21. Giovannucci E: Diet, body weight, and colorectal cancer: a summary of the epidemiologic evidence, *J Women's Health* 12:173-182, 2003.
22. Michels KB and others: Prospective study of fruit and vegetable consumption and incidence of colon and rectal cancers, *J Natl Cancer Inst* 92:1740-1752, 2000.
23. Alberts DS and others: Fecal bile acid concentrations in a subpopulation of the wheat bran fiber colon polyp trial, *Cancer Epidemiol Biomarkers Prev* 12:197-200, 2003.
24. Chi E and others: Dairy foods, calcium, and colorectal cancer: a pooled analysis of 10 cohort studies, *J Natl Cancer Inst* 96:1015-1022, 2004.
25. Baron JA and others: Calcium supplements for the prevention of colorectal adenomas, *N Engl J Med* 340: 101-107, 1999.
26. Reid ME and others: Smoking exposure as a risk factor for prevalent and recurrent adenomas, *Cancer Epidemiol Biomarkers Prev* 12:1006-1011, 2003.
27. Schoen RE, Weissfeld JL, Kuller LH: Are women with breast, endometrial, or ovarian cancer at increased risk for colorectal cancer? *Am J Gastroenterol* 89:835-842, 1994.
28. Weinberg DS, Newschaffer CJ, Topham A: A risk for colorectal cancer after gynecologic cancer, *Ann Intern Med* 131:189-193, 1999.
29. Sargent C, Murphy M: Colorectal cancer, *Nursing 2003* 33:36-41, 2003.
30. Grodstein F, Newcomb PA, Stampfer MJ: Postmenopausal hormone therapy and the risk of colorectal cancer: a review and meta-analysis, *Am J Med* 106:574-582, 1999.
31. Janjan NA and others: The colon and rectum. In Cox JD, Ang KK, editors: *Radiation oncology, rationale, technique, results*, ed 8, St Louis, 2003, Mosby.
32. Martinez ME, Giovanncucci E, Alberts DS: Prevention of colorectal cancer: epidemiologic evidence and chemoprevention. In Willett CG, editor: *Cancer of the lower gastrointestinal tract*, Hamilton, 2001, B.C. Decker.

33. Martinez ME and others: Pronounced reduction in adenoma recurrence associated with aspirin use and a polymorphism in the ornithine decarboxylase gene, *PNAS* 100:7859-7864, 2003.
34. Giovanncucci E and others: Aspirin and the risk of colorectal cancer in women, *N Engl J Med* 333:609-614, 1995.
35. Healthy People 2010. Washington, D.C., US Department of Health and Human Services 2000.
36. Smith RA, Cokkinides V, Eyre HJ: American cancer society guidelines for the early detection of cancer 2004, *CA Cancer J Clin* 54:41-52, 2004.
37. Rao KV, Goodin S: Prevention and management of colorectal cancer in women, *J AM Pharm Assoc* 41:585-595, 2001.
38. Donovan JM, Syngal S: Colorectal cancer in women: an underappreciated but preventable risk, *J Womens Health* 7:45-48, 1998.
39. Collins JF and others: Accuracy of screening for fecal occult blood on a single stool sample obtained by digital rectal examination: a comparison with recommended sampling practice, *Ann Intern Med* 142:81-85, 2005.
40. Mandel JS and others: Reducing mortality from colorectal cancer by screening for fecal occult blood. Minnesota Colon Cancer Control Study, *N Engl J Med*, 328:1365-1371, 1993.
41. Bell J: Q & A Readers forum, *Advance Imaging Oncol Admin* 14:24-25, 2004.
42. Benson AB III and others: 2000 update of American Society of Clinical Oncology colorectal cancer surveillance guidelines, *J Clin Oncol* 18:3586-3588, 2000.
43. Burke W and others: Engaging women's interest in colorectal cancer screening: a public health strategy, *J Women's Hlth Gend Based Med* 9:363-371, 2000.
44. O'Malley AS and others: Patient and provider barriers to colorectal cancer screening in the primary care safety-net, *Prev Med* 39:56-63, 2004.
45. Subramanian S and others: Adherence to colorectal screening guidelines: a review, *Prev Med* 38:536-550, 2004.
46. Green PM, Kelly BA: Colorectal cancer knowledge, perceptions, and behaviors in African Americans, *Cancer Nurs* 27:207-215, 2004.
47. Busch S: Elderly African American women's knowledge and belief about colorectal cancer, *The ABNF Journal*, 14:99-103, 2003.
48. Dibble SL, Roberts SA: Improving cancer screening among lesbians over 50: results of a pilot study, *Oncol Nurs Forum* 30:E71-E79, 2003.
49. Holmes-Rovner M and others: Colorectal cancer screening barriers in persons with low income, *Cancer Pract* 10: 240-247, 2002.
50. Hull SK and others: The practice of quality: incorporating high-yield strategies into the daily reality of medical practice, *NC Med J* 65:275-280, 2004.
51. Frank-Stromborg M, Cohen RF: Assessment and interventions for cancer detection. In Yarbro CH and others, editors: *Cancer nursing principles and practice*, Boston, 2000, Jones and Bartlett.
52. O'Connell JB and others: Colorectal cancer in the young, *Am J Surg* 187:343-348, 2004.
53. Compton CC, Greene FL: The staging of colorectal cancer: 2004 and beyond. *CA Cancer J Clin* 54:295-308, 2004.
54. Enker WE: Designing the optimal surgery for rectal carcinoma, *Cancer* 78:1947-1950, 1996.
55. McCormink D, Kibbe PJ, Morgan SW: Colon cancer: prevention, diagnosis, treatment, *Gastroenterol Nurs* 25: 204-211, 2002.
56. Ott MJ, Pierue JP: Surgery of primary colon and rectal cancer. In Willett CG, editor: *Cancer of the lower gastrointestinal tract*, Hamilton, 2001, B.C. Decker.
57. Wolmark N, Fischer B: An analysis of survival and treatment failure following abdominoperineal and sphincter-saving resection in Dukes' B and C rectal carcinoma, *Ann Surg* 204:480-489, 1986.
58. Waldman AR, Crane ME: Surgical aspects of colon cancer. In Berg DT, editor: *Contemporary issues in colorectal cancer*, Boston, 2001, Jones and Bartlett.
59. Iannitti DA and others: Hepatic radiofrequency ablation, *Arch Surg* 137:422-427, 2002.
60. Anthony T and others: The association of pretreatment health-related quality of life with surgical complications for patients undergoing open surgical resection for colorectal cancer, *Ann Surg* 238:690-696, 2003.
61. Gosselin TK: Radiation therapy. In Berg DT, editor: *Contemporary issues in colorectal cancer*, ed 1, Boston, 2001, Jones and Bartlett.
62. Minsky BD and others: Combined modality therapy of rectal cancer: decreased acute toxicity with the preoperative approach, *J Clin Oncol* 10:1218-1224, 1992.
63. Sauer R and others: Preoperative versus postoperative chemoradiotherapy for rectal cancer, *N Engl J Med* 35: 1731-1740, 2004.
64. Minsky BD: The role of adjuvant radiation therapy in the treatment of colorectal cancer, *Hematol Oncol Clin North Am* 11:679-697, 1999.
65. Lewis WG and others: Potential disadvantages of post-operative adjuvant radiotherapy after anterior resection for rectal cancer: a pilot study of sphincter function, rectal capacity and clinical outcome, *Int J Colorectal Dis* 10: 133-137, 1995.
66. National Comprehensive Cancer Network: NCCN clinical practice guidelines for rectal cancer—v.1.2005 On the Web at www.nccn.org/professionals/physician_gls/PDF/rectal.pdf.
67. National Comprehensive Cancer Network: NCCN clinical practice guidelines for colon cancer—v.1.2005 On the Web at www.nccn.org/professionals/physician_gls/PDF/colon.pdf.
68. Alektiar KM and others: High-dose-rate intraoperative brachytherapy for recurrent colorectal cancer, *Int J Radiat Oncol Biol Phys* 48:219-226, 2000.
69. Gosselin-Acomb TK: Intraoperative radiation therapy. In Bruner DW, Haas ML, Gosselin-Acomb TK, editors: *Manual for radiation oncology nursing practice and education*, ed 3, Pittsburgh, 2004, Oncology Nursing Society.
70. Schaffer M and others: Feasibility and morbidity of combined hyperthermia and radiochemotherapy in recurrent rectal cancer-preliminary results, *Onkologie* 26:120-124, 2003.
71. Anscher MS and others: A pilot study of hyperthermia continuous infusion 5-fluorouracil, external microwave hyperthermia, and external beam radiotherapy for treatment of locally advanced, unresectable, or recurrent rectal cancer, *Int J Radiat Oncol Biol Phys* 47:719-724, 2000.

72. Meta-analysis Group in Cancer: Efficacy of intravenous continuous infusion of fluorouracil compared with bolus administration in advanced colorectal cancer, *J Clin Oncol* 16:301-308, 1998.
73. Meta-analysis Group in Cancer. Modulation of fluorouracil by leucovorin in patients with advanced colorectal cancer: an updated meta-analysis, *J Clin Oncol* 22:3766-3775, 2004.
74. Saltz LB and others: Irinotecan plus fluorouracil and leucovorin for metastatic colorectal cancer. Irinotecan Study Group, *N Engl J Med* 343:905-914, 2000.
75. Andre T and others: Oxaliplatin, fluorouracil, and leucovorin as adjuvant treatment for colon cancer, *N Engl J Med* 350:2343-2351, 2004.
76. Gamelin E and others: Clinical aspects and molecular basis of oxaliplatin neurotoxicity: current management and development of preventative measures, *Semin Oncol* 29:21-33, 2002.
77. Sorich J and others: Oxaliplatin: practical guidelines for administration, *Clin J Oncol Nurs* 8:251-256, 2004.
78. Spencer-Cisek PA: The role of growth factors in malignancy: a focus on the epidermal growth factor receptor, *Semin Oncol Nurs* 18(Suppl 2):13-19, 2002.
79. Mitchell EP: Therapeutic update, *Curr Top Colorectal Cancer* 1:2-3, 2004.
80. Fernando N, Hurwitz HI: Inhibition of vascular endothelial growth factor in the treatment of colorectal cancer, *Semin Oncol* 30(Suppl 3):159-165, 2003.
81. Hurwitz HI and others: Bevacizumab plus irinotecan, fluorouracil, and leucovorin for metastatic colorectal cancer, *N Engl J Med* 350:2335-2342, 2004.
82. Goetz MP, Grothey A: Developments in combination chemotherapy for colorectal cancer, *Expert Rev Anticancer Ther* 4:627-637, 2004.
83. Schwartz RN, Blanke CD, Pesko LJ: Targeted therapies in the treatment of colorectal cancer: what managed care should know, *J Manag Care Pharm* 10(Suppl S-b): S2-S13, 2004.
84. Wood LS and others: Molecular targets for treating colorectal cancer. In Wood LS and others, editors: *Targeting colorectal cancer: novel approaches to patient care*, Pittsburgh, 2004, Oncology Education Services.
85. Tabernero J and others: Targeted therapy in advanced colon cancer: the role of new therapies, *Ann Oncol* 15(Suppl 4):iv55-iv62, 2004.
86. Oliveria SA and others: Treatment and referral patterns for colorectal cancer, *Medical Care* 42:901-906, 2004.
87. Matasar MJ and others: Management of colorectal cancer in elderly patients: focus on the cost of chemotherapy, *Drugs Aging* 21:113-133, 2004.
88. Amersi F, Stamos MJ, Ko CY: Palliative care for colorectal cancer, *Surg Oncol Clin N Am* 13:467-477, 2004.
89. Bender CM and others: Chemotherapy-induced nausea and vomiting, *Clin J Oncol Nurs* 6:94-102, 2002.
90. Arbuckle RB, Huber SL, Zacker C: The consequences of diarrhea occurring during chemotherapy for colorectal cancer: a retrospective study, *Oncologist* 5:250-259, 2000.
91. Hauer-Jensen M, Wang J, Denham JW: Bowel injury: current and evolving management strategies, *Semin Radiat Oncol* 31:357-371, 2003.
92. Coia, LR, Myerson RJ, Tepper JE: Late effects of radiation therapy on the gastrointestinal tract, *Int J Radiat Biol Phys* 31:1213-1236, 1995.
93. Thaler-DeMers D: Intimacy issues: sexuality, fertility, and relationships, *Semin Oncol Nurs* 17:255-262, 2001.
94. Chorost MI and others: Sexual dysfunction, informed consent and multimodality therapy for rectal cancer, *Am J Surg* 179:271-274, 2000.
95. Rozmovits L, Zieland S: Expressions of loss of adulthood in the narratives of people with colorectal cancer, *Qual Health Res* 14:187-203, 2004.
96. Klemm P, Miller MA, Fernsler J: Demands of illness in people treated for colorectal cancer, *Oncol Nurs Forum* 27:633-639, 2000.
97. Bui LL and others: Interest and participation in support group programs among patients with colorectal cancer, *Cancer Nurs* 25:150-156, 2002.
98. Gosselin-Acomb T, Tinnen R: A pilot study to determine the nutritional needs of radiation patients, *Oncol Nurs Forum* 32:184 (abstract), 2005.
99. Balducci L, Extermann M: Management of cancer in the older person: a practical approach, *Oncologist* 5:224-237, 2000.
100. DeMarco MF and others: Comorbidity and colorectal cancer according to subsite and stage: a population-based study, *Eur J Cancer* 36:95-99, 2000.
101. Kurtz ME and others: Predicators of depressive symptomatology of geriatric patients with colorectal cancer: a longitudinal view, *Support Care Cancer* 10:494-501, 2002.
102. Office of Cancer Survivorship: National Cancer Institute. On the Web at http://dccps.nci.gov/ocs/ocs_factsheet.pdf.
103. Colorectal Facts: American Cancer Society. On the Web at www.cancer.org, type in "What are the key statistics for colon and rectum cancer?" in the search box.
104. Mullens AB and others: Coping after cancer: risk perceptions, worry, and health behaviors among colorectal cancer survivors, *Psycho-Oncology* 13:367-376, 2004.
105. Trentham-Dietz A and others: Health related quality of life in female long-term colorectal cancer survivors, *Oncologist* 8:342-349, 2003.
106. Sapp AL and others: Social networks and quality of life among female long-term colorectal cancer survivors, *Cancer* 15:1749-1758, 2003.
107. The State of Health Care Quality 2004: Industry trends and analysis, National Committee for Quality Assurance, Washington, D.C. On the Web at www.ncqa.org/communications/SOMC/SOHC2004.pdf.
108. Adams VR, DeRemer D, Holdsworth MT, editors: Guide to cancer chemotherapeutic regimens 2004, New York, 2004, McMahon Publishing Group.

CHAPTER

10 Non-Hodgkin's Lymphoma

Lisa Holland Downs and Carrie Tompkins Stricker

INTRODUCTION

The non-Hodgkin's lymphomas (NHLs) are a heterogeneous group of malignancies consisting of diverse pathologic characteristics, natural histories, and patterns of response to therapy. The central process in all NHLs is the malignant transformation which originates within a B or T lymphocyte at a certain point in its cellular development and is subsequently passed on to each daughter cell, thereby creating a clonal expansion of malignant lymphocytes.[1] Approximately 85% of NHL arise from B cells, with the remainder being of T cell type.[2] Although lymphomas usually arise in lymph nodes, they may occur in extranodal sites, and many lymphomas undergo a leukemic phase during which malignant lymphocytes are present in the bloodstream. Using a combination of morphologic features, clinical information, and immunologic and genetic studies, at least 20 types of non-Hodgkin's lymphoma are now recognized as distinct clinical entities.

From a clinical perspective, non-Hodgkin's lymphomas can be categorized by median into "indolent" or low-grade lymphomas (survival measured in years), "aggressive" or intermediate-grade lymphomas (survival measured in months) and "highly aggressive" or high-grade lymphomas (survival measured in weeks), based on usual duration of survival in untreated or palliatively treated patients. NHL constitutes nearly 90% of all lymphomas, and is differentiated from Hodgkin's disease by the absence of the multinucleated Reed-Sternberg cells that are the distinguishing hallmark of Hodgkin's disease.[1]

EPIDEMIOLOGY

The incidence of NHL is strongly linked to socioeconomic status, and rates in the US are among the highest in the world.[1] Non-Hodgkin's lymphoma has increased in incidence by 81% in the US between 1973 and 1996, and most other Western nations report similar trends of increasing incidence.[1,3] In 2005 there will be an estimated 56,390 new cases of NHL and 19,200 deaths, decreased from 24,400 deaths in 2002.[4] NHL is the fifth most common cancer among both women (29,070 cases projected in 2005) and men, and the seventh most common cause of cancer deaths (10,150) in women.[4] Encouragingly, the relative 5-year survival rate in the US has increased significantly from 47% from 1974 to 1976 to 59% in the 1995-2000 period.[3,4]

The incidence of NHL rises with age, and increases markedly from the ages of 20 to 79 years. A woman's probability of developing NHL increases from a rate of 1 in 1,147 from birth to age 39 to a rate of 1 in 100 between ages 60 and 79.[4] NHL incidence is greater in men than women, both in the US and worldwide.[4,5] Caucasians are affected more often than African Americans, and African Americans more often than Asians.[1,3] However, African Americans have not benefited from the markedly improved relative survival rates experienced by whites. Five-year survival rates in African Americans have only increased from 49% to 51% in the period from 1974-1976 to the 1995-2000 period, compared to the 12% absolute increase in survival observed in Caucasians during this same time.[4]

ETIOLOGY AND RISK FACTORS

Pathogenesis

As with all cancers, somatic genetic mutations are central to the pathogenesis of NHL, and chromosomal translocations have been confirmed in up to 90% of all NHL types.[1] Translocations and other genetic errors, such as chromosomal deletions and mutations, lead to uninhibited growth of malignant cells. These genetic mutations at times precipitate the activation of oncogenes, which promote malignant lymphocyte growth, and may also inactivate tumor suppressor genes. The integrity of the immune system plays a critical role in the suppression and development of NHL as these genetic errors are occurring.

Risk Factors

Viral Pathogens

Although there are many risk factors associated with the development of NHL, a clear and comprehensive understanding of its etiology remains elusive. Chronic immunosuppression, chronic antigenic stimulation, and conditions and factors which cause damage to lymphocyte DNA all appear to play a significant role in the pathogenesis of NHL. Certain pathogens have been associated with an increased risk for NHL. A number of external and environmental factors have been inconsistently linked to an increased risk of NHL, including exposure to certain chemical and agricultural agents, increased dietary fat intake, and blood transfusions.[6] Finally, female reproductive factors, including exposure to exogenous estrogens and menstrual and reproductive patterns may modify risk of NHL, but this line of investigation is too premature to draw definitive conclusions.[5-7]

Current evidence best supports the following explanation of the pathogenesis of NHL.[1] Chronic antigenic stimulation, most commonly due to host exposure to or infection with pathogens, results in proliferation of B cells intended to fight off the offending antigen. However, as the number of B lymphocytes undergoing replication grows, the potential for random genetic errors increases, leading to the potential for development of malignant lymphocytes. Furthermore, T lymphocyte response may become down-regulated in response to antigenic stimulation. The subsequent immunosuppressive state renders the body less able to resist and eliminate the malignant lymphocytes. Finally, other independent factors that cause immunosuppression may further contribute to the body's ability to resist the development of NHL.

A number of pathogens have been implicated in the development of NHL, an effect likely resulting from their stimulation of the antigenic response described above, as well as possibly a result of insertion of viral DNA following infection of normal lymphocytes.[1] Pathogens linked to NHL include hepatitis C virus (HCV), human T-cell lymphotrophic virus type I (HTLV-1), Epstein-Barr virus (EBV), *Helicobacter pylori*, human immunodeficiency virus (HIV), human herpesvirus 8 (HHV-8), simian virus 40, *Borrelia burgdorferi*, and malaria.[1,8] In the case of HIV, chronic antigenic stimulation combines with significant immunosuppression, resulting in a markedly increased risk of NHL of up to 250-fold in individuals with acquired immunodeficiency syndrome (AIDS).[1] In addition, individuals with HCV have been shown to be at increased risk for NHL,[9-11] and treatment of HCV has induced remission of NHL in HCV-infected individuals in two case series.[12,13] Certain pathogens are associated with specific subtypes of NHL. For example, infection with *H. pylori* increases the risk of gastric mucosa-associated lymphoid tissue (MALT) lymphoma, but not other lymphoma types. Similarly, HTLV-1 is strongly implicated in the development of adult T-cell leukemia/lymphoma.[1]

Immunosuppression

Immunosuppression is the strongest and most consistently validated factor predisposing for the development of NHL. Since the immune system is the first line of defense against abnormal lymphocytes, immunosuppression undermines the body's ability to suppress these aberrant cells, thereby contributing to the development of NHL. Both primary and acquired immunodeficiencies may increase risk for NHL.[1] Many cases of NHL in individuals with secondary immunodeficiency are associated with the presence of EBV infection.[1]

HIV. Infection with HIV is a salient example of an acquired immunodeficiency that increases one's risk of developing NHL. A significant proportion of the increase in the incidence of intermediate- and high-grade NHL in the past two decades is related to the dramatic increase in AIDS-associated lymphomas as the number of individuals affected with HIV has escalated during this period.[1] The risk of most NHL in individuals with HIV is inversely proportional to their CD4 cell counts.[8] Fortunately, the increasing prescription and effectiveness of combined highly-active antiretroviral therapy (HAART) has markedly reduced the rate of HIV lymphomas, with a 42% drop in incidence reported between 1992-1996 and 1997-1999.[1]

Organ Transplant. Individuals undergoing solid organ and bone marrow transplants are at increased risk for the development of NHL as a result of chronic secondary immunodeficiency.[1] The risk in solid organ transplant is staggering and appears to be related to the degree of pharmacologic immunosuppression. The relative risk of developing NHL may be as much as 67 times higher than in individuals who have not undergone organ transplant, and up to 5% of cardiac transplant patients develop NHL.

Other Conditions. Other medical conditions that may place individuals at higher risk include autoimmune disorders such as systemic lupus erythematosus (SLE), rheumatoid arthritis, and celiac disease.

Because blood transfusions not only confer an increased risk of viral transmission but can also cause temporary immunosuppression, a number of studies have examined their role as a risk factor for NHL. Evidence is conflicting. Several cohort studies have reported up to a 3.5 times greater risk, but case-control studies have not validated these findings.[1]

Radiation

A number of environmental and iatrogenic exposures have been associated with increased risk for NHL. Controversy remains as to whether or not exposure to ionizing radiation is a risk factor for NHL. However, radiation for both Hodgkin's lymphoma and ankylosing spondylitis has been clearly associated with a higher incidence of NHL, and an increased incidence of NHL has been noted in individuals exposed to ionizing radiation in both Hiroshima and Chernobyl.

Chemicals/Pesticides

Occupational and other exposure to certain chemicals and solvents may increase the risk for NHL.[14] Such agents include benzenes, herbicides and pesticides, asbestos, arsenic, and chemicals involved in the production of rubber. Hair dyes have also been implicated as a risk factor for lymphoma, but recent epidemiologic studies found no relationship with current dye formulations.[15,16]

Other Risk Factors

Heredity may also play a role in the development of certain types of NHL. Clusters of multiple NHL cases within families may account for up to 5% of all NHL cases; however, family members' similar environmental exposures could also explain this phenomenon.[1] In general, individuals who have close family members with a history of NHL or other lymphoproliferative disease experience an increased risk of NHL of 2.5- to 4 fold.[1]

Finally, dietary and other modifiable factors have been examined as risk factors for NHL.[14] Unlike their role in the development of other cancers, tobacco and alcohol do not appear to increase the risk of NHL. However, evidence from a number of epidemiologic studies suggests that increased consumption of animal protein and fat may slightly increase risk for NHL, but there is significant inconsistency among findings.[6] Further study is needed before definitive conclusions can be drawn.

CLASSIFICATION AND IMMUNOBIOLOGY

Classification Systems

Classification of NHL has been a source of confusion for both pathologists and clinicians. While some NHL types are readily identifiable and pathologically distinct, others are difficult to distinguish and are vulnerable to subjectivity in pathologic interpretation.[17] The goal of a classification system is to enable the reliable and reproducible identification of clinically distinct types of lymphomas in a format that is readily applicable to clinical practice.

Classification for non-Hodgkin's lymphoma has evolved over time as laboratory hematopathologic techniques have become more sophisticated. Classification systems for lymphoma have been in use for over 30 years; the most widely used include the Kiel classification,[18] the Working Formulation,[19] the Revised European American Lymphoma classification,[17] and the World Health Organization (WHO)[20] systems.

Kiel

The Kiel classification system was developed in Germany in 1974, and was the first system to be adopted.[18] The Kiel system, updated in both 1988 and 1992, split lymphomas into broad categories of B- and T-cell malignancies.[21-23] This system was based on the idea that malignant lymphomas occur at different levels of lymphocyte maturation, and that NHL could therefore be classified based on normal lymphocyte counterparts.

National Cancer Institute Working Foundation

Around this time, two other major classification systems were developed in the US, the Lukes-Collins classification and the Rappaport classification. These were organized based on tumor histology, which is the study of cells and cell structure.[24] By the early 1980s, six major NHL classification systems were available. Due to the confusion and inconsistency generated by these varying classification systems, the National Cancer Institute (NCI) sponsored an international study to enable correlation between the various classification systems and to promote consistency in NHL diagnosis and in communication between clinicians and researchers.[19] As a result of this study, which reviewed the records and pathology of 1175 cases of NHL, the NCI Working Formulation was developed in 1982.[18] The Working Formulation (WF) enabled translation between the various other classification systems.

In the US, the WF was promptly adopted for NHL classification upon its development. In the WF, lymphomas are broadly grouped into low, intermediate and high grades based on clinical behavior when treated palliatively.[18] The WF classifies lymphomas by histopathology (examination of the cell type and its characteristics) and does not employ immunophenotypic or genetic characterization using flow cytometry or cytogenetic techniques. The WF divides the lymphomas into two histologic groups, follicular or diffuse, based on the architecture of the involved node. Nodal architecture is determined by how the pattern of cells is distributed. In follicular lymphomas, the malignant cells are lumped together in a circular pattern. In diffuse lymphomas, the malignant lymphocytes are spread throughout the biopsy specimen. Within each of these two broad architectural groups, lymphomas are further classified as either small cell or large cell type, based on the size of the predominant malignant cell. The appearance of small cells is further described as either lymphocytic, cleaved cell or noncleaved cell. Large cells are categorized as large cell or large cell immunoblastic type. Lymphomas that have both small and large malignant cells are categorized as mixed lymphomas.

In spite of its strengths and widespread adoption, the Working Formulation has significant limitations. The WF has not been updated since 1988 and therefore does not include more recently described B-cell lymphomas and certain T-cell lymphomas.[25] Moreover, it is not based on recent immunologic techniques which are critical to contemporary NHL diagnosis. Finally, certain NHL subtypes could not be translated between the WF and the Kiel system, the predominant classification system used at the time in Europe.[23]

Revised European American Lymphoma (REAL)

Given the limitations of contemporary classification systems, the Revised European American Lymphoma (REAL) classification system was developed in 1994 by the International Lymphoma Study Group (ILSG), a consensus group of

19 hematopathologists from the US and Europe (Table 10-1).[17] The ILSG developed the REAL classification with a straightforward goal: to categorize the types of NHL that could be reliably recognized at the time using available morphologic, immunologic, and genetic techniques. Due to this diagnostic specificity, the REAL system categorization produced NHL subgroups with largely similar clinical presentations and natural histories. The REAL classification is based on cell differentiation and cell lineage, and therefore separates lymphomas into T- and B-cell NHL subtypes as well as into subgroups characterized by precursor or by mature cells.[16] A novel feature of the REAL system is its inclusion of clinical features in defining distinct types of lymphomas, such as site of origin, aggressiveness, and prognosis.[20] As seen in Table 10-1, the REAL classification groups NHL into categories of indolent, aggressive, and highly aggressive lymphomas, terminology which is widely used in clinical practice and medical literature today. These categories correspond to the low-, intermediate-, and high-grade categories

Table **10-1** REVISED EUROPEAN-AMERICAN LYMPHOMA (REAL) CLINICAL GROUPING OF CURRENTLY RECOGNIZED NON-HODGKIN'S LYMPHOMAS

I. Indolent Lymphomas (untreated survival measured in years)	
Indolent Disseminated Lymphoma/Leukemias	
B-cell Neoplasms	***T/NK-cell Neoplasms***
• B-cell CLL/small lymphocytic lymphoma • Lymphoplasmacytic lymphoma • Splenic marginal zone lymphoma/SLVL • Hairy cell leukemia	• T-cell CLL • Large granular lymphocyte leukemia
Indolent Extranodal Lymphomas	
B-cell Neoplasms	***T/NK-cell Neoplasms***
• Extranodal marginal zone lymphoma/MALT lymphoma	• Mycosis fungoides
Indolent Nodal Lymphomas	
B-cell Neoplasms	***T/NK-cell Neoplasms***
• Nodal marginal zone B-cell lymphoma • Follicular center cell lymphoma, grade I and grade II	
II. Aggressive Lymphomas (untreated survival measured in months)	
B-cell Neoplasms	***T/NK-cell Neoplasms***
• Follicular center cell lymphoma, grade III • Mantle cell lymphoma • Diffuse large B-cell lymphoma	• Peripheral T-cell lymphoma • Anaplastic large cell lymphoma
III. Highly Aggressive Lymphomas (untreated survival measured in weeks)	
B-cell Neoplasms	***T/NK-cell Neoplasms***
• Precursor B-lymphoblastic leukemia/lymphoma • Burkitt's and Burkitt's-like lymphoma	• Precursor T-lymphoblastic leukemia/lymphoma • Adult T-cell leukemia/lymphoma (HTLV I+)

CLL, Chronic lymphocytic leukemia; *T/NK*, T/natural killer; *SLVL* = splenic lymphoma with villous lymphocytes; *MALT*, gastric mucosa-associated lymphoid tissue; *HTLV*, human T-cell lymphotrophic virus.

of the WF.[16] Individual NHL types included in each of these categories will be discussed in great detail in the section on treatment later in this chapter.

World Health Organization

The newest classification system is the World Health Organization (WHO) system. The WHO classification system improves upon the REAL system by enabling it to be refined and updated as hematopathologic and genetic techniques evolve.[20] The WHO is the first lymphoma classification system to be widely accepted for use on an international level and is the system most widely used today in clinical practice, research, and medical communication, both in the US and Europe.[23]

Pathology and Diagnostic Techniques

Histopathology, the process of examining cell appearance and structure, is one major technique used to identify and categorize NHL into the classification systems discussed above. Immunophenotyping is an additional method; it uses flow cytometry to detect cell surface and cytoplasmic markers on normal and malignant lymphocytes. Molecular genetic analysis enables the identification of somatic genetic mutations through cytogenetics, polymerase chain reaction (PCR) testing, Southern blot analysis, and/or fluorescence in-situ hybridization (FISH) testing.[2]

Lymphoma cells often retain the phenotypic markers of the normal lymphocyte counterparts from which they have arisen, thereby rendering immunophenotyping a valuable diagnostic technique for NHL. Phenotypic cell surface and cytoplasmic markers are associated with stages of normal lymphocyte development and can be also used to identify the corresponding stage from which malignant cells have arisen. The antigen markers used to immunophenotype normal and malignant lymphocytes have been assigned cluster designation (CD) numbers based on monoclonal antibody reactivity. Some important antigenic markers are listed in Table 10-2.

Identification of normal lymphocyte counterparts is useful not only in aiding classification but also in understanding the clinical behavior of NHL. Specific NHL subtypes often behave quite similarly to the normal lymphocytes from which they have arisen, particularly in B-cell NHL.[20] For example, immature lymphocytes proliferate quite rapidly, as do lymphomas which arise during this developmental stage. It is therefore useful to discuss normal lymphocyte development in order to better understand NHL diagnosis and clinical behavior.

Table **10-2** Important CD Antigens in Lymphocytes and Lymphoid Neoplasms

Cell Type	Antigen	Distribution/Function
T cell	CD2	Pan-T cell marker; E rosette
T cell	CD3	Pan-T cell marker; associated with T cell antigen receptor
T cell & B cell	CD5	Pan-T cell marker Subset B cell marker (CLL)
T cell	CD7	Pan-T cell marker
T cell	CD8	Suppressor and cytotoxic T cell subset marker
T cell	CD4	Helper/inducer T cell subset marker
B cell	CD19	Early pan-B cell marker
B cell	CD20	Later pan-B cell antigen
Granulocyte and monocyte	CD15	Marker for Reed-Sternberg cell
T and B cells	CD30	Marker for Reed-Sternberg cell and anaplastic large cell lymphoma

Immunophenotyping: Normal and Malignant Lymphocytes

Normal Lymphocyte Development

In normal B lymphocyte development, the earliest B cells are bone marrow lymphoblasts that possess rearranged immunoglobulin heavy chain genes and express common acute lymphoblastic leukemia antigen (CALLA), CD10, and intranuclear terminal deoxynucleotidyl transferase (TdT). With maturation to a pre-B cell, cytoplasmic μ chains appear and TdT is lost; most cases of B-precursor acute lymphoblastic leukemia arise from these immature cells.[25] The cell becomes an immature B cell when immunoglobulin M (IgM) appears on the surface membrane and CALLA is lost. Burkitt's lymphoma/leukemia arises from this immature B cell stage. Because cell growth and proliferation is very rapid during these initial phases of normal lymphocyte development, NHL, which arises during this phase of development, tends to behave very aggressively and demonstrate very rapid mitotic rates.

When surface immunoglobulin D (IgD) is expressed in addition to IgM, the cell has become a mature B cell. From this point forward, any and all development and maturation of the normal B lymphocyte is driven by antigen exposure. These developmental events triggered by antigen exposure occur in the follicles, or germinal centers, of lymph nodes. Most follicular and diffuse B-cell lymphomas arise from mature, antigen-activated B cells. Waldenstrom's macroglobulinemia, multiple myeloma, and hairy cell leukemia arise from cells near the latest or final stages of B-cell development, during terminal differentiation.[2]

Mantle zone B cells appear to have a different life cycle than other types of B lymphocytes. They express CD5, a pan-T cell marker, in addition to B cell phenotypic markers. Chronic lymphocytic leukemia and mantle cell NHL arise from these CD5-positive (+) nonfollicular lymphocytes.

Malignant Lymphoma Phenotypes

In normal T lymphocyte development, the earliest T cells are bone marrow and thymic lymphoblasts that express the transferrin receptor (T9), TdT, and pan-T cell markers such as CD2-E rosette receptor. T-cell acute lymphoblastic leukemia and T-cell lymphoblastic lymphomas possess this immunophenotype. As with B-cell malignancies, T-cell malignancies arising at this stage of development tend to proliferate rapidly and behave very aggressively. Early T cells mature to cortical thymocytes, whereupon T9 and TdT are lost and cells coexpress CD4 and CD8. Some cases of lymphoblastic lymphoma possess this immunophenotype.[2]

With completion of maturation, T cells become committed to either the CD4 (helper) or CD8 (suppressor) phenotype. At this stage of development, T lymphocytes are noted to have a mature or postthymic phenotype, also called a peripheral T cell phenotype because T lymphocytes are predominantly circulating outside the thymus at this stage. This phenotype characterizes the peripheral T-cell lymphomas.[2] In addition to either CD4 or CD8, the pan-T cell markers CD2, CD3, and CD5 are also expressed on all mature peripheral blood T cells. On encountering an antigen, mature T cells transform into T immunoblasts, which are large cells with prominent nucleii and basophilic cytoplasm. T immunoblasts are TdT-negative, in contrast to T lymphoblasts, which are TdT-positive. The neoplastic counterpart of the T immunoblast is T-immunoblastic lymphoma.[25]

Molecular Genetic Analysis

Molecular genetic analysis is another method used in the identification and classification of NHL, since these malignancies are often associated with nonrandom chromosomal changes. Molecular genetic analysis is employed to detect the presence of clonal immunoglobulins in B-cell NHL, and to detect T cell antigen receptor gene rearrangement in T-cell NHL. Malignant transformation initially occurs in a single B or T lymphocyte, and all daughter cells therefore possess the identical pattern of gene rearrangement, indicating clonality. In contrast, although benign lymphoid proliferations also possess gene rearrangements, these are not identical from one cell to the next. Clonal gene rearrangement can be detected by Southern blot analysis if a clonal population comprises

1% or more of cells examined. PCR analysis for clonal gene rearrangement is considerably more sensitive and can detect 1 in 10^5-10^6 cells.[2] Most recently, FISH is being used to detect gene rearrangements. FISH is particularly useful when low numbers of cells are available for testing, such as with fine-needle aspiration.[26]

A number of specific chromosomal changes are associated with particular NHL subgroups. Some of the most common are listed in Table 10-3. The diagnosis of many types of NHL is markedly enhanced by testing for these translocations, which may also aid in predicting prognosis.[27] For example, most cases of Burkitt's lymphoma are associated with a translocation of the eighth and fourteenth chromosomes, t(8;14); or, less commonly, t(2;8) or t(8;22).[28] All three translocations involve juxtaposition of the *c-myc* proto-oncogene on chromosome 8 with a portion of a gene coding for the immunoglobulin molecule.[29] This juxtaposition allows the cells carrying the translocation to proliferate more freely, resulting in clonal expansion of these malignant lymphocytes.[25]

In the follicular lymphomas, t(14;18) is observed in about 85% of cases and is also observed in approximately 30% of diffuse B-cell NHLs. This translocation results in juxtaposition of the *bcl-2* proto-oncogene on chromosome 18 with the immunoglobulin heavy chain locus on chromosome 14. Increased *bcl-2* expression confers resistance to apoptosis, which is the process of normal cellular death.[30]

Approximately 50% of mantle cell lymphomas have a t(11;14) translocation involving rearrangement of the *cyclin D1 (CCND1)* gene on chromosome 11, which results in elevated *cyclin D1* expression. The site of chromosomal breakage on chromosome 11 is called bcl-1. The *cyclin D1* gene encodes a protein important in cell cycle regulation and appears to contribute to lymphomagenesis by shortening the G_1 growth phase of the cell cycle.[30]

Most recently, rearrangement of the *bcl-6* proto-oncogene at the end of chromosome 3 (3q27) has been observed in about 30% of cases of B-cell diffuse large cell lymphoma.[31] *Bcl-6* encodes a regulatory nuclear protein important in cell differentiation and development. Rearrangement of the *bcl-6* gene correlates with extranodal lymphoma as well as a favorable clinical outcome.[32]

CLINICAL PRESENTATION

Clinical presentation of NHL is quite diverse. NHL may be diagnosed in individuals with few subtle signs or symptoms, as well as conversely in individuals who have evident and rapidly progressive signs and symptoms. The most common presentation of NHL is the presence of one or more enlarged and nontender peripheral lymph nodes. Often individuals will first be seen with enlarged lymph nodes that wax and wane. This clinical picture may cause a delay in diagnosis, since it is common to treat patients with one or more courses of antibiotics before proceeding with diagnostic testing. Enlarged lymph nodes that do not resolve for a period of 6 weeks should be biopsied.[33]

Only 20% of individuals present with systemic B symptoms, which include night sweats, fever, and/or weight loss of greater than 10% of body weight. The clinical presentation of NHL further depends on the site(s) involved. For example, individuals with central nervous system (CNS) disease may have apathy, confusion, seizures, and/or mental status changes.[33] Patients with large mediastinal tumors can have shoulder pain, dyspnea upon exertion (DOE), and/or chest pain.

Table **10-3** COMMON CHROMOSOMAL ABNORMALITIES IN NHL

Lymphoma Type	Cytogenetics	Oncogene
Burkitt's	t(8;14) t(2;8) t(8;22)	*c-myc*
Follicular	t(14;18)	*bcl-2*
Mantle cell	t(11;14)	*bcl-1*
Diffuse large cell	3q27	*bcl-6*

Table 10-4 Ann Arbor Staging System of NHL[34-37]

STAGE I	Involvement of a single lymph node region (I) or a single extralymphatic organ or site (IE).
STAGE II	Involvement of two or more lymph node regions on the same side of the diaphragm (II), alone or with localized involvement of an extralymphatic organ or site (IIE).
STAGE III	Involvement of lymph node regions on both sides of the diaphragm (III), alone or with localized involvement of an extralymphatic organ or site (IIIE) or spleen (IIIS) or both (IIISE).
STAGE IV	Diffuse or disseminated involvement of one or more extralymphatic organs with or without associated lymph node involvement.

All patients are subclassified A or B to indicate the absence or presence, respectively, of unexplained weight loss of more than 10% body weight, unexplained fever with temperatures more than 38° C, and/or night sweats.

STAGING AND PROGNOSTIC DETERMINATION

Ann Arbor Staging System

In addition to the histologic type of NHL, prognosis and approach to therapy depend on the extent of disease present at diagnosis. Clinical staging is the process of determining the extent of disease. The Ann Arbor staging system (see Table 10-4) was originally developed for use in staging Hodgkin's disease[34] and has frequently been applied in NHL staging, although with significant limitations.[35] For example, although the distinction between stage III and stage IV disease is critical in determining therapy for Hodgkin's disease, the treatment of stage III and stage IV disease is generally the same in NHL, and the prognostic difference between stage III and stage IV aggressive NHL is becoming less important with current therapy.[35,36] In addition, the Ann Arbor system does not address other important prognostic features for the aggressive NHLs such as age, performance status, serum lactate dehydrogenase (LDH), and extent of extranodal involvement.[36,37]

International Prognostic Index

The International Prognostic Index (IPI) is a more useful model for predicting 5-year survival rates for aggressive NHL and has become the standard.[35] The IPI identifies four risk groups based on age, Ann Arbor tumor stage, LDH level, performance status, and number of extranodal disease sites. Negative prognostic clinical features include age greater than 60 years, serum LDH 1 × normal, poor performance status (Eastern Cooperative Oncology Group 2-4), stage III or stage IV disease, and more than one site of extranodal involvement.[35] (See Box 10-1.)

Once the diagnosis of NHL is suspected, a full staging evaluation begins. The process of staging involves a series of tests that is somewhat specific to each patient. The goal of the staging evaluation is to determine the type, location, and extent of the lymphoma, thereby allowing the clinician to individually tailor the treatment.

Excisional Biopsy

The most critical diagnostic test is an excisional biopsy, during which an entire lymph node or a portion of a mass is removed. An excisional biopsy is invaluable, since fine-needle aspirate

Box 10-1 International Prognostic Index Prognostic Factors

PROGNOSTIC FACTORS IN AGGRESSIVE LYMPHOMAS

1. Age
2. Tumor stage (Ann Arbor)
3. LDH level
4. Performance status
5. Number of extranodal sites

(FNA) or core biopsy alone does not allow for optimal differentiation of the various lymphomas.[38] Although not yet in routine use, power Doppler ultrasound is a novel imaging technique that can be used to guide the selection of a lymph node for biopsy.[39] Power Doppler ultrasound has been shown to not only increase the likelihood of making an accurate diagnosis of malignancy, but also to decrease patient-specific complications such as pain, numbness, and unsatisfactory scarring.[39] Currently, most excisional biopsies are performed intraoperatively under either local or general anesthesia, and rebiopsy is sometimes necessary for findings that are unequivocal or inconsistent with the clinical picture.

Complete Staging Workup

After the diagnosis of NHL is made, the staging evaluation includes a detailed history and physical with attention to systemic symptoms, lymph node areas, and the spleen and liver, as well as computed tomography (CT) scans of the chest, abdomen, and pelvis, with or without the neck. Examination of Waldeyer's ring, which consists of the palatine, pharyngeal, and lingual tonsils encircling the pharynx, is necessary in staging gastrointestinal lymphomas. Either unilateral or bilateral bone marrow biopsy is often undertaken to evaluate for bone marrow involvement by malignant lymphocytes. Laboratory studies on the blood are necessary, and includes complete blood count (CBC), LDH, comprehensive metabolic panel with an albumin level, and a β-2 microglobulin level. Some patients will need to undergo lumbar puncture (LP), depending on the type and location of the NHL and the patient's symptoms. For example, patients with highly aggressive lymphomas are at higher risk for CNS involvement; therefore, an LP should be performed in these individuals for staging.[29] Depending on the patient's symptoms and the results of prior tests, an magnetic resonance imaging (MRI) scan may be needed to visualize areas such as the spine.

Positron emission tomography

Positron emission tomography (PET) scanning has been recently adopted into widespread use for staging of NHL. PET scan has replaced the gallium-67 scan as well as staging laparotomy in most cases. PET scans are more sensitive in detecting subclinical sites of NHL, because this imaging technique detects metabolic changes that are indicative of malignancy, at times even before a mass or enlarged lymph node can be clinically detected. PET provides useful diagnostic and staging information in all the aggressive and highly aggressive lymphomas, and is playing an increasing role in the evaluation of many of the low-grade lymphomas as well.[40]

TREATMENT OF NON-HODGKIN'S LYMPHOMAS

Treatment for NHL varies greatly based on type and stage. Therapy is guided broadly by the lymphoma grade (low-, intermediate-, or high-grade), as well as by the specific NHL type and stage of disease. However, treatment plans should be tailored to individual patients. Age, stage, presence of comorbid illnesses, and even religion and culture can influence treatment decisions.

Highly Aggressive Lymphomas

The highly aggressive B-cell lymphomas and Burkitt's and Burkitt's-like lymphoma, as well as lymphoblastic lymphoma, are uncommon diseases which together account for about 10% of non-Hodgkin's lymphomas classified by the WF. These lymphomas are staged and managed differently from the more common aggressive lymphomas.

Burkitt's/Burkitt's-like Lymphoma/Leukemia

Burkitt's lymphoma/leukemia (BLL) was originally called small noncleaved cell lymphoma in earlier US and European classification systems, and L3 acute lymphoblastic lymphoma in individuals with greater than 25% bone marrow involvement. The WHO classification currently denotes Burkitt's lymphoma/leukemia as a single NHL entity.[29] BLL is characterized by an extremely rapid proliferation rate, and its hallmark diagnostic feature is the presence of overexpression of the *c-myc* gene due to various translocations including t(8:14).[41] BLL is most often staged using the St. Jude/Murphy staging system, which incorporates clinically significant features such as number and extent of extranodal disease sites, as well as the presence of either CNS disease or bone marrow involvement greater than 25%, each of which automatically upgrades BLL to stage IV. Since these features are not part of the Ann Arbor staging system, this system is much less frequently used for staging of BLL.[29]

BLL is most commonly a disease of children and young adults, occurring predominantly in the first two decades of life. In adults it is often associated with immunodeficiency, and is 2 to 3 times more likely to occur in men than in women.[17] There are three clinical types of BLL: endemic, sporadic, and immunodeficiency BLL.[29] Endemic BLL develops most frequently in young children in equatorial Africa and often involves the jaw and other facial bones.[17] Sporadic BLL accounts for about 1% to 2% of all adult NHLs in the US and Europe and occurs predominantly in extranodal locations, most frequently presenting as an abdominal tumor. Immunodeficiency BLL occurs most frequently in individuals infected with the HIV virus and, interestingly, occurs most frequently in individuals whose CD4 cell counts exceed 200/mcl.[29] All BLL variants typically present with bulky disease and elevated LDH and uric acid levels. Bone marrow and CNS involvement are present, respectively, in up to 38% and 17% of adult cases. Although bone marrow and CNS involvement have long been considered to confer a poor prognosis, the use of increasingly aggressive regimens, which include CNS-penetrating therapies, are rendering these cases increasingly curable.[29] The most effective regimens used in treating BLL result in cure in almost all patients who have limited disease, and in a high proportion of patients with extensive disease.

The mainstay of treatment for BLL is intensive combination chemotherapy using agents such as cyclophosphamide, vincristine, methotrexate, doxorubicin, and cytarabine. Given the rapid growth rate of BLL, which has a doubling time of approximately 25 hours, critical treatment strategies include fractionated doses of chemotherapy and administration methods that maintain serum concentrations of chemotherapy for 48 to 72 hours. The most common treatment regimens for BLL have been successful in achieving complete remission (CR) rates of 61% to 92%, and 1- to 5-year disease-free survival (DFS) rates of 60% to 86%. CR is typically obtained within 4 to 6 weeks of initiation of chemotherapy.[29] Several different chemotherapeutic treatment approaches have been successful, including short-course cytoreductive induction chemotherapy such as the Vanderbilt regimen,[42] cytoreductive induction regimens followed by additional courses of intensive combination chemotherapy (German B-cell non-Hodgkin's lymphoma regimen,[43] French LMB protocols[44]), and prolonged administration of intensive combination chemotherapy without a defined induction period (Stanford regimen,[45] CODOX-M/IVAC,[47] hyper-CVAD,[47] R-Hyper-CVAD[48]).

Each of these regimens involves the administration of chemotherapy on 2 or more days of a 21-day cycle, and most also cyclically alternate exposures to non–cross-reactive agents. CNS prophylaxis is mandatory for the treatment of all adult cases of BLL, and the above regimens accomplish this through the administration of intrathecal and/or high dose intravenous (IV) methotrexate and/or cytarabine. There is no role for prophylactic CNS irradiation in the above regimens, as it increases the risk of severe neurotoxicity without conferring a concomitant improvement in outcome.[29] Finally, stem cell transplant in first complete remission has not been shown to improve clinical outcomes over those observed with brief-duration intensive chemotherapy regimens such as those listed above.[29]

In BLL, primary refractory disease (that which does not respond to initial therapy) and relapse are particularly challenging clinical situations for which the optimal treatment strategy remains unknown. The administration of salvage chemotherapy with non–cross-resistant agents induce few, if any, remissions.[29] In one trial, autologous stem cell transplant (ASCT) was effective in a proportion of individuals: 37% who had chemosensitive disease and 7% with chemotherapy-resistant disease were alive 3 years following transplantation.[49] Allogeneic stem cell transplant (SCT) does not appear to be more effective than ASCT, and there appears to be no graft-versus-lymphoma effect in BLL. Therefore, experts currently recommend participation in clinical trials as the preferred treatment for individuals with relapsed or primary refractory BLL, although ASCT may be considered for individuals with chemosensitive disease.[49]

Lymphoblastic lymphoma

Lymphoblastic lymphoma (LL) is a high-grade malignancy that accounts for approximately 2% to 4% of adult NHL. LL is more common in men than women and occurs in both children and adults.[51] The average overall age of individuals with LL is around 30 years. The vast majority of cases are of T cell origin, but 5% to 20% of cases originate from B lymphocytes. LL commonly manifests with large subdiaphragmatic and/or a bulky mediastinal adenopathy, usually accompanied by significant clinical symptoms ranging from cough and shortness of breath to respiratory distress and superior vena cava syndrome. As in BLL, CNS involvement is not uncommon, with an incidence up to 20% in LL. Bone marrow involvement greater than 25% defines a leukemic phase in lymphoblastic lymphoma and may cause LL to be diagnostically indistinguishable from lymphoblastic leukemia.[47]

Historically, LL was treated with traditional lymphoma regimens such as cyclophosphamide, adriamycin, vincristine, and prednisone (CHOP) in combination with asparaginase. Long-term prognosis was poor, with a median survival of 17 months in one national series of patients.[51] In the 1990s, adding prolonged systemic maintenance chemotherapy and CNS prophylaxis or treatment with intrathecal chemotherapy improved prognosis, with a 3-year DFS rate of 56% in one study.[52]

Current aggressive treatment of LL has improved survival rates for this malignancy, and CNS prophylaxis and treatment remains an essential component of LL therapies. A common therapeutic strategy involves the administration of induction-consolidation combination chemotherapy, followed by maintenance chemotherapy over months to years, along with mediastinal irradiation for individuals with mediastinal masses.[53] One example of this approach utilizes hyper-CVAD (cyclophosphamide, adriamycin, vincristine, decadron alternating with high dose methotrexate and cytarabine) for 8 cycles with growth factor and prophylactic antibiotic support, followed by maintenance therapy with 6-mercaptopurine, vincristine, methotrexate, and prednisone for 2 to 3 years. Mediastinal irradiation is included for individuals with mediastinal masses. The hyper-CVAD regimen may also be modified to include an additional cycle with cytarabine and an anthracycline.

In one series of 33 patients with LL receiving this regimen at a median follow-up time of 4 years, 67% of patients were alive without disease.[54] Slightly inferior results have been reported when LL is treated with protocols for acute lymphoblastic leukemia, which include multiple phases of chemotherapy including induction, consolidation, reinduction, and maintenance therapy with non–cross-reactive agents, as well as CNS prophylaxis with intrathecal methotrexate and cytarabine.[55] Longer maintenance therapy may improve the outcome with these leukemia protocols.[54]

ASCT has not been shown to significantly improve survival of individuals with LL in first complete remission when compared to current intensive therapy.[56] Nonetheless, both autologous and allogeneic SCTs have been performed in these individuals.[50] Risk factors have not been shown to reliably predict prognosis in individuals with LL, making it difficult to determine which patients would be most likely to benefit from SCT in first remission.[53] The role of transplant for LL in first remission remains unclear.[50] However, both allogeneic and autologous transplants remain options for treatment of refractory LL as well as relapsed LL, once remission has been regained with salvage chemotherapy.

Aggressive Lymphomas

The aggressive lymphomas, which are comprised of diffuse large B-cell lymphoma (DLBL), follicular large cell lymphoma (grade 3), primary mediastinal large cell lymphoma, peripheral T-cell lymphoma, and anaplastic large cell lymphoma, are all generally treated in a similar fashion. DLBL provides an excellent model for investigating therapies for aggressive NHL, and results from these trials are generally adopted in the treatment of all aggressive lymphomas. CHOP is generally accepted as standard therapy, based on a large intergroup study carried out in the early 1990s by the Southwest Oncology Group (SWOG) and the Eastern Cooperative Oncology Group (ECOG). This trial compared other more intensive regimens to CHOP.[57] Previously untreated patients with stages II to IV aggressive lymphomas were randomized to one of four treatment arms, and no differences in failure-free survival (FFS) and overall survival (OS) were seen in the CHOP arm, along with less toxicity and death. Given these findings and the ease and cost-effectiveness of administration, CHOP has become the standard therapy for these diseases.

Although the OS at 5 years in the CHOP group was only 36% at the conclusion of this pivotal study, clinically significant differences were observed in subgroups of individuals stratified by the IPI. This model resulted in four risk categories with four very different 5-year survival statistics: low risk (0-1 risk factors) = 73% OS; low to intermediate risk (2 risk factors) = 51%; high intermediate risk (3 risk factors) = 43%; and high risk (4-5 risk factors) = 26%.[58] Nonetheless, the globally low OS rates clearly indicated a need for significant improvement in therapy for aggressive NHL.

Initial Therapy

CHOP chemotherapy. In 1997, a chimeric monoclonal antibody against CD20, rituximab (Rituxan, Genentech) was approved by the FDA for use in B-cell lymphoma; it has proven to be an active agent that improves outcomes in the treatment of DLBL. Rituximab depletes B cells by inducing apoptosis, antibody-dependent cellular cytotoxicity, and complement-mediated cytotoxicity.[59,60] Rituximab is typically an extremely tolerable therapy with minimal side effects. The major potential complication is risk for an infusion reaction. While common during the first infusion, reactions are mild and self-limiting in the vast majority of patients, as long as pretreatment with acetaminophen and diphenhydramine is administered.

Rituximab + Chemotherapy. Rituximab has been combined with chemotherapy in an attempt to improve survival in DLBL, as this combination appears to be synergistic.[61] A randomized study done by the Group d'Etude des Lymphomes de l'Adulte (GELA) compared CHOP plus Rituximab (RCHOP) with CHOP alone in older adults with previously untreated large B-cell NHL. Superior response rates, OS, and event-free survival (EFS) were demonstrated in the RCHOP group, without concomitant increase in toxicity.[62] Recent long-term follow-up documented a continued improvement in survival rates over time in the RCHOP patients.[63]

A larger (N=632) US intergroup study also compared CHOP to RCHOP in previously untreated elderly patients with DLBL.[64] This study was also designed to secondarily evaluate whether or not prolonged maintenance therapy with Rituximab could improve outcomes over standard duration RCHOP therapy in individuals who responded to initial therapy. Patients who received RCHOP in combination did better; however, no differences were seen between groups who received Rituximab as part of initial chemotherapy as opposed to maintenance therapy. In summary, the addition of Rituximab to CHOP in any fashion results in superior survival rates in the elderly. A large (n=824) randomized study confirmed these superior outcomes in younger patients, establishing RCHOP as standard therapy for all individuals with DLBL.[65]

Dose-intense chemotherapy has also been investigated as treatment for DLBL, and shows promising early results. Two recent studies have shown better OS rates with dose intensification strategies as compared to standard therapy. A SWOG trial first evaluated dose-intense CHOP (CHOP-DI): cyclophosphamide 1600 mg/m^2, doxorubicin 65 mg/m^2, and vincristine 1.4 mg/m^2) given every 14 days for six planned cycles, with filgrastim as white blood cell (WBC) growth factor support. This CHOP-DI regimen produced an improvement of 14% compared to historical survival rates in prior SWOG studies.[66] Second, the German NHL-B1 trial compared four arms as follows: standard CHOP every 14 days, CHOP every 21 days, CHOEP (CHOP with etoposide 100 mg/m^2 days 1-3) every 14 days, and CHOEP every 21 days. Patients over 60 years old experienced better OS in the arm with CHOP every 14 days; however, toxicities were also increased.[67,68] Despite these promising results, dose-intense regimens are not yet recommended for standard therapy outside of clinical trials.[58,69]

Finally, ASCT is under investigation as part of first-line therapy for DLBL. Although a recent trial found that ASCT in this setting did not improve outcome as compared to standard chemotherapy,[69] a recent international consensus conference concluded that high-dose therapy with stem cell support may benefit patients in the high-risk IPI category.[70] An ongoing intergroup study in the US is attempting to answer this question.

Early-Stage Disease and Radiation Therapy. Primary treatment for patients with aggressive lymphomas varies according to stage of disease. As first demonstrated in the late 1980s, patients who have low-stage, nonbulky disease without B symptoms experience favorable results with a shorter course of chemotherapy combined with involved field radiation therapy (RT). An overall response rate of 99% and a 30-month DFS rate of 84% were demonstrated.[71] A later SWOG study established that patients with low-stage, low-risk disease experience superior outcomes, including decreased toxicity, with CHOP for three to four cycles followed by involved field radiation, as compared to eight cycles of chemotherapy alone.[72] RCHOP now replaces CHOP in this combined modality approach. However, individuals with stage I and stage II aggressive lymphoma who have bulky disease show similar survival data to those with stage III or stage IV and thus are treated similarly. Bulky disease was defined as having a mediastinal mass larger than one third the transthoracic diameter of the chest on chest x-ray study or masses greater than 10 cm.

Refractory and Recurrent Disease

Autologous Stem Cell Transplant. Initial therapy for aggressive lymphomas can be curative, but it falls short of this goal in a significant number of patients. As many as 40% to 60% of patients either relapse or are initially refractory to anthracycline-containing therapies.[73] ASCT provides the possibility of cure in a proportion of these individuals, with approximately 50% of these individuals enjoying long-term disease-free survival after ASCT. The pivotal Parma trial demonstrated an EFS rate of 51% in the transplant group as compared to 12% in the group who received chemotherapy alone.[74] In an attempt to further improve outcomes with ASCT, novel conditioning regimens are being tested. Conditioning regimens are the cytotoxic agents given to ablate the bone marrow before reinfusion of stem cells. A phase I/II trial evaluated the use of an ASCT conditioning regimen of iodine-131 (I-131) tositumomab (Bexxar) radioimmunotherapy followed by chemotherapy with etoposide and cyclophosphamide in patients with relapsed indolent or aggressive NHL.[75] The OS and progression-free survival (PFS) were better in both groups at 2 years when compared historically to trials using total body irradiation (TBI)-based conditioning regimens. A phase I study revealed no added toxicity with the addition of I-131 tositumomab as compared to high-dose carmustine, etoposide, cytarabine, and melphalan,[76] and another phase II study of this approach is currently underway.

Radioimmunotherapy. Unfortunately, a number of patients do not meet the selection criteria for ASCT. Patients who are not eligible for transplant include those with significant organ dysfunction, poor performance status, older adults with significant comorbidities, and individuals whose disease is not chemotherapy-sensitive. For individuals who either cannot undergo or who are not cured by ASCT, alternative strategies are under investigation. Radioimmunotherapy is one such approach that has demonstrated promising results. Yttrium-90 ibritumomab tiuxetan (Zevalin) is an active treatment for patients who are ineligible for ASCT for relapsed or refractory disease.[77] It has also been administered safely to patients after ASCT,[78] if used with caution concerns that these individuals would experience unacceptable toxicity are decreased.

In summary, the treatment of choice for aggressive lymphomas is chemotherapy with RCHOP, with or without RT depending on the stage and size of the disease. Individuals who relapse or are refractory to initial therapy should be considered first for ASCT. For those who are either ineligible for or relapse following transplant, radioimmunotherapy appears to be an effective treatment option. In spite of this multitude of treatment options, a proportion of patients will still not be cured. These individuals can be treated either palliatively or be placed on a clinical trial aimed at cure. Current clinical trials are focusing on targeted therapies such as other radioimmunotherapeutic agents,[79] other monoclonal antibodies such as epratuzumab,[80] and other novel therapies such as genasense, gallium nitrate, and anti-vascular endothelial growth factor (anti-VEGF) agents. Although these agents have begun to show promising activity, investigation is too premature to determine their place in the treatment of aggressive lymphoma.

Mantle Cell Lymphoma

Mantle cell lymphoma (MCL) is a distinct entity that has recently been classified as an aggressive NHL, despite its earlier classification as an indolent lymphoma in the REAL system.[2] MCL comprises approximately 6% of the non-Hodgkin's lymphomas.[81] MCL cells express the pan-B cell antigens CD19, CD20, CD22, and CD5 along with surface IgM and IgD. Over 90% of MCL possesses a unique and reliable cytogenetic marker, t(11:14), which results in overproliferation of cyclin D1 and leads to excessive B cell proliferation. Many patients with MCL have gastrointestinal tract (GI) involvement, and an upper GI series and colonoscopy should therefore be part of MCL staging. Although MCL is generally considered to be an aggressive lymphoma, it can behave quite indolently in some individuals and is highly aggressive in others. Individuals with MCL typically experience low response rates and short remission durations with current therapies. The median survival is 3 to 4 years.[82] This disease currently remains incurable, and there is no clear standard approach to treatment.

Initial Therapy. The approach to treatment of MCL depends greatly on the age of the patient and his or her expected tolerance of aggressive therapy. Various chemotherapeutic agents have been used for MCL, but none have significantly improved durable clinical outcomes. Off-protocol regimens such as chlorambucil, cyclophosphamide, vincristine, and prednisone (CVP), and CHOP can be used in patients not eligible for aggressive treatment. These regimens induce both partial responses (PRs) and complete response, but provide little benefit with respect to long-term survival.[83] Rituximab therapy alone induces response rates of approximately 30%. When anthracycline-based therapy is added to rituximab, the response rate increases to 95%.[81]

The hyper-CVAD regimen, designed by a group of oncologists from M.D. Anderson Cancer Center, is commonly used in aggressive first-line treatment strategies for MCL. Hyper-CVAD induction chemotherapy, followed by ASCT with a cyclophosphamide and TBI-based conditioning regimen, has demonstrated promising efficacy in MCL as compared to CHOP therapy alone. In previously untreated subjects, this approach can produce OS rates over 90% and 3-year EFS rates of 72%, whereas previously treated individuals have much poorer outcomes, with survival rates of 25% for OS and 17% for EFS.[84] When tested with reduced cytarabine dosing in adults over 65 years, rituximab plus hyper-CVAD (R-hyper-CVAD) produced comparable efficacy and manageable but clinically significant, toxicity.[85] More recently R-hyper-CVAD has demonstrated comparable rates of response and survival (EFS and OS) to those seen with hyper-CVAD plus ASCT.[82] Long-term follow up for these patients will need to be done to assess long-term disease free survival to compare the two treatment approaches.

The use of novel conditioning regimens before ASCT is another promising form of therapy for MCL. Combination radioimmunotherapy and chemotherapy with I-131 tositumomab and high-dose etoposide and cyclophosphamide chemotherapy has shown remarkable and durable response rates approaching 100% in one small (n=16) study in relapsed or refractory MCL.[86]

Relapsed or Refractory MCL. For patients with relapsed or refractory MCL, treatment strategies are continuously evolving. One promising therapeutic strategy is nonmyeloablative allogeneic transplantation. Nonmyeloablative transplants utilize chemotherapy-based conditioning regimens in doses that do not completely ablate the bone marrow, followed by reinfusion of stem cells from related or unrelated donors. In patients with relapsed or refractory MCL, OS rates of 85% have been observed, with DFS rates approaching 100% at 24.6 months.[87]

Finally, novel biologic therapeutic strategies are being tested in MCL. The use of bortezomib, a proteasome inhibitor,[88] and combination thalidomide/rituximab treatment[89] are two such approaches currently under investigation. The role of these and other novel treatments will continue to evolve as oncologists persist in addressing the challenge of improving outcomes in this complicated, poor-prognosis NHL.

Indolent (Low-Grade) Lymphomas

Overview

At present, no consensus exists as to the best treatment approach for individuals with indolent NHL. The development and evaluation of therapies for indolent lymphoma currently represents the largest and most diverse body of investigation in NHL. There are many types of indolent lymphomas that will not be discussed in this chapter. Some have curative therapies that are standard, for example mucosa associated lymphoid tissue (MALT) lymphomas of the stomach. These can be cured with either a gastectomy or RT. The discussion will be limited to the area where most of the research is being conducted as a model to discuss therapeutic options. The majority of research is being conducted in follicular lymphoma, which is the second most common type of NHL. As of yet, no treatment strategy has been shown to be curative for a significant proportion of individuals with indolent NHL, making ongoing investigation imperative. Patients with indolent lymphomas, particularly follicular NHL, frequently experience repeated remissions with multiple sequential treatments, but these remissions become progressively shorter over time. The life span of individuals with indolent NHL has been previously reported to be 8 to 10 years; however, this statistic does not reflect the recent explosion of novel, highly efficacious therapies. In addition, great variability exists among patients with follicular NHL, with some patients enjoying very prolonged remissions of 10 or more years, whereas others remain in remission for months or less. The major challenge of treating these patients lies in strategically devising stepwise treatment plans that will allow the use of the multiple available therapies throughout the patient's disease trajectory.

Individuals with stage I or stage II disease constitute the only subgroup of indolent NHL patients for whom standard initial therapy currently exists. For this small number of patients, involved field RT is standard treatment; it yields long-term relapse rates of 54% at 15 years and 56% at 25 years.[90] Combination chemotherapy plus involved field RT appear to provide superior response rates in stage I/II indolent NHL, with 10-year OS rates of 82%.[91] These two treatment approaches are currently being compared in randomized clinical trials. Finally, in selected patients with stage I and stage II follicular lymphoma, deferral of therapy is appropriate and does not compromise outcomes.[92]

For the majority of individuals with indolent NHL who have stage III or stage IV disease, treatment options are broadly diverse, ranging from no initial therapy (watch and wait) to intensive chemotherapy and even to allogeneic SCT. Radioimmunotherapy is another treatment strategy that intuitively seems promising for the treatment of indolent NHL, since it is a systemic therapy without significant life-threatening toxicity. Clinical trials are currently investigating this approach in individuals with indolent NHL.[93] The plethora of treatment strategies for indolent NHL is discussed below.

Careful Observation (Watch and Wait)

Most patients (85%) with indolent lymphoma are first seen with disease that is stage III or stage IV. Advanced-stage indolent lymphoma may initially need no treatment at all. The *watch and wait* approach is used frequently for patients with stage III or stage IV low-volume indolent NHL. One study compared immediate treatment versus watch and wait, and overall and cause-specific survival rates were no different between the two groups after 16 years of follow-up.[94] Individuals with indolent NHL who are followed with careful observation often do not require treatment for 2 to 3 years or longer.[93,95] Similar results have been seen when watch and wait is compared to combination chemotherapy, and response rates are excellent at time of progression, exceeding 80% with a median remission duration of greater than 4 years.[96] The watch and wait strategy allows the clinician to gauge an individual's lymphoma in terms of the indolence or aggressiveness of its behavior. Such observation significantly contributes to the ease and effectiveness of treatment decision making in indolent NHL.

When patients and physicians chose the watch and wait option, diligence in monitoring for progression becomes imperative. Patients must follow a rigorous schedule of visits with their oncologists for physical examination and lab work, which should include a CBC, metabolic panel, and measurement of LDH level. Changes in these values should precipitate a more detailed evaluation. CT scans are also a very important monitoring tool and are often performed 2 to 4 times annually for ongoing assessment of disease status. Once the tempo of the individual's disease has been established, the frequency of testing can be decreased in patients with stable disease. One particular concern during careful observation is the potential for indolent NHL to transform into aggressive lymphoma. Signs and symptoms that may alert the clinician to transformation include a markedly elevated LDH level, rapidly enlarging lymph node(s), and the development of B symptoms. Biopsy should be performed immediately in these patients to evaluate for transformation, which if diagnosed requires urgent, aggressive treatment.

Chemotherapy

Once a decision has been made to pursue treatment, chemotherapy is commonly used as first-line therapy in indolent NHL. Both single-agent and combination chemotherapy regimens are commonly used, including regimens with low toxicity potential as well as intensive chemotherapy. The majority of indolent lymphomas are sensitive to chemotherapy in this setting, and therefore initial chemotherapy should be tailored to the individual patient and the expressed goals of treatment. Chemotherapy has historically included the use of chlorambucil alone; cyclophosphamide, vincristine, and prednisone in combination (CVP); and fludarabine-based regimens. Attempts to cure patients with CHOP chemotherapy have also been undertaken, but these efforts have proven unsuccessful.[97] CHOP alone has not been demonstrated to be curative therapy for patients with indolent NHL in any significant numbers.

Fludarabine-based regimens are very active in follicular NHL, and have demonstrated high response rates and molecular remissions in which malignant follicular lymphocytes are no longer detectable using molecular genetic analysis.[93,98] Unfortunately, fludarabine is not an ideal agent for first-line therapy for a number of reasons. Fludarabine may induce a number of clinically significant toxicities, particularly high rates of infection when used in combination with cyclophosphamide.[99] This combination induces prolonged decreases in CD4 and CD8 T cells, which requires the prophylactic use of acyclovir and sulfamethoxazole/trimethoprim during and for months after the cessation of treatment. These toxicities are particularly unfortunate, as other fludarabine-based regimens have not yielded remissions as durable as those seen with this combination.[93] Furthermore, use of fludarabine can lead to poor subsequent mobilization of stem cells, which individuals may eventually require for ASCT, particularly if their disease transforms into an aggressive NHL. Finally, the development of autoimmune processes has been associated with the use of fludarabine, including SLE, autoimmune hemolytic anemia, and autoimmune thrombocytopenia.[100,101]

Rituximab

Rituximab is commonly employed in the treatment of indolent lymphoma, both as initial therapy and in patients with relapsed and refractory disease. Response rates are approximately 67% in patients who are chemotherapy-naïve, and response rates are approximately 50% in relapsed or refractory indolent NHL.[93] Maintenance therapy with rituximab has also been evaluated for indolent NHL; it achieves prolongation of remission as long as 12 to 19 months, respectively, both in individuals who have received prior treatment and those who are treatment-naïve.[102] The comparative benefit of prophylactic administration of maintenance rituximab, versus retreatment at time of progression, is not yet known.[103] A randomized clinical trial is ongoing.

Rituximab in combination with chemotherapy has also been investigated in the treatment of indolent NHL. Two studies adding rituximab to CHOP show promising results, with response rates as high as 95%, approximately half of which were complete responses. Remissions appear to last for 2 years and beyond in a majority of patients.[104] Longer follow-up of these studies will determine whether or not RCHOP has curative potential. Furthermore, the addition of maintenance rituximab following CVP chemotherapy has significantly improved progression-free survival (58% versus 34%) at 4.5 years when compared to observation after CVP in a phase III study.[105]

Despite its efficacy in the treatment of both indolent and aggressive NHL, rituximab is associated with the development of resistance to therapy. One strategy for attempting to overcome resistance is the use of rituximab in combination with interleukin-2. This strategy may enhance antibody-dependent cytotoxicity, but requires further evaluation in clinical trials.[93]

Immunotherapy

The addition of immunotherapy to common chemotherapy regimens has been examined in individuals with indolent NHL. Multiple studies of interferon-α as adjuvant therapy have yielded conflicting results.[106] Interferon-α is not commonly used in the US, in part due to the significant fatigue and flu-like symptoms which render this treatment intolerable for many individuals. Other agents currently under investigation include anti-CD22 (epratuzumab) and anti-CD80 monoclonal antibody.[93]

Radioimmunotherapy

Radioimmunotherapy (RIT) agents have been available since 2001. The first FDA-approved agent was yttrium-90 ibritumomab tiuxetin (Zevalin), and I-131 tositumomab became clinically available in 2003. Like rituximab, these agents are monoclonal antibodies that are administered intravenously and target the CD20 lymphocyte surface markers. However, these agents attach to the CD20 marker and deliver a targeted dose of RT. Both are effective in the treatment of indolent NHL and can be safely and easily administered to carefully selected patients in treatment settings that follow appropriate radioprotection precautions. These agents are effective in producing longer remissions than many prior agents utilized in indolent NHL therapy, and may even hold potential for cure.

Yttrium-90 ibritumomab tiuxetan is a high energy beta (β)-ray emitter.[107] In the pivotal trial of this agent in relapsed or refractory CD20+ follicular or transformed NHL, the overall response rate was 80%, with a CR rate of 30%, and a median duration of response of 14 months.[108] The response rate for subjects with disease refractory to rituximab was a remarkable 74%, although a shorter duration of response was seen in these individuals.[109] Yttrium therapy is dosed based on body weight (0.4 μCi/kg), with a dose reduction (0.3 μCi/kg) for platelet counts below 100,000.[107] Patients who are overweight or obese may be at a disadvantage with this therapy, since a maximum dose of 32 μCi is allowed.[107] Minimal radiation precautions are required with its use because of the short distance (5 mm) traveled by beta particles, and family members' exposure is similar to that of background radiation.[110] Nonetheless, condoms should be used for sexual intercourse for 7 days following treatment, and caregivers should be instructed not to handle or come in close contact with the patient's waste.[110,111]

I-131 tositumomab emits both β and gamma (γ) rays. A multicenter pivotal trial demonstrated its efficacy in relapsed or refractory CD20+ follicular or transformed NHL, with overall response rates of 65%, a CR rate of 20%, and a 6.5-month median duration of response.[112] In treatment-naïve individuals, overall and complete response rates of 95% and 75%, respectively, have been documented, with no evidence of disease progression in 62% of subjects at a 5-year follow-up.[113] To achieve appropriate levels of radiation exposure, dosimetry is used to ensure a total body irradiation dose of 75 cGy of I-131 tositumomab. Patients do emit γ rays after treatment, and therefore must follow post–treatment guidelines for limiting secondary exposure to nontreated individuals. Patients must be able and willing to follow these guidelines in order to receive I-131 tositumomab, and must also take thyroid-protective agents during and after therapy.[114]

Both currently available radioimmunotherapy agents are well tolerated. Complete blood counts should be obtained on a weekly basis, because myelosuppression, including neutropenia and thrombocytopenia, is common. Although myelosuppression is often mild, colony-stimulating factors or transfusions may be necessary. The nadir predictably occurs 7 to 9 weeks after therapy. RIT patients experience an increased risk of secondary leukemia and myelodysplastic syndrome (MDS); however, it is unclear how much of this risk is due to RIT as opposed to prior chemotherapy and RT treatments.[93]

The use of RIT in combination with chemotherapy is currently under investigation. CHOP followed by I-131 tositumomab has been shown to be superior to CHOP alone, with CR rates of 60% and 39%, respectively, and 80% of subjects remaining in remission at the 2-year follow-up.[115] A large US intergroup trial is presently underway to assess the difference between RCHOP and CHOP I-131 tositumomab.

Patient selection for both the RIT drugs is quite specific. Individuals who have undergone stem cell transplantation are excluded, as are those who have severely hypocellular bone marrow (less than 15%) or bone marrow with more than 25% involvement by lymphoma. Doses can be reduced for mild thrombocytopenia, but individuals with platelet counts of less than 100,000 are generally not eligible. Individuals who have received prior fludarabine-based therapy are at risk for prolonged and more severe toxicities.

Novel radioimmunotherapy agents currently under development and investigation include Y-90-eptatuzumab (radiolabeled anti-CD22) and HLA-DR 10-β.[93] The concomitant or tandem administration of radiolabeled monoclonal antibodies holds potential as another therapeutic strategy. However, such strategies first require further investigation.

Vaccines

Vaccines continue to be investigated in the treatment of indolent NHL. Lymphoma-specific vaccines are typically created from a patient's individual tumor. Specific idiotypes are produced that, when injected into the patient in vaccine form, enable the individual's immune system to respond by recognizing and targeting tumor-specific antigens. The development of an antiidiotype reaction is associated with longer remissions as compared to individuals who do not develop this reaction.[116] A promising NCI trial demonstrated the ability of vaccination to induce molecular remission following chemotherapy-induced clinical remission. Three phase III trials are currently underway to assess to use of antiidiotype vaccines in follicular lymphoma.[93]

Autologous Stem Cell Transplantation

A multitude of studies have attempted to determine the best approach to integration of ASCT into the treatment of relapsed follicular lymphoma. These trials have tested varying preparative regimens, sources of hematopoietic cells, and techniques for purging the autologous stem cells (autograft) of contamination by malignant lymphocytes. Only one prospective randomized trial has been undertaken to evaluate ASCT in relapsed follicular NHL. This trial, conducted by the European Bone Marrow Transplant Registry (EBMTR), was called the CUP trial because it compared conventional chemotherapy to high-dose chemotherapy followed by either an *u*npurged or *p*urged autograft.[117] ASCT was superior in terms of both progression-free and overall survival at 2 years, with rates of 55% and 71%, respectively, as compared to 26% and 46% with conventional chemotherapy. Unfortunately, this study was closed after enrollment of 140 patients because of slow accrual, and too few patients were available to evaluate the role of purging. Nonetheless, this trial demonstrated the safety and efficacy of ASCT in chemosensitive relapsed follicular lymphoma.

A number of small nonrandomized studies have evaluated the efficacy of ASCT as consolidation therapy for follicular lymphoma in first remission. These studies have yielded conflicting results, although no studies to date have demonstrated inferior outcomes with ASCT in first remission.[118,119] Two European phase III randomized trials by the GELA and GOELAMS (Groupe Ouest Est pour l'Etude des Leucemies Aigues et des Maladies du Sang) groups have compared conventional chemotherapy to ASCT. The GELA used unpurged stem cells, and the GOELAMS used purged stem cells. An interim analysis of the first 136 patients on the GOELAMS trial revealed a superior 4-year PFS rate of 61% in the ASCT arm, as opposed to 27% in those receiving conventional chemotherapy, although OS was equivalent.[120] Neither study has yet reached its endpoint; therefore, ASCT in first remission for follicular NHL has not yet been shown to have definitive benefit.

Allogeneic Stem Cell Transplantation

While allogeneic stem cell transplantation is very effective at inducing prolonged remissions in indolent lymphoma, its use has been limited by unacceptable rates of toxicity accompanied by an inability to produce complete cures.[121] A study by the International Bone Marrow Transplant Registry (IBMTR) compared allogeneic stem cell transplant to ASCT in follicular NHL, and found a significantly decreased relapse rate of only 20% in the allogeneic transplant arm.[122] Unfortunately, high rates of early treatment-related mortality led to a markedly decreased rate of long-term OS in these individuals. As with MCL, nonmyeloablative allogeneic transplantation is currently being investigated as a therapeutic strategy for indolent NHL. Nonmyeloablative transplants have the potential to decrease treatment-related mortality while maintaining the therapeutic benefits of allogeneic SCT. As with many evolving therapies for NHL, further clinical trials must be conducted to determine if and how to best integrate non-myeloabative transplants into treatment strategies for indolent lymphomas.

REFERENCES

1. Fisher SG, Fisher RI: The epidemiology of non-Hodgkin's lymphoma, *Oncogene* 23(38):6524-6534, 2004.
2. Skarin AT, Dorfman DM: Non-Hodgkin's lymphomas: current classification and management, *Cancer J Clin* 47(6):351-372, 1997.
3. Jemal A and others: Cancer statistics, 2002, *Cancer J Clin* 52(1):23-47, 2002.
4. Jemal A and others: Cancer Statistics, 2005. *Cancer J Clin* 55(1):10-30, 2005.
5. Nelson RA, Levine AM, Bernstein L: Reproductive factors and risk of intermediate- or high-grade B-cell non-Hodgkin's lymphoma in women, *J Clin Oncol* 19(5): 1381-1387, 2001.
6. Purdue MP and others for Canadian Cancer Registries Epidemiology Research Group: Dietary factors and risk of non-Hodgkin lymphoma by histologic subtype: a case-control analysis, Cancer Epidemiol Biomarkers Prevent 13(10):1665-1676, 2004.
7. Zhang Y and others: Menstrual and reproductive factors and risk of non-Hodgkin's lymphoma among Connecticut women, Am J Epidemiol 160(8):766-773, 2004.
8. Little RF: AIDS-related non-Hodgkin's lymphoma: etiology, epidemiology, and impact of highly active antiretroviral therapy, *Leukemia Lymphoma* 44(Suppl 3): S63-68, 2003.
9. Engels EA and others: Hepatitis C virus infection and non-Hodgkin lymphoma: results of the NCI-SEER multi-center case-control study, *Int J Cancer* 111(1):76-80, 2004.
10. Negri E and others: B-cell non-Hodgkin's lymphoma and hepatitis C virus infection: a systematic review, *Int J Cancer* 111(1):1-8, 2004.
11. Matsuo K and others: Effect of hepatitis C virus infection on the risk of non-Hodgkin's lymphoma: a meta-analysis of epidemiological studies, *Cancer Sci* 95(9):745-752, 2004.
12. Svoboda J and others: Regression of advanced non-splenic marginal zone lymphoma after treatment of hepatitis C virus infection, *Leukemia Lymphoma* 2005, in press.
13. Vallisa D and others: Role of anti-hepatitis C virus (HCV) treatment in HCV-related, low-grade, B-cell, non-Hodgkin's lymphoma: a multicenter Italian experience, *J Clin Oncol* 23(3):468-473, 2005.
14. Chiu BC, Weisenburger DD: An update of the epidemiology of non-Hodgkin's lymphoma, *Clin Lymphoma* 4(3): 161-168, 2003.

15. Tavani A and others: Hair dye use and risk of lymphoid neoplasms and soft tissue sarcomas, *Int J Cancer* 113(4): 629-631, 2005.
16. Zhang Y and others: Hair-coloring product use and risk of non-Hodgkin's lymphoma: a population-based case-control study in Connecticut, *Am J Epidemiol* 159(2): 148-154, 2004.
17. Harris NL and others: A revised European-American classification of lymphoid neoplasms: a proposal from the International Lymphoma Study Group, *Blood* 84(5): 1361-1392, 1994.
18. Lennert K: Morphology and classification of malignant lymphomas and so-called reticuloses, *Acta Neuropathol* Suppl 6:1-16, 1975.
19. National Cancer Institute-sponsored study of classifications of non-Hodgkin's lymphomas: summary and description of a working formulation for clinical usage, The Non-Hodgkin's Lymphoma Pathologic Classification Project, *Cancer* 49(10):2112-2135, 1982.
20. Isaacson PG: The current status of lymphoma classification, *Br J Haematol* 109(2):258-266, 2000.
21. Lennert K: [Non-Hodgkin's lymphomas: principles and application of the Kiel classification], *Verhandlungen der Deutschen Gesellschaft fuer Pathologie* 76:1-13, 1992.
22. Stansfeld AG and others: Updated Kiel classification for lymphomas, [erratum appears in *Lancet* 1(8581):372, 1988], *Lancet* 1(8580):292-293, 1988.
23. Uppenkamp M, Feller AC: Classification of malignant lymphoma, *Onkologie* 25(6):563-570, 2002.
24. Armitage JO: Treatment of non-Hodgkin's lymphoma, *N Engl J Med* 328(14):1023-1030, 1993.
25. Skarin AT, Dorfman DM: Non-Hodgkin's lymphomas: current classification and management, *Cancer J Clin* 47(6): 351-372, 1997.
26. Gong Y and others: Evaluation of interphase fluorescence in situ hybridization for the t(14;18)(q32;q21) translocation in the diagnosis of follicular lymphoma on fine-needle aspirates: a comparison with flow cytometry immunophenotyping, *Cancer J Clin* 99(6):385-393, 2003.
27. Lestou VS and others: Multicolour fluorescence in situ hybridization analysis of t(14;18)-positive follicular lymphoma and correlation with gene expression data and clinical outcome, *Br J Haematol* 122(5):745-759, 2003.
28. Fisher RI: Overview of non-Hodgkin's lymphoma: biology, staging, and treatment, *Semin Oncol* 30 (2 Suppl 4):3-9, 2003.
29. Blum KA, Lozanski G, Byrd JC: Adult Burkitt leukemia and lymphoma, *Blood* 104(10):3009-3020, 2004.
30. Foon KA, Fisher RI: Lymphomas. In Beutler E and others, editors: Williams Hematology, ed 6, New York, 2001, McGraw-Hill.
31. Offit K and others: Rearrangement of the bcl-6 gene as a prognostic marker in diffuse large-cell lymphoma. [see comment], *N Engl J Med* 331(2):74-80, 1994.
32. Lossos IS and others: Expression of a single gene, BCL-6, strongly predicts survival in patients with diffuse large B-cell lymphoma, *Blood* 98(4):945-951, 2001.
33. Theodossiou C, Schwarzenberger P: Non-Hodgkin's lymphomas, *Clin Obstet Gynecol* 45(3):820-829, 2002.
34. Carbone PP and others: Report of the Committee on Hodgkin's Disease Staging Classification, *Cancer Res* 31(11): 1860-1861, 1971.
35. A predictive model for aggressive non-Hodgkin's lymphoma. The International Non-Hodgkin's Lymphoma Prognostic Factors Project, *N Engl J Med* 329(14):987-994, 1993.
36. Rosenberg SA: Validity of the Ann Arbor staging classification for the non-Hodgkin's lymphomas, *Cancer Treat Rep* 61(6):1023-1027, 1977.
37. Denham JW And others: The follicular non-Hodgkin's lymphomas—II. Prognostic factors: what do they mean? *Eur J Cancer* 32A(3):480-490, 1996.
38. Hehn ST, Grogan TM, Miller TP: Utility of fine needle aspirate as a diagnostic technique in lymphoma, *J Clin Oncol* 22(15):3046-3052, 2004.
39. Picardi M and others: Randomized comparison of power Doppler ultrasound-directed excisional biopsy with standard excisional biopsy for the characterization of lymphadenopathies in patients with suspected lymphoma, *J Clin Oncol* 22(18):3733-3740, 2004.
40. Elstrom R and others: Utility of FDG-PET scanning in lymphoma by WHO classification, *Blood* 101(10): 3875-3876, 2003.
41. Kasamon YL, Swinnen LJ: Treatment advances in adult Burkitt lymphoma and leukemia, *Curr Opin Oncol* 16(5): 429-435, 2004.
42. McMaster ML and others: Results of treatment with high intensity, brief duration chemotherapy in poor prognosis non-Hodgkin's lymphoma, *Cancer* 68(2):233-241, 1991.
43. Hoelzer D and others: Improved outcome in adult B-cell acute lymphoblastic leukemia, *Blood* 87(2):495-508, 1996.
44. Soussain C and others: Small noncleaved cell lymphoma and leukemia in adults. A retrospective study of 65 adults treated with the LMB pediatric protocols, *Blood* 85(3): 664-674, 1995.
45. Bernstein JI and others: Combined modality therapy for adults with small noncleaved cell lymphoma (Burkitt's and non-Burkitt's types), *J Clin Oncol* 4(6):847-858, 1986.
46. Mead GM and others: An international evaluation of CODOX-M and CODOX-M alternating with IVAC in adult Burkitt's lymphoma: results of United Kingdom Lymphoma Group LY06 study, [erratum appears in *Ann Oncol* 13(12):1961, 2002 Note: Norbert, P [corrected to Pescosta, N]], *Ann Oncol* 13(8):1264-1274, 2002.
47. Thomas DA and others: Hyper-CVAD program in Burkitt's-type adult acute lymphoblastic leukemia, *J Clin Oncol* 17(8):2461-2470, 1999.
48. Cabanillas ME and others: Outcome with hyper-CVAD and rituximab in Burkitt (BL) and Burkitt-like (BLL) leukemia/lymphoma. Paper presented at American Society of Clinical Oncology Annual Meeting, 2003.
49. Sweetenham JW and others: Adult Burkitt's and Burkitt-like non-Hodgkin's lymphoma—outcome for patients treated with high-dose therapy and autologous stem-cell transplantation in first remission or at relapse: results from the European Group for Blood and Marrow Transplantation, *J Clin Oncol* 14(9):2465-2472, 1996.
50. Levine JE and others: A comparison of allogeneic and autologous bone marrow transplantation for lymphoblastic lymphoma, *Blood* 101(7):2476-2482, 2003.
51. Nathwani BN and others: Lymphoblastic lymphoma: a clinicopathologic study of 95 patients, *Cancer* 48(11): 2347-2357, 1981.
52. Coleman CN and others: Treatment of lymphoblastic lymphoma in adults, *J Clin Oncol* 4(11):1628-1637, 1986.

53. Hoelzer D, Gokbuget N: Treatment of lymphoblastic lymphoma in adults, *Baillieres Best Pract Clin Haematol* 15(4):713-728, 2002.
54. Thomas DA and others: Outcome with the hyper-CVAD regimens in lymphoblastic lymphoma, *Blood* 104(6): 1624-1630, 2004.
55. Hoelzer D and others: Outcome of adult patients with T-lymphoblastic lymphoma treated according to protocols for acute lymphoblastic leukemia, *Blood* 99(12):4379-4385, 2002.
56. Sweetenham JW and others: High-dose therapy and autologous stem-cell transplantation versus conventional-dose consolidation/maintenance therapy as postremission therapy for adult patients with lymphoblastic lymphoma: results of a randomized trial of the European Group for Blood and Marrow Transplantation and the United Kingdom Lymphoma Group, *J Clin Oncol* 19(11): 2927-2936, 2001.
57. Fisher RI and others: Comparison of a standard regimen (CHOP) with three intensive chemotherapy regimens for advanced non-Hodgkin's lymphoma, *N Engl J Med* 328 (14):1002-1006, 1993.
58. Fisher RI, Miller TP, O'Connor OA: Diffuse aggressive lymphoma, *Hematology* 221-236, 2004.
59. Cheson BD: CHOP Plus rituximab—balancing fact and opinion, *N Engl J Med* 346(4):280-282, 2002.
60. Reff ME and others: Depletion of B cells in vivo by a chimeric mouse human monoclonal antibody to CD20, *Blood* 83(2):435-445, 1994.
61. Demidem A and others: Chimeric anti-CD20 (IDEC-C2B8) monoclonal antibody sensitizes a B cell lymphoma cell line to cell killing by cytotoxic drugs, *Cancer Biother Radiopharmaceut* 12(3):177-186, 1997.
62. Coiffier B and others: CHOP chemotherapy plus rituximab compared with CHOP alone in elderly patients with diffuse large-B-cell lymphoma. [see comment], *N Engl J Med* 346(4):235-242, 2002.
63. Coffier B and others: Long-term results of the GELA study, RCHOP vs. CHOP in elderly patients with diffuse large B-cell lymphoma, *Blood* 104(11):Abstract #1383, 2004.
64. Habermann TM and others: Rituximab-CHOP versus CHOP with or without maintenance rituximab in patients 60 years of age and older with diffuse large B-cell lymphoma: an update, *Blood* 104(11):Abstract #127, 2003.
65. Pfreundschuh M and others: Randomized intergroup trial of first line treatment for patients ≤ 60 years with diffuse large B-cell non-Hodgkin's lymphoma with a CHOP-like regimen with or without the anti-CD20 antibody rituximab—early stopping after the first interim analysis [abstract #6500]. *Proceedings of the Annual Meeting Amer Soc Clin Oncol* 23:556a, 2004.
66. Blayney DW and others: Dose-intense chemotherapy every 2 weeks with dose-intense cyclophosphamide, doxorubicin, vincristine, and prednisone may improve survival in intermediate- and high-grade lymphoma: a phase II study of the Southwest Oncology Group (SWOG 9349) *J Clin Oncol* 21(13):2466-2473.
67. Pfreundschuh M and others: Two-weekly or 3-weekly CHOP chemotherapy with or without etoposide for the treatment of elderly patients with aggressive lymphomas: results of the NHL-B2 trial of the DSHNHL, *Blood* 104(3):634-641, 2004.
68. Wunderlich A and others: Practicability and acute haematological toxicity of 2- and 3-weekly CHOP and CHOEP chemotherapy for aggressive non Hodgkins lymphoma: results form the NHL-B Trial of the German High-Grade Non Hodgkins Lymphoma Study Group (DSHNHL), *Ann Oncol* 14(6):881-893, 2003.
69. Kaiser U and others: Randomized study to evaluate the use of high-dose therapy as part of primary treatment for "aggressive" lymphoma, *J Clin Oncol* 20(22):4413-4419, 2002.
70. Shipp MA and others: High-dose CHOP as initial therapy for patients with poor-prognosis aggressive non-Hodgkin's lymphoma: a dose-finding pilot study, *J Clin Oncol* 13(12): 2916-2923, 1995.
71. Connors JM and others: brief chemotherapy and involved field radiation therapy for limited-stage, histologically aggressive lymphoma, *Ann Int Med* 107(1):25-30, 1987.
72. Miller TP and others: Chemotherapy alone compared with chemotherapy plus radiotherapy for localized intermediate- and high-grade non-Hodgkin's lymphoma, *N Engl J Med* 339(1):21-26, 1998.
73. Kewalramani T and others: Rituximab and ICE as second-line therapy before autologous stem cell transplantation for relapsed or primary refractory diffuse large B-cell lymphoma, *Blood* 103(10):3684-3688, 2004.
74. Philip T and others: Autologous bone marrow transplantation as compared with salvage chemotherapy in relapses of chemotherapy-sensitive non-Hodgkin's lymphoma, *N Engl J Med* 333(23):1540-1545, 1995.
75. Press OW and others: A phase I/II trial of iodine-131-tositumomab (anti-CD20), etoposide, cyclophosphamide, and autologous stem cell transplantation for relapsed B-cell lymphomas, *Blood* 96(9):2934-2942, 2000.
76. Vose J and others: Phase I trial of iodine-131 tositumomab with high-dose chemotherapy and autologous stem cell transplantation for relapsed non Hodgkin's lymphoma, *J Clin Oncol* 23(3):461-467, 2005.
77. Morschhauser F HD and others: Yttrium-90 ibritumomab tiuxetan (Zevalin) for patients with relapsed/refractory diffuse large B-cell lymphoma not appropriate for autologous stem cell transplantation: results of an open label phase II trial, *Blood* 104(11):abstract #130, 2004.
78. Jacobs S and others: Evaluation of yttrium 90 (90y) ibritumomab tiuxetan (zevalin) in patients with non-Hodgkins lymphoma (NHL) having previously received autologous stem cell transplant (ASCT), paper presented at *Am Soc Hematol Annual Meeting* 2004.
79. Heeger S and others: Radioimmunotherapy of B-lineage non-Hodgkin's lymphoma using anti-CD19 and anti-CD20 conjugates, *J Clin Oncol* 22(14S):abstract #2625, 2004.
80. Chatal J and others: Radioimmunotherapy in non-Hodgkin's lymphoma (NHL) using a fractionated schedule of DOTA-conjugated, 90Y-radiolabeled, humanized anti-CD22 monoclonal antibody, epratuzumab, *J Clin Oncol* 22(14S):abstract #2545, 2004.
81. Kauh J And others: Mantle cell lymphoma: clinicopathologic features and treatments, *Oncology (Huntingt)* 17(6): 879-891, discussion 896-898, 2003.
82. Hagemeister FB: Mantle cell lymphoma: non-myeloablative versus dose-intensive therapy, *Leukemia Lymphoma* 44(Suppl 3):S69-75, 2003.
83. Densmore JJ, Williams ME: Mantle cell lymphoma, *Curr Treat Options Oncol* 4(4):281-287, 2003.

84. Khouri IF and others: Hyper-CVAD and high-dose methotrexate/cytarabine followed by stem-cell transplantation: an active regimen for aggressive mantle-cell lymphoma, *J Clin Oncol* 16(12):3803-3809, 1998.
85 Romaguera JE and others: Untreated aggressive mantle cell lymphoma: results with intensive chemotherapy without stem cell transplant in elderly patients, *Leukemia Lymphoma* 39(1-2):77-85, 2000.
86. Gopal AK and others: High-dose chemo-radioimmunotherapy with autologous stem cell support for relapsed mantle cell lymphoma, *Blood* 99(9):3158-3162, 2002.
87. Maris MB and others: Allogeneic hematopoietic cell transplantation after fludarabine and 2 Gy total body irradiation for relapsed and refractory mantle cell lymphoma, *Blood* 104(12):3535-3542, 2004.
88. Schenkein D: Proteasome inhibitors in the treatment of B-cell malignancies, *Clin Lymphoma* Jun 3(1):49-55, 2002.
89. Kaufmann H and others: Antitumor activity of rituximab plus thalidomide in patients with relapsed/refractory mantle cell lymphoma, *Blood* 104(8):2269-2271, 2004.
90. Peterson P, Gospodararowitz M, Tsang R: Long term outcome in stage I and II follicular lymphoma following treatment with involved field radiation therapy alone, *Proc Am Soc Clin Oncol Ann Meeting* 23:561, 2004.
91. Seymour JF and others: Long-term follow-up of a prospective study of combined modality therapy for stage I-II indolent non-Hodgkin's lymphoma, *J Clin Oncol* 21(11):2115-2122, 2003.
92. Advani R, Rosenberg SA, Horning SJ: Stage I and II follicular non-Hodgkin's lymphoma: long-term follow-up of no initial therapy, *J Clin Oncol* 22(8):1454-1459, 2004.
93. Winter J, Gascoyne R, Besien K: Low-grade lymphoma, *Hematology* 203-220, 2004.
94. Ardeshna KM and others: Long-term effect of a watch and wait policy versus immediate systemic treatment for asymptomatic advanced-stage non-Hodgkin lymphoma: a randomised controlled trial, *Lancet* 362(9383):516-522, 2003.
95. Morabito F and others: Prospective study of indolent non-follicular non-Hodgkin's lymphoma: validation of Gruppo Italiano per lo studio dei linfomi (GISL) prognostic criteria for watch and wait policy, *Leukemia Lymphoma* 43(10):1933-1938, 2002.
96. Young RC, and others: The treatment of indolent lymphomas: watchful waiting v aggressive combined modality treatment. Seminars in Hematology. Apr.; 25 (2suppl 2): 11-6. 1998.
97. Dana BW and others: Long-term follow-up of patients with low-grade malignant lymphomas treated with doxorubicin-based chemotherapy or chemoimmunotherapy, *J Clin Oncol* 11(4):644-651, 1993.
98. Hagemeister F and others: The role of mitoxantrone in the treatment of indolent lymphomas, *Oncologist* 10:150-159, 2005.
99. Hochster HS and others: Phase I study of fludarabine plus cyclophosphamide in patients with previously untreated low-grade lymphoma: results and long-term follow-up—a report from the Eastern Cooperative Oncology Group, *J Clin Oncol* 18(5):987-994, 2000.
100. Gonzalez H and others: Severe autoimmune hemolytic anemia in eight patients treated with fludarabine, *Hematologic Cell Therapeut* 40(3):113-118.
101. Leach M and others: Autoimmune thrombocytopenia: a complication of fludarabine therapy in lymphoproliferative disorders, *Clin Labor Haematol* 22(3):175-178, 2000.
102. Ghielmini M and others: Prolonged treatment with rituximab in patients with follicular lymphoma significantly increases event-free survival and response duration compared with the standard weekly x 4 schedule, *Blood* 103(12):4416-4423, 2004.
103. Hainsworth J and others: Maximizing therapeutic benefit of rituximab: maintenance therapy versus re-treatment at progression in patients with indolent non-Hodgkin's lymphoma—a randomized phase II trial of the Minnie Pearl Cancer Research Network, *J Clin Oncol* 23(6): 1088-1095, 2005.
104. Czuczman MS and others: Prolonged clinical and molecular remission in patients with low-grade or follicular non-Hodgkin's lymphoma treated with rituximab plus CHOP chemotherapy: 9-year follow-up [erratum appears in *J Clin Oncol* 23(1):248, 2005], *J Clin Oncol* 22(23):4711-4716, 2004.
105. Hochster H and others: Results of E1496: A phase III trial of CVP with or without maintenance rituximab in advanced indolent lymphoma (NHL) [abstract #6502], *J Clin Oncol* 22(14S):6502, 2004.
106. Rohatiner A and others: A meta-analysis of randomized studies evaluating the role of interferon alpha as treatment for follicular lymphoma [abstract #1053], *Proc Am Soc Clin Oncol Ann Meeting* 21:264a, 2002.
107. Zimmer AM: Logistics of radioimmunotherapy with yttrium 90 ibritumomab tiuxetan (Zevalin), *Semin Nucl Med* 34(1 Suppl 1):14-19, 2004.
108. Witzig TE and others: Randomized controlled trial of yttrium-90-labeled ibritumomab tiuxetan radioimmunotherapy versus rituximab immunotherapy for patients with relapsed or refractory low-grade, follicular, or transformed B-cell non-Hodgkin's lymphoma, *J Clin Oncol* 20(10):2453-2463, 2002.
109. Witzig TE and others: Treatment with ibritumomab tiuxetan radioimmunotherapy in patients with rituximab-refractory follicular non-Hodgkin's lymphoma, *J Clin Oncol* 20(15):3262-3269, 2002.
110. Zhu X: Radiation safety considerations with yttrium 90 ibritumomab tiuxetan (Zevalin), *Semin Nucl Med* 34 (1 Suppl 1):20-23, 2004.
111. Byar K: Educating patients about radioimmunotherapy with yttrium 90 ibritumomab tiuxetan (Zevalin), *Sem Oncol Nurs* 20(1 Suppl 1):20-25, 2004.
112. Kaminski MS and others: Pivotal study of iodine I 131 tositumomab for chemotherapy-refractory low-grade or transformed low-grade B-cell non-Hodgkin's lymphomas [see comment], *J Clin Oncol* 19(19):3918-3928, 2001.
113. Kaminski MS and others: 131I-tositumomab therapy as initial treatment for follicular lymphoma *N Engl J Med* 352(5):441-449, 2005.
114. Vose JM: Bexxar: novel radioimmunotherapy for the treatment of low-grade and transformed low-grade non-Hodgkin's lymphoma, *Oncologist* 9(2):160-172, 2004.
115. Press OW and others: A phase 2 trial of CHOP chemotherapy followed by tositumomab/iodine I 131 tositumomab for previously untreated follicular non-Hodgkin lymphoma: Southwest Oncology Group Protocol S9911, *Blood* 102(5):1606-1612, 2003.

116. Weng WK and others: Clinical outcome of lymphoma patients after idiotype vaccination is correlated with humoral immune response and immunoglobulin G Fc receptor genotype [erratum appears in *J Clin Oncol* 23(1):248, 2005], *J Clin Oncol* 22(23):4717-4724, 2004.
117. Schouten HC and others: High-dose therapy improves progression-free survival and survival in relapsed follicular non-Hodgkin's lymphoma: results from the randomized European CUP trial, *J Clin Oncol* 21(21): 3918-3927, 2003.
118. Horning SJ and others: High-dose therapy and autologous bone marrow transplantation for follicular lymphoma in first complete or partial remission: results of a phase II clinical trial, *Blood* 97(2):404-409, 2001.
119. Sanz-Rodriguez, C and others: Chemotherapy plus interferon alpha-2b vs high-dose therapy for response consolidation in low grade non Hodgkin's lymphoma: results of a retrospective case control study [abstract], *Blood* 96:791a, 2000.
120. Colombat, P and others: Value of autologous stem cell transplantation in first line therapy of follicular lymphoma with high tumor burden: first results of the randomized GOELAMS 064 trial [abstract], *Blood* 98:861a, 2001.
121. van Besien K and others: Allogeneic bone marrow transplantation for low-grade lymphoma, *Blood* 92(5): 1832-1836, 1998.
122. van Besien K and others: Autologous vs allogeneic transplantation for follicular lymphoma: report from the IBMTR and ABMTR, paper presented at *Am Soc Clin Oncol Annual Meeting*, 2002.

UNIT III

Physical and Psychosocial Response to Cancer Treatment

CHAPTER

11 Osteoporosis and Cancer

Suzanne M. Mahon

Osteoporosis may be defined as a disorder of decreased bone mass, microarchitectural deterioration, and fragility fractures. Fragility fractures can occur in the absence of trauma or following minimal trauma. Bone strength is a result of bone quality and bone density. Bone strength is compromised in osteoporosis. The emotional and physical toll on patients and their families and the financial toll for health care are staggering. Women, in particular, are at risk for osteoporosis as they age. As more and more women complete therapy for malignancy and become long-term survivors of cancer, there is an increasing population of women at risk for other complications related to osteoporosis. Nurses who provide tertiary prevention care for patients who are long-term survivors of malignancy need to take direct steps to assess, prevent, and provide early intervention to prevent further suffering associated with osteoporosis. This chapter will provide an overview of the pathophysiology and treatment of osteoporosis in women who are survivors of cancer.

EPIDEMIOLOGY AND SCOPE OF THE PROBLEM

Osteoporosis is the most common bone disease in humans. Current estimates suggest that one out of every two Caucasian women will experience an osteoporotic fracture during her lifetime.[1] The National Osteoporosis Foundation (NOF) estimates that 20% of postmenopausal Caucasian women in the US have osteoporosis and an additional 52% have low bone density at the hip. In the whole population of the US, more than 7.8 million women have osteoporosis and an additional 21.8 million women have low bone density of the hip.[2]

African American women are also affected by osteoporosis. Even though they achieve a higher peak bone mass, they still lose bone density at the same rate as Caucasians.[1,2] Therefore, African American women are also at risk for osteoporosis, although the effects may be seen approximately a decade later than for Caucasian women. Significant risk for developing osteoporosis has been reported in all age groups; thus all women, especially as they age, should consider themselves at risk for developing osteoporosis.

There are an estimated 1.5 million osteoporotic fractures annually in the US.[1] This includes over 700,000 vertebral fractures, 250,000 distal forearm fractures, and 300,000 hip fractures.

Osteoporosis has significant economic consequences. The cost of fractures in the US was $17 billion in 2001, with hip fractures accounting for over one third of the total cost.[1,3] Among women 45 years old and older, hip fractures account for over half of all osteoporosis-related hospital admissions in the US.

The social costs of osteoporosis are even higher. Sixty percent of women older than 80 years have vertebral compression fractures, suggesting that these are the most common osteoporotic fractures. Vertebral compression fractures are associated with height loss, limited range of motion, muscle weakness, a protruding abdomen, and thoracic kyphosis.[4] Vertebral fractures resulting from osteoporosis cause pain, debilitation, and impairment. These fractures can limit an individual's ability to perform activities of daily living, restricting function in employment as well as in social and recreational activities.

Once a woman experiences two or more vertebral fractures, osteoporosis begins to have a noticeable impact on emotional functioning. High levels of anxiety result from a very real fear of future fractures and can lead to inactivity, depression, and diminished self-esteem.[1,5,6]

Mortality associated with osteoporosis is also significant. Most mortality is related to hip fractures. Men and women are 2 to 5 times more likely to die during the first 12 months after a hip fracture as compared with people of the same age and sex in the general population without hip fractures.[1,4] Virtually all patients are hospitalized after a hip fracture. The average length of hospitalization is between 20 and 30 days. Almost half of all patients with hip fractures in the US are discharged to an institution, and more than one third are rehospitalized during the year following the fracture. At 2 months after hospital discharge, fewer than 30% of patients have regained their prefracture walking ability and only about 25% have recovered their previous capacity to perform physical activities of daily living.[2,4]

These figures represent a staggering health problem. A relatively small body of systematic data is available on the exact risk and incidence of osteoporosis in survivors of cancer, but there is concern that this may be an important health problem for many. Most data about cancer and osteoporosis have been collected on women with a history of breast cancer. From a public health perspective, the number of women with a near-normal life expectancy who reach menopause after a diagnosis of localized breast cancer will continue to increase as a result of early diagnosis and improved therapy. It is estimated there are at least 2 million women in the US alone who are living with a history of breast cancer; more than 80% of these have been alive for at least 5 years.[7,8] These women face several decades of estrogen deficiency because current medical opinion is that, in general, estrogen replacement therapy (ERT) is contraindicated in this population. These figures do not consider the number of women who are successfully treated for other malignancies, although there is much less by way of systematic data available for these populations.

Patients who have been successfully treated for malignancy should not have to suffer the morbidity and mortality associated with osteoporosis just because they may not be candidates for ERT. Awareness of recent improvements in diagnostic and treatment modalities can prevent the devastating effects of osteoporosis in these cancer survivors.

PATHOPHYSIOLOGY OF OSTEOPOROSIS

An understanding of normal bone remodeling is necessary to appreciate the pathophysiology of osteoporosis. Bone remodeling consists of phases of resorption and formation. These events are coupled and occur in bone remodeling units. The bone remodeling unit consists of osteoblasts and osteoclasts. The osteoclasts are the bone cells responsible for bone resorption, and the osteoblasts are responsible for bone formation. The osteoclasts will create a cavity in the bone called the resorption pit that will subsequently be filled by osteoblasts. The rate at which this process occurs is bone turnover.

In osteoporosis, the coupling of the bone remodeling unit is impaired. The resorption pit created by the osteoclast is not completely refilled by the osteoblast. This results in a net deficit of total bone formation. Ultimately, this results in lower bone mass.

Peak bone mass is achieved between ages 30 and 35. Women who are premenopausal lose approximately 0.3% of their skeleton per year.[4] Immediately after the menopause, the lack of estrogen causes an accelerated bone loss for the first 5 to 10 years. After this period there is a gradual but continual loss of bone. This loss of bone mass can increase bone fragility and make the bone more susceptible to fracture. At menopause, or for every year that women are amenorrheic or oligomenorrheic, they will lose 2% of their skeleton.[4] The sites for fracture most associated with low bone mass and osteoporosis include the distal forearm, the hip, and the vertebrae.[1-3]

RISK FACTORS FOR OSTEOPOROSIS

All women have some risk for developing osteoporosis and sustaining a fracture. This risk increases steadily after menopause, especially if the patient remains estrogen-deficient. Risk for osteoporosis and subsequent fracture is definitely higher in some groups of women. Identification and early detection of women at higher risk for developing osteoporosis is critical to providing more effective management. A number of factors contribute to low bone mass as shown in Box 11-1. Risk factors for osteoporosis and increased fracture risks that are particularly significant in long-term survivors of malignancy include estrogen deficiency and certain medications used in the treatment of malignancy.

Estrogen deficiency

Estrogen deficiency is one of the most significant contributors to low bone mass in postmenopausal women. Estrogen deficiency is thought to affect both the osteoclasts and osteoblasts.[9] Estrogen deficiency can cause rapid loss of bone immediately after menopause. Menopause may occur naturally, surgically following the removal of both ovaries, or medically following the administration of some medications and in particular chemotherapeutic agents.

Chemotherapeutic agents that are often used in the treatment of breast and gynecologic malignancies that are associated with gonadal dysfunction and an earlier menopause include cyclophosphamide, methotrexate, 5-fluorouracil, and adriamyacin.[6,9] At least 50% of the women receiving these agents will have a premature chemotherapy-induced menopause. Cyclophosphamide is known to be directly toxic to the ovaries. The risk of ovarian injury and failure is related to the age of the patient at the time of treatment, the cumulative dose of the drug administered, and the duration of therapy. Ovarian failure is almost always irreversible after the age

Box 11-1 Risk Factors for Osteoporosis[1,3,5]

GENETIC
Caucasian or Asian ethnicity
Family history of osteoporosis
Small body frame (less than 127 lbs)

LIFESTYLE FACTORS
Smoking
Inactivity
Nulliparity
Excessive exercise (causing amenorrhea)
Estrogen deficiency
Early surgical menopause
Early natural menopause
Late menarche

NUTRITIONAL FACTORS
Milk intolerance
Life-long low dietary intake
Vegetarian diet
Excessive alcohol intake
Consistently high protein intake

MEDICAL DISORDERS
Anorexia nervosa
Thyrotoxicosis
Cushing's syndrome
Type I diabetes
Rheumatoid arthritis
Prolactinoma
Hemolytic anemia, hemochromatosis, and thalassemia

MEDICATIONS
Thyroid replacement medications
Glucocorticoids for more than three months
Chemotherapeutic agents
Gonadotropin-releasing hormone agonist or antagonist therapy
Anticonvulsant therapy
Long-term heparin use
Extended tetracycline use
Diuretics producing calciuria
Phenothiazine derivatives
Cyclosporin
Tamoxifen (premenopausal use)
Progesterone (parenteral, long-acting forms)

of 42.[9] A premature menopause that is related to the use of these agents results in these women being estrogen-deficient at a younger age. Since adjuvant chemotherapy is becoming a standard treatment for premenopausal women with both node-negative and node-positive breast cancer, chemotherapy-induced menopause will be seen more frequently.

The administration of ERT to women with malignancies that are thought to have a hormonal etiology (such as breast or endometrial cancer) is very controversial. Most of these women will not receive ERT. The studies that address the use of ERT in women diagnosed with breast and endometrial cancer are scarce and preliminary.[10] Follow-up time is short. Prospective studies are being conducted, but it will be many years before definitive results are available. At present the decision of whether ERT should be used is made on a very individual basis and only after the expected benefits and potential consequences (including an early recurrence) are discussed.

Questions regarding the safety of ERT in women without breast cancer are emerging. The Women's Health Initiative (WHI) has shown that ERT has been associated with an increased risk of coronary heart disease, stroke, venous thromboembolic disease, and invasive breast cancer.[11-13] Further data has shown that ERT has failed to prevent mild cognitive impairment. Therefore many women, especially those who are considered to be at higher risk for developing breast and/or endometrial cancer, will often choose to not take ERT. The estrogen deficiency in these women also places them at significant risk for developing osteoporosis and fracture.

Medications that Contribute to Bone Loss

Although many medications are associated with bone loss, as shown in Box 11-1, nurses need to be particularly aware of medications used in the treatment of malignancy that increase bone loss. There are a number of drugs which have a negative effect on the skeletal system. High-dose methotrexate decreases bone mass as a result of an increase in bone resorption and inhibition of bone formation. Doxorubicin has been shown to cause a decrease in the trabecular bone volume.[9]

Tamoxifen, which is commonly used in the management of breast cancer, is an estrogen antagonist with weak agonist activity. Most of the studies that have studied the effect of tamoxifen on bone remodeling in women with breast cancer have had a small sample size. Measurement of bone mineral density (BMD) in women with breast cancer suggests that tamoxifen exerts a neutral or estrogenic effect on bone such that bone mass is preserved in postmenopausal women.[8] In premenopausal women, tamoxifen has been shown to cause bone loss in the spine and hip, since it has a weaker effect than the genuine estrogens.[9] More recently, aromatase inhibitors are being used in the adjuvant treatment of breast cancer. These agents may be associated with an increased risk of fracture risk in postmenopausal women.[9]

Glucocorticoid use, particularly long-term and at high doses (at least 7.5 mg daily of prednisone or its equivalent for at least 6 months), is associated with significant bone loss and increased risk for fracture. Glucocorticoids appear to affect osteoblast function, impair calcium absorption, and impair gonadal function which all contribute to increased bone loss.[1,5,9]

History of Previous Fracture

Women diagnosed with cancer may also have other comorbid conditions that place them at risk for developing osteoporosis. A history of a previous osteoporotic fracture is also a significant risk factor for future fractures. Women with a single previous vertebral fracture experience subsequent spine fractures at a rate 2.6 to 3.0 times greater than women without previous fractures, independent of bone mass.[1,2] Women with a low bone mass and one previous fracture at baseline have a 25-fold increased risk of subsequent spine fractures as compared to women with high bone mass and no previous fractures.[11]

Two thirds of all vertebral fractures are asymptomatic.[1,4] For this reason a comprehensive history and physical assessment are critical. A seemingly benign act such as reaching for dishes in the cabinet, weeding the garden, or carrying a child can result in a fragility vertebral fracture. A fragility fracture is an atraumatic fracture sustained from a fall of standing height or less.[3] It is not uncommon for long-term survivors of cancer to experience a fragility fracture without prior warning or symptoms.

Clinical Implications of Risk Assessment

It is impossible to accurately predict BMD based on risk factors.[1,3,4] Consequently, most risk factors (as outlined in Box 11-1) are not adequate predictors of fracture risk. These risk factors do indicate women who might benefit from further diagnostic evaluation for osteoporosis. Further, the NOF has initiated guidelines for the evaluation of osteoporosis in women (Box 11-2).[1] Medicare will reimburse for bone densitometry in the presence of estrogen deficiency and vertebral abnormalities, for evaluation of response to ongoing therapy for osteoporosis, during long-term steroid use, and for secondary osteoporosis. Routine screening for osteoporosis prophylaxis is not currently covered.[14]

Other clinical assessments which should be incorporated into routine follow-up of women include a height measurement. This should be compared with previous measurements, if available, or self-reports to determine if height has been lost. Significant loss of height (2 inches or more) may indicate the presence of one or more vertebral fractures and is suggestive of osteoporosis and the need for further diagnostic evaluation.[1,3]

Box 11-2 Indications for Osteoporosis Evaluation[1,14]

- All women ages 65 and over regardless of risk factors
- Younger women with one or more risk factors (estrogen deficiency, vertebral abnormalities, long-term steroid therapy, primary hyperparathyroidism)
- Younger postmenopausal women on approved osteoporosis therapy to evaluate the effectiveness of the therapy
- Postmenopausal women who are first seen with fractures as a means to confirm the diagnosis of osteoporosis and assess disease severity.

PRIMARY PREVENTION OF OSTEOPOROSIS

Ideally, primary prevention measures to reduce the risk of developing osteoporosis are initiated in adolescence and continue through life. All women should receive information about these prevention practices regardless of whether or not they have a diagnosis of osteoporosis. The goals of osteoporosis prevention include optimizing bone mass and preserving skeletal integrity.[1,3] These measures include adequate calcium and vitamin D intake, regular weight-bearing exercise, smoking cessation, limiting alcohol intake, and pharmacologic therapy when appropriate.

Calcium Intake

Calcium is essential for maintaining a healthy skeleton. It is a mineral found in many foods, and adequate calcium intake is important because the human body cannot produce calcium. Even after reaching full skeletal growth, a diet with adequate calcium intake is important because the body loses calcium daily through shed skin, nails, hair, swear, feces, and urine. When the diet does not contain enough calcium to perform these activities, calcium is taken from the bones, which are the storage area for calcium. An adequate calcium intake will not completely protect a person against bone loss caused by estrogen deficiency, physical inactivity, smoking, alcohol abuse, or medical problems or treatments including chemotherapy.[1]

In providing advice about calcium intake, the intent is to ensure the body has sufficient calcium to maintain calcium balance. Women who do not attain an average peak bone mass as a young adult may be at higher risk for osteoporosis in the future.[13] Calcium can reduce the rate of bone loss at or after the menopause. The NOF has recommended 1,200 mg of elemental calcium daily for women 51 years of age and older.[1]

The best source of calcium is the diet.[1,13] Calcium supplements can be added to ensure that the daily calcium requirement is met. The amount needed from a supplement depends on how much calcium is consumed from dietary sources. Table 11-1 provides a list of the calcium content of a variety of foods. Women should be encouraged to add dietary items higher in calcium content to their diets. This list can also be used to calculate the approximate daily intake of dietary calcium.

Calcium exists only in combination with other substances. Several different calcium compounds are used in supplements including calcium carbonate, calcium phosphate, and calcium citrate. Each of these compounds contains different amounts of elemental calcium, which is the actual amount of calcium in the supplement. Consumers must read the label carefully to determine how much elemental calcium the supplement actually provides. When selecting a supplement the consumer needs to consider tolerance, convenience, cost, and availability.

Calcium, whether consumed in the diet or as a supplement, is best absorbed by the body when it is taken several times a day in amount of 500 mg or less.[1] In some patients, supplements lead to side effects including constipation and gas. Often these side effects can be avoided with the addition of increased fiber and fluids. Increasing the amount of supplementation by 250 mg each week until the amount of daily supplementation is reached may also improve tolerance. If an individual cannot tolerate one preparation or form of calcium, it may be necessary to try a different type.

Table **11-1** DIETARY SOURCES OF CALCIUM[1,3,13]

Source	Calcium (in mg)
Yogurt (1 cup)	400
Low-fat dry milk ({1/4} cup)	375
Ricotta cheese ({1/2} cup)	350
Evaporated milk ({1/2} cup)	350
Sardines (3 oz)	324
Milk shake (10 oz)	319
Milk (1 cup)	300
Swiss cheese (1 oz)	275
Soft-serve ice milk (1 cup)	275
Cheese pizza ({1/4} of a 12-inch pizza)	232
Salmon (canned with bones, 3 oz)	203
Cheddar cheese (1 oz)	200
Fortified orange juice (8 oz)	200
Tofu (4 oz)	154
Shrimp (1 cup)	147
Spaghetti with meatballs (1 cup)	124
Dried beans (cooked, 1 cup)	100
Greens ({1/2} cup)	100
Broccoli ({1/2} cup)	89
Cottage cheese ({1/2} cup)	75
Nuts ({1/4} cup)	75

Vitamin D Intake

A vitamin D deficiency can easily be overlooked. Vitamin D helps to ensure that calcium is absorbed from the gastrointestinal tract.[1,3] A vitamin D deficiency can cause a secondary hyperparathyroidism, which will increase bone turnover and increase bone loss. A vitamin D deficiency may also impair mineralization and cause osteomalacia. Vitamin D is synthesized naturally following approximately 10 minutes of daily exposure to natural sunlight, and is also found in eggs, butter, and milk. Most multivitamins contain 400 international units, and some calcium supplements also contain vitamin D.

Exercise

In adults the amount, duration, and intensity of exercise that is optimal for preserving bone mass is unknown. Two types of exercises are important for building and maintaining bone mass and density. These include weight-bearing and resistance exercises. Weight-bearing exercises are those in which bones and muscles work against gravity. These include any exercise in which the feet and legs are bearing the body's weight. Examples include jogging, walking, stair climbing, dancing, and soccer. Resistance exercises use muscular strength to improve muscle mass and strengthen bone. These usually include some type of weight lifting. Further, exercise does have cardiovascular benefit, and may improve agility and therefore improve the patient's ability to break or prevent a fall.[1,13]

Estrogen Replacement Therapy

For decades, ERT was used to treat menopausal symptoms and was considered a preventive agent for osteoporosis. Results of the WHI have demonstrated a reduced risk of vertebral and nonvertebral fractures with ERT use for postmenopausal women without osteoporosis.[15,16] In summary, the WHI suggests that administration of ERT for 5.2 years reduced the risk of vertebral and hip fractures by one third and the risk of all fractures decreased by almost one fourth. The safety of ERT was also examined in the study, and the WHI concluded that because of the adverse risk-to-benefit ratio, it could not be recommended for the prevention of osteoporosis. The effects of ERT on fractures in women with osteoporosis have not been evaluated. Given the results of this large study, fewer women are using ERT, and therapy for the prevention and treatment of osteoporosis has shifted toward the use of antiresorptive medications such as bisphosphonates.

SCREENING AND DIAGNOSTIC EVALUATION FOR OSTEOPOROSIS

Low bone mass is the single most accurate predictor of increased fracture risk.[1,2] The identification of persons at higher risk for developing osteoporosis is critical, so they can be referred for further diagnostic evaluation and treatment when indicated. Nurses should remember that women who have survived cancer are probably at higher risk for developing osteoporosis because of estrogen deficiency and medications used in treatment of these malignancies. For these women, a discussion of osteoporosis and bone densitometry and possibly referral for further evaluation is appropriate, especially for women who are in long-term follow-up.[8] The risk of osteoporosis is high enough in premenopausal women diagnosed with cancer who underwent cytotoxic therapy associated with cessation of menses to consider ordering a baseline evaluation.[6]

Definition of Osteoporosis

The current definition of osteoporosis is dependent on bone mass and/or the presence of a fragility fracture. BMD is expressed as standard deviations (SD) from the mean. The World Health Organization suggests the following definitions for osteoporosis based on BMD measurement at the spine, hip, or wrist in Caucasian postmenopausal women.[17] Normal BMD is a value for BMD within 1 SD of the young adult reference mean. Low bone mass (osteopenia) is defined as a BMD value between 1.0 and 2.5 SD below the young adult mean. Osteoporosis is defined as a BMD value more than 2.5 SD from the young adult mean. Severe or established osteoporosis is defined as a BMD greater than 2.5 SD below the young adult mean in the presence of one or more fragility fractures. A 75-year-old woman's bone mass will always be compared to a 30-year-old woman's bone mass (young adult mean) to determine fracture risk.

Dual Energy X-Ray Absorptiometry

The most common method of measuring bone mass and currently the "gold standard" is dual energy x-ray absorptiometry (DXA). DXA subjects the patient to a radiation exposure that is equivalent to one tenth the exposure of a chest x-ray.[3,14]

DXA can be used to measure BMD in the spine, hip, or wrist, which are the most common sites for osteoporotic fractures. A DXA measurement can be completed in less than 15 minutes.

DXA scanners typically include a table on which the patient is positioned and beneath which the x-ray source is located on a moving support. The x-ray source moves and projects the photon beam through a collimator and through the patient. The images are projected on a separate computer and display system.

In addition to the assessment of bone health and making choices about pharmacologic management of osteoporosis, other benefits to DXA have been reported. Knowledge of one's BMD often influences decisions about lifestyle modifications including exercise, diet, and calcium/vitamin D supplementation, as well as compliance with recommended pharmacologic treatments.[11]

Other Methods to Detect Osteoporosis

Other methods to determine BMD include quantitative computerized tomography (QCT), peripheral DXA (pDXA), radiographic absorptiometry, ultrasound, and single x-ray studies. T-scores are often higher when measured at peripheral sites such as the heel or finger, so relying on pDXA may underestimate osteoporosis.[11] QCT measures trabecular and cortical bone densities and is most commonly used in the spine. Access to this equipment is often limited. Ultrasound assesses bone in the heel, the tibia, the patella, or other peripheral sites where the bones are relatively superficial. Measurements are not generally as precise as those obtained with DXA. Since greater than 30% of bone must be lost to determine osteopenia by routine x-ray exam, this method is not used to determine bone density.[4] Radiographs can be used, however, to determine the presence of vertebral fractures and confirm fractures at other sites.

Markers of bone turnover in the serum or urine are also sometimes used to help assess risk of fracture and response to therapy. None is a substitute for DXA, and all are subject to considerable biologic availability.[3] The most commonly used biochemical bone markers are collagen cross-links (pyridinoline), bone-specific alkaline phosphatase, and N-telopeptide and C-telopeptide.[11]

Implications of Low Bone Mass

Once low bone mass has been determined, secondary causes must be ruled out. The major conditions contributing to decreased bone mass include genetics traits, lifestyle factors, nutritional factors, medical disorders, and certain medications (see Box 11-1). Whenever possible, the underlying cause of osteoporosis should be corrected. Low bone mass in the population of oncology patients may also be related metastatic lesions.

PHARMACOLOGIC MANAGEMENT OF OSTEOPOROSIS

The primary goals of pharmacologic therapy for osteoporosis are to increase bone mass, to stop or reverse bone loss, and to reduce the incidence of fractures. Currently, there are several medications approved by the Food and Drug Administration (FDA) for the prevention and/or treatment of osteoporosis. These medications are described in Table 11-2. Making direct comparisons across agents is sometimes difficult because of a lack of direct head-to-head trials of treatments for osteoporosis.[17-20] Comparisons between drugs are often derived from metaanalyses in which the baseline characteristics of the populations studied are different and there are overlapping confidence intervals for evaluating the effect of treatment.[20]

Selective Estrogen Receptor Modulators

Selective estrogen receptor modulator (SERM) agents act like estrogen on bone and antiestrogen on the breast. Two common SERMs seen in clinical practice are tamoxifen citrate and raloxifene (Evista). Raloxifene, like tamoxifen citrate, has been shown to prevent or reduce the risk of breast cancer in women at average risk of breast cancer.[18] Tamoxifen increases bone mass and reduces the frequency of fractures in postmenopausal women, but probably not to the extent that raloxifene does.[13] The National Surgical Adjuvant Breast and Bowel Project Study of Raloxifene and Tamoxifen (STAR) Trial seeks to better define the effectiveness of these medications in preventing osteoporosis.

The American Society of Clinical Oncology (ASCO) notes that there are reservations about using raloxifene following 5 years of tamoxifen adjuvant therapy in women with breast cancer, because raloxifene has limited activity against advanced breast cancer when used after tamoxifen, and 10 years of tamoxifen administration has been associated with more recurrences than stopping tamoxifen after 5 years.[21]

Bisphosphonates

The bisphosphonates inhibit bone resorption through uptake by osteoclasts. Alendronate (Fosamax) and risedronate (Actonel) have both been FDA-approved for the prevention and treatment of osteoporosis. Both of these agents have the advantage of being available in an oral preparation taken once a week and are considered

Table 11-2 MEDICATIONS USED IN THE PREVENTION AND TREATMENT OF OSTEOPOROSIS[1,3,11,17-20]

Medication (brand name)	Route/Dose	Effectiveness	Side Effects	Nursing Implications
Alendronate (Fosamax)	Treatment: 10 mg PO once daily or 70 mg PO once weekly Prevention: 5 mg PO once daily or 35 mg PO once weekly	• Reduces incidence of spine, hip, wrist fractures by 50% over 3 yr in patients with prior spine fracture • Reduces incidence of spine fractures by 48% over 3 yr in patients without prior spine fracture	• Esophageal ulcer, dysphagia, gastritis and/or abdominal pain, dyspepsia • Musculoskeletal pain	• Take tablet upon rising with 6 to 8 oz plain water • Do not lie down until after first meal • Wait at least 30 min before taking food, beverage, or other medications
Risedronate (Actonel)	Prevention and Treatment: 5 mg PO once daily or 35 mg PO once weekly	• Reduces incidence of spine fractures by 41%-49% • Reduces incidence of other-than-spinal fractures by 36% over 3 yr in patients with prior spine fracture	• Diarrhea, abdominal pain, nausea, belching, colitis • Headache, dizziness • Arthralgia, bone pain, leg cramps	• Take tablet upon rising with 6 to 8 oz plain water • Do not lie down until after first meal • Wait at least 30 min before taking food, beverage, or other medications
Calcitonin (Miacalcin)	Treatment: 200 international units every intranasally, one nostril per day	• Reduces vertebral fracture risk in postmenopausal women with osteoporosis by 33%	• Nausea, vomiting, epigastric distress • Dizziness • Nasal mucosal alterations, sinusitis	• Instruct patient on need for periodic nasal evaluations for nasal mucosal alterations • Careful instruction on pump assembly and nasal introduction of drug • Patients should alternate nostrils daily
Raloxifene (Evista)	Prevention and Treatment: 60 mg PO once	• Reduces fracture risk daily by 68% the first yr • Reduces fracture risk 36% at 4 yr • Reduces risk of estrogen-dependent breast cancer by 65% over 4 yr	• Hot flashes • Deep vein thrombosis • Migraine • Vaginitis, urinary tract infection • Arthralgia, myalgia	• May be taken with or without food • Avoid prolonged immobilization and movement restrictions because of increased risk of venous thromboembolic events • Report any pain in calves, swelling in legs, acute migraines, sudden chest pain, and shortness of breath, or vision changes.

Mg, Milligrams; *PO,* by mouth; *oz,* ounces; *yr,* year(s); *min,* minute(s).

first-line agents for the prevention and treatment of postmenopausal osteoporosis.[20] The most significant side effect associated with these agents is gastrointestinal irritation.

Calcitonin

Calcitonin is a hormone secreted by the thyroid gland that works an antiresorptive agent by inhibiting osteoclastic function. Calcitonin is FDA-approved for the treatment of osteoporosis in women with low bone mass who are at least 5 years past menopause. Calcitonin has been available in the US for over 30 years in its injectable form.

The intranasal form of calcitonin has been available since October 1995. When given by the intranasal route it has been shown to increase spinal bone mass in postmenopausal women with established osteoporosis but not in early postmenopausal women.[13] There is no evidence that calcitonin will increase BMD at the hip.

Estrogen Replacement Therapy

In the past, ERT has been recommended for the prevention of osteoporosis. The WHI study has changed prescribing patterns.[11,12,22,23] ERT is still an option for women experiencing menopausal symptoms, especially hot flashes. The publication of risks of breast cancer, and lack of protection against cardiovascular disease and dementia associated with ERT, has caused many women to rethink the decision as to whether to use ERT. The prevention of osteoporosis alone is probably not sufficient reason to use ERT, and women require sufficient counseling to make an informed decision about the safety and efficacy of ERT.[22,23] Further, many women with cancer, especially those with breast and endometrial malignancies, should not take ERT because of the risks for malignancy associated with exogenous estrogen use.[21]

IMPLICATIONS FOR NURSES

Oncology nurses need to include an assessment for osteoporosis for their perimenopausal and postmenopausal female patients. Particular care should be given so as to not overlook this potential problem in women whose long-term prognosis is favorable and who may have other risk factors for developing osteoporosis.

Assessment

As the issue of osteoporosis gains more public attention, patients may have more questions about their risk for developing osteoporosis. Little is known about the attitudes and concerns of women with hormone-dependent malignancies and concerns related to estrogen deficiency. Clearly, oncology nurses cannot overlook this concern their patients have, whether they verbalize the concern or not.

A variety of tools have been developed to assist in the assessment of risk of developing osteoporosis, as well as instruments that assess knowledge regarding osteoporosis and its treatment. These instruments have been used in both clinical and research settings.[24]

The Osteoporosis Assessment Questionnaire is a 71-item self-report questionnaire that has been used with persons with nonvertebral fractures.[25] The Osteoporosis Functional Disability Questionnaire is a self-administered 59-item instrument that has demonstrated reliable correlation with objective measures of spinal changes caused by osteoporosis.[26] The Osteoporosis Quality of Life Questionnaire is a 30-item instrument that is administered as an interview. It is reported to detect improvements or deterioration in persons with osteoporosis.[27] The Osteoporosis Targeted Quality of Life Survey has also been used to assess quality of life and has been translated into several languages.[28] The European Foundation for Osteoporosis has developed a specific tool for persons with vertebral fractures that includes questions on pain, physical function, general health, and psychologic function.[29]

There is also a tool available to measure patients' knowledge of osteoporosis called the Facts on Osteoporosis Quiz.[30] This instrument contains 20 questions with a content validity index of 0.7 and an internal consistency reliability rating of 0.76 and has been documented as suitable for those with a 6th-grade reading level.

In addition to assessment of risk and knowledge regarding osteoporosis, nurses must also assess dietary and exercise habits. Clearly, better tools are needed to assess both issues. Some find the pedometer a reasonable means to assess general walking. Diet histories are more challenging to record. Many researchers use an average from a 3-day diet record because it is thought to yield more reliable data on actual nutrient intake.[31] Other factors that should routinely be included in the assessment of osteoporosis include DXA results, height, and weight. These assessment data are necessary to properly interpret information about risk to women and to guide them in making choices about further screening or diagnostic testing, prevention strategies, and possible treatment modalities.

Patient Education

Education regarding osteoporosis should also be a significant component of cancer screening and early detection programs. Women who seek cancer screening services often have questions about the risks and benefits of ERT. This information is usually included in education about breast and endometrial cancer prevention. This discussion needs to be a balanced one that includes a comprehensive discussion of the strengths and limitations of ERT. In particular, consideration for further evaluation for osteoporosis should be given to women who decide not to take ERT. Assessment for osteoporosis can easily be included with the cancer risk assessment and provides a foundation for education about women's health and well-being. This education can be supplemented by written materials.

Nurses can incorporate assessment of osteoporosis into routine visits to follow up women who have survived cancer. Women who have a higher risk for development of osteoporosis should be counseled about the importance of diagnostic evaluation.

Many oncology patients may mistakenly believe that osteoporosis is the same as a bony metastasis. Oncology nurses need to provide clear education that normal bone remodeling and hypercalcemia and/or metastatic lesions associated with malignancy are two entirely different physiologic processes that have different implications for treatment and long-term survival.

Many long-term survivors of cancer may question why attention is now being given to osteoporosis. It is important to inform these women that historically, little could be done to medically manage osteoporosis and so, in most cases, evaluation for osteoporosis was not viewed as relevant. With the development of bisphosphonates and other types of medications, new hope is available to prevent fractures and treat this disease and ultimately improve the long-term quality of life for women with osteoporosis. Patients may also experience some hope and a sense of reassurance regarding their malignancy, if the focus of the discussion is on a complication related to long-term survival.

Nurses can also be key providers of education about what to expect when a patient is scheduled for bone density testing. During DXA a woman will be asked to undress if she is wearing clothes with metal parts such as zippers or snaps, or underwire bras. The examination using DXA usually takes about 5 to 10 minutes per site (hip, spine, or forearm). The radiation exposure with a DXA examination is equivalent to one tenth of a chest radiograph. To image the spine the patient will be asked to lie flat on her back on the imaging table. To further stabilize the spine, the patient is asked to elevate her legs on a foam wedge. To image the hip, the patient is again asked to lie flat on her back, and the hip is immobilized by using a brace on the ankle. The gold standard is to image by DXA one hip and the spine at the same appointment. Patients may also be asked to not take their calcium supplements several days before imaging to decrease the probability of false-positive result, because unabsorbed calcium in the GI tract will falsely elevate BMD. A history of previous fractures at the hip or spine will compromise the results, and a thorough history should be elicited before the examination so alternate or peripheral sites can be considered for evaluation. Peripheral sites include the wrist, the calcaneus, or the phalanges. No special preparation is needed before imaging these sites.

If a woman is diagnosed with osteoporosis or bone loss, options for medical management must be discussed. Some women are not candidates to take bisphosphonates. These include women with a history of esophageal disorders or an inability to sit upright for at least 30 minutes. Women with a history of hypocalcemia, kidney diseases, or an allergy to alendronate or residronate will not be candidates for this type of therapy. Nurses can offer clarification about how to take medications correctly (see Table 11-2).

Nurses also need to obtain a dietary history and provide education about dietary sources of calcium (see Table 11-1) and vitamin D and differences in calcium supplements. Calcium supplements should be selected based on their content of elemental calcium, which can be determined by carefully reading the label. Encouraging patients to engage in weight-bearing exercise should also be included in patient counseling.

Many women will be distressed if they are diagnosed with osteoporosis. Nurses must emphasize that a low BMD does not mean a fracture will occur, but that the risk is higher. Patients should continually be encouraged and reminded that there are things they can do to help reduce their risk of a fracture related to osteoporosis. Providing education may be one means of support. For those at significant risk for fracture, education about ways to prevent fracture is important, as shown in Box 11-3.[32,33]

Box 11-3 Prevention of Falls in Persons with Osteoporosis[32,33]

- Keep living environment well lit
- Remove clutter from floors
- Remove throw rugs
- Make sure shoes fit well and do not pose a tripping hazard
- Correct hearing and vision problems; make sure glasses are clean and hearing aids are functioning
- Seek evaluation and modification of medications that might affect balance or coordination
- Use assistive devices such as walkers or canes to maintain balance
- Limit alcohol intake
- Install railings on stairs and in tub, shower, and toilet areas
- Ensure that there are nonslip surfaces in tubs and shower
- Keep most commonly used items in easy reach
- When outdoors, watch for wet or slippery surfaces; be especially careful when getting in and out of vehicles, when in crowds, and when walking near curbs
- Ask for assistance when needed
- Stay physically and socially active to prevent further loss of function

Research

Nurses must continue to engage in research that identifies women at risk for osteoporosis, as well as research that develops interventions that prevent or delay the development of osteoporosis and prevent complications from falls. Ways to promote adherence to dietary, medication, and exercise regimens are undoubtedly needed.[34]

Clearly, osteoporosis is an emerging concern for long-term survivors of cancer that cannot be ignored. Oncology nurses should not underestimate the important role they will play in helping to identify women at higher risk for developing osteoporosis. This includes the development of comprehensive systems to document both assessment data and educational interventions.[35] The early identification and management of osteoporosis can ultimately improve and promote the long-term quality of life for these women.

REFERENCES

1. National Osteoporosis Foundation: *Physician's guide to prevention and treatment of osteoporosis*, Washington D.C., 2004, National Osteoporosis Foundation.
2. Sris ES and others: Identification and fracture outcomes of undiagnosed low bone mineral density in postmenopausal women: results from the National Osteoporosis Risk Assessment. *JAMA*, 286:2815-2822, 2001.
3. Kleerekoper M, Siris E, McClung M: *The bone and mineral manual*, San Diego, 1999, Academic Press.
4. Lane JM, Russell, L, Safdar K: Osteoporosis, *Clin Orthop* 1(372):139-150, 2000.

5. Sullivan MP, Sharts-Hopko NC: Preventing the downward spiral, *AJN* 100(8):26-33, 2000.
6. Ganz, PA: Long-term complications after primary therapy of breast cancer, *ASCO Spring Educational Book* 19:393-399, 2000.
7. American Cancer Society: *Cancer facts and figures – 2004,* Atlanta, 2004, American Cancer Society.
8. Burstein HJ, Winer EP: Primary care: primary care for survivors of breast cancer, *N Engl J Med* 343(15):1086-1094, 2000.
9. Pfeilschifter J, Diel IJ: Osteoporosis due to cancer treatment: pathogenesis and management, *J Clin Oncol* 18(7): 1570-1593, 2000.
10. Pritchard, KI: Estrogen, tamoxifen, and raloxifene: decisions in practice hormone replacement therapy, *ASCO Spring Educational Book* 21:673-681, 2002.
11. Bilezikian JP and others: The state of the art in the management of osteoporosis, *Clinician,* 22(3):1-18, 2004.
12. Pritchard KI: Impact of the Women's Health Initiative (WHI) on the practicing oncologist: putting the WHI results into perspective, *ASCO Spring Educational Book* 23:543-549, 2004.
13. Chlebowski RT: Menopausal hormone therapy and breast, colon, and gynecologic cancer risk: Women's Health Initiative results, *ASCO Spring Educational Book* 23: 550-555, 2004.
14. Gosfield E, Bonner FJ: Evaluating bone mineral density in osteoporosis, *Am J Phys Med Rehab* 79(3):283-291, 2000.
15. Rossouw JE and others: Risks and benefits of estrogen plus progestin in healthy postmenopausal women: principal results from the Women's Health Initiative randomized controlled trial, *JAMA* 288:321-333, 2002.
16. Cauley JA and others: Effects of estrogen plus progestin on risk of fracture and bone mineral density: the Women's Health Initiative randomized trial, *JAMA* 290:1729-1738, 2003.
17. World Health Organization Study Group on Assessment of Fracture Risk and its Application to Screening for Postmenopausal Osteoporosis. *Assessment of fracture risk and its application in screening for postmenopausal osteoporosis,* Geneva, 1994, World Health Organization.
18. Spratto GR, Woods AL: *2004 Edition PDR nurse's drug handbook,* Clifton Park, NY, 2004, Thompson Delmar Learning.
19. Cauley JA: Prevention and treatment of osteoporosis with raloxifene, estrogen, alendronate, and risedronate, *ASCO Spring Educational Book* 21:663-666, 2002.
20. Cranney A: Treatment of postmenopausal osteoporosis, *BJM* 327:355-356, 2003.
21. Hillner BE and others: American Society of Clinical Oncology 2003 update on the role of bisphosphonates and bone health issues in women with breast cancer, *J Clin Oncol,* 21:4042-4057, 2003.
22. Hendrix SL: Menopausal hormone therapy informed consent, *Am J Obstet Gynecol* 189(4):S31-S36, 2003.
23. Warren MP: A comparative review of the risks and benefits of hormone therapy regimens, *Am J Obstet Gynecol* 190: 1141-1167, 2004.
24. Morris R, Masud T: Measuring quality of life in osteoporosis, *Age Ageing* 30:371-373, 2001.
25. Cantarelli FB and others: Quality of life in patients with osteoporosis fractures: cultural adaptation, reliability and validity of the Osteoporosis Assessment Questionnaire, *Clin Exp Rheumatol* 17:547-551, 2001.
26. Helmes E And others: A questionnaire to evaluate disability in osteoporotic patients with vertebral compression fractures, *J Gerontol* 50:M91-M98, 1995.
27. Osteoporosis Quality of Life Study Group: Measuring quality of life in women with osteoporosis, *Osteoporos Int* 7:478-487, 1997.
28. Chandler JM and others: Quality of life in patients with vertebral fractures: validation of the Quality of Life Questionnaire of the European Foundation for Osteoporosis, *Osteoporos Int* 10:150-160, 1999.
29. Badia, X and others: Development of the ECOS-16 clinical questionnaire for the assessment of the quality of life in patients with osteoporosis, *Med Clin* 114:68-75, 2000.
30. Ailinger RL, Lasus H, Braun MA: Revision of the Facts on Osteoporosis Quiz, *Nurs Res* 52(3):198-202, 2003.
31. Lindsey AM and others: Postmenopausal survivors of breast cancer at risk for osteoporosis: nutritional intake and body size, *Cancer Nurs* 25(1):50-56, 2002.
32. Viale PH, Yamamoto DS: Bisphophonates: expanded roles in the treatment of patients with cancer, *Clin J Oncol Nurs* 7(4):393-401, 2003.
33. Ebersole P, Hess P, Luggen AS: *Toward healthy aging,* ed 6, St. Louis, 2004, Mosby.
34. Waltman NL and others: Testing an intervention for preventing osteoporosis in postmenopausal breast cancer survivors, *J of Nurs Scholarship* 35(4):333-338, 2003.
35. deVillers MJ: Documentation of preventive education and screening for osteoporosis. *Outcomes Manage* 7(1):28-32, 2003.

CHAPTER

12 Lymphedema

Jane M. Armer

IMPACT AND PREVALENCE

Lymphedema (LE) is both an acute and a chronic condition in which significant and persistent swelling occurs with an abnormal accumulation of protein-rich fluid.[1,2] Both the physical and psychosocial consequences of lymphedema can be severe. Lymphedema occurs when there is a disruption of lymphatic channels, most commonly from surgery and/or radiation therapy, and has been commonly associated with patients undergoing node dissection for cancer treatment. Lymph node dissections (LNDs) are common oncologic procedures that are performed for the treatment of a variety of solid tumors.[3,4] LE may occur more frequently in patients with certain cancers because surgeons routinely perform more extensive LND of the upper and/or lower extremity to manage and stage the disease.

Among breast cancer survivors alone, some 400,000 to 800,000 women in the US may be affected by LE during their lifetimes. Among the tens of thousands of people in this country who develop lymphedema annually, LE is cited as not only the most frequent cancer treatment effect, but also the most serious.[5] Lymphedema is the greatest concern of cancer survivors, except for cancer recurrence. The swelling associated with LE often causes discomfort and disability that result from loss of range of motion.[1,2,6] Also, it often causes cellulitis and lymphangitis later, predisposing patients to recurrent infections.[7] Hull[5] noted that LE has a wide-ranging impact on the survivor's daily life. Specifically, (a) sleeping is disturbed because of an inability to comfortably position the swollen limb; (b) carrying heavy items becomes difficult; (c) many forms of exercise, even walking, cannot be performed as easily; and (d) the fit and comfort of clothing become problematic. Thus, the physical problems associated with LE affect a wide range of daily activities and significantly impact quality of life in years of cancer survivorship. Unfortunately, neglect of LE by health professionals has not only meant that many persons go undiagnosed and fail to receive basic risk reduction information, it has also inhibited the development of effective physiologic and psychosocial interventions.

PATHOPHYSIOLOGY RELATED TO CANCER TREATMENT

The main cause of lymphedema after cancer treatment is the interruption of the lymphatic pathways due to lymph node resection.[2,8] Surgery involving staging and management of the cancer through removal of lymph nodes damages the lymph vessels that form the main evacuation route for the return of lymphatic fluid to the central part of the body.[8] The surgically damaged lymph vessels are further injured by radiation and subsequent radiation fibrosis. When the affected lymph vessels and the nonoperative vessels attempt to take on the workload of the damaged vessels, the active transport of the lymph fluid from the (potentially) affected limb is further compromised. The inadequate lymphatic drainage of the limb results in limb swelling. The remaining functional lymphatics may also be at risk for damage by postoperative infection. Recurrent infections over time pose a risk for increasing lymphatic damage and may lead to life-threatening infections such as septicemia.[7]

In some treatment plans, surgical management of the cancerous tumor involves not only lymph node sampling or dissection, but removal of tissue in the limb itself, as in the case of melanoma of the arm or leg.[3] In such cases, the affected limb may have an even greater predisposition to development of LE, since the lymph vessels draining the limb, and lymph nodes of the groin or axilla, are resected and are functioning suboptimally. In addition to the surgical interruption of the lymphatic pathways, three categories of factors may influence development of LE: treatment-related, disease-related, and patient-related factors (further discussed later).[4]

The literature on current LE incidence following cancer treatment is sparse, considering this is a condition which affects hundreds of thousands of cancer survivors.[5] The literature that exists is largely focused on breast cancer LE because that is the leading women's cancer, affecting some 200,000 women annually in the US alone, and associated with some 2 million survivors.[5] Even in this relatively more widely studied area, the reported findings on LE incidence and prevalence are inconclusive, thus hindering the development of effective interventions to reduce LE risk and progression.

All cancer survivors with dissection of or treatment involving the lymph nodes, including both surgical and radiation approaches, have a lifetime risk for developing LE, though current data for LE incidence and prevalence are far from complete and provide only a crude estimate of risk. It has been noted that breast cancer lymphedema studies with the shortest follow-up (12 months) report the lowest incidence (6%),[8] while studies with the longest follow-up have the highest incidence. Similar trends are noted in a review of the melanoma literature,[3] with the lowest lymphedema rates (upper and lower extremity) noted in studies that examined patients 6 months after surgery,[9] whereas the highest incidence (67%, lower-extremity lymphedema) had the longest follow-up (20 years).[10] High rates (44%) were also noted when lymphedema was defined as "swelling lasting more than 6 months."[11]

Although researchers know relatively little about current incidence of LE in women's cancers, there is reason to believe that LE may occur even more often in patients with certain cancers such as melanoma than in breast cancer patients, because of the extent of LND performed and the physiology associated with the lymphatic system of the lower extremity, which is a common site of disease.[3] Some of these same issues apply to those treated for gynecologic cancers with radical hysterectomy, in which the LND is extensive and surgery may be followed by radiation.[12] To date, research has been limited in physiologic aspects of LE and is even more limited in psychosocial areas.

MEASUREMENT AND DIAGNOSIS OF LYMPHEDEMA

Measurement and quantification of LE has been problematic despite the fact that various methods have been used to measure limb volume (LV).[9,13-16] Circumferences (limb girth measurements) and volume measurements by water displacement (the "gold standard" of volume measurements) or infrared laser perometry (now applied experimentally in LE settings) are three clinical assessment approaches for LE. Volume measurement using water displacement has historically been regarded as the most sensitive and accurate measure; however, clinicians rarely use this cumbersome and messy approach.[17,18] Exemplifying measurement discrepancies in the scientific literature, 2 of 25 melanoma studies Cormier and colleagues reviewed[3] used water displacement alone[19] or in combination with circumference measurements.[20] Circumference measurements were utilized in five of the studies.[10,14,21-23] The remaining 15 studies reported on lymphedema in melanoma patients using clinical definitions with no objective measurement criteria. Clinically, and often in research studies as well, subjective observation is the basis of the judgment about presence of LE.[24,25]

Similar discrepancies are seen in the LE diagnostic criteria used in the studies reported in the literature. For example, in one melanoma study in which significant lymphedema was defined as greater than a 1-inch difference between the affected and the unaffected limb, lymphedema was reported in 80% of patients 5 years after surgery.[10] Two other studies reported rates of 21% to 26% when 2 to 4 cm^2[21] or 3 to 4.5 cm^2[22] differences were used as criteria.

Perhaps the most common clinically applied objective criterion for diagnosis has been a finding of a 2-cm or greater difference in arm (or leg) circumference (or a 200-ml limb volume difference [LVD]) between affected and unaffected limbs.[1,26] LE can be categorized as mild, moderate, or severe. Three stages are identified:[1] grade I, in which pitting occurs upon application of pressure and edema reverses with limb elevation; grade II, in which the edematous limb becomes larger and harder and no longer pits under pressure; and grade III, in which swelling worsens and skin changes occur—the skin may become very thick and develop huge folds associated with elephantiasis. LE also may be classified as acute (lasting less than 6 months) or chronic (lasting longer than 6 months).[27]

Measurement Issues in Lymphedema

The ideal volumetric measurement for LE would be easy to use, accessible, quick, noninvasive, hygienic, inexpensive, reliable, quantifiable, usable at the bedside, suitable for any portion of the limb, and able to provide information on shape.[17,28] Existing measures that are easy to use and inexpensive have limited reliability and do not address the functional impact of LE.[28] Limb volume measurements must be done routinely, preoperatively, and also at follow-up. Currently, there is no standard clinical protocol (a clinical gold standard) that is easy to use, noninvasive, and reliable for the measurement of the affected limb in the clinical setting.[18]

Although *water displacement* has been regarded as the sensitive and accurate gold standard for volume measurement in the laboratory setting, it is little used clinically because it is cumbersome and messy. It is usually applied to a certain part of the limb and does not provide data about localization of the edema or the shape of the extremity.[17,18] It can be difficult for the patient to assume a comfortable and appropriate position for repeated measurements. Moreover, a standard deviation of 25 ml for repeated measures of the arm has been reported by Swedborg.[17,29] Finally, water displacement is contraindicated in patients with open skin lesions and infections.

Circumferences at various points of a body part are used most frequently to quantify LE, but several problems exist.[28] Limits for acceptable difference between repeated circumferential measurements of the normal adult arm, forearm, and wrist are 0.2 cm,[30] a standard rarely met clinically. Measurement variance in the adult leg is even greater, because of limb size and shape and positioning issues. Although circumferences may appear to be simple measures, control of reliability both in single measurers and among different measurers is difficult. Volume calculations assume a circular circumference, which is seldom the case. This systematic methodologic error yields a slightly higher volume than the true value. Studies report correlations with water displacement ranging from 0.70 to 0.98.[17,18] Because of its irregular shape, circumference of the hand (and foot) is an inaccurate way of determining volume. There are severe limitations for both these methods when skin damage exists. Handling of the extremity and contact with equipment raise hygienic concerns.[17] The circumference method is time-consuming and requires considerable experience.

The *Perometer 400T/350S* (Juzo, Cuyahoga Falls, Ohio) is an optoelectronic volumetry (OEV) device developed to meet the need for a quick, hygienic, and accurate method of limb volume calculation. It works similarly to computer-assisted tomography but uses infrared light instead of x-rays.[17] Light sources (two arrays of infrared-emitting diodes at right angles to each other) are placed along two sides of a 46 × 46 cm frame with corresponding light sensors (two arrays of infrared-detecting diodes) opposite the light sources.[17,18] The array of 360 light beams is emitted perpendicular to the axis of and sequentially along the limb. Where the path of the beams is interrupted by the limb, the receivers in the limb's shadow are not lit, allowing the OEV to calculate a precise transection. Dimensions along the x- and y-axes are measured to an accuracy of 10^{-4} m.[17] Transections are measured every 3 mm and summed to the volume by a computer.[17]

The Perometer 400T/350S has a standard deviation with repeated measures of 8.9 ml, less than 0.5% of the arm volume.[17,18] In addition, the volume and transection of any part of the limb can be measured, the shape of the limb or limb segment can be displayed, and accurate calculations of change in volume can be made in seconds. To date, testing of the Perometer 400T/350S on limbs with LE had been limited to Europe and largely to the horizontal leg unit, but has shown very promising results.[18,31] Its potential application for baseline LV and follow-up measurements of limb volume change (LVC) is promising.

Symptom Experience

Frequently, the patient's subjective experience of sensation changes is the first sign of LE, sometimes occurring before observable LVC. Research into symptom experience reveals that certain symptoms (swelling, heaviness, and numbness) differentiate between women with breast cancer LE and healthy women.[32] When these three symptoms were used to examine a group of survivors with and without LE at the 2-cm circumferential difference, swelling and heaviness differentiated group membership (c statistic = 0.952).[32] In an earlier preliminary analysis of this second set of data, participants who were breast cancer survivors with LE experienced more symptoms than those without limb swelling at the recognized criterion.[33] It is recommended that LV measurements routinely be accompanied by symptom assessment.

FACTORS AFFECTING LYMPHEDEMA

In 2004, van der Veen and colleagues[4] reported on the following treatment, disease, and patient factors affecting LE development in the 245 breast cancer survivors they assessed: metastatic lymph nodes (odds ratio [OR] = 2.60, 95% confidence interval [CI], 1.43-4.75); axillary/superclavicular radiography in combination with chest or breast radiography (OR = 2.53, 95% CI, 1.38-4.64); dominant operative side (OR = 1.97, 95% CI, 1.09-3.55); trauma to the affected arm (e.g., burns or puncture wounds; OR = 7.23, 95% CI, 1.45-20.58); overweight (body mass index [BMI] ≥25; OR = 2.45, 95% CI, 1.34-4.47); and menopause (OR = 3.15, 95% CI, 1.07-9.28).

Axillary/superclavicular radiography, arm injury, and positive lymph nodes have been reported by others as associated factors, but menopause and surgery on the dominant side have not yet been reported by other researchers. Limb trauma and weight gain have been anecdotally associated with increased incidence of LE in the literature. On the other hand, van der Veen[4] found no association with limb swelling when examining the following factors: radiography dose; radiography to the chest wall and to the breast; number of resected lymph nodes; kind of surgery; chemotherapy; side of surgery; tumor stage; number of pathologic lymph nodes; tumor localization; age; and smoking.[4]

In 2003, Tada and colleagues[12] reported LE incidence among 694 gynecologic cancer patients (endometrial, cervical, and ovarian) with LND: 189 (27%) had lower extremity LE. Logistic regression to identify independent risk factors for lower extremity LE revealed the following: paraaortic LND in ovarian cancer patients (OR: 2.75, 95% CI: 1.11-6.78) and postoperative radiotherapy in uterine cancer patients (OR: 1.63, 95% CI: 1.08-2.46) were statistically significant factors related to LE. The study classified patients into three degrees of risk categories depending on cancer site, postoperative radiotherapy, and paraaortic LND.

Based on an extensive literature search performed on over 1,900 references on primary and secondary lymphedema, Weiss[34] abstracted 200 research reports that cited the incidence of lymphedema from any cause and collected the relevant findings into a matrix including the reference, cause of lymphedema, appropriate statistic, number of cases, year of treatment, length of study, and lymphedema measurement used. The majority of the estimates relate to breast cancer treatment protocols, but the survey includes pelvic and inguinal treatment protocols, as well as other cancers. The wide range of reported findings is concluded to be due to changing cancer diagnostic procedures and treatment protocols during the timeframe of the studies, lack of standard LE measurement and grading criteria, prolonged course of toxicity, therapeutic interventions during the study, variation in physicians' viewpoints and knowledge, inadequate contemporary documentation, selection criteria of patients for study, and nonuse of actuarial estimates.[34] The researcher suggests the reported occurrence of lymphedema is dependent on patient genetic predisposition, the patient's general health and lymphatic system health, the nature and extent of lymphatic trauma, and lack of a standard clinical definition of the condition.

Weiss[34] concludes in his summary that reports of LE onset vary as a function of the method of LE measurement and the causative therapeutic procedure. For example, toxic effects of radiation therapy do not become fully evident until many years after treatment. Using sensitive lymphoscintigraphic measures of lymphedema, Campisi[35] shows early LE effects of breast cancer treatment at 3 to 6 months (range <1 to 24). The delayed effects of radiotherapy were demonstrated by Pierquin[36] with median LE onset at 7 months (range 2 to 37) with surgery alone, 12 months (range 1 to 52) with surgery and radiation, and 25 months (range 6 to 156) months with radiation alone. Other researchers demonstrate medians for LE onset between 1 and 2 years, with maximum times of onset of 3 to 10 years for mixed cohorts.[34]

Swelling after breast cancer treatment can occur at a number of sites, and the restriction of measurements to one particular site such as the forearm, the upper arm, or the entire arm and hand results in an underestimation of the incidence of lymphedema.[34] Further, arm swelling may account for only about half of the patient-reported swelling.[37] Other reported sites for treatment-related swelling include the breast, the chest, the axilla, and the back. However, measurement of these sites is very challenging, and therefore incidence remains largely unreported. Breast lymphedema incidences of 70% using measurement of dermal swelling have been demonstrated,[38] whereas clinical examination detects only 35% in the same cohort.[34]

Similarly Armer[39] reported a variance in LE incidence based on four measurement and LE definitional approaches, in a preliminary analysis of data from an ongoing NIH-funded longitudinal study. Results were reported as a series of four survival analyses using the four common definitions of lymphedema: 200-ml volume difference; 10% limb volume change; 2-cm limb girth difference; and self-reported LE signs and symptoms.

Using volume change estimated by perometry to define LE, the estimated rate of LE at 6 months was about 24% (95% CI: 17%, 32%), while the rate at 1 year was about 42% (95% CI: 31%, 53%).

Using 10% volume change to define LE in the same sample, the estimated rate of LE at 6 months was about 8% (95% CI: 2%, 13%) while the rate at 1 year was about 21% (95% CI: 12%, 30%).

In the third analysis, the criteria of 2-cm difference at any location along the arm was applied, where the difference could be either between sides within a visit or could be between the same location (including the same side) at a visit as compared to preoperative baseline. Based on the 2-cm definition, the estimated rate of LE at 6 months was about 46% (95% CI: 36%, 56%) while the rate at 1 year was about 70% (95% CI: 60%, 79%). In the fourth analysis, self-reported signs and symptoms were used to assess LE. Following a definition based on earlier work,[32] the researchers looked for the reported symptoms of heaviness or swelling, either "now" or "in the past" as the definition of LE. Using symptom report, the estimated rate of LE at 6 months was about 19% (95% CI: 11%, 26%) while the rate for 1 year was about 40% (95% CI: 30%, 59%). Although the "true" incidence of LE is unknown, it is clear that LE incidence estimation varied based on the definition and measurement approach applied.

From a historical perspective, changes in the application of breast cancer surgery and radiotherapy over the last 50 years have resulted in a shift in the reported incidence of lymphedema, since each therapy has a different associated morbidity.[34] Halsted radical mastectomies with and without radiotherapy, the standard until the 1970s, resulted in upper limb LE rates of 22% to 44%, based on Weiss's review.[34] With the application of the modified radical mastectomy with and without radiotherapy in the 1970s and 1980s, lymphedema rates fell to 19% to 29%.[40] The 1990s brought breast-conserving surgery with and without radiotherapy from a small percentage of procedures to approximately half of the surgeries performed,[41] with a further drop in upper limb LE rates to 7% to 10%,[40,47] as summarized by Weiss.[34]

Weiss[34] further reports that lymphedema of the breast started to receive attention in 1982; Kissin[42] reported clinical rates of 8% and Clarke[43] rates of 41% using skin measurements. Recent reports estimate the rates of LE of the breast at 1% to 9% based on subjective reporting,[44,45] 10% to 19% based on clinical examination,[44,46] and 23% to 48% by clinical examination[38] and 28%-70% based on skin thickness measurement including ultrasound in the same sample, depending on surgery and nodal status.[38]

Lower limb LE rates are likewise a strong function of the extent of the surgery and radiation used for treatment of reproductive and pelvic cancers, as well as lower limb melanomas.[34] Whereas there are several different methods commonly used to evaluate upper limb swelling, there are relatively few methods reported to measure lower limb swelling. Lower limb LE often is reported in medical records only when it is severe enough that compression is not adequate to treat it, or it causes disability.[34] Reported lower limb LE following groin dissection ranges from zero[48] to 60% to 80%,[10,49,50] with many reports between these extremes.[34]

A literature review of reported LE following treatment of selected sites of women's cancers[25] reported LE incidence in lower extremities: following vulvectomy it ranged from 1.5% to 69%; after cervical cancer it ranged from 10% to 41%; and after melanoma with groin dissection it ranged from 21% to 49%. In this review, ovarian cancer was rarely associated with reported LE, except in end-stage disease and abdominal carcinomatosis. Few data were found on LE in endometrial cancer.

Cormier and colleagues systematically reviewed the literature[3] and found a total of 25 studies performed between 1972 and 2004 pertaining to melanoma and LE.[9,11,13-16,20,24,51-55] As with the reported incidence of postsurgical lymphedema for breast cancer patients,[8,56] the reported incidence of lymphedema in patients with melanoma varies widely, with reported rates ranging from 2% to 67%. The disparity likely relates to the heterogeneity of the reports, as discussed earlier.

Based on his literature review, Weiss[34] reports that the incidence of LE of the genitals, a particularly troublesome cancer treatment effect, has been reported as 2% to 5%[57,58] and 18% (combined with lower limb LE).[59] A finding important for clinicians to note, genital lymphedema among users of pneumatic pumps on the lower limb has been reported at 43%.[34,60]

RISK REDUCTION IN WOMEN'S CANCERS

Although common medical assumptions imply LE is not a problem of the present or future because of modern procedures such as sentinel lymph node biopsy (SLNB) and breast conservation surgical approaches, the latest data reported in 2003 and 2004 reveal LE occurrence at a significant level of concern in spite of these improved techniques. Two national cooperative clinical trials are now in design and approval stages, aimed at investigating LE occurrence and prevention in breast cancer patients (Cancer and Leukemia Group B [CALGB]; American College of Surgeons Oncology Group [ACOSOG]), evidence that clinicians recognize the continuing breadth and impact of this post–treatment complication on survivors' quality of life.

Clinicians and researchers report modest estimates of LE following breast cancer surgery even for SLNB-only patients.[8,33,61] This group with node-negative (SLNB-only) disease represents the group at lesser risk for LE, and this LE occurrence is commonly reported by clinical observation rather than objective limb measurement,[62] posing a high probability of underrepresentation of the condition. Further, current protocols require further nodal dissection for node-positive disease, meaning that SLNB alone may not complete the cancer management plan.

A 2003 study by Deutsch and Flickinger[63] reports incidence of LE at 7% at 6-month follow-up after postlumpectomy radiotherapy (n = 265). In the same year, Coen and colleagues[64] estimated up to a 10% 10-year risk of developing LE (highest with axillary irradiation), as compared to a 26% prevalence reported by Voogd and colleagues[65] in a sample of women receiving axillary lymph node dissection (ALND) but no axillary radiation in the Netherlands; 28% in a group (n = 240) undergoing ALND at 18+ months after surgery in Turkey by Ozaslan and Kuru;[66] and a prevalence of 38% self-reported postsurgical arm or hand swelling (n = 145) by Geller and colleagues.[62] A 2004 study by van der Veen and colleagues[4] similarly reports an incidence of 24% swelling at more than 2.5 cm increase following axillary dissection among 245 breast cancer patients treated in Belgium.

LE among breast cancer patients, even using the lowest estimates of its incidence, affects hundreds of thousands of women and represents a major societal problem. It is hoped that newer cancer treatment approaches will reduce the long-term treatment effects of the past such as LE.[67] Indeed, it is believed that a lower percentage of breast cancer patients without radiation or surgery to the axilla will develop LE; however, the risk of LE following treatment of breast cancer still exists.[8,33,61,68] Postsurgical infection or radiation skin reaction (even in radiation to the breast), as well as comorbid conditions and cotreatment effects such as seroma,[69] may increase risk of LE. Even in radiation treatment directed toward the breast alone, not directed at the axilla, some radiation scatter may have an impact on the axillary lymphatics. Although chemotherapy or hormonal therapy is not known to cause LE, some studies and clinical practice guidelines[70-75] hint at association of weight gain during treatment with risk of LE; chemotherapy and hormonal therapy are known to affect fluid balance changes. It is conservatively estimated that 20 to 40 of every 100 persons (or 1 in 4) treated for breast cancer with contemporary treatment modalities will experience LE in their lifetimes.[8] Indeed, in Armer's cross-sectional study, 39% of the 103 women returning for follow-up after breast cancer treatment (mean time since diagnosis = 36 months) had a 2-cm or greater circumferential difference between the affected and unaffected limbs at one or more points.[33]

Over the past decade, breast conservation techniques, most often coupled with radiotherapy, have been used widely in an effort to diminish unpleasant, lasting side effects (such as LE) long associated with more radical treatments.[67] Similar medical optimism regarding reduction in LE has been associated in recent years with the advent of SLNB procedures that spare the cancer patient the more invasive and traumatic axillary (or groin) lymph node dissection.[67] However, preliminary observations and data indicate that LE incidence following breast conservation surgical methods, such as lumpectomy and partial mastectomy combined with radiotherapy, may be equal to (or in fact greater than) the incidence following traditional surgical treatment (mastectomy with or without radiation).[34,67,68]

The impact of SLNB on LE occurrence is not yet known because too little time has elapsed to observe LE that may occur up to 20 years after treatment.[8] It is important to note current protocols continue to call for ALND in node-positive disease; thus, a large cohort of women continue to require axillary dissection—alone or in addition to SLNB.[33,61,67,74] Indeed, SLNB in combination with lumpectomy is typically followed by radiation therapy—again (even if limited to the breast) incurring additional LE risk. Both breast conservation techniques and SLNB are generally components of a program of treatment including radiotherapy to the breast and/or axilla.[67,74] Since radiation exposure is associated with trauma to the lymphatic system, risk for LE likely continues for women who undergo state-of-the-art treatment modalities. Through increased measurement accuracy, LE incidence and prevalence following current therapeutic treatment approaches for breast cancer will be better understood, and more informed decisions about risk factors, treatment interventions, and recovery will be made. In addition, appropriate sampling decisions can be made for the next stage of intervention research.

Because there is currently no cure for LE, prevention—more accurately described as risk reduction—is the first major goal. The focus of risk reduction is minimizing injury or damage to the involved extremity. Over the past 15 years, the National Lymphedema Network (NLN) has taken a lead in educating professionals and patients about risk reduction for LE development and progression.[72] In the absence of evidence-based research, the NLN's classic 18 steps to LE prevention have been carefully reviewed by Ridner[75] in validation of the pathophysiologic basis for the risk reduction guidelines. In 2005, these 18 steps were reviewed and revised by the NLN Medical Advisory Committee and renamed "LE Risk-Reduction Practices." Precautions recommended by the NLN for those at risk of upper or lower extremity LE are detailed in Box 12-1.[72] Although based on practitioners' best clinical knowledge,[75] unfortunately even rigorous adherence to these guidelines does not prevent LE in all cases. For those who do develop LE from weeks to years after cancer treatment, the focus is on life-long self-management, as further discussed in the following section (see also Tables 12-1, 12-2, and Box 12-2).

TREATMENT AND SELF-MANAGEMENT

Management of LE is both multifaceted and multidisciplinary.[3,26,70] A range of clinical approaches with varying levels of success in LE management has been reported in the literature.[1,25,75-81] Treatment options are broadly categorized as classic (or traditional) conservative or nontraditional surgical.[26] In general, nontraditional surgical approaches, with varying levels of success reported and accompanied by some controversy, are reserved for refractory cases of LE that have been painful and distressing.[25] Certain classic comprehensive approaches in therapy and self-management, such as complete decongestive physiotherapy (including manual lymph drainage, bandaging, exercise, and meticulous skin care), have become the standard in managing LE.[1,77-81] Tables 12-1, 12-2, and Box 12-2 outline professional guidelines in LE management, various LE treatment approaches, and nursing strategies to foster LE self-management.

A comprehensive scientific literature review by the Cochrane Breast Cancer Group[81] substantiates the deficit in randomized clinical research examining LE therapies: studies of adequate design rigor, sample size, and follow-up are lacking. Early detection and intervention hold the greatest promise of reducing this widespread condition.[68,70] Further identification of epidemiologic and clinical factors associated with risk and incidence will provide the necessary foundation for preventive intervention.

It is noted here that tumors arising in the lymphatic tissue sometimes cause LE, requiring treatment of the malignant tumors, a scenario to be ruled out before LE is diagnosed as secondary to cancer treatment.[82] Treatment in this case generally is chemotherapy or hormone treatment targeting the tumor, rather than LE-specific treatment. In addition, in rare cases LE may be associated with angiosarcoma, a very serious cancer which may be life-threatening. These tumors require targeted therapy as a priority, with potential incorporation of the comprehensive LE treatment approaches listed above as palliative therapy.[71,83,84]

Lymphedema treatment and management are challenging. Many of the most promising LE management techniques are time-consuming, very difficult to accomplish by the patient alone, and may be vulnerable to incomplete patient compliance without strong support and practical assistance from family or friends. As noted in the following section, the special challenges of women's multiple roles, including the traditional role of caregiver to young and old family members, and occupational responsibilities may further complicate the design and implementation of a successful LE self-management plan of care.

Box 12-1 Lymphedema Risk Reduction Practices

Position Paper of the National Lymphedema Network

By NLN Medical Advisory Committee; Approved by the NLN Board of Directors: 07/01/2005; Expires: 07/01/2007

I. SKIN CARE—AVOID TRAUMA/INJURY AND REDUCE INFECTION RISK

- Keep extremity clean and dry.
- Apply moisturizer daily to prevent chapping/chafing of skin.
- Pay attention to nail care; do not cut cuticles.
- Protect exposed skin with sunscreen and insect repellent.
- Use care with razors to avoid nicks and skin irritation.
- If possible, avoid punctures such as injections and blood draws.
- Wear gloves while doing activities that may cause skin injury (e.g., gardening, working with tools, using chemicals such as detergent).
- If scratches/punctures to skin occur, wash with soap and water, apply antibiotics, and observe for signs of infection (e.g., redness).
- If a rash, itching, redness, pain, increased skin temperature, fever or flu-like symptoms occur, contact your physician immediately.

II. ACTIVITY/LIFESTYLE

- Gradually build up the duration and intensity of any activity or exercise.
- Take frequent rest periods during activity to allow for limb recovery.
- Monitor the extremity during and after activity for any change in size, shape, tissue, texture, soreness, heaviness, or firmness.
- Maintain optimal weight.

III. AVOID LIMB CONSTRICTION

- If possible, avoid having blood pressure measured on the at risk arm.
- Wear loose-fitting jewelry and clothing.

IV. COMPRESSION GARMENTS

- These should be well-fitting.
- Support the at-risk limb with a compression garment for strenuous activity (e.g., weight-lifting, prolonged standing, running).
- Wear a well-fitting compression garment for air travel.

V. EXTREMES OF TEMPERATURE

- Avoid exposure to extreme cold, which can be associated with rebound swelling or chapping of skin.
- Avoid prolonged (>15 minutes) exposure to heat, particularly hot tubs and saunas.
- Avoid immersing limb in water temperatures above 102° F.

VI. ADDITIONAL PRACTICES SPECIFIC TO LOWER-EXTREMITY LYMPHEDEMA

- Avoid prolonged standing or sitting.
- When possible, avoid crossing legs.
- Wear proper, well-fitting footwear.

NLN ♦ 1611 Telegraph Ave. Suite 1111 ♦ Oakland, CA 94612 ♦ Tel: 510-208-3200 ♦ Fax: 510-208-3110 Infoline: 1-800-541-3259 ♦ Email: nln@lymphnet.org ♦ Online: www.lymphnet.org.
Retrieved from www.lymphnet.org/riskreduction/riskreduction.htm. Accessed January 4, 2006.

Table **12-1** MANAGEMENT GUIDE FOR CHRONIC EDEMA BY THE BRITISH LYMPHOLOGY SOCIETY

Group	Clinical Evaluation	Intervention	Health Care Provider
Group 1: persons at risk	No clinical signs of edema One or more risk factors, e.g., lymphatic abnormalities, cancer treatment, chronic venous insufficiency, immobility, trauma to lymphatics	Education, information, and advice Prompt referral to appropriate practitioner if required	All health care practitioners
Group 2: persons with mild and uncomplicated edema	Edema with excess limb volume <20% No trunk, head, or genital swelling Healthy skin Tissues soft and pitting No arterial insufficiency or malignancy	Education, information, and advice Daily self maintenance program: skin care, exercise, simple lymphatic drainage, compression garments Long-term monitoring and prompt referral to appropriate specialist practitioner if required	Practitioners liaison with key worker who may be a nurse, physical therapist, occupational therapist, or other with appropriate education in all aspects of the LE maintenance program
Group 3: persons with moderate to severe, complicated edema	Edema with excess limb volume >20% with one or more of the following: Trunk, head, or genital edema Distorted limb shape Skin problems Evidence of active but controlled malignancy, arterial and/or venous insufficiency, current acute inflammatory episode, lymphorrhoea	Education, information, and advice Treatment plan which may include multilayer LE bandaging, manual lymph drainage, isotonic exercises, skin care, compression garments Referral to others members of the health care team Transfer to maintenance program as required	Specialist LE practitioner with appropriate education in specialist skills such as multilayer bandaging, manual lymphatic drainage, exercise

Continued

Table 12-1 Management Guide for Chronic Edema by the British Lymphology Society—cont'd

Group	Clinical Evaluation	Intervention	Health Care Provider
Group 4: persons with edema and advanced disease	Edema associated with advanced disease Common symptoms are trunk and/or midline edema, lymphorrhoea, tension in the tissues, impaired mobility and function, pain, infection	Education, information, and advice Emphasis on optimizing quality of life Daily treatment program which may include skin care, support and positioning of the limb, appropriate exercises, simple lymphatic drainage Specialist interventions such as manual lymphatic drainage, modified multilayer bandaging, compression garments, appliance to aid mobility and function	Practitioner with appropriate education in specialist skills and palliative care

LE, Lymphedema.
Adapted from: British Lymphology Society: Chronic oedema population and need, 2001, www.lymphoedema.org/bls/index.html; Williams, A: An overview of non-cancer related chronic oedema—a UK perspective, 2003, www.worldwidewounds.com/2003/april/Williams/Chronic-Oedema.html.

SELF-MANAGEMENT OF LYMPHEDEMA

Because LE tends to be a lifelong and chronic condition, appropriate self-management of LE is critical to the prevention of complications and other untoward effects that diminish functional abilities and quality of life related to cancer LE survivorship. There are many factors that are believed to affect women's risk for onset of LE:[2,8,12,26,53,54,67-69,85] personal and historical characteristics such as age, weight, and infection; comorbidities such as diabetes; treatment-related factors such as axillary (or groin) dissection and radiation; and complications such as infection, seroma, and tumor location and staging. However, patient compliance has been identified as the most important factor in *treating and managing* LE.[70,86] Even so, little is known about factors influencing patient compliance and the factors that promote effective self-management strategies for LE symptoms. As noted, many of the most promising LE management techniques (Tables 12-1 and 12-2 and Box 12-2) are time-consuming and complex and may be very difficult to accomplish by the patient herself; without strong support and practical assistance from family or friends, their completion may be at risk.

In one recent study, the most frequently reported LE symptom self-management strategy was "no action."[33] One breast cancer survivor with moderately severe LE in her dominant limb reported she was unable to comply with the bandaging regime when her husband traveled or was too tired to assist her. It was evident that the patient experienced difficulties with both social support and problem solving, which negatively influenced her LE symptom management—and ultimately, the limb swelling and her functional health status.

Table 12-2 LYMPHEDEMA TREATMENT APPROACHES INCLUDING EFFECTIVENESS AND IMPLICATIONS

Treatment	Effectiveness	Aging Implications
Limb elevation	Effective in acute (early) LE when swelling is reversible; not effective for chronic (later) LE	Elevation of limb on soft pillow while at rest may increase comfort. Avoid long periods of immobility.
Diuretics	Not effective for protein-rich LE May be effective for systemic or vascular non–protein-rich edema	Diuretics may be prescribed for other comorbid conditions associated with fluid retention. Adequate oral fluid intake is essential. Systemic dehydration will affect development of fibrosis from protein-rich lymph fluid in interstitium. Weight fluctuations will affect limb measurements for LE diagnosis and assessment of treatment efficacy. Bilateral measurements over time are recommended.
Comprehensive (complex, complete) decongestive physiotherapy (therapy) (CDP, CDT): Manual lymph drainage, bandaging and compression garments, exercise, and meticulous skin care (inclusive)	Highly effective; comprehensive program of specialized manual lymph drainage to stimulate lymphatic function locally, regionally, and systemically; regimen of bandaging and day time compression, exercise and skin care; usually specified period of intensive treatment until maximal limb volume reduction achieved, followed by continuing self-care program, sometimes with occasional "boosts" of intensive treatment; optimal dosing (length of each treatment (60-90 minutes, scheduled daily vs. 3 times a week, for periods of 3-4 to 6 weeks); not yet established by rigorous research	Appropriate and potentially effective for all ages following medical assessment. Assess for contraindications such as congestive heart failure and swelling due to thrombus. Routine daily self-management includes: self-massage manual lymph drainage (MLD); daytime compression and night-time bandaging/compression; exercise (conditioning, flexibility and monitored strength-building with individualized repetition and weight limits); and skin care. Assistance may be required with MLD to back and shoulder, skin inspections, application of lotion, bandaging, and donning of garments.
Compression sleeve	Effective for maintaining limb volume when properly fitted and periodically replaced (every 6 months); alone not generally effective for reduction	Proper fitting and regular replacement of garments is essential for maintenance. Weight changes may affect proper fit.
Sequential pressure device/pump	Mixed efficacy; not currently first line of treatment recommended by the National Lymphedema Network; further damage to lymphatics possible with inappropriate use/pressure	Not recommended. Sensory changes may increase risk of tissue injury and exacerbation of LE. If used, must be under close supervision of a therapist.

Continued

Table **12-2** Lymphedema Treatment Approaches Including Effectiveness and Implications—cont'd

Treatment	Effectiveness	Aging Implications
Exercise	Effective for management and reduction of swelling with carefully individualized exercise plan, with limb appropriately compressed, avoiding extreme repetitions, excessive weights, and extreme temperatures	Important component of LE self-management program to maintain strength and conditioning, enhance independence, and maintain ADLs.
Infection control	Essential and highly effective; prevention and early treatment most effective; history of cellulitis, lymphangitis, erysipelas, septice mia denotes higher risk for infection; may require standing prescription for antibiotics	Infection risk may be increased because of comorbidites. Signs and symptoms of infection may be diminished because of autoimmune changes. Increased vigilance is essential.
Skin integrity	Essential and highly effective: prevention of skin breaks; skin cleansed with mild soaps and moisturized with pH-neutral lotions	Increased vigilance in maintaining meticulous skin care and observing for skin changes is essential. Sensory changes may impair detection of skin breaks and infection; visual inspection using mirror to view back and shoulder is recommended. pH-neutral moisturizing lotions should be used to decrease dryness and skin breaks.
Benzopyrones	Unproven effectiveness (no randomized double-blinded placebo clinical trials); not FDA-approved; discontinued in Australia following deaths resulting from liver disease	Not recommended for LE treatment for persons of any age, and particularly not for persons with other comorbid conditions.

LE, Lymphedema; *ADLs,* activities of daily living.
Adapted from Armer JM: Lymphedema. In Dow KH: *Contemporary issues in breast cancer,* ed 2, Sudbury, MA: 2004, Jones & Bartlett.

LE support groups are one tool for effective education, peer support, and problem solving. Unfortunately, support groups and training in practical problem solving are not yet readily available to all patients. Along with other patient education resources, LE support groups are listed by state at the website of the National Lymphedema Network.[72] In total, there were 134 LE support groups listed for all 50 states in 2005, down from approximately 150 in 2002 (retrieved from www.lymphnet.org/support.html on July 16, 2005).[72]

As discussed in the following section, the special challenges of women's multiple roles may further complicate the design and implementation of a successful LE self-management plan of care. Tables 12-12, 12-32, and Box 12-2 outline professional guidelines in LE management, various LE treatment approaches, and nursing strategies to foster LE self-management. Box 12-3 lists

Box 12-2 Nursing Strategies to Foster Lymphedema Self-Management

Nursing strategies to enhance self-management of post–breast cancer lymphedema (LE) among cancer survivors include the following:

1. Review LE pathophysiology and NLN Risk Reduction Practices; ensure that the patient has printed materials at the appropriate reading-level and in easy-to-read font to review at home and contact information for follow-up for future questions (National Lymphedema Network, 2005; http://www.lymphnet.org/nlnriskreduction.pdf; Ridner, 2002).
2. Ask patients about LE or "limb swelling" and other LE signs and symptoms: patients may not volunteer information unless asked directly. Instruct patient to report immediately to her health provider any changes in limb swelling or other signs and symptoms, such as the sensations of heaviness and aching, and skin changes such as redness, rash, or increased temperature.
3. Facilitate referral to a certified manual lymph drainage (MLD) therapist (nurse, physical therapist, occupational therapist, or massage therapist with specialized training and certification in comprehensive decongestive physiotherapy [CDP]) for LE assessment, intensive treatment, and teaching on self-management (National Lymphedema Network, 2005; www.lymphnet.org/resource.html).
4. Although optimal treatment benefits are seen with early intervention, with appropriate therapy improvement can be seen even after substantial time of swelling. Encourage patients to report early symptoms of acute LE and request referral for treatment; also encourage those with chronic LE to request assessment and treatment referral.
5. Monitor patients closely when LE occurs. Teach patients the importance of intensive self-monitoring of swelling and skin to prevent complications such as infection and functional impairment, to maintain independence.
6. Be alert to risk of repeated infections in the patient who has experienced a single infection. Patients with repeated localized infections and history of regionalized or systemic infections should be evaluated for standing orders for antibiotics (prescription to be filled at earliest sign of infection or medication kept on hand to start immediately at earliest signs of infection). Review with the patient her first observations of the previous infection(s) and appropriate early interventions. When traveling, access to antibiotics must be maintained.
7. Do not dismiss even a seemingly minor injury. The body's normal ability to deal with increased circulation in an area of tissue injury has been impaired by changes in the lymphatic system. Even minor cellular breakdown and repair may stress a lymphatic system in delicate balance and lead to LE and further complications.
8. Assess psychosocial concerns as well as the physical and functional changes. Self-image and self-esteem, social support, and problem solving may be affected by the acute and long-term demands of dealing with LE risk and management; the patient is now forced to contemplate a future of dealing with not only the life-threatening chronic condition of breast cancer but also LE. Refer as appropriate to individual, family, and group counseling resources.
9. Explore perceived barriers to self-management and compliance and provide resources for problem solving. Help the person to review problem solving strategies that have worked successfully in the past, as with management of another chronic condition or an earlier life change. Share strategies specific to LE management that have been reported as successful by patients encountering similar issues related to self-management and compliance. Encourage attendance at a professionally supported LE support group. Refer patients to the National Lymphedema Network (NLN) organization, informing them about their quarterly publication and web site (Box 12-1; National Lymphedema Network, 2005; http://www.lymphnet.org).

Continued

Box 12-2 NURSING STRATEGIES TO FOSTER LYMPHEDEMA SELF-MANAGEMENT—CONT'D

10. Assist patients to assess personal short-term and long-term goals and place self-management actions in the context of these self-concordant goals. For example, a woman might have goals such as caring for a grandchild or great grandchild on occasional overnight visits, or even for to provide daily child care while the parents work; or to live to see the child or grandchild graduate from high school. This woman may be further motivated to manage her LE to reduce life-threatening complications such as infection and functional impairments that would limit her own independence and ability to assist in caring for family members.
11. Suggest that patients wear a medical alert bracelet noting LE and other important health history. Ensuring proper care of the at-risk limb (no blood pressure monitoring, intravenous fluids, or blood draws on the affected limb) during emergencies, health care visits, and hospitalizations will further reduce risk of LE and related complications. LE bracelets and necklaces are available at a modest price by mail from the NLN (http://www.lymphnet.org).

Adapted from Armer JM: Lymphedema. In Dow KH: *Contemporary issues in breast cancer, ed 2,* Sudbury, MA: 2004, Jones & Bartlett.

Box 12-3 SELECTED INTERNET RESOURCES ON LYMPHEDEMA MANAGEMENT

National Lymphedema Network
www.lymphnet.org
National Cancer Institute
ww.nci.nih.gov/cancerinfo/pdq/supportivecare/lymphedema

selected Internet websites for LE education for patients, families, and health professionals.

SPECIAL CONSIDERATIONS

Women's Roles

Coping with the time-consuming and sometimes complex treatment and self-management strategies essential for preventing complications associated with cancer treatment-related LE, over and beyond the surveillance required for cancer management itself, can be daunting. A recent group of qualitative studies by family studies scientist Radina and colleagues has examined how post–breast cancer LE affected women's roles. The first of these studies examined coping with the chronic illness of post–breast cancer LE and the impact of LE on women's family roles.[87] In this study, an ethnographic approach was used to investigate how LE affects women and their families in terms of task completion and family functioning. The Family Adjustment and Adaptation Response (FAAR) Model was used to interpret findings. These indicate that families who are more flexible in modifying daily tasks and who have preexisting resources for coping with stressors have more positive outcomes than do those families who are rigid and cope with stressors poorly.

A second qualitative study took a resiliency approach to examining how LE onset and its related stressors affect women and their families.[88,89] Data included interviews with survivors from a prior study used as secondary data, in-depth interviews with survivors and health professionals, and observations of an LE support group. The Resiliency Model of Family Stress, Adjustment, and Adaptation guided the investigation. Three particular stressors were found (modification of daily tasks, reminder of breast cancer, and frustration with medical professionals) that contributed to the vulnerability of these families. The resiliency of the survivors and their families were characterized as Adjustment, Adaptation, or Crisis.

The third study explored women's experiences of off-time life course transitions from caregivers to care recipients as a result of post–breast cancer LE.[90] Life course theory was used as a template to guide analyses. Preliminary key findings include two themes related to participants' predominant concerns: not wanting to be a burden to others and living an independent lifestyle. The findings from these three studies collectively inform the understanding of women's perceptions of the impact of LE on their lives and family functioning. Insight into the impact of the shift of the woman's role because of LE-related functional changes from caregiver to care recipient, an often off-time transition, is an essential component of an individualized plan of care. Further, considering and incorporating personal, family, and occupational responsibilities into the plan for life-long self-management of LE is key to successful adaptation and quality of life.

Age-related Lymphedema Differences

Older breast cancer survivors, the largest demographic group of the most prevalent cancer to affect women, may particularly be at risk of LE and likewise at higher risk of underdiagnosis and undertreatment.[5,91] The vulnerability to diminished social support and problem-solving capacity may be even greater for the older breast cancer survivor, who may be single, widowed, or caring for a frail spouse. Daily assistance with LE management activities such as overnight bandaging and manual lymph drainage to hard-to-reach areas of the shoulder and back (see Table 12-2), and occasional needs such as transportation to health care appointments, therapy, and garment-fitting appointments may further tax an already stressed social support system or be perceived by the aging person as a further threat to independence and autonomy in the later years. The younger cancer survivor may be balancing career, home management, and family caregiving responsibilities, in addition to time-consuming self-care activities.

A secondary data analysis by Armer and Fu[91] of LE-associated symptoms and bilateral limb girth measurements in 103 breast cancer survivors found that women younger than 60 years of age reported a greater number of symptoms than survivors older than age 60, although a higher percentage of older women had bilateral circumferential differences greater than 2 cm. Sensory changes of aging, comorbidities, varying treatment protocols for older breast cancer survivors (possibly based on tumor grade, stage of disease, or comorbidities), and cultural expectations of aging symptoms unrelated to LE may affect the older woman's symptom report. Likewise, current conservative treatments such as lumpectomy coupled with SLNB and radiation in lieu of mastectomy without radiation in younger women may be associated with increased sensations after treatment.

UPPER EXTREMITY, LOWER EXTREMITY, BREAST, AND TRUNK EDEMA

Women's cancer treatments are associated with little-studied LE of the trunk, including the breast, the chest, the axilla, and the back, as well as the extremities. As challenging as limb measurements are, measurement of these trunk sites is even more challenging, and therefore incidence remains largely unreported. As Weiss[34] noted, breast LE incidences ranged from 35% to 70% (depending on use of clinical examination or dermal swelling measurements).[38] Women with pelvic surgery and radiation may also be affected by genital LE, another area difficult to objectively assess and treat. Further, gynecologic and other cancers treated with groin dissections and pelvic radiation, which potentially impact lymph drainage, may carry higher risk of LE of the lower extremity than the LE risk in upper extremities associated with cancers in which the axilla is dissected or radiated. It is known from the existing literature that the incidence and prevalence of LE in breast cancer (likely vastly underestimated) are higher than that of many other cancers, but many clinicians believe the rates of LE associated with gynecologic cancers and melanoma are even higher, as a result of required surgical approaches, adjunct radiation, and the physiology of the lower extremity.[3,34]

There are several tasks that are crucial to the development of intervention research directed at LE prevention, early detection, treatment, and symptom management: investigations with consideration of the strengths and challenges of the roles of women as affected by LE; examination of age-related and cancer-specific differences in LE experiences that follow cancer treatment; increased precision in LE measurement to establish its current incidence and prevalence among cancer survivors; and identification of protective mechanisms.[92]

IMPLICATIONS FOR EDUCATION, PRACTICE, AND RESEARCH

Education

Lymphedema is a major problem affecting a significant number of women treated for cancer. Some 400,000 to 800,000 breast cancer survivors alone in this country, the majority over age 60, may be affected by LE during their lifetimes. Over the years, both professional and self-care actions in management of LE in the US have been limited and little studied. To date, nursing and medical school curricula have had limited content related to LE etiology and management.

Lymphedema is a potential and significant problem for all cancer survivors. Understanding of the special needs of older and younger women at risk for or managing LE after cancer has been overlooked. In addition to the symptoms and physiologic risks, the associated challenges may also lead to psychosocial distress after treatment. Although researchers have documented the psychologic sequelae of cancer treatment,[56] little is known about such issues in survivors with LE. A conclusion by Maunsell and colleagues still stands: "The impact of lymphedema problems on patient quality of life has not been quantitatively assessed."[93] This research has been hampered by the traditional view that quality of life is less important than the eradication of cancer and detection of recurrence.

Unfortunately, lack of attention to LE by health professionals has not only meant that many persons go undiagnosed and fail to receive basic preventive information,[94] but has also hindered the development of effective psychosocial and physiologic therapeutic interventions.

It is important that nurses and other health care providers understand the physical, functional, and psychosocial impact of the chronic nature of LE among women treated for cancer. Management of treatment effects such as LE among oncology patients constitutes a lifetime concern. Awareness of the potential impact of LE on the individual and family is an important first step in the development of an effective individualized intervention to assist women to manage and adjust to the chronic condition of LE that follow cancer. Through appropriate early LE intervention and self-management, the psychosocial and functional autonomy and independence of the woman surviving cancer can be maximized, thereby maintaining and enhancing quality of life in the years of survivorship.

For cancer survivors, knowledge is power: educating patients about risk-reduction behaviors, self-monitoring of symptoms and limb changes, and self-management of LE is a key aspect of a plan of lifelong self-management of lymphedema that follows cancer treatment.

Practice

In 2001 the British Lymphology Society[95] published a matrix of educational and treatment needs of persons with varying grades of chronic LE, from those at risk to those with advanced disease.[96] The principles have application to those at risk of cancer-related LE, as well as those challenged to manage LE following cancer treatment. It is important to note that persons may shift from one level to another as limb swelling changes, requiring professional treatment or only self-management depending on stability, progression, and acute occurrences such as trauma or infection. Table 12-1 displays the criteria for each group and details of the treatment required.[96] Further, the guidelines establish the role of the generalist (nurse or other health care provider not specialized in LE) and the lymphedema specialist (nurse, physical therapist, occupational therapist, or other health professional with specialized LE training) in the management of LE. As noted, since LE is a lifelong chronic condition, patient education and patient compliance with best practices in LE management are key to optimal outcomes in cancer survivorship and quality of life.

Assessment of limb volume change (LVC) following breast cancer treatment cannot be accurately carried out without a pretreatment limb baseline measurement.[97] Limb volume measurements must be done routinely, preoperatively, and also at follow-up. Optimally, this measurement would be done before surgery when other "preop" activities are carried out (e.g., physical assessment, lab tests, electrocardiogram, chest x-ray, and anesthesia assessment). Alternatively, data could be gathered immediately after surgery. The greatest disadvantage to forgoing the preop measurement is that surgical edema may cloud the baseline measurements taken immediately after surgery.[97] By definition, acute LE lasts less than 6 months,[27] but delaying treatment to allow spontaneous resolution of edema (surgical or lymphatic) may predispose to a less favorable LE outcome.[68-70] Only with passage of time can surgical edema be differentiated from early-onset (acute or chronic) LE. A useful step in differentiating generalized surgical edema from postoperative LE is the assessment of bilateral LV both at baseline and at follow-up. If both limbs have increased by a similar percentage of volume or circumferences in the follow-up period, this is an indication of overall fluid retention rather than isolated lymph congestion in the affected limb. This LVC is likely to be associated with a body weight increase as well. Comparison of the affected limb volume with the contralateral limb volume provides evidence of LVC associated with LE, with certain caveats, as discussed below.[97]

It has long been assumed (although not always spoken or written) that the limbs are symmetrical and of similar, if not identical, volume. Indeed, the basis of LE diagnosis leading to eligibility for third-party payment for LE treatment is the underlying assumption that the two limbs are symmetrical in circumferences and volume. As noted earlier, the most common criteria for LE diagnosis are a 2-cm circumferential difference or a 200 ml LVD (affected versus nonaffected limbs). These criteria are based on the underlying—but erroneous—assumption that the limbs are symmetrical and identical in volume. When this assumption is challenged and the potential of asymmetry considered, the next assumption is that the dominant limb is larger than the nondominant limb—and this LVD that is due to dominance is sometimes estimated to be as high as 200 ml. In preliminary measurement studies, LVDs as large as to 160 ml have been noted between healthy limbs[98] and in some few cases (3 of 10 initial participants), nondominant limbs have been found to have larger volume than dominant limbs.[98] These incidental findings provide further justification for the bilateral baseline limb measurements. Further, continued bilateral measurements over time are necessary to assess LVC during follow-up, since it is important as part of the differential diagnosis to note whether volume change has occurred in the affected limb alone or in both limbs.

Research

Early detection and intervention hold the greatest promise of reducing the widespread condition of cancer-related LE.[68-70] The range of findings in the literature reflects inconsistent criteria for defining lymphedema, small studies, retrospective analyses, and short follow-up.[3,8,34,70,92] It is necessary to clearly identify epidemiologic and clinical factors associated with risk and incidence to build a foundation for preventive interventions. Before developing effective interventions to prevent and manage LE, it is necessary to (1) measure limb volume (LV) change (LVC) accurately and reliably, (2) determine the incidence and prevalence of LE and associated symptoms across time, (3) examine coping and self-management strategies, as well as the frequency and impact on daily living of LE symptoms, and (4) identify mechanisms that reduce the severity and progression of LE, improve self-management strategies, and enhance psychosocial adjustment and functional health status of patients with LE.[92] Examination of genetic and personal characteristics influencing risk of LE development, before the cancer treatment itself, will illuminate understanding of the pathophysiologic processes associated with LE.

Rigorously developed longitudinal research has the potential to influence LE clinical practice guidelines for persons undergoing treatment for cancer. Findings from such studies have potentially widespread clinical applications in developing and testing a protocol for consistent, accurate, noninvasive, and labor- and cost-effective measurement of the lymphedematous limb. Potential application is considerable for both upper and lower extremity LE attributable to surgery, radiation, and other adjunct treatment for malignancy including breast, melanoma, gynecologic, and other cancers involving lymph node dissection and irradiation. Moreover, research examining the psychosocial links between protective mechanisms, LVC, coping effectiveness, and psychosocial outcomes/functional health status will lead to a more complete understanding of the consequences of LE, and subsequently to more appropriate care. In addition, identification of potential protective mechanisms could greatly inform clinical treatment and preventive interventions.[99] Accurate and consistent anthropometric measurements are essential to scientific evaluation of the effectiveness of LE treatments, as well as to sound clinical assessment of disease management and progression.

Comparisons of LE incidence and treatment effectiveness across multiple sites, therapeutic modalities, and patient characteristics are necessary to better understand this complex issue.[97] It becomes increasingly imperative that clinicians and researchers across disciplines collaborate to establish multisite research programs focused on incidence and prevalence of post–breast cancer treatment LE, with the aim of developing multisite randomized intervention programs. Applying rigorous measurement protocols, assessing symptom experience, and establishing databases on bilateral preoperative LV for comparison purposes is essential to create the necessary foundation for intervention studies. This will offer an opportunity to better target risk factors for development of LE and improve post–treatment quality of life.

SUMMARY

To date, no single reliable and valid method for routinely assessing limb volume differences in the clinical setting is available in this country. Therefore, LE symptoms are often underreported or unsolicited. The result is that LE in women treated for cancer is underdiagnosed and undertreated, leaving a large number of women with untoward outcomes and compromised quality of life. When one takes a life span perspective, the impact of chronic LE is viewed as being far more life-changing than the acute treatment for cancer itself. Among women of all ages the onset and chronic nature of LE represent a daily, distressful reminder of the cancer and its life-changing impact.

Of 2 million women with breast cancer in the US, at least one in four is likely to have LE within 11 years[8] and experience a wide range of potentially debilitating outcomes as a result. This risk of LE may be significantly higher for women treated for other cancers affecting lymphatic drainage from the lower extremities. At this point, much remains unknown about the measurement, incidence, and correlates of LE, including effective and ineffective health care self-management strategies. For cancer survivors, knowledge is power: educating patients about risk-reduction behaviors, self-monitoring of symptoms and limb changes, and self-management of LE is a key aspect of a plan of life-long self-management of lymphedema that follows cancer treatment. With such a plan, quality of life in the years of cancer survivorship can be maximized.

REFERENCES

1. Casley-Smith JR: Modern treatment of lymphoedema, *Mod Med Aust* 5:70-83, 1992.
2. Mortimer PS: The pathophysiology of lymphedema, *Cancer* 83(suppl):2798-2802, 1998.
3. Cormier JN and others: Lymphedema in melanoma patients, *Nat Lymphedema Net LymphLink* 17:1-2, 27, 2005.
4. van der Veen P and others: Lymphedema development following breast cancer surgery with full axillary resection, *Lymphology* 37:206-208, 2004.
5. American Cancer Society: Cancer Facts and Figures, Atlanta, GA, 2004, American Cancer Society.
6. Hull MM: Functional and psychosocial aspects of lymphedema in women treated for breast cancer, *Innov Breast Cancer Care* 3:97-100, 117-118, 1998.
7. Olszewski WL: Inflammatory changes of skin in lymphedema of extremities and efficacy of benzathine penicillin administration, *Natl Lymphedema Net LymphLink* 8:1-2, 1996.
8. Petrek JA, Heelan MC: Incidence of breast carcinoma-related lymphedema, *Cancer* 83(suppl):2776-2781, 1998.

9. Wrone DA and others: Lymphedema after sentinel lymph node biopsy for cutaneous melanoma: a report of 5 cases, *Arch Dermatol* 136:511-514, 2000.
10. Papachristou D, Fortner JG: Comparison of lymphedema following incontinuity and discontinuity groin dissection, *Ann Surg* 185(January):13-16, 1977.
11. Beitsch P, Balch C: Operative morbidity and risk factor assessment in melanoma patients undergoing inguinal lymph node dissection, *Am J Surg* 164:462-466, 1992.
12. Tada H, Sasaki H, Teramukai S: Para-aortic lymph node dissection as a risk factor related to the lower leg lymphedema after lymph node dissection in gynecological malignancies, *Proc Am Soc Clin Oncol Annual Meeting* 461, 2003.
13. Serpell JW and others: Radical lymph node dissection for melanoma, *ANZ J Surg* 73:294-299, 2003.
14. Lawton G, Rasque H, Ariyan S: Preservation of muscle fascia to decrease lymphedema after complete axillary and ilioinguinofemoral lymphadenectomy for melanoma, *J Am Coll Surg* 195:339-351, 2002.
15. Hughes TM, A'Hern RP, Thomas JM: Prognosis and surgical management of patients with palpable inguinal lymph node metastases from melanoma, *Br J Surg* 87:892-901, 2000.
16. Stevens G and others: Locally advanced melanoma: results of postoperative hypofractionated radiation therapy, *Cancer* 88:88-94, 2000.
17. Petlund CF: Volumetry of limbs. In Olszewski WI, editor: *Lymph stasis: pathophysiology, diagnosis and treatment,* Boston, 1991, CRC Press.
18. Tierney Sand others: Infrared optoelectronic volumetry, the ideal way to measure limb volume, *Eur J Vas Endovas Surg* 12:412-417, 1996.
19. James JH and others: Lymphoedema following ilio-inguinal lymph node dissection, *Scand J Plast Reconstr Surg* 16:167-171, 1982.
20. Baas PC and others: Groin dissection in the treatment of lower-extremity melanoma. Short-term and long-term morbidity, *Arch Surg* 7:281-286, 1992.
21. Urist MM and others: Patient risk factors and surgical morbidity after regional lymphadenectomy in melanoma patients, *Cancer* 51:2152-2156, 1983.
22. Karakousis CP, Heiser MA, Moore R:. Lymphedema after groin dissection, *Am J Surg* 145:205-208, 1983.
23. Holmes EC and others: A rational approach to the surgical management of melanoma, *Ann Surg* 186:481-490, 1977.
24. Strobbe LJ and others: Positive iliac and obturator nodes in melanoma: survival and prognostic factors, *Ann Surg Oncol* 6:255-262, 1999.
25. Wright JD and others: Lower extremity lymphedema, *Women's Oncol Rev* 2:269-276, 2002.
26. Meek AG: Breast radiotherapy and lymphedema, *Cancer Suppl* 83:2788-2797, 1998.
27. National Cancer Society: Lymphedema, retrieved 10/14/05 from www.cancer.gov/cancerinfo/pdq/supportivecare/lymphedema/healthprofessional. Accessed October 14, 2003.
28. Gerber LH: A review of measures of lymphedema, *Cancer Suppl* 8312:2803-2804, 1998.
29. Swedborg I: Volumetric estimation of the degree of lymphedema and its therapy by pneumatic compression, *Scand J Rehab Med* 9:131, 1977.
30. Callaway CW and others: Circumferences. In: Lohman TG, Roche AF, Martorell R, editors: *Anthropometric standardization reference manual,* Lohman TG, Roche AF, Martorell R (Eds.), Champaign, Illinois, 1988, Human Kinetics Books.
31. Stanton AW and others: Validation of an optoelectronic limb volumeter (perometer), *Lymphology* 30:77-97, 1997.
32. Armer JM and others: Prediction of breast cancer lymphedema based on Lymphedema and Breast Cancer Questionnaire (LBCQ) symptom report, *Nurse Res* 52: 370-379, 2003.
33. Armer JM, Whitman M: The problem of lymphedema following breast cancer treatment: prevalence, symptoms, and self-management, *Lymphology* 35(suppl):153-159, 2002.
34. Weiss B: Incidence of lymphedema: a literature review summary, *Nat Lymphedema Net LymphLink* 17:12, 27, 2005.
35. Campisi C and others: [Lymphedema secondary to breast cancer treatment: possibility of diagnostic and therapeutic prevention], *Italian Ann Ital Chir* 73:493-498, 2002.
36. Pierquin B, Mazeron JJ, Glaubiger D: Conservative treatment of breast cancer in Europe: report of the Groupe Européan de Curiethérapie, *Radiother Oncol* 6:187-198, 1986.
37. Bosompra K and other: Swelling, numbness, pain, and their relationship to arm function among breast cancer survivors: a disablement process model perspective, *Breast J* 8:338-348, 2002.
38. Rönkä RH and others: Breast lymphedema after breast conserving treatment, *Acta Oncol* 43(Sept):551-557, 2004.
39. Armer, JM, Stewart, BR: A Comparison of Four Diagnostic Criteria for Lymphedema in a Post-Breast Cancer Population. *Lymphatic Research and Biology, 3*(4), 208-217, 2005.
40. Schünemann H, Willich N: Lymphoedema nach Mammakarzinom—physikalische und medikamentose Therapien, [Lymphatic edema after breast carcinoma—physical and drug therapies], *Zeitschrift für Onkologie* 32:56-60, 2000.
41. Yoshimoto M and others: Improvement in the prognosis of Japanese breast cancer patients from 1946 to 2001—an institutional review, *Jpn J Clin Oncol* 34:457-462, 2004.
42. Kissin MW and others: The inadequacy of axillary sampling in breast cancer, *Lancet* 1:1210-1212, 1982.
43. Clarke D and others: Breast edema following staging axillary node dissection in patient with breast carcinoma treated by radical radiotherapy, *Cancer* 49: 2295-2299, 1982.
44. Fehlauer F and others: Long-term radiation sequelae after breast-conserving therapy in women with early-stage breast cancer: an observational study using the LENT-SOMA scoring system, *Int J Rad Oncol Biol Phys* 55: 651-658, 2003.
45. Højris I and others: Late treatment-related morbidity in breast cancer patients randomized to postmastectomy radiotherapy and systemic treatment versus systemic treatment alone, *Acta Oncol* 39:355-372, 2000.
46. Goffman TE and others: Lymphedema of the arm and breast in irradiated breast cancer patients: risks in an era of dramatically changing axillary surgery, *Breast J* 10:405-411, 2004.
47. Senofsky GM and others: Total axillary lymphadenectomy in the management of breast cancer, *Arch Surg* 126: 1336-1342, 1991.

48. Coblentz TR, Theodorescu D: Morbidity of modified prophylactic inguinal lymphadenectomy for squamous cell carcinoma of the penis, *J Urol* 168:1386-1389, 2002.
49. Balzer K, Schonebeck I: Edema after vascular surgery interventions and its therapy, *German Z Lymphol* 17:41-47, 1993.
50. James JH: Lymphoedema following ilio-inguinal lymph node dissection, *Scand J Plast Reconstr Surg* 16:167-171, 1982.
51. Karakousis CP, Driscoll, DL: Positive deep nodes in the groin and survival in malignant melanoma, *Am J Surg* 171:421-422, 1996.
52. Karakousis CP, Driscoll DL: Groin dissection in malignant melanoma, *Br J Surg* 82:1771-1774, 1994.
53. Shaw JH, Rumball EM: Complications and local recurrence following lymphadenectomy, *Br J Surg* 77:760-764, 1990.
54. Ames FC, Singletary SE: Cutaneous malignancies of the trunk and lower extremities. In Johnson DE, Ames FC, editors: Groin dissection, Chicago, 1985, Year Book Medical Publishers.
55. Ingvar C, Erichsen C, Jonsson PE: Morbidity following prophylactic and therapeutic lymph node dissection for melanoma—a comparison, *Tumori* 6:529-533, 1984.
56. Passik SD, McDonald MV: Psychosocial aspects of upper extremity lymphedema in women treated for breast carcinoma, *Cancer* 83(suppl):2817-2820, 1998.
57. Gaarenstroom KN and others: Postoperative complications after vulvectomy and inguinofemoral lymphadenectomy using separate groin incisions, *Int J Gynecol Cancer* 13: 522-527, 2003.
58. Nelson BA and others: Complications of inguinal and pelvic lymphadenectomy for small squamous cell carcinoma of the penis: a contemporary series, *J Urol* 172:494-497, 2004.
59. Lieskovsky G, Skinner DG, Weisenburger T: Pelvic lymphadenectomy in the management of carcinoma of the prostate, *J Urol* 124:635-638, 1980.
60. Boris M, Weindorf S, Lasinski B: The risk of genital edema after external pump compression for lower limb lymphedema, *Lymphology* 31:15-20, 1998.
61. Armer JM and others: Lymphedema following breast cancer treatment, including sentinel lymph node biopsy, *Lymphology* 37:73-91, 2004.
62. Geller BM and others: Factors associated with arm swelling after breast cancer surgery. *J Womens Health* 12:921-930, 2003.
63. Deutsch M, Flickinger JC: Arm edema after lumpectomy and breast irradiation, *Am J Clin Oncol* 26:229-231, 2003.
64. Coen JJL and others: Risk of lymphedema after regional nodal irradiation with breast conservation therapy, *Int J Radiat Oncol Biol Phys* 55:1209-1215, 2003.
65. Voogd AC and others: Lymphoedema and reduced shoulder function as indicators of quality of life after axillary lymph node dissection for invasive breast cancer, *Br J Surg* 90:76-81, 2003.
66. Ozaslan C, Kuru B: Lymphedema after treatment of breast cancer, *Am J Surg* 187:69-72, 2003.
67. Pressman PI: Surgical treatment and lymphedema, *Cancer Suppl* 83:2782-2787, 1998.
68. Rockson SG: Precipitating factors in lymphedema: myths and realities, *Cancer Suppl* 83:2814-2816, 1998.
69. Porock D: Impact of seroma on the development of radiation skin reactions, paper presented at the International Society for Nurses in Cancer Care, 12th International Conference, London, UK. 2002.
70. Petrek JA, Pressman PI, Smith RA: Lymphedema: current issues in research and management, *Can J Clin* 50:292-307, 2000.
71. Harris SR and others: Clinical practice guidelines for the care and treatment of breast cancer lymphedema, *Can Med Assoc J* 164;191-199, 2001.
72. National Lymphedema Network: Lymphedema risk reduction practices, retrieved 1/4/06 from www.lymphnet.org/riskreduction/riskreduction.htm.
73. Yap KP and others: Factors influencing arm and axillary symptoms after treatment for node negative breast carcinoma, *Cancer* 97:1369-1375, 2003.
74. Nattinger AB and others: Relation between appropriateness of primary therapy for early-stage breast carcinoma and increased use of breast-conserving surgery, *Lancet* 356:1148-1153, 2000.
75. Ridner SH: Breast cancer lymphedema: pathophysiology and risk reduction guidelines, *Oncol Nurse For* 29: 1285-1293, 2002.
76. Humble CA: Lymphedema: incidence, pathophysiology, management, and nursing care, *Cont Educ* 22:1503-1509, 1995.
77. Mason M: The treatment of lymphoedema by complex physical therapy, *Aust Physiother* 39:41-45, 1993.
78. Rockson SG, Miller LT, Senie R: Workgroup III. Diagnosis and management of lymphedema, *Cancer Suppl* 83: 2882-2885, 1998.
79. Casley-Smith JR and others: Treatment for lymphedema of the arm—the Casley-Smith method, *Cancer Suppl* 83: 2843-2863, 1998.
80. Hutzschenreuter PO and others: Post-mastectomy arm lymph-edema: treated by manual lymph drainage and compression bandage therapy, *Phys Med Rehabil* 1: 166-170, 1991.
81. Badger C and others: Physical therapies for reducing and controlling lymphedema of the limbs, *Cochrane Database of Systematic Reviews* 4, CD003141, 2004, Oxford, UK, Cochrane Breast Can Group.
82. De Roo T: Analysis of lymphoedema as first symptom of a neoplasm in a series of 650 patients with limb involvement, *Radiologia Clinica* 45:236-241, 1967.
83. Fialka-Moser V and others: Cancer rehabilitation. Particularly with aspects of physical impairments, *J Rehab Med* 35:153-162, 2003.
84. Kiyohara T and others: Spindle cell angiosarcoma following irradiation therapy for cervical carcinoma, *J Cutaneous Pathol* 29:96-100, 2002.
85. Ridner SH: Symptom clusters occurring with lymphedema after breast cancer, *Disser Ab Int* 64:DAIB, 2003. (UMI No. 3113289)
86. Rose KE, Taylor HM, Twycross RG: Long-term compliance with treatment in obstructive arm lymphedema in cancer, *Palliat Med* 5:52-55, 1991.
87. Radina ME, Armer JM: Post-breast cancer lymphedema and the family: a qualitative investigation of families coping with chronic illness, *J Fam Nurse* 7:281-299, 2003.
88. Radina ME, Armer JM: Surviving breast cancer and living with lymphedema: resiliency among women and their families, *J Fam Nurse* 10:485-505, 2004.

89. Radina ME, Armer JM: "I'll do it myself": the experiences of self-reliant women coping with post-breast cancer lymphedema, paper presented at the First Montreal International Lymphedema Congress, Montréal, Quebec, (Manuscript in review). May, 2003.
90. Radina ME, Armer JM: The experiences of self-reliant women coping with post-breast cancer lymphedema: preliminary results, poster presented at the conference Moving Research into Practice: Chronic Disease & Missouri Women, Columbia, MO. May, 2003.
91. Armer JM, Fu M: Age differences in post-breast cancer lymphedema signs and symptoms, *Cancer Nurs* 28: 200-207, 2005.
92. Armer JM, Heppner PP, Mallinckrodt B: Post breast cancer treatment lymphedema: the hidden epidemic, *Scope Phlebo Lymphology* 9:334-341, 2004.
93. Maunsell E, Brisson J, Deschenes L: Arm problems and psychological distress after surgery for breast cancer, *Can J Surg* 36:315-320, 1993.
94. Tobin MB: The psychological morbidity of breast cancer-related arm swelling: psychological morbidity of lymphoedema, *Cancer* 72:3248-3252, 1993.
95. British Lymphology Society: Chronic oedema population and need. On the Web at www.lymphoedema.org/bls/index.html, 2001.
96. Williams A: An overview of non-cancer related chronic oedema—a UK perspective, available at: http://www.worldwidewounds.com/2003/april/Williams/Chronic-Oedema.html. Accessed December 27, 2004.
97. Armer J M: The problem of post-breast cancer lymphedema: impact and measurement issues, Can Invest 23(1):76-83, 2005.
98. Armer JM: Nursing measurement of lymphedematous limbs, National Institutes of Health (NIH;NINR), August 2000-August 2001(unpublished data).
99. Armer JM: Prospective nursing study of breast cancer lymphedema: National Institutes of Health (NIH;NINR), August 2000-April 2006.

CHAPTER

13 Aches, Pain, and Neuropathy

Judith Kehs Much

OVERVIEW

Pain continues to be one of the most feared and problematic areas facing both cancer patients and caregivers. In a prospective analysis of symptoms of 1,000 advanced cancer patients referred to palliative care (45% of whom were female), pain ranked number one in the top ten most prevalent symptoms. Eighty-four percent of the patients experienced pain. Younger age was associated with more pain and a variety of other symptoms. No gender-related pain differences were found.[1]

There are distinctive types of pain described in the literature, and the experienced clinician has seen them all: nociceptive, inflammatory, neuropathic, and functional pain. The reality is, in any given patient, one can see a variety of pain types and etiologies, both in cancer-related pain and pain unrelated to cancer.[2-4]

Nociceptive pain can be described as a key early warning system serving a protective function. A vital physiologic function, nociceptive pain occurs only in the presence of noxious stimuli. Nociceptive pain is comprised of the processes of transduction from the source, conduction and transmission of the impulse, and perception.[5]

Inflammatory pain is an adaptive mechanism that occurs if damage happens in spite of nociceptive defense. The body shifts from the goal of protecting to the goal of promoting healing of the injured tissues. Inflammatory pain accomplishes this goal by increasing sensitivity in the affected area, where there would not normally be pain. Because of the pain, individuals generally do not use the affected part as they typically would, so that healing can occur. The pain decreases as healing occurs.[5]

Neuropathic and functional pain are not adaptive but are a response either to injury to the peripheral or the central nervous system (neuropathic) or to abnormal operation of the nervous system (functional).[5]

In functional pain, no neurologic deficits can be detected. This pain is due to abnormal responsiveness or function of the nervous system in which heightened gain or sensitivity amplifies symptoms. Examples of painful conditions that may fit into this category include fibromyalgia, irritable bowel syndrome (IBS), some forms of noncardiac chest pain, and tension-type headaches. These types of pain have increased frequency among women.[6] It is unknown why the central nervous systems of some of these patients exhibit hyperresponsiveness.

There is a better understanding of the roles of various neurotransmitters (γ-aminobutyric acid [GABA], glutamate), neuropeptides (substance P), nerve growth factor, *N*-methyl-D-aspartate (NMDA) receptor and excitatory amino acids.[5,7-8] This knowledge is beginning to lead to more targeted therapies. However, as mechanisms of pain are becoming more clear the question remains: what is known about the pain of the women who comprise 48% of the estimated new cancer cases of cancer?[9]

GENDER-BASED-BASED DIFFERENCES IN PAIN

Researchers have long suspected that there are gender-based-based differences in pain presentation, treatment, and response, but even today, clear answers remain elusive. Much of what is known about gender differences comes from the study of nonmalignant pain.

In 1996, Unruh reviewed the literature on pain and gender-based-based differences and drew conclusions regarding the reasons for purported "gender differences" in pain.[10] In her work, a review of 310 studies from 1970-1994, she cautions students of gender and pain that gender is rarely the primary focus of pain research; instead it is typically included as a socio-demographic variable. Historically, many outcomes were reported as gender-based differences without statistical significance attached. Uneven distribution within samples obscured or exaggerated outcomes related to gender distinctions. Many of the studies had methodologic problems. In spite of these shortcomings, her literature review found that women are more likely than men to experience a variety of recurrent pains. They may also have more severe pain that lasts longer than their male counterparts. Women seek more health care related to pain than men and are more verbal about their pain. Unruh also noted gender-based-related differences in the literature regarding how the health care establishment treated pain.[10] Historically, it was believed that women should be given smaller doses of analgesics. Even as late as 1994, women were given less pain medication than men for the same type of pain.[11,12]

Unruh cited the need for more research in the following areas: (1) gender-based variation in biologic mechanisms of pain; and (2) psychologic and sociologic factors contributing to the expression of pain behaviors and the meaning of pain.[11]

Berkley drew similar conclusions in her review of gender differences in pain to those of Unruh. She found data to support the view that women have lower pain threshold and tolerance, are able to better discriminate between painful sensations, and report pain ratings than their male counterparts.[8] She found gender-based differences in acute surgical pain, chronic nonmalignant pain, and cancer pain. In addition, she found differences based on gender-based in response to analgesics. However, given the many interacting variables in the data—for example, what is being measured; where, when and how measures are taken; who is being measured and of what age; which pain is the object of investigation; and so on—she also concluded that is difficult to draw meaningful conclusions. She specifies that only a few conclusions should be drawn: (1) women have more morbidity and greater use of health care (much of this can be accounted for in obstetric and gynecologic issues); (2) women do report more multiple or recurrent pains then men, especially in certain regions of the body at certain ages; and (3) the reasons for the differences might be explained by gender-based differences in reproductive organs, gender-based differences in the temporal features of hormones (estrogen, progesterone, and testosterone), and gender-based differences in action of substances such as GABA, serotonin, dopamine, thyroid-stimulating hormone and others.[8]

In a more recent review 6 years later, Fillingim reported similar conclusions.[6] Experimentally, women typically report lower pain threshold and tolerance and higher pain ratings then men. The prevalence of disability with pain is greater among women as compared with men. Clinically, women are at greater risk for routine, day-to-day pain. Several chronic pain conditions are more frequently seen in women (e.g., fibromyalgia, rheumatoid arthritis, and osteoarthritis). Again, the reasons for these differences may be indirectly related to gender. Women will have a greater awareness of pain and will more readily report pain. Fillingim believed it was possible to determine whether there was a self-selection bias creating the appearance of gender-based differences that resulted from men with less pain not making themselves known to the health care community.

At the time of Fillingim's review, additional theories were being postulated regarding the reasons for gender-related pain differences. Biologic theorists believe that genetic and hormonal influences, as well as gender-based differences in brain anatomy and function, create the differences in pain and treatment response. Evolutionary theorists believe that survival benefit explains differences in pain behaviors. Social learning theorists believe that gender differences are learned though modeling and reinforcement. Others believe there is a familial or genetic basis for pain, such as can be seen with headache and fibromyalgia.[6]

In 2003, Fillingim and colleagues examined the characteristics of chronic back pain as a function of gender and opioid use.[13] They enrolled a sample of 240 patients with pain in the lower back, upper back, and neck regions. Thirty-five percent of the patients were female. Enrollees were classified as either opioid or non–opioid users by self-report and record review. Opioid use was found to be associated with greater self-reported disability and poorer function in both men and women. Women using opioids had less affective distress. Women reported greater pain than men, but opioid use was not associated with greater pain severity.[13]

In a cross-sectional descriptive study by Yates, 205 hospitalized patients were assessed for the presence and severity of pain.[14] Women were significantly more likely to report high levels of pain (46.8%) than men (20.3%). Differences in severity of pain between age groups were not seen. Interestingly, in this study, women indicated they were less willing to ask for help with their pain to the nursing staff, whereas they were more likely than men to speak with their doctors about pain. For both men and women, the most commonly reported effect of pain was reduced mobility (64.3%). Patients stated that pain affected their ability to sleep (59%) and made them feel worried (57.3%) and exhausted (53.9%). There were no significant differences between genders in the reported psychologic impact of pain.[14]

In another study looking at gender-based-differences, 640 patients in the US undergoing total hip arthroplasty, or replacement (THA), were evaluated for pain and functional status, which was measured at time of THA through 1 year after surgery. At time of THA, women were more likely to report severe pain with walking and needing assistance with walking, housework, and grocery shopping. These differences persisted after adjustment for comorbidities. Men could walk greater distances. At 1 year, women continued to be more likely to need assistance with walking and could only walk shorter distances.[15]

Conversely, in a recent study of 716 subjects (63% female) that investigated gender-based differences in chronic pain, Marcus found that men had greater pain severity, constancy, and more days of pain per week than women.[16] Men also had higher levels of disability. These results differ from other reported studies. The author postulated that gender-related differences might differ among different pain categories.[16]

In the cancer literature, assessment of chronic cancer pain and gender is even more complicated because there are more intervening variables that may account for the pain and the differences (e.g., stage of disease, symptoms that accompany disease and its treatment). The type of cancer and mechanism for pain seem to be more predictive of similarities and differences in pain than gender-based.[12]

In 2000, Mercandante evaluated prevalence of pain types and severity in 181 patients with advanced cancer.[17] Pain differed along gender-based lines in relation to the type of pain. Somatic pain was more common in men, whereas women experienced more visceral pain. Neuropathic pain was seen in equal frequencies.[17]

In Esnaola's 2002 study of the treatment of patients with locally recurrent rectal cancer (LRRC), pain and quality of life (QOL) were assessed.[18] The results revealed pain to be a common problem in LRRC when palliative treatment included either surgical or nonsurgical methodology. Female gender, pelvic/sciatic pain at presentation, total pelvic exenteration, and bony resection were associated with higher rates of moderate to severe pain. Women had more severe pain and lower QOL at time of recurrence. After palliative treatment, women also had worse QOL and had significantly lower physical well-being scores. Pain at presentation of recurrence was an independent predictor of pain after treatment.[18]

In 2003, Avemark and others reported the data from a descriptive study with self-report questionnaires that evaluated experiences of pain, energy, mood, appetite, and sleep in cancer patients receiving palliative care in their homes.[19] The study, which involved daily paperwork for 4 weeks, was completed by 27 patients. Pain was measured using visual analog scales. Over the 4-week period, women experienced significantly more pain than men. There were gender-based differences in the correlation of pain and QOL indicators. Men had an overall lower QOL than women as measured by energy, mood, appetite, and sleep.[19]

MEANING OF PAIN

The concept of pain is linked to and described in terms of suffering, giving it strong cognitive and emotional components.[5]

In 1999, Moore and Spiegel compared how African American and Caucasian women with metastatic breast cancer used guided imagery for pain control.[20] They reported that guided imagery was used as a vehicle to help manage anxiety and pain in this group of women, who were seen as being left behind by the medical establishment's emphasis on cure and prevention. The technique was used to help to reestablish the connection between the body and mind, which had been disrupted by cancer and its pain. These illness narratives help in understanding the meaning of pain and in communicating cultural patterns and can offer a window into the individual's search for meaning in the experience.[20]

The meaning of pain helps to differentiate pain experienced in the experimental setting from that in the clinical setting. In her review article evaluating experimental versus clinical differences between the genders in the experience of pain, Vallerand reported that clinical pain differed from experimentally-induced pain because clinical pain was accompanied by concerns including death, ill health, and disability.[21]

In a study using semistructured interviews to investigate the meaning of pain in patients with metastatic bone pain, Coward spoke with 10 men (most of whom had prostate cancer) and 10 women (most of whom had breast cancer) who had bone pain.[22] The presence of pain was seen as a metaphor for the recurrence of cancer and meant the treatments were not effective. The experience elicited fear and uncertainty in the participants regarding their ability to control the cancer. Women in the study had an average of four pain locations, while men had an average of three. In both groups, the presence of pain interfered with their work and pleasure activities, and family relationships.[22]

In this same study, Coward found that most participants, to maintain normalcy and not worry others, did not tell others about their pain unless it was necessary. Men were more likely than women to take their medication as directed. Many individuals held back on taking medication for fear that if they were too comfortable, they might "overdo" and hurt themselves further. Side effects of medications were a concern in both groups. The presence of pain with movement decreased an individual's mobility. No significant gender-based differences were found in her sample.[22]

In an investigation regarding gender's effect on the appraisal of pain and coping, Unruh found that when plagued with chronic nonmalignant pain, women show more concern about the effects of pain on their lives.[10] Women reported pain in greater amount and intensity than men. Unruh found that tension was one of the leading causes of pain in women. For women, the interference in usual activities was a major component of the effects of chronic pain: it caused them to be upset by not being able to do what they normally would do. In attempt to minimize disruption of these activities, women sought help for managing pain more quickly than men.[11] Women reported more problem solving, behavioral distraction, positive self-statements, and palliative behaviors, as well as more social support, as compared with men. Women sought medical care for the pain more frequently than men. Interestingly, Unruh also postulated that the gender of the interviewer may have an impact on the responses, especially from men.[10]

Given the small sample sizes and the small numbers of studies, more research is clearly needed to determine if there are gender differences related to pain meaning.

DESCRIPTORS

Do gender differences exist in the manner in which patients describe their pain? Clinicians generally ask patients to describe their pain in terms of intensity (mild, moderate, or severe) quality (sharp, burning, or dull), duration (transient, intermittent, or persistent) and referral (superficial or deep, or localized or diffuse). Until recently, there has been no systematic inquiry regarding possible differences in terms/descriptors used to describe and differentiate nociceptive pain from neuropathic pain.

Wilkie and others described the predictive validity (ability) of words in the McGill Pain Questionnaire.[23] In the study, 123 patients, predominantly with lung cancer, were provided with the 78 pain descriptors from the questionnaire and were asked to indicate the corresponding pain site for each word. Subjects indicated their pain location on the questionnaire. Information about their cancer and treatment data were abstracted from medical records. Each pain site was classified by etiology as either nociceptive or neuropathic. Location of the pain and the descriptors attributed to that pain were examined for differences. Of the 437 pain sites identified, 343 were described as nociceptive (75%) and 114 (25%) as neuropathic.[23]

Descriptors associated with nociceptive pain were found to be the following: lacerating, stinging, heavy, and suffocating. However, because of infrequent word selection, the sensitivity for these words to predict nociceptive pain was poor (6% to 9%). The following words were found describe neuropathic pain: throbbing, aching, numb, tender, punishing, pulling, tugging, pricking, penetrating, miserable, and nagging. A number of descriptors that were not included in the neuropathic pain list had previously been thought to describe this kind of pain: burning, shooting, blasting, tingling, itching, and cold. These descriptors, once thought to be uniques to neuropathic pain were used to describe both neuropathic and nociceptive pain and as such were not used as unique neuropathic descriptors.[23]

Wilkie found some gender-based differences. A significantly higher proportion of women selected gnawing (21% vs. 5%), dull (31% vs. 15%) and heavy (23% vs. 6%) as descriptors for their pains, whereas men selected shooting (34% vs. 16%), sharp (48% vs. 28%) and tingling (20% vs. 0%). However, there were no differences in gender or age in pain ratings or intensity scores in this sample.[23]

TYPES OF PAIN IN WOMEN

Aches

The concept of post–chemotherapy "rheumatism"[19] was first reported in 1993 in a variety of retrospective and clinical case reports by a number of authors.[24-28] Reportedly, symptoms described as myalgias, arthralgias, arthritis, periarticular swelling, and tenosynovitis usually occurred 2 to 16 months after completing chemotherapy. Reports were cited in connections with breast and ovarian cancer and non-Hodgkin's lymphoma and include the agents cyclophosphamide, doxorubicin, methotrexate, 5-flurouracil, and tamoxifen.[25,29]

Non–Cancer Breast Pain

For women it is important to remember that breast pain exists outside of the diagnosis and treatment of breast cancer. In her review of the literature on nonmalignant breast pain, Berry reported the prevalence rate to be up to 70% of women. The experience of pain for those women lasted an average of 5 to 14 days per month. Breast pain is reported to be both cyclical and noncyclical. When breast pain is cyclical (67% of all breast pain), it is usually bilateral and generally resolves with menopause. Noncyclical breast pain (26%) usually occurs in the fourth or the fifth decade, can be either unilateral or bilateral, and is described as sharp or burning. Also, the pain spontaneously resolves but is not associated with menopause. Chest wall pain accounts for 7% of all breast pain and can occur at any age. It is often associated with costochondritis or cervical nerve compression. Chest wall pain is usually unilateral and medial to the breast and is associated with deep inspiration.[30]

Cancer-Related Breast Pain

Certainly, cancer itself is a factor in the presence or absence of pain. In an analysis of the Nurses Health Study data (both NHS and NHS2), researchers explored changes in physical and psychosocial function before and after breast cancer by age at diagnosis. Almost 1,100 women in the study were diagnosed with breast cancer between 1992 and 1997. Young age predicted a variety of functional losses, including greater levels of bodily pain, in comparison to those of middle age or the elderly with breast cancer. This factor was not correlated with severity of illness or treatment.[31]

Breast Surgery Pain

A number of authors have investigated the type and intensity of ongoing pain associated with various breast surgical interventions.

In 1995, Kwekkenboom reported two distinct pain syndromes in patients having mastectomy for breast cancer: phantom breast pain and postaxillary dissection pain.[32] She reviewed nine papers on pain after axillary dissection, which affects the arm, hand, chest wall, and shoulder on the surgical side. Pain of this type is related to nerve damage and consists of shooting pain, pins and needles sensations, and numbness. The pain can be mild to intense and begins shortly after surgery, often lasting years thereafter. Phantom breast pain is similar to other phantom limb pains reported in the literature. This pain is also neuropathic in nature. Four of the studies reviewed addressed this type of pain. The incidence of this pain is likely to be underreported. The nature of the pain is sharp and shooting, and it lasts a few seconds to minutes at a time. Onset is usually noted within 3 months of surgery and may persist for years.[32]

Breast pain in sequel to conservative breast cancer surgery was reported by Kornguth et al.[33] Specifically the authors investigated pain on return mammograms in women who had breast surgery and compared their pain with that of women receiving mammograms who did not have breast surgery. Additionally, the women in the breast cancer surgery group had an evaluation of the pain in the treated breast as opposed to the untreated one. The researchers found significantly greater pain (41%) in the treated breast than in the untreated breast regardless of radiation therapy. Women who had breast cancer treatment had 32% more pain as compared with controls. Interestingly, there was more pain in the untreated breast of women who had had breast cancer surgery as compared with controls. Pain at the time of the last mammogram predicted pain in both the treated and untreated breasts. It is unknown if these women were experiencing a chronic breast pain syndrome after their surgery. Coping strategies and perceived effectiveness of coping ability did not correlate with the degree of pain.[33]

In a study examining sensory morbidity associated with sentinel lymph node biopsy (SLNB), Temple and others concluded both that improvement in sensation associated with the surgery reached its peak by 3 months after surgery and that younger women had more problems regardless of the type of surgery performed.[34] Axillary lymph node dissection (ALND) was associated with sensory symptoms reported as more severe than in the SLNB group. Radiation therapy and surgery on the dominant side were not found to be factors in symptom severity. Although the SLNB group was found to have about half the morbidity of the ALND group, the morbidity associated with SLNB was greater than had been assumed.[34]

In a later study investigating the prevalence of distress in women who received surgical treatment for breast cancer, Baron documented prevalence of 18 sensations and concluded that the overall prevalence of distress was lower for individuals who had SLNB than for those undergoing the more traditional ALDN.[35] In the study, 294 patients were followed for 2 years after surgery. The most prevalent sensation for SLNB at baseline was tenderness; after 2 years it was still the most prevalent sensation. The tenderness was rated as either severe or distressing in 4% and 5% of the patients respectively. Soreness and twinges were also experienced in this population. For ALND there was significantly more tightness, numbness, pain, and stiffness at baseline. Tightness, numbness, pulling, and tingling remained significantly more prevalent at 24 months for those with ALND than for the women who had SLNB. For ALND, numbness was the most severe sensation at baseline (40%) and 24 months (20%).

The authors concurred with earlier research that noted that the most notable improvement in symptoms occurred during the first 3 months. This can have implications for patient teaching. Young women (under age 50) in the study reported more sensations both at baseline and 24 months than older women. Of the 80 women who had undergone mastectomy, as many as 50% reported phantom breast and nipple sensations at some time after surgery.[35]

Colorectal Surgery Pain

In a small study of patients with locally recurrent colorectal cancer, 15 being treated with nonsurgical palliation and 30 with resection, Esnaola assessed pain and QOL. Pain was correlated with decreased QOL.[18] Patients with nonsurgical palliation reported moderate to severe pain beyond the third month of treatment, and their QOL decreased accordingly. Patients who underwent resection of their tumors had mild to moderate levels of pain during first 3 years after surgery (especially after bony resection), with QOL slowly improving during this time. Long-term survivors (more than 3 years postoperatively) had minimal pain and good QOL. Female gender, pelvic/sciatic pain at presentation, total pelvic exenteration, and bony resection were associated with higher rates of moderate to severe pain. Women reported significantly worse QOL after treatment. Pain at presentation, occurring in 40% of subjects, was an independent predictor of pain following treatment.[18]

Lymphedema Pain

Lymphedema can occur after either surgery or radiation therapy as treatment for breast cancer. If left untreated, lymphedema can progress to cause pain, loss of function, and disability. Bosompra and others conducted 148 interviews to investigate the relationships between breast surgery and other treatments and the functional arm and shoulder limitations experienced afterward.[36] The women were asked to rate the intensity and frequency of their pain as well as location of the pain and the functioning of the arm. The predominant surgery was lumpectomy (69%), and the median number of lymph nodes removed was 16 (range 1 to 60). Information was collected about other treatments in addition to surgery. Pain intensity and frequency levels were generally low, but when pain occurred it was reported as moderate to severe in the affected arm (14%), chest wall/breast tissue area (14%), or axilla (13%). Numbness in the trunk corresponded to swelling in the trunk and extremities and, in addition, to increased intensity and frequency of pain. Presence of pain and numbness and increased intensity and frequency were inversely proportional to the ability to use the arm.[36]

As the application of cancer therapies continues to evolve into the outpatient setting, researchers are concerned that outpatient surgeries may leave people to recover on their own away from their health care providers. Uncontrolled pain may interfere with the postoperative recovery process.

Chemotherapy-Related Pain

Oncologic treatment is unique in its damage to the peripheral sensory neurons. The precise mechanisms are unknown, and there may be as many mechanisms for damage as there are agents causing the damage. Animal data are beginning to show similar syndromes in animals after exposure to these chemotherapy agents, and the mechanisms are becoming clearer.[37]

The leading sites of new cancers in women include breast, lung and bronchus, colon and rectum, and gynecologic (i.e., uterine and ovary) cancers.[9] Antineoplastic agents involved in these treatments often cause pain related to neurotoxic side effects. Although data are not available regarding gender-based differences in the toxicities of these drugs, because of their frequent use, these effects are of significant consequence for women with cancer.

The vinca alkaloids, platinums, and taxanes are the most important drugs inducing peripheral neuropathy. Neurotoxicities are clearly related to either cumulative dose or dose intensity, or both. The presence of existing neuropathy due to other comorbidities places a person at higher risk.

Cisplatin produces paresthesias and numbness at cumulative doses of greater than 400 mg/m^2, with symptoms often occurring 2.5 to 5.5 months after treatment has stopped. Sensory large fibers are affected, resulting in a loss of proprioception and an ataxic gait. Patellar and ankle reflexes usually disappear. Motor function, however, is spared. Pin and temperature sensation may be only mildly affected. Nerve conduction studies show decreased sensory nerve action potentials and prolonged sensory distal latencies.[38-39]

At postmortem, high concentrations of cisplatin have been found in the dorsal root ganglia cells, and so it is postulated to result in axonal changes secondary to the neuronal damage.[40] A recent study conducted by the Canadian Sociobehavioural Research Network and the National Cancer Institute of Canada Clinical Trials Group examined toxicity and quality of life of 152 patients from a randomized trial of either paclitaxel and cisplatin or cyclophosphamide and cisplatin. The most common symptom during and shortly following chemotherapy was neurosensory loss. Motor weakness and gastrointestinal pain were indicators for change in global quality of life.[41]

Carboplatin is less neurotoxic than cisplatin, but if given in high doses it can cause sensory neuropathy. Another platin analog, oxaliplatin, induces both acute and chronic neurotoxicity. Acute neurotoxicity occurs 30 to 60 minutes after infusion and disappears within days. Once it appears at all, it is likely to appear with each subsequent infusion. In up to 15% of individuals given the drug, the dose-limiting toxicity of this drug is the transient, acute, and predominantly sensory peripheral neuropathy, which is cumulative. Sensory ataxia and dysesthesias of the limbs, mouth, throat, and larynx occurs and are sometimes associated with muscular cramps or spasms exacerbated by cold. Symptoms develop in up to 97% of patients within a few minutes and resolve spontaneously. Cumulative or chronic neurotoxicity changes are identical to the cisplatin-induced neuropathies, although the mechanism of action differs. Cumulative toxicity is manifested by increased difficulty with activities of daily living (ADLs). Toxicity is most likely due to alterations in the kinetics of sodium channel inactivation resulting in the interference with axonal ion conductance and neural excitability.[42-44]

The vinca alkaloids include natural (vincristine and vinblastine) and synthetic (vindesine and vinorelbine) products. In vinblastine, bone marrow toxicity precedes neurotoxicity, which is manifested by loss of deep tendon reflexes. The neurotoxicity of vincristine is both central and peripheral. Peripheral nervous system symptoms are frequent and are thought to be caused by inhibition of fast axonal transport by microtubules. Paresthesias in fingers and toes are initial symptoms and are followed by loss of ankle reflexes. Occasionally one can see loss of vibratory sense, but weakness can also occur, usually of extensor muscles of the wrist and dorsiflexors of the toes.[45] Neuropathy usually resolves in a few months.

A recent report of a trial including vinorelbine and vinblastine in women with taxane-refractory breast cancer revealed significant neurotoxicity.[46] In the trial, 301 women were assigned to receive either pegylated liposomal doxorubicin versus vinorelbine or mitomycin-C plus vinblastine. Thirty-seven percent of the women who received pegylated lipsomal doxorubicin had palmar-plantar erythrodysesthesia (18% with grade 3 toxicity and 1% with grade 4 toxicity). The incidence of neuropathy was 11% with vinorelbine.

The neuropathies of paclitaxel can be either central or peripheral. Peripheral neuropathy is responsible for the pain. Paclitaxel works by promoting formation of microtubules and preventing their depolymerization, resulting in many rigid microtubules that accumulate in the nerves. Because they are defective, the microtubules inhibit axonal transport.[47] The predominant side effects from the process include sensory signs and symptoms. These paresthesias (numbness and pain in feet and hands) usually begin shortly after treatment (48 to 72 hours) after a cumulative dose of 100-200 mg/m^2 or can be insidious in onset. This large fiber sensory neuropathy is characterized by pain, numbness, and tingling. Up to 60% of all individuals receiving taxanes will experience some sort of neuropathy.[48] Difficulties with ADLs can occur. Patients can experience unsteadiness when walking, especially in the dark. Muscle weakness is usually mild. Deep tendon reflexes disappear. When paclitaxel is administered at high doses (250 mg/m^2) with granulocyte-colony stimulating factor (G-CSF), neuropathy is dose-limiting. Proximal muscle weakness can also occur and resolves spontaneously. Acute arthralgias and myalgias in the legs commonly occur 2 to 3 days after administration and last for 2 to 4 days.

Reduction in the neuropathy and pain of paclitaxel therapy can be achieved by dose modification as is seen in a recent study by Bolis.[49] In the study, 502 women with advanced ovarian cancer received 6 cycles of treatment consisting of either standard-dose (175 mg/m^2) or high-dose (225 mg/m^2) paclitaxel with carboplatin. The lower-dose treatment was as effective in treating the cancer as the higher-dose therapy and was associated with much less neuropathy (grade 2 toxicity of 13.2% as opposed to 28.9%, and grade 3 toxicity of 0.8% as opposed to 6.2%, respectively). Myalgias occurred in less than half of the patients and did not differ by treatment.[49]

In the recently reported large Intergroup trial, dose-dense chemotherapy with combinations and sequences of doxorubicin (Adriamycin or "A"), cyclophosphamide (Cytoxan or "C") and paclitaxel (Taxol or "T") was evaluated in node-positive primary breast cancer. Side effects between groups were not significant since 5% of the patients reported grade 3 myalgias and arthralgias across all treatments. The only grade 4 toxicities, occurring in two patients, were reported on the conventional 3-week arm AC+T. Severe neurotoxicities were rare, but were more prevalent in the concurrent group (AC+T) than the sequential regimens (A+C+T)(4% vs. 2%).[50]

When using paclitaxel, neuromuscular toxicities are frequently the dose-limiting toxicity for 1- to 3-hour infusions. Incidence of myalgias and arthralgias closely approximates or surpasses sensory neuropathy.[51] No correlations have been found between myalgias/arthralgias and patient parameters such as age, sex, height, prior chemotherapy, renal or hepatic function, or sites of metastatic disease.[52] At equivalent doses, the length of infusion does not predict incidence of myalgias and arthralgias.[26,53-54]

The neuropathy of docetaxel is usually mild to moderate and involves paresthesias and loss of deep tendon reflexes and vibratory sense. Proximal motor weakness can develop. Palmar/plantar erythrodysesthesia, the very painful "hand/foot" syndrome, can develop. Hand-foot syndrome is also a side effect of capecitabine therapy.

Sensory peripheral neurotoxicity is a rare but painful side effect of treatment with cytarabine and ifosfamide. Risk factors include high doses, frequent administration, and radiation therapy preceding the use of methotrexate.

Many of the biologic therapies are associated with a flu-like syndrome including myalgias that typically occurs shortly after initial dosing and lasts 4 to 8 hours.

Analgesics

A number of researchers have investigated the concept of pain caused by pain medicine itself. Specifically, opioid-induced abnormal sensitivity has much in common with neuropathic pain and has been observed in patients and animals. Animal data supports the theory that repeated administration of opioids results in tolerance (desensitization) as well as sensitization. Sensitization can exacerbate and confuse the picture of tolerance, which in turn decreases the analgesic efficacy.[55-59] There are data at this time to support the theory of gender-based differences in this area.

GENDER-BASED DIFFERENCES RELATED TO INTERVENTIONS

Investigating cancer patients' knowledge about pain and its management, Yeager evaluated a convenience sample of 369 adult oncology outpatients from 16 ambulatory care settings.[60] Of this group, 200 subjects had cancer-related pain and 169 were pain-free. Patients with pain knew more about pain and its management than those without pain, but even those patients with pain had scores below 60% on knowledge. Older patients had less knowledge than younger patients. Patients with more education and higher reported pain intensity scores had more knowledge of pain and pain management. Women had more knowledge about pain and pain management than did men.[60]

A report detailing patient satisfaction with pain management in small communities sheds light onto what patients expect from their disease and their providers in terms of management of their pain. In all 114 inpatients and outpatients were studied regarding their cancer-related or acute postoperative pain and their satisfaction with its management. Interestingly, the inpatients (68) were mostly women and less than 60 years old, while outpatients were predominantly men older than 60. Even though the patients reported satisfaction with their pain management, they simultaneously reported presence of a high level of pain.[61] Specifically, 90% of inpatients reported postoperative pain and 100% of outpatients had cancer-related pain. The inpatients expected and had a higher intensity of pain. The inpatients expected more pain relief than outpatients. Outpatients were more concerned about costs and communicating their pain than were inpatients. Both groups expected to have higher degrees of pain intensity than they would be able to tolerate. In addition, their expectation of pain relief was higher than what they experienced.[61]

In a study highlighting the need for continuing education of medical professionals, Green queried a random selection of 368 physicians licensed in Michigan who provide clinical care for acute postoperative and patients with cancer pain.[62] More than 50% of the physicians surveyed reported providing pain care frequently for postoperative pain as opposed to less than 20% for cancer pain. More than 75% reported that their goal was to provide at least adequate pain relief in both types of pain syndromes. Respondents were provided with clinical scenarios. The physicians more frequently chose the optimal pain management response for men following prostatectomy than for women following myomectomy. They also chose optimal pain management response for metastatic prostate cancer more frequently than for metastatic breast cancer. The authors hypothesized that the variability in treatment contributes to the undertreatment of pain, and the degree of undertreatment might differ by patient characteristics including gender. Most physicians believed it was appropriate to refer for cancer and terminal pain to pain specialists, and more would refer a male than a female. Those physicians who were younger or with better education in pain management provided better treatment.[62]

Prevention

Many chemotherapeutics given to women for their cancers can result in neurotoxicity. Research into prevention of neurotoxicities associated with chemotherapy is in its infancy. There is anecdotal evidence in the literature to support that there are treatments that can provide protection against the neurotoxic effects of some chemotherapy agents.[37,43,63-70] There is no literature illustrating the case for or against gender-based differences in these effects.

Pharmacologic

There are simply few data to support gender-based-based differences in pharmacologic interventions for cancer pain. A discussion of some of the issues can illustrate some of the opportunities in this area.

Advanced understanding of mechanisms of neuropathic pain has not led to effective mechanism-based therapies. The NMDA receptor has been a key target for new therapies, but the results of the trials have been disappointing. Treatments believed to act by restoration of endogenous inhibitory systems include drugs that mimic descending or local inhibitory pathways (clonidine, tricyclic antidepressants, opioids, GABA agonists)[7] and nonpharmacologic techniques such as transcutaneous electrical nerve stimulation (TENS), spinal cord stimulation, acupuncture, massage, and therapeutic massage. TENS units have failed to show efficacy in trials for chronic pain.[71] Where there is ongoing neural injury, pain is likely to be caused by activation of primary afferent nociceptors. When injury is not ongoing, impulses of pain are thought to be generated by either spontaneous activity of the nervous system, and/or lowered threshold in damaged nociceptors or in neurons involved in central pain production. In ongoing injury to the nervous system, the pain is more likely to respond to opioids and antiinflammatory medications, whereas older injuries are more responsive to antidepressants and anticonvulsants. Failure to make this distinction is the reason that some interventions are not thought to be effective.[72] Despite improvements in therapy, up to 30% of patients may have intractable pain.[7]

Finding specific mechanisms in individual patients is difficult. The US Food and Drug Administration has approved drugs for only two neuropathic pain syndromes: trigeminal neuralgia (carbamazepine) and postherapeutic neuralgia (gabapentin and the 5% lidocaine patch). First-line pharmacologic therapies have been established based on evidence from clinical trials on multiple types of neuropathic pain with similar results.[4,73] They include tricyclic antidepressants, gabapentin, topical lidocaine, tramadol, and opioids. In general, pharmacologic agents should be used for their intended effect and one can capitalize on side effects. One should not call a drug a failure until it has been titrated to effect and given an adequate trial.

For cancer pain, opioids are the mainstay of treatment. Opioids, quite successful in the treatment of nociceptive pain, historically have been reported to be less successful in treating neuropathic pain. Selection of opioids is dependent on prior exposure to opioids and which other drugs a patient is taking.[74] Recent systematic review of 16 randomized trials of patients with chronic nonmalignant pain did not show any evidence to support any one opioid over another, either for length of action, safety, or functional outcome.[75] In these trials, gender was not a factor in choice of opioid treatment.

Are there gender-based differences in treatment response? If so, these can lead to targeted interventions?

Hepatic metabolism of opioids has been linked to gender-related differences in response. Metabolism depends on the presence of microsomal enzymes located in the smooth endoplasmic reticulum of the liver, and genetic factors are believed to be determinants of the efficiency in this activity.[12]

Based on their review of literature from 1966-1998, and their own work with oral surgery, Miaskowski and Levine suggest that certain opioids are better for treating the pain of women.[76] They found that κ-opioids (pentazocine, nalbuphine, butorphanol although effective for women, were relatively ineffective in treating postoperative oral surgery pain in men. They found no differences in effectiveness of μ-opioids.[76]

How, then, does one choose? A number of considerations should be examined before choosing an opioid. They include general, pharmacologic, genetic, and economic considerations.

General considerations are whether the patient has drug allergies, a history of previous adverse events with drugs, and adequate renal/hepatic clearance. The drug must also be evaluated for its metabolites and whether or not they are active. Thoughtful consideration must be given to the respiratory effects if combined with other CNS depressants. The clinician must review drug history and monitor current medications, being alert to drugs using the same pathway. Discussion with a pharmacist or use of a drug interaction program can be important.[4]

Pharmacologic considerations include knowing the patients' prior experience with opioids. This is especially true in the elderly. Diminished plasticity in older patients may make them more sensitive to drug effects.[4] Systemic changes related to aging may cause an alteration in the perception of pain. Decreased numbers of opioid receptors may lead to increased sensitivity to opioids in the elderly. Changes in the glomerular filtration rate, reduction in cytochrome P450 activity, and hypoalbuminemia can all lead to changes in absorption and metabolism of opioids in the elderly. That, coupled with issues related to polypharmacy, leads experts to recommend nonpharmacologic therapies in these individuals if possible. If it is necessary to treat with opioids, lower doses and longer dose intervals should be used.[77] Evaluation must also take place to determine the ability of the individual, no matter what the age, to maintain the treatment regimen.[4]

Pharmacogenic considerations are becoming more important. Some individuals are "slow metabolizers"; that is, they express less active or inactive enzymes (P450 system) needed for biotransformation of drug into active state. Probably the best-known example is with codeine, in which individuals who are slow metabolizers show no response to the drug. Currently, there are no routine screenings for these genetic polymorphisms.

Economic information is also very important. Can the patient afford the drug? If the patient buys the drug, is he or she able to pay for other important things in life such as food, insurance, caregiver costs, and costs of side effects management?[4]

Little attention has been paid by the oncology community to the effects seen in the nonmalignant pain literature of prolonged opioid therapy; that is, therapy lasting years in duration. Literature also exists in the nonmalignant pain population regarding failure of opioids to produce adequate analgesia in pain syndromes.

Most data on failure to achieve analgesia and adverse effects are derived from subjects who are addicts. In 2003, Ballantyne reviewed the concepts of opioid tolerance, opioid-induced pain sensitivity, hormonal changes, and immune modulation and the clinical implications of each.[59]

Tolerance is the pharmacologic phenomenon that develops over time with repeated use of the drug, which results in the need to increase the dose of the drug to achieve an equianalgesic effect. Tolerance is a physiologically adaptive process at the cellular level that involves down-regulation (either reduction in turnover rate and number of opioid receptors) or desensitization of opioid receptors or both. This process seems linked to the NMDA receptor cascade.[77]

In patients receiving prolonged opioid therapy, increased expression of the endogenous opioid dynorphin has been noted in the spinal cord dorsal horn and is associated with enhanced pain sensitivity. Although the mechanism is unclear, electrophysiology suggests that the NMDA receptor is involved. Repeated administration of drug results in tolerance (desensitization) as well as sensitization. Sensitization can exacerbate and confuse the picture of tolerance, which in turn can decrease the analgesic efficacy.[55] Therefore, apparent tolerance can be related to pharmacologic opioid tolerance, opioid-induced abnormal pain sensitivity, or disease progression. Unfortunately, in clinical practice today it is not possible to distinguish between pharmacologic tolerance and abnormal pain sensitivity. This phenomenon may in part explain, whatever the reason, why some patients fail to achieve adequate levels of analgesia even in the face of increasing amounts of opioids.

Opioids given over long periods can influence at least two hormonal systems: the hypothalamic-pituitary-adrenal axis (HPA) and the hypothalamic-pituitary-gonadal (HPG) axis. Morphine has been reported to progressively decrease cortisol levels in adults. In animal models showing effects on the HPG axis, there is modulation of hormonal release (an increase in prolactin and a decrease in luteinizing hormone, follicle-stimulating hormone, testosterone, and estrogen). The effect is likely dose-related. Clinically, the effect is also seen in a majority of men receiving intrathecal opioids for chronic nonmalignant pain. These men benefit from replacement testosterone. In heroin addicts the effect is that of decreased libido, aggression, amenorrhea or irregular menses and galactorrhea. Studies are needed to address these issues, which may be clinically relevant in cancer patients.[59] Since women also take opioids for extended periods of time, this population must also be studied.

Preclinical evidence indicates that opioids alter the development, differentiation, and function of immune cells. Both the innate and adaptive systems are affected. Opioid-related receptors are on immune cells. Animal studies point to prolonged exposure being more likely to suppress immune function than abrupt withdrawal. Different opioids may have different effects on immune suppression. Clinical evidence is lacking because studies have not been done in humans.[59]

Interventional

Most patients with cancer who have chronic pain achieve good pain relief with standard and adjuvant analgesics (90%). The others are resistant to conventional modalities and may need interventional techniques. These techniques are used in conjunction with standard pain management therapies and are often used when disease is more aggressive.

There are two general types of interventions, surgical and anesthetic. In his recent review of interventional technologies, Sloan reviews these modalities.[78] Gender has not been investigated as a factor in the effectiveness of these therapies.

Psychoeducational

There is some evidence to support the use of psychoeducational interventions for pain management for women—more because women were included in studies, and less because of specific interventions designed and detailed for women. The opportunity for much nursing research exists in this area.

Efficacy for educational pain education intervention was tested in a trial of underserved minority patients by Anderson and others.[79] The intervention targeted African Americans and Hispanic Americans randomized within their minority. In the trial, 97 individuals participated. Eligibility included a cancer diagnosis, socioeconomic disadvantage, and Eastern Cooperative Oncology Group (ECOG) performance status less than or equal to 2. Pain was rated as greater than 4 on the Brief Pain Inventory (BPI). The intervention group received a culture-specific video and book on pain management. The control group received a video and booklet on nutrition. Outcomes included pain intensity, changes in quality of life, perceived pain control, functional status, analgesic use, and physician pain assessment at 2 to 10 weeks after the intervention.

All subjects, regardless of randomized group, received "standard" pain management information usually given by the staff. Physicians were blinded to patient assignments. Results indicated that at least half of the time, physicians underestimated the individual's pain needs including pain needs and analgesic requirements. Results showed that the educational intervention did not affect quality of life, perceived pain control, or functional status. Pain intensity ratings decreased over time but were not statistically significant for both groups. The authors felt that educational programs alone are not sufficient. Unfortunately, although important because of the population studied, there was no evaluation done on gender-related differences.

In her recent review of 25 psychoeducational intervention studies, Devine found reasonably strong evidence for relaxation-based cognitive-behavioral interventions, education about analgesic usage, and supportive counseling.[80] These interventions cannot serve as a substitute for pharmacologic interventions but can serve as adjuncts. In the sample, 68% of the studies had more women than men in the samples. Seven of the studies (28%) included only women. However in no instance was there a separate analysis for gender. The most frequent interventions were relaxation-based (either alone or in combination with visualization, self-selected music therapy, or hypnosis). A statistically significant, homogeneous, moderate to large beneficial effect on pain was found. In educational interventions a statistically significant small to moderate beneficial effect was found. When relaxation plus other treatment (distraction, self massage, problem solving, positive affirmation, cognitive reappraisal, goal setting, education, or supportive counseling) was looked at, when aggregated there was no effect on pain. Supportive counseling plus other content was found to have a small to moderate effect.[80]

Published subsequent to the metaanalysis by Devine is an interventional study by Helgeson and colleagues.[81] In the study 312 women with breast cancer within 3 months of their diagnosis were randomized to education (79), peer discussion (74), combination (82), or control (77) groups. Each large group was divided into small groups (about 8 to 12 women). The education group had eight weekly meetings lasting about 45 minutes where an expert made a presentation on topics, followed by a brief question-and-answer period. The goal of education was to provide expert information and enhance women's control over their illness experience. The peer discussion group also met weekly for 8 times (60 minutes each) and was facilitated by an advanced practice oncology nurse and a social worker. The goal of the peer group was to have discussion on feelings, and self-disclosure (determined by group members). The combined group had an educational lecture followed by a 1-hour discussion group.

Results as measured by the Short-Form 36 (SF-36) Health Survey, showed that members of the education group had statistically greater vitality, less bodily pain, and greater physical function than the control group members. The education group also had better scores than the peer discussion group on mental health, vitality, and social functioning. These differences were maintained at 3 years, and there is no effect in the discussion group alone.[81] The findings suggest that educational sessions held during treatment can have long-term effects on quality of life and long-term adjustment to disease for women with breast cancer.

In a more recent study by Vallerand and colleagues, educational strategies for advanced pain management were directed at nurses instead of patients.[82] A two-tiered educational program focused on basic and advanced pain management strategies (e.g., pharmacologic options, assertive communication skills) of homecare nurses. The nurses in the intervention group had a significant increase in knowledge, a more positive attitude toward pain management, fewer perceived barriers to pain management, and increased perceived control over pain. The effect has lasted 24 months. Preliminary data from patients are showing a significant decrease in pain scores when the patients were cared for by nurses who had the intervention.[82] It is unknown if the patient data, when published, will be analyzed for gender-based differences.

Given and colleagues reported on the effectiveness of cognitive-behavioral intervention administered by nurses, which focused on symptom management.[83] They studies 237 patients from comprehensive and community centers, who were randomly assigned to intervention (a problem solving approach directed at those symptoms that reached a threshold) or conventional care. The target outcome was symptom severity. Intervention patients reported significantly lower symptom severity at 10 and 20 weeks. Gender had no effect, nor did age, site, or stage of cancer, or supportive medications.[83]

Complementary Therapy

Recently there have been publications looking at the effect of complementary medicine (CAM), some of which shows promise in pain management.[84] Data exist to support the efficacy of acupuncture, mind-body therapy, and, potentially, massage therapy. Some of the studies have indicated that these modalities have efficacy in women.

Acupuncture (stimulation of certain points in the body by a needle or pressure) was shown to be effective in the first randomized trial of auricular acupuncture for neuropathic cancer pain. End points for efficacy were based on absolute decrease in pain intensity measured 2 months after randomization using the Visual Analog Scale (VAS). Patient eligibility included patients in pain and a VAS score of 30 mm or more after analgesic treatment appropriate for both intensity and type of pain for at least a month. There was a statistically significant decrease in pain (36%). Women comprised 69% of the treatment group.[85] There was no analysis of the data by gender.

Reflexology, one type of massage therapy, has been shown to be effective in significantly reducing pain in breast cancer patients. This was confirmed in a larger study with a variety of hospitalized cancer patients.

In a quasi-experimental, pre/post, crossover trial consisting predominantly of female cancer patients on regularly scheduled opioids and adjuvant medications, reflexology was performed. Foot reflexology is massage that targets points on the foot believed to correspond to parts of the body. The intervention in the study was foot reflexology to both feet for 30 minutes total (by a certified reflexologist); there was a control condition for each patient. Variables included anxiety and pain. There was a significant decrease in anxiety. Breast cancer patients experienced a significant decrease in pain after reflexology based on three pain measurements. Pain types were somatic and visceral.[86]

In a larger study of 87 cancer patients (the majority of whom were women), a 10-minute foot massage (5 minutes per foot) had significant, immediate effect on perceptions of pain, nausea, and relaxation on VAS.[87] Again with a quasi-experimental design, the study had subjects have massage on two occasions, and they acted as their own control on a third occasion. Massage was found to be statistically significant. No significant gender-based differences were found.

National Institutes of Health Technology Assessment panel found strong evidence for relaxation techniques reducing chronic pain and for hypnosis relieving cancer-related pain. Evidence for effectiveness of cognitive-behavioral techniques and biofeedback in relieving chronic pain was moderate.[4]

SUMMARY

For over 2 decades, researchers have been investigating gender-related pain differences. Few researchers have delved into cancer pain in women. Opportunities abound for nurse researchers and health care providers to further investigate this area. Questions remain regarding the specifics of gender differences in pain mechanisms, pain experience, and pain behavior. The influence of role-based and societal expectations on and the meaning of pain in the experience of cancer pain in women must be determined. Gender determined differences in interventions (i.e., pharmacologic, interventional, psychoeducational, and complementary) have to be further explored in a rigorous fashion. The influence of genetics must also be explored. Health care professionals' response to women in pain as opposed to men in pain requires examination, looking for influence of stereotyping on pain management interventions. Investigations of women with cancer from culturally diverse populations and of various ages are desperately needed. Full understanding of neurotoxicities of various cancer therapies and gender related differences regarding pathophysiology, prevention, and treatment require exploration.

Until this information is known, it is the professional's obligation to contribute to the accrual to trials researching these areas, listen to patients regardless of gender, and assess and treat their pain aggressively.

REFERENCES

1. Walsh D, Donnelly S, Rybicki L: The symptoms of advanced cancer: relationship to age, gender and performance status in 1000 patients, *Supportive Care Cancer* 8:175-179, 2000.
2. Farrar JT, Portenoy RK: Neuropathic cancer pain: the role of adjuvant analgesics, *Oncology* 15(11):1435-1442, 2001.
3. Mendell JR Sahenk Z: Painful sensory neuropathy, *N Engl J Med* 348:1243-1255, 2003.
4. Fine PG, Miaskowski C, Paice JA: Meeting the challenges in cancer pain management, *J Support Oncol* 2(6 Suppl 4): 5-22, 2004.
5. Woolf C: Pain: Moving from symptom control toward mechanism-specific pharmacologic management, *Ann Intern Med* (140):441-451, 2004.
6. Fillingim R: Sex-related influences on pain: a review of the mechanisms and clinical implications, *Rehab Psychol* 48(3): 165-174, 2003.
7. Chen H and others: Contemporary management of neuropathic pain for the primary care physician, *Mayo Clin Proc* 79(12):1533-1545, 2004.
8. Berkley K: Sex differences in pain, *Behav Brain Sci* 20: 371-380, 435-513, 1997.
9. American Cancer Society. *Cancer Facts and Figures 2005.* Atlanta: American Cancer Society; 2005. On the Web at www.cancer.org.
10. Unruh A: Gender variations in clinical pain experience, *Pain* 65:123-167, 1996.
11. Unruh AM, Ritchie J, Merskey H: Does gender affect appraisal of pain and pain coping strategies? *Clin J Pain* 15:31-40, 1999.
12. Anderson KO and others: Pain education for underserved minority cancer patients: a randomized controlled trial, *J Clin Oncol* 22(24):4918-4925, 2004.
13. Fillingim RB and others: Clinical characteristics of chronic back pain as a function of gender and oral opioid us, *Spine* 28(2):143-150, 2003.
14. Yates P and others: The prevalence and perception of pain amongst hospital in-patients, *J Clin Nurs* 7(6):521-530, 1998.
15. Holtzman J, Saleh K, Kane R: Gender differences in functional status and pain in a Medicare population undergoing elective total hip arthroplasty, *Med Care* 40(6):461-470, 2002.
16. Marcus D: Gender differences in chronic pain in a treatment seeking population, *J Gender Specific Med* 6(4):19-24, 2003.
17. Mercandante S and others: Factors influencing opioid response in advanced cancer patients with pain followed at home: the effects of age and gender, *Support Care Cancer* 8:123-130, 2000.
18. Esnaola NF and others: Pain and quality of life after treatment in patients with locally recurrent rectal cancer, *J Clin Oncol* 20(21):4361-4367, 2002.
19. Avemark CB, Ericsson KE, Ljunggren G: Gender differences in experienced pain, mood, energy, appetite, and sleep by cancer patients in palliative care, *Vard I Norden* 23 (67): 42-46, 2003.
20. Moore RH, Spiegel D: Uses of guided imagery for pain control by African-American and white women with metastatic breast cancer, *Integrative Med* 2(2/3):115-126, 1999.

21. Vallerand A: Gender differences in pain, *Image J Nurs Scholarship* 27(3):235-237, 1995.
22. Coward DD, Wilkie DJ: Metastatic bone pain: meanings associated with self-report and self-management decision making, *Cancer Nurs* 23(2):101-108, 2000.
23. Wilkie DJ, Huang H-J, Reilly N, Cain KC: Nociceptive and neuropathic pain in patients with lung cancer: a comparison of pain quality descriptors, *J Pain Symptom Manage* 22(5): 899-910, 2001.
24. Abu-Shakra M and others: Cancer and autoimmunity: autoimmune and rheumatic features in patients with malignancies, *Ann Rheum Dis* 60:433-440, 2001.
25. Loprinzi CL, Duffy J, Ingle JN: Postchemotherapy rheumatism, *J Clin Oncol* 11:768-770, 1993.
26. Smith D: Additional cases of postchemotherapy rheumatism, *J Clin Oncol* 11:1625-1626, 1993.
27. Michl I, Zielinski CC: More postchemotherapy rheumatism, *J Clin Oncol* 11:2051-2052, 1993.
28. Raderer M, Scheithauer W: Postchemotherapy rheumatism following adjuvant therapy for ovarian cancer, *Scand J Rheumatol* 23:291-292, 1994.
29. Creamer P and others: Acute inflammatory polyarthritis in association with tamoxifen, *Br J Rheumatol* 33:583-585, 1994.
30. Berry J: Breast pain: all that hurts is not cancer, *Am J Nurse Pract* 5(4):9-10, 15-18, 2001.
31. Kroenke CH and others: Functional impact of breast cancer by age at diagnosis, *J Clin Oncol* 22(10):1849-1856, 2004.
32. Kwekkenboom K: Postmastectomy pain syndromes, *Cancer Nurs* 19(1):37-43, 1995.
33. Kornguth PJ and others: Mammography pain in women treated conservatively for breast cancer, *J Pain* 1(4):268-274, 2000.
34. Temple LKF and others: Sensory morbidity after sentinel lymph node biopsy and axillary dissection: a prospective study of 233 women, *Ann Surg Oncol* 9(7):654-662, 2002.
35. Baron RH and others: Eighteen sensations after breast cancer surgery: a two year comparison of sentinel lymph node biopsy and axillary lymph node dissection, *Oncol Nurs Forum* 31(4):691-698, 2004.
36. Bosompra K and others: Swelling, numbness, pain, and their relationship to arm function among breast cancer survivors: a disablement process model perspective, *Breast J* 8(6):338-348, 2002.
37. Paice J: Mechanisms and management of neuropathic pain in cancer, *J Support Oncol* 1(2):107-120, 2003.
38. Lomonaco M and others: Cisplatin neuropathy: clinical course and neurophysiological findings, *J Neurol* 239: 199-204, 1992.
39. Riggs J and others: Prospective nerve conduction studies in cisplatin therapy, *Ann Neurol* 23:92-94, 1988.
40. Gregg RW and others: Cisplatin neurotoxicity: the relationship between dosage, time, and platinum concentration in neurologic tissues and morphologic evidence of toxicity, *J Clin Oncol* 10:795-803, 1992.
41. Butler L and others: Determining the relationship between toxicity and quality of life in an ovarian cancer chemotherapy clinical trial, *J Clin Oncol* 22(12):2461-2468, 2004
42. Adelsberger H and others: The chemotherapeutic oxaliplatin alters voltage-gated Na (+) channel kinetics on rat sensory neurons, *Eur J Pharmacol* 406:25-32, 2000.
43. Lersch C and others: Prevention of oxaliplatin-induced peripheral sensory neuropathy by carbamazepine in patients with advanced colorectal cancer, *Clin Colorect Cancer* 2(1):54-58, 2002.
44. Fracasso PM and others: Phase II study of oxaliplatin in platinum-resistant and refractory ovarian cancer: a Gynecologic Group Study, *J Clin Oncol* 21(15):2856-2859, 2003.
45. DeAngelis LM and others: Evolution of neuropathy and myopathy during intensive vincristine/cortico steroid chemotherapy for non-Hodgkins lymphoma, *Cancer* 67:2241-2246, 1991.
46. Keller AM and others: Randomized phase III trial of pegylated liposomal doxorubicin vs vinorelbine or mitomycin—c plus vinblastine in women with taxane-refractory advanced breast cancer, *J Clin Oncol* 22(19): 3893-3901, 2004.
47. Verstappen CCP and others: Neurotoxic complications of chemotherapy in patients with cancer: Clinical signs and optimal management, *Drugs* 63(15):1549-1563, 2003.
48. Preston F: Neuropathies and myalgias-arthralgias associated with taxane therapy, *Innov Breast Cancer Care* 5(3):66-68, 2000.
49. Bolis G and others: Paclitaxel 175 or 225 mg/meters squared with carboplatin in advanced ovarian cancer: a randomized trial, *J Clin Oncol* 22(4):686-690, 2004.
50. Citron ML and others: Randomized trial of dose-dense versus conventionally scheduled and sequential versus concurrent combination chemotherapy as postoperative adjuvant treatment of node-positive primary breast cancer: first report of Intergroup Trial C9741/Cancer and Leukemia Group B Trial 9741, *J Clin Oncol* 21(8):1431-1439, 2003.
51. Garrison JA and others: Myalgias and arthralgias associated with paclitaxel: incidence and management, *Oncology* 17(2):271-277, 2003.
52. Kunitoh H and others: Neuromuscular toxicities of paclitaxel 210 mg/m^2 by 3 hr infusion, *Br J Cancer* 77: 1686-1688, 1998.
53. Eisenhauer EA and others: European-Canadian randomized trial of paclitaxel in relapsed ovarian cancer: high dose versus low dose and long vs short infusion, *J Clin Oncol* 12:2654-2666, 1994.
54. Hainsworth JD and others: One hour paclitaxel plus carboplatin in the treatment of advanced non-small cell lung cancer: results of a multicentre, phase II trial, *Eur J Cancer* 34:654-658, 1998.
55. Mao J: Opioid-induced abnormal pain sensitivity: implications in clinical opioid therapy, *Pain* 100:213-217, 2002.
56. Mao J and others: Chronic morphine induces downregulation of spinal glutamate transporters: implications in morphine tolerance and abnormal pain sensitivity, *J Neurosci* 22:8312-8323, 2002.
57. Mao J and others: Neuronal apoptosis associated with morphine tolerance: evidence for an opioid-induced neurotoxic mechanism, *J Neurosci* 22:7650-7661, 2002.
58. Giffard RG, Morgan RL: Cell death in the central nervous system: Therapeutic possibilities? *Reg Anesth Pain Med* 25:22-25, 2000.
59. Ballantyne JC, Mao J: Opioid therapy for chronic pain, *N Engl J Med* (349):1943-1953, 2003.
60. Yeager KA and others: Differences in pain knowledge in cancer patients with and without pain, *Cancer Practice* 5(1):39-45, 1997.

61. Corizzo CC, Baker MC, Henkelmann GC: Assessment of patient satisfaction w pain management in small community inpatient and outpatient settings, *Oncol Nurs Forum* 27(8): 1279-1286, 2000.
62. Green CR, Wheeler JRC: Physician variability in the management of acute postoperative and cancer pain: A quantitative analysis of the Michigan experience, *Pain Med* 4(1):8-20, 2003.
63. Boyle FM, Wheeler HR, Shenfield GM: Glutamate ameliorates experimental vincristine neuropathy, *J Pharmacol Exp Ther* 279:410-415, 1996.
64. Cascinu S and others: Neuroprotective effect of induced glutathione on oxaliplatin-based chemotherapy in advanced colorectal cancer: randomized, double-blind, placebo-controlled trial, *J Clin Oncol* 20:3478-3483, 2002.
65. Vahdat LT and others: Reduction of paclitaxel induced peripheral neuropathy with glutamine. In *37th Annual Meeting of the American Society of Clinical Oncology*, San Francisco, Calif., May 12-15, 2001 (abstract 1562).
66. Savarese D, Boucher J Corey B: Glutamine treatment of paclitaxel induced myalgias and arthralgias [letter to the editor], *J Clin Oncol* 16:3918-3919, 1998.
67. Laine-Cessac P and others: Acute oxaliplatin neurotoxicity dramatically improved with intravenous calcium and magnesium salts, *Therapie* (Paris) 53:183, 1998 (abstract 132).
68. Penz M and others: Subcutaneous administration of amifostine: a promising therapeutic option in patients with oxaliplatin-related peripheral sensitive neuropathy, *Ann Oncol* 12:421-422, 2001.
69. Mariani G and others: Oxaliplatin induced neuropathy: could gabapentin be the answer? *Proc Am Soc Clin Oncol* 19:609a, 2000 (abstract 2397).
70. Eckel F and others: Prevention of oxaliplatin induced neuropathy by carbamazepine: a pilot study, *Dtsch Med Wochenschr* 127:78-82, 2002.
71. Carroll D and others: Transcutaneous electrical nerve stimulation (TENS) for chronic pain, *Cochrane Database System Rev* 3(CD003222), 2001.
72. Manfredi PL and others: Neuropathic pain in patients with cancer, *J Palliat Care* 19(2):115-118, 2003.
73. Dworkin RH and others: Advances in neuropathic pain: diagnosis, mechanisms, and treatment recommendations, *Arch Neurol* 60:1524-1534, 2003.
74. Chou R, Clark E, Helfand M: Comparative efficacy and safety of long-acting oral opioids for chronic non-cancer pain: a systematic review, *J Pain Symptom Manage* 26: 1026-1048, 2003.
75. Miaskowski C, Levine JD: Does opioid analgesia show a gender preference for females? *Pain Forum* 8(1):34-44, 1999.
76. Balducci L: Management of cancer pain in geriatric patients, *J Support Oncol* 1(3):175-191, 2003.
77. Mitchell JM, Basbaum AI, Fields HL: A locus and mechanism of action for associative morphine tolerance, *Nat Neurosci* 3:47-53, 2000.
78. Sloan P: The evolving role of interventional pain management in oncology, *J Support Oncol* 2:491-506, 2004.
79. Anderson KO and others: Pain education for underserved minority cancer patients: a randomized controlled trial, *J Clin Oncol* 22(24):4918-4925, 2004.
80. Devine E: Meta-analysis of the effect of psychoeducational interventions on pain in adults with cancer, *Oncol Nurs Forum* 30(1):75-89, 2003.
81. Helgeson VS and others: Long term effects of educational and peer discussion group interventions on adjustment to breast cancer, *Health Psychol* 20:387-392, 2001.
82. Vallerand AH and others: Improving cancer pain management by homecare nurses, *Oncol Nurs Forum* 31(4):809-816, 2004.
83. Given C and others: Effect of a cognitive behavioral intervention on reducing symptom severity during chemotherapy, *J Clin Oncol* 22(3):507-516, 2004.
84. G, Cassileth BR, Yeung KS: Complementary therapies for cancer-related symptoms, *J Support Oncol* 2(5):419-429, 2004.
85. Alimi D and others: Analgesic effect of auricular acupuncture for cancer pain: a randomized, blinded, controlled trial, *J Clin Oncol* 21(22):4120-4126, 2003.
86. Stephenson NLN, Weinrich SP, Tavakoli AS: The effects of foot reflexology on anxiety and pain in patients with breast and lung cancer, *Oncol Nurs Forum* 27(1):67-72, 2000.
87. Grealish L, Lomasney A, Whiteman B: Foot massage: a nursing intervention to modify the distressing symptoms of pain and nausea in patients hospitalized with cancer, *Cancer Nurs* 23 (3):237-243, 2000.

CHAPTER

14 Chronic Wounds

Patrick McNees

INTRODUCTION

Skin is the largest organ. Yet when skin and cancer are considered, it is most often in the context of skin cancer. Indeed, skin may be the organ of least concern, and skin integrity is often taken for granted until anomalies develop. Unfortunately, those anomalies develop all too often. Because of differential incidence rates for certain types of cancer (e.g., breast cancer), women with cancer may be at greater risk for developing chronic, nonhealing wounds than men with cancer.

This chapter neither specifically focuses on skin cancer nor limits discussion to the side effects of cancer treatment on skin. While skin effects from disease and treatment are presented, the overriding focus of this chapter is on women with cancer and the development, management, and treatment of chronic wounds.

Chronic wounds may be differentiated from acute wounds by etiology and/or healing characteristics. Put simply, acute wounds typically heal in a matter of days or weeks. Chronic wounds do not typically heal in such a short period and can exist for months or even the remainder of one's life.[1] Chronic wounds can be associated with a variety of etiologies including radiation, skin cancers, fistulae, nonhealing surgical wounds, dermatitis, vasculitis, and burns. However, the most common chronic wounds are pressure ulcers, diabetic/neuropathic ulcers, and other lower extremity ulcers due to venous and arterial insufficiency.[1]

Although a complete discussion of the skin physiology is unnecessary and beyond the scope of this chapter, a brief reminder of the structure and function of skin provides a foundation on which the chapter will be built. Skin performs three main functions: (1) sensation, (2) protection, and (3) temperature control. When compromised there is increased morbidity and mortality risk. The degree of that risk is typically associated with the severity of the wound condition.

OVERVIEW

This chapter will focus on chronic wounds. The next section will address risk assessment; that is, the risk of developing a chronic wound. One reason for performing risk assessments is to determine the likelihood that a patient will develop a wound. However, ascertaining substantial risk does little to help the patient in the absence of prevention efforts. Thus a section of the chapter is devoted to activities beyond assessing risk: in other words, to prevention efforts. One's best efforts to prevent wounds are not always successful. When wounds develop the formulation of treatment efforts should be premised on comprehensive and reliable wound assessments. A part of the chapter will be devoted to assessment issues that should be addressed and alternatives for addressing those issues. Wound treatment can involve surprising subtleties, yet there are only a few questions that should govern fundamental wound treatment.

Those questions are reviewed in a section of the chapter devoted to treatment. The final section addresses some special considerations for skin care and wound treatment for women with cancer.

RISK OF DEVELOPING A CHRONIC WOUND

Beyond treatment side effects, a number of patient conditions increase the probability that patients will develop chronic wounds. Barbara Braden, Nancy Bergstrom, and their colleagues have identified six patient characteristics that affect the risk of a patient developing one of more pressure ulcers: (1) sensory perception, (2) moisture, (3) activity, (4) mobility, (5) nutrition, and (6) friction and shear.[2] Each of these six factors or subscales included in the Braden Scale for Pressure Ulcer risk will be discussed briefly. However, before addressing each factor it is important to understand the scoring logic for the scale.

For scoring purposes, consider a subscale for each of the six factors. Five of the six subscales are scored on a 1- to 4-point scale. The friction and shear subscale is scored on a 1 to 3 scale. The total risk score is derived by summing the subscale scores. Lower Braden Scale scores are associated with greater risk of developing a pressure ulcers, with 6 representing the lowest score possible and 23 representing the highest possible score. Table 14-1, reflecting differential risk based on five different score ranges, is derived from Ayello and Braden.[3]

Sensory perception

The sensory perception factor addresses the patient's ability to respond meaningfully to pressure-related discomfort. In general, the risk of developing a pressure ulcer increases as a function of the patient (1) not being able to respond to verbal commands, (2) not being able to communicate his or her discomfort or needs, and (3) not being able to discriminate pain. If the patient responds to verbal commands and has no sensory deficit that would limit ability to feel and/or communicate pain or discomfort, there is little risk from this factor. This would be reflected as a score of 4 on the Braden Scale. However, the fact that other factors may increase the risk of developing a wound should be noted.

If the patient responds to verbal commands but cannot consistently communicate discomfort or the need to be turned, there is increased risk of developing a wound. Even if there is adequate communication ability, if the patient has sensory impairment that limits ability to feel pain or discomfort in one or two extremities, there is increased risk of developing a wound, resulting in a Braden Score of 3 for this item.

Responding only to painful stimuli, and not being able to communicate discomfort except by moaning or restlessness, indicates an even higher risk level. If the patient's condition prevents feeling pain over one half of the body, risk is also increased. If any of these conditions describe the patient's condition a Braden score of 2 would recorded.

Unresponsiveness to painful stimuli resulting from a low state of consciousness or sedation or limited ability to feel pain over most of the body reflects the highest level of risk and would be scored as a 1.

Moisture

The presence of moisture increases the likelihood that a pressure ulcer will develop. The extent to which moisture places a patient at risk depends on the degree to which the skin is exposed to moisture. If the patient is normally dry, there is

Table **14-1** DIFFERENTIAL RISKS FOR DEVELOPMENT OF A CHRONIC WOUND[3]

Risk Level	From	To
No risk	19	23
At risk	15	18
Moderate risk	13	14
High risk	10	12
Very high risk	9	6

little additive risk for developing a wound (a score of 4). If the patient is occasionally moist, there is an increased risk (a score of 3); and if the patient is often moist, there is even more risk (a score of 2). Constant moisture places the person at the greatest risk (a score of 1).

Activity

The degree of physical activity a patient exhibits relates negatively to the risk of developing a pressure ulcer. Patients who walk frequently are at little additional risk. Patients who walk occasionally but for short distances and who spend the majority of time in a chair or in bed are at increased risk. Persons who are chair-fast are at even greater risk. Patients confined to bed are at the greatest risk.

Mobility

The ability to control and change body position is an important factor contributing to pressure ulcer risk. If the patient is able to make frequent changes in position without assistance, little additional risk is incurred. If the patient makes frequent but slight changes body or extremity position independently, there is some additional risk (that is, the Braden score for this item is 3). If the person only makes occasional, slight changes, additional risk is indicated. Complete immobility reflects the greatest degree of risk.

Nutrition

Nutrition is not only a factor in establishing pressure ulcer risk but may also be a factor in delayed wound healing. In terms of risk, little additional risk is noted if the patient eats most meals and rarely refuses to eat, thus requiring no supplements. If the patient is on a tube-feeding or total parenteral nutrition (TPN) regimen that, in theory at least, meets nutritional requirements, risk is increased. The patient who is not receiving tube feeding or TPN but who eats over one half of most meals including 4 servings of protein, only occasionally refuses a meal, and will usually accept a supplement when offered, is also at slightly elevated risk.

If the adequacy of nutrition is questionable, risk is increased even more. Situations in which nutrition is probably inadequate include the following: the patient rarely eats a complete meal or eats only about a half of the food offered; protein intake includes only three servings per day; and the patient is receiving less than an optimum amount of a liquid diet or tube feeding.

The patient at highest risk is on nothing-by-mouth status (NPO) and/or is maintained on clear liquids or intravenous fluids (IVs) for more than 5 days. These patients also include those who never eat a complete meal and rarely eat even one half of any food offered. Patients who eat only two servings of protein, take fluids poorly, or do not take dietary supplements would also be included in this highest risk category.

Friction and shear

Risk of developing a pressure ulcer is affected by the manner in which the skin contacts sheets, chairs, or other materials and devices. All other items on the Braden Scale have a scoring range from 1 to 4. The Friction and Shear item has a scoring range of 1 to 3. Thus, each of the other five items on the Braden Scale has the possibility of contributing 17.4% of the total risk score. The friction and shear item contributes a maximum of 13% to the total score.

If there is no apparent problem, there is little additional risk indicated (score equals 3). This means that the patient moves in bed or chair independently and has sufficient muscle strength to lift up completely during a move. Potential problems incur higher risk. Such patients may move feebly or require some assistance. During a move, skin may slide against the sheets, chair, or other materials and devices. These patients may occasionally slide down in chairs or in bed. Patients at highest risk require moderate to maximum assistance in moving. Complete lifting without the patient sliding against sheets is impossible. Such patients frequently slide down in chairs or in bed, requiring frequent repositioning; and spasticity, contractures, or agitation can lead to almost constant friction.

To summarize, the Braden Scale yields specific subscale scores for six domains. These subscale scores can be summed into a total score. In general, the lower the subscale score, the higher the risk for developing a pressure ulcer.

Diabetic Cancer Patients

The foregoing discussion focused on risk factors associated with the development of pressure ulcers. Neuropathy, often associated with cancer patients who also have diabetes, frequently decreases sensation in the lower extremities, thus increasing the chance of a wound developing. The American Diabetic Association (ADA) recently published a position statement regarding the prevention of chronic wounds in diabetic patients.[4] Identified risk factors included having diabetes for 10 years or more; male sex; poor glucose control; and cardiovascular, retinal, or renal complications. Additionally, foot deformity or limited joint mobility places patients at 12 times the risk for developing a chronic wound as patients who have intact protective sensation and no deformity or joint immobility.[5] A previous wound pathology places the patient at 36 times the risk for wound development.[5]

Several factors place diabetic patients at increased risk for foot, partial limb, or limb amputation. Acute Charcot's arthropathy (neuropathic osteoarthropathy) is a progressive condition affecting the musculoskeletal system.[5] The diabetic patient with a foot infection or ischemia is at the highest level of risk for amputation. The ADA lists the following foot-related conditions associated with increased risk of amputation:[4]

- Peripheral neuropathy with loss of protective sensation
- Altered biomechanics in the presence of neuropathy
- Evidence of increased pressure (erythema, hemorrhage under a callus)
- Bony deformity
- Peripheral vascular disease (decreased or absent pedal pulses)
- History of ulcers or amputation
- Severe nail pathology

Arterial ulcers

Typically occurring on the lower extremities, arterial (ischemic) ulcers can occur in cancer patients who are diabetic and those who are not diabetic but have peripheral vascular disease.[5] Smoking, high blood pressure, coronary artery disease, stress, hyperlipidemia, diabetes, obesity, and increasing age have been identified as risk factors.

Venous ulcers

Goldstein and colleagues have identified several factors that increase the likelihood of the development of leg ulcers of venous origin.[6] The factors include chronic venous insufficiency, varicose veins, arteriovenous (AV) fistula, and poor calf muscle pump. Such wounds are the most prevalent lower leg wounds and can be very difficult to heal.

Other lower leg ulcers in cancer patients

Leg ulcers may also be caused by squamous cell carcinoma (SCC). It has been suggested that certain factors may predispose individuals to SCC. Among those factors are burn scars, chronic infection or ulceration, and discoid lupus.[7]

In general, risk assessment is essential for identifying persons at risk for developing debilitating wounds. However, identifying risk is only one part of a two-part equation. Risk assessment alone has never prevented a wound.

PREVENTION

Consider the purpose for performing a wound risk assessment. It has been suggested that a risk assessment scale is a screening tool designed to help identify patients who might develop a wound.[3] Indeed, there are a plethora of tools and scales addressing pressure ulcers including Braden[2], Norton,[8] Gosnell,[9] Knoll,[10] and Waterlow[11] scales. The typical lecturer's response to the question of why one performs pressure ulcer risk assessments is, "to determine individuals who are at risk for developing pressure ulcers." Although this is certainly one role of risk assessments, there are others.

McNees, Braden, and Ovington have suggested that while the total score allows determinations of the general level of risk, the profile of subscale scores provides the basis for identifying ways of reducing risk and preventing wound development.[12] However, the development of a coherent detailed prevention plan may require more information that can be ascertained from the subscale scores.

Consider a patient who has the following Braden Scale scores: sensory perception = 3; moisture = 2; mobility = 3; activity = 2; nutrition = 2, and; friction/shear = 2. The total score would be 14, placing the patient at moderate risk for developing a wound. How might this risk be reduced? Risk is reduced by altering the conditions that are reducing the subscale scores. For example, consider the moisture item. A score of 2 indicates that the patient is often moist. However, to determine what should be done about the moisture, one needs to understand the source. Perhaps the person is incontinent. If so, is it fecal incontinence, urinary incontinence, or both? Does the incontinence occur during the day, at night, or both? If fecal incontinence is involved, are stools well formed or loose? These questions are being asked to illustrate how the subscale score may trigger further assessment needs. The answers to each of these questions affect specific elements of an effective prevention plan.

The most common preventive strategy for wounds that are of venous origins is compression and limb elevation. In cases of arterial compromise, patients should avoid situations that increase vascular constriction. Controlling risk factors such as smoking, high blood pressure, coronary artery disease, stress, and obesity will decrease the likelihood of wound development.

The ADA's position statement regarding chronic wounds specifies an annual foot examination as the cornerstone of prevention efforts.[4] According to the ADA this exam includes assessment of protective sensation, foot structure and biomechanics, vascular status, and skin integrity. If risk factors are present, examinations should be performed more frequently. If the patient has neuropathy, foot examinations should be performed at every visit to a health care professional. Such examinations are particularly important for diabetic patients with cancer, since other factors associated with cancer and cancer treatment may increase the difficulty of wound healing if a wound develops. Several strategies have identified by the ADA to reduce the probability of a wound developing:

- Maintain glycemic levels as near normal as possible.
- Cease smoking.
- Refer to a foot care specialist.
- If neuropathy or increased plantar pressure is present, use well-fitting walking or athletic shoes.
- Educate patients on the implications of sensory loss and ways to substitute other sensory modalities (hand palpation, visual inspection) for surveillance of early problems.
- If increased plantar pressure is present (i.e., erythema, warmth, callus, or measured pressure), use footwear that cushions and redistributes pressure.
- Callus can be debrided with a scalpel.
- Extra-wide shoes may be necessary for people with bony deformities.

ASSESSING CHRONIC WOUNDS

In spite of best risk assessment and prevention efforts, wounds develop. Wound assessment has been said to be the foundation for maintaining and evaluating a therapeutic plan of care.[13] Bates-Jensen points out that adequate baseline wound assessment is necessary for ensuring that the plan of care is appropriate and effective.[14] McNees goes further and suggests that the cornerstone of incremental improvements in health care practice is standardized assessment.[15] He argues that the absence of commonly accepted assessment protocols and a universal language for describing salient conditions affects clinical decision making and adherence to practice guidelines, and diminishes one's ability to ascertain the relationship between treatment and effects as well as whether there have been status changes between assessments.

Wound assessments should reliably reflect changes in wound status since the last assessment. The assessment should also provide information essential to formulating a wound management/treatment plan.

van Rijswijk suggests the rationale and frequency of reassessment and monitoring are affected by the overall patient condition, wound severity, patient care environment, the goal of care, and the plan of care.[13] In general, wounds are classified according to etiology and depth.[13] The Krasner/van Rijswijk classification algorithm discriminates between surgical wounds and nonsurgical wounds. Both surgical and nonsurgical wounds can be acute or chronic. Incisions, excisions, and skin graft donor sites are examples of acute surgical wounds. Examples of chronic surgical wounds include dehisced or infected wounds. Acute nonsurgical wound are exemplified by mild burns, abrasions, and skin tears. As suggested previously, chronic nonsurgical wounds include pressure ulcers, leg ulcers (e.g., venous ulcers, arterial ulcers), and foot ulcers (e.g., diabetic ulcers). Regardless of etiology, wounds are also classified by depth. Such wounds as blisters are considered superficial wounds. Partial thickness wounds include donor sites and stage II pressure ulcers. Punch biopsies and stage III or stage IV pressure ulcers are examples of full thickness wounds. While each system varies for wounds of different etiologies, early attempts to classify wounds utilized staging or grading protocols.

The Agency for Health Care Policy and Research (now Agency for Healthcare Research and Quality) guidelines outline the following "stage" classification system for pressure ulcers.[16]

Stage 1

Nonblanchable erythema of intact skin, the heralding lesion of skin ulceration. In individuals with darker skin, discoloration of the skin, warmth, edema, induration, or hardness may also be indicators. A stage I pressure ulcer is an observable pressure-related alteration of intact skin, whose indicators may include changes as compared to the adjacent or opposite area on the body in one or more of the following: skin temperature (warmth or coolness), tissue consistency (firm or boggy feel), and/or sensation (pain, itching). The ulcer appears as a defined area of persistent redness in lightly pigmented skin, whereas in darker skin tones the ulcer may appear with persistent red, blue, or purple hues.

Stage 2

Partial thickness skin loss involving epidermis, dermis, or both. The ulcer is superficial and presents clinically as an abrasion, blister, or shallow crater.

Stage 3

Full thickness skin loss involving damage to or necrosis of subcutaneous tissue that may extend down to, but not through, the underlying fascia. The ulcer presents clinically as a deep crater with or without undermining of adjacent tissue.

Stage 4

Full thickness skin loss with extensive destruction, tissue necrosis, or damage to muscle, bone, or supporting structures (e.g., tendon, joint capsule). Undermining and the development of sinus tracts also may be associated with stage 4 pressure ulcers.

Although such a staging system yields a general idea as to the severity of a pressure ulcer, there are two major problems in using such a system to support clinical decision making and tracking wound status changes. Put simply, the staging system does not provide sufficient information to allow judgment as to how the wound should be treated or whether it has been treated appropriately. For example, although it is possible to determine whether there is a wound cavity, it is not possible to determine whether the cavity should be filled with a product that hydrates the wound bed or one that absorbs excess moisture.

Staging a pressure ulcer and accounting at the same time for wound status changes over time is also problematic. As a wound becomes more severe, dermis, fat, and muscle are lost. However, as wounds heal, granulation tissue fills the cavity before reepithelialization occurs. In brief, wounding and healing are two different processes, each possessing very different characteristics. Thus a stage 3 pressure ulcer that is healing cannot become a stage 2 wound. In fact, it is a "healing" stage 3 pressure ulcer until there is complete reepithelialization, at which time it becomes a healed stage 3 wound.

The problems with "reverse staging" or "back-staging" have been articulated by the National Pressure Ulcer Advisory Panel and others.[17-20] Bates-Jensen provided one of the first examples of an assessment alternative that quantitatively described the status of salient physiologic wound characteristics.[21] Bates-Jensen's *Pressure Sore Status Tool (PSST)* evaluates 13 anatomic wound characteristics on a 5-point scale, with a score of 5 representing the most serious rating for a particular characteristic and 1 representing the least serious. The *Pressure Sore Status Tool* was subsequently renamed the *Bates-Jensen Wound Assessment (BWAT)* after it was validated for use with wounds other than pressure ulcers. Wound characteristics addressed in the BWAT include size (wound area), depth, wound edges, undermining/tunneling, type of necrotic tissue, amount of necrotic tissue, type of exudates, amount of exudates, skin coloration surrounding the wound, peripheral edema, peripheral induration, granulation tissue, and epithelialization.

Even though the PSST/BWAT was the first empirically-based chronic wound assessment tool, it remains the most comprehensive. It has been argued that a disadvantage in using the BWAT is the amount of time it takes to administer.[22] Other tools for assessing pressure ulcers include the Sussman Wound Healing Tool,[23] Sessing Scale,[24] Wound Healing Scale,[25] and the Pressure Ulcer Scale for Healing (PUSH).[26]

The purposes for assessing a wound are to ascertain changes in wound status over time and to aid the formulation of treatment or management alternatives.

TREATING CHRONIC WOUNDS

It can be difficult to find a clinician who thinks he or she might not know how to treat wounds. The principles of wound treatment that result in superior outcomes have been known for decades. Still, less effective methods too frequently remain the treatment of choice.

Jones and Harding have said, "Moist wound healing is considered to be the ideal environment for optimal wound healing."[27] While considerable work arguably preceded his work, George Winter's porcine studies, published in 1962, provided a remarkably clear illustration of the healing differences in wounds exposed to air and left to scab as compared to those kept moist by polythene.[28] In brief, it was shown that when scabs form, new epithelium has to burrow beneath the scab. Thus, the scab acts as a barrier to the epidermal cells. Wounds kept moist by polythene had no such barrier, and the epidermis proceeded to grow without hindrance. In over 4 decades since Winter's seminal publication, the literature documenting the effects of moist wound healing has grown to the point that it is no longer a topic of debate among wound experts.

It is somewhat ironic that when considering wound treatment, many clinicians continue to think primarily of gauze use. Gauze has played a role in medical care for over a century, being used in a variety of ways and impregnated with a variety of substances. A common procedure involves saturating gauze with water or saline, applying the wet bandage to a wound, and allowing it to dry. The adverse effects of using wet-to-dry gauze in wound treatment were documented over 20 years ago.[29] Yet gauze use continues, and general-purpose gauze is marketed under at least 48 different brands.[30] Using standardized assessment and care protocols that predominantly relied on principles of moist wound healing and advanced non–gauze dressings, Bolton and colleagues reported wound healing rates for 767 wounds that were superior to prior healing rates reported in the literature.[31] These results build on and support the considerable evidence accumulated from prior studies regarding the effects of standardized assessment and treatment using principles of moist wound healing. The computerized algorithm used in Bolton and colleagues' study was sophisticated; and yet, only a few fundamental elements of effective treatment exist.

Despite the many nuances of wound treatment, three principles should guide most wound care considerations: (1) clean the wound bed; (2) pack the cavity with an appropriate primary dressing, and (3) cover the wound with an appropriate secondary dressing. In turn, in addressing these basics there are a few fundamental questions that should guide practice: Is the wound bed clean? What type of necrosis (if any) is present? Does a cavity exist? Is the wound bed wet (heavily exuding), moist, or dry (virtually no exudates)?

What is the condition of the surrounding skin? Are there signs of infection?

Clean Wound Beds

One of the goals of care is a clean wound bed. This involves the removal of all inflammatory foreign bodies. Cleansing with water, saline, or commercial wound cleansers is one alternative. Irrigation of the wound bed can be accomplished with a bulb syringe, by delivering fluid through a syringe and needle or catheter, or an irrigation device. Cleaning should typically occur with each dressing change.

Types of Necrosis Present

A plan for removing necrotic tissue should be devised. Debridement choices fall into four categories: (1) autolytic, (2) enzymatic, (3) surgical, and (4) mechanical. *Autolytic debridement* typically involves use of an occlusive or semiocclusive cover dressing to allow lytic enzymes present in the wound fluid to "naturally" debride the necrosis. *Enzymatic debridement* employs specific enzymes that act on eschar, protein, and nucleic acids.[32] *Surgical* or *sharp debridement* should be performed by a qualified clinician and is the fastest and most effective way to remove devitalized necrotic tissue.[32] If infection is present, surgical or sharp debridement should be considered as the method of choice. *Mechanical debridement* involves applying wet gauze to a wound, then allowing it to dry. When removed, the dried gauze adheres to the necrosis. Unfortunately, gauze does not discriminate devitalized tissue from granulation tissue or normal tissue, which may also be removed with equal effectiveness. Mechanical debridement can be painful and result in bleeding.

If hard, black eschar characterizes the type of necrotic tissue and autolytic or enzymatic debridement is being used, cross-hatching the eschar with a scalpel should be considered. This procedure will allow moisture to better penetrate the eschar.

Existence of a Cavity

If the wound is full thickness and a cavity exists, the cavity should be filled. In considering the optimal filler, it should be remembered that maintaining a moist wound environment should be a goal of care. Thus, if the wound is wet and highly exudating, a product that absorbs moisture should be considered. Such products in include alginates and hydrofibers. If the wound bed is dry and there is little or no exudate, a hydrating agent, such as a hydrogel, should be considered.

Condition of the Surrounding Skin

The condition of the skin surrounding the wound can affect the choice of the cover dressing. For example, adhesive dressing edges should not be placed over macerated skin. Redness surrounding the wound or streaks emanating from the wound can indicate infection.

Signs of Infection

While infection is confirmed by laboratory results (e.g., more than 105 organisms per gram of tissue or the presence of specific organisms such as streptococci), clinicians should observe for other signs of possible infection. Such signs include edema, warmth surrounding the wound, pain in the wound, erythema, a foul odor, and purulent drainage (National Pressure Ulcer Advisory Panel, www.npuap.org/woundinfection.html). If necrosis is present and the wound is infected, surgical, sharp, or some other form of rapid debridement should be considered.

SKIN AND WOUND CARE FOR WOMEN WITH CANCER

Skin and wound care for cancer patients is often considered in the context of palliative care.[33] For such patients, mobility, activity, sensory loss, and a myriad of other factors are often issues, and the risk of developing pressure ulcers is high. Unfortunately, comorbid conditions that may delay wound healing are frequently present in this population.

Skin care is also frequently considered in the context of side effects to treatment.[34] Radiotherapy may result in acute skin reactions such as local irritation, erythema, dry flaky skin, and moist sloughing of the epidermal layers.[35]

Radiation as a cumulative process has side effects beyond fatigue. Skin irritation, itchiness, redness, shininess, soreness, peeling, blistering, swelling, hyposensation, and hypersensation can all be side effects. Avoid direct sun.[34] Ellen Sitton[36] provides an excellent review of the side effects of skin changes in radiation oncology. Among the recommendations for reducing the symptoms to irradiated skin she suggests are the following:

- Protect the skin from sun exposure.
- Avoid mechanical irritants such as scratching, wash with hands rather than a wash cloth, avoid tape, and shave with an electric razor and not a blade razor.
- Reduce use of chemical irritants. Use mild soap. Avoid the use of detergents. Use mild detergent to wash clothing.
- Avoid thermal irritants. Use lukewarm water. Avoid exposure to temperature extremes.
- Keep skin folds dry.
- Wear cotton clothing.
- Prevent infection.

Belcher has identified several major categories of chemotherapy-related cutaneous toxicity that may result in skin anomalies: these include alopecia, hyperpigmentation, photo-sensitivity, extravasation injury, and hypersensitivity reactions.[37] Specific skin conditions such as redness, rashes, itching, peeling, dryness, acne, and increased sun sensitivity are common during chemotherapy. Certain medications may cause the skin to darken. Certain IV-administered drugs can cause rather serious problems if leakage occurs.[38]

Chemotherapy can also affect the risk of developing wounds. For example, paclitaxel and carboplatin can cause damage to nerve endings in fingers and toes, resulting in possible numbness.[34] If such conditions occur in women with diabetes, the likelihood of neuropathic foot ulcers' developing may be increased.

Thus when considering wound care, cancer patients and those providing care to them face special issues and challenges. However, the fundamental issues of appropriate skin and wound care are the same. Assess risk in a methodical fashion using a reliable and valid risk assessment instrument and protocol. Use the information gleaned from the risk assessment to inform a prevention plan that reduces the probability of developing a wound. If a wound develops, use standardized assessment to describe the wound status and to inform the treatment plan. Use evidence-based treatment practices. Monitor healing progress, and change treatment strategies if the wound is not healing. This four-part paradigm was previously used to describe the conditions necessary for incrementally improving international health care practice.[13] The paradigm is also applicable to considerations of skin and wound care for women with cancer.

REFERENCES

1. Kane D: Chronic wound healing and chronic wound management. In Krasner DL, Rodeheaver GT, Sibbald RG, co-editors: *Chronic wound care: a clinical source book for healthcare professionals,* ed 3, Wayne, Penna., 2001, HMP Communications.
2. Bergstrom N and others: The Braden Scale for predicting pressure ulcer risk, *Nurs Res* 36(4):205-210, 1987.
3. Ayello EA, Braden B: How and why to do pressure ulcer risk assessment, *Adv Skin Wound Care* 15(3):125-132, 2002.
4. American Diabetes Association: Preventive foot care in diabetes, *Diabetes Care* 27:S63-S64, 2004.
5. Colburn L: Prevention of chronic wounds. In Krasner DL, Rodeheaver GT, Sibbald RG, co-editors: *Chronic wound care: a clinical source book for healthcare professionals,* ed 3, Wayne, Penna., 2001, HMP Communications.
6. Goldstein, DR and others: Differential diagnosis: assessment of the lower extremity ulcer: is it arterial, venous or neuropathic? *Wounds* 10(4):125-131, 1998.
7. Bowman PH, Hogan DJ: Leg ulcers: a common problem with sometimes uncommon etiologies, *Geriatrics* 54(3):43, 47-48, 50 passim, 1999.
8. Norton D: Norton Scale for decubitus prevention, *Krankenpflege* 34(1):16, 1980.
9. Gosnell DJ: An assessment tool to identify pressure ulcers, *Nurs Res* 22(1):55-59, 1973.
10. Towey AP, Erland SM: Validity and reliability of an assessment tool for pressure ulcer risk, *Decubitus* 1(2): 40-48, 1988.
11. Waterlow J: Pressure ulcer scores: a risk assessment card, *Nurs Times* 81(48):49-55, 1985.
12. McNees P, Braden B, Ovington L: Beyond risk assessment: elements for pressure ulcer prevention, *Ostomy Wound Manage* 44(Suppl):51S-58S, 1998.
13. van Rijswijk L: Wound assessment and documentation. In Krasner DL, Rodeheaver GT, Sibbald RG, co-editors: *Chronic wound care: a clinical source book for healthcare professionals,* ed 3, Wayne, Penna., 2001, HMP Communications.
14. Bates-Jensen BM: Chronic wound assessment, *Nurs Clin North Am* 34(4):799-845, 1999.
15. McNees MP: International systems to support incremental improvement in healthcare. In Davidson P, editor: *Best practices series: healthcare information systems,* London, 1999, Auerbach.

16. Bergstrom N and others: Treatment of pressure ulcers, Clinical Practice Guideline, No. 15, AHCPR Publication No. 95-0652, Rockville, MD, 1994, U.S. Department of Health and Human Services, Public Health Service, Agency for Health Care Policy and Research.
17. Maklebust J: Policy implications of using reverse staging to monitor pressure ulcer status, *Adv Wound Care* 10(5): 32-35, 1997.
18. Baranoski S, Ayello EA: *Wound care essentials: practice principles,* Springhouse, PA, 2004, Lippincott.
19. Maklebust J: Perplexing questions about pressure ulcers, *Decubitus* 5(4):15, 1992.
20. Xakellis G, Frantz RA: Pressure ulcer healing: What is it? What influences it? How is it measured? *Adv Wound Care* 10(5):20-26, 1997.
21. Bates-Jensen B: New pressure ulcer status tool, *Decubitus* 3(3):14-15, 1990.
22. Woodbury MG and others: Pressure ulcer assessment instruments: a critical appraisal, *Ostomy Wound Manage* 45(5):42-45, 1999.
23. Sussman, C: Presenting a draft pressure ulcer scale to monitor healing, *Adv Wound Care* 10(5):92, 1997.
24. Ferrell BA, Artinian BM, Sessing D: The Sessing Scale for assessment of pressure ulcer healing, *J Am Geriatr Soc* 43(1):37-40, 1995.
25. Krasner D: Wound healing scale, Version 1.0: a proposal, *Adv Wound Care* 10(5):82-85, 1997.
26. Thomas DR and others: Pressure ulcer scale for healing: derivation and validation of the PUSH tool. The PUSH Task Force, *Adv Wound Care* 10(5):96-101, 1999.
27. Jones V, Harding K: Moist wound healing. In Krasner DL, Rodeheaver GT, Sibbald RG, co-editors: *Chronic wound care: a clinical source book for healthcare professionals,* ed 3, Wayne, Penna., 2001, HMP Communications.
28. Winter GD: Formation of the scab and the rate of epithelialization of superficial wounds in the skin of the young domestic pig, *Nature* 193:293-294, 1962.
29. Alvarez OM, Mertz PM, Eaglstein WH: The effects of occlusive dressings on collagen synthesis and re-epithelialization in superficial wounds, *J Surg Res* 35(2):142-148, 1983.
30. Ovington L, Peirce B: Wound dressings: form, function, feasibility and facts. In Krasner DL, Rodeheaver GT, Sibbald RG, co-editors: *Chronic wound care: a clinical source book for healthcare professionals,* ed 3, Wayne, Pennsylvania, 2001, HMP Communications.
31. Bolton L, McNees MP, van Rijswijk L: Wound-healing outcomes using standardized assessment and care in clinical practice, *J Wound Ostomy Continence Nurs* 31(2):65-71, 2004.
32. Dolynchuk K: Debridement. In Krasner DL, Rodeheaver GT, Sibbald RG, co-editors: *Chronic wound care: a clinical source book for healthcare professionals,* ed 3, Wayne, Pennsylvania, 2001, HMP Communications.
33. BM, Early L, Seaman S: Skin disorders. In Ferrell BR, Coyle N, editors: *Textbook of Palliative Care,* Oxford, 2001, Oxford University Press.
34. Hartman, LC, Loprinzi, CL: *Mayo Clinic guide to women's cancer,* Rochester, Minn, 2005, Mayo Clinic Health Information.
35. Naylor W, Laverty D, Mallett J: *The Royal Marsden Hospital handbook of wound management in cancer care,* Oxford, 2001, Blackwell Science.
36. Sitton E: Managing side effects of skin changes and fatigue. In Dow KH and others: *Nursing care in radiation oncology,* ed 2, Philadelphia, 1997, W.B. Saunders.
37. Belcher AE, Selekof JS: Skin care for the oncology patient. In Krasner DL, Rodeheaver GT, Sibbald RG, co-editors: *Chronic wound care: a clinical source book for healthcare professionals,* ed 3, Wayne, Pennsylvania, 2001, HMP Communications.
38. Bellenir K: *Cancer sourcebook for women,* ed 2, Detroit, 2002, Omnigraphics.

CHAPTER

15 *Anxiety and Depression*

Patricia A. Carter

INTRODUCTION AND OVERVIEW

The diagnosis and treatment of cancer may be associated with increased anxiety and depression;[1-3] however, the extent and severity of these symptoms have varied greatly among the patient populations in different studies. For example, in a sample of 170 patients with newly diagnosed cancer, 50% met the criteria for anxiety, depression or both, 1 year after diagnosis; 25% in the second, third, and fourth years; and 15% in the fifth year. Of patients with recurrence, 45% experienced depression, anxiety, or both within 3 months of diagnosis.[4] In a study of patients with epithelial ovarian cancer, 21% of the patients scored above the clinical cut-off for the Center for Epidemiological Studies Depression Scale (greater than 16) placing them at increased risk for clinical depression.[5] In contrast, Berard[6] found rates of depressive disorder to be 14% among samples of patients with breast cancer, head and neck cancer, and lymphoma. This variation may be the result of methodologic difference between studies.

Irrespective of the true prevalence, a diagnosis of cancer is a stressful event that often generates a great deal of fear and uncertainty; therefore symptoms of anxiety and depression are not surprising. Sanson-Fisher and colleagues[7] found that psychologic needs made up 5 of the 10 highest unmet supportive care needs in a survey of 888 people undergoing treatment for cancer.

This chapter will focus on depression and anxiety in cancer patients. Literature describing depression and anxiety in cancer patients will be presented, along with a discussion of the etiology and risk factors for depression and anxiety in this population. A discussion of ways to prevent and treat depression and anxiety is presented next. The final sections of this chapter present special considerations for elderly clients and implications for nursing.

While it is rarely specifically stated in this chapter, the information presented here has been derived from studies primarily conducted with female participants. The exceptions are noted where they occur. A concerted effort was made to include studies with women diagnosed with cancers other than breast cancer; however, a majority of studies exploring anxiety and depression have been conducted with breast cancer populations.

Background Relating to Anxiety and Depression

Depression is an important and neglected problem in cancer patients.[8] Previous studies have estimated the prevalence of depression in cancer patients to be as high as 50%.[1-3,9] Depression has substantial impact on the quality of life of cancer patients and may lead to a reduction in compliance with medical treatment and poorer outcomes from treatment.[10] Yet studies show that psychiatric disorders commonly go unrecognized and untreated in cancer patients.[11,12] Several factors contribute to this lack of acknowledgment of psychologic symptoms in cancer patients. These factors are discussed in detail in the treatment and management section of this chapter.

Why is depression in cancer patients a concern? After all, it is "normal" to feel depressed following a diagnosis of cancer. One answer to this question is that comorbid psychologic conditions can have an impact on patients' treatment and recovery. Depression can result in greater pain and poorer physical and social functioning.[13] Depression can also affect both the severity and number of side effects, and can lead to greater anxiety and fatigue experienced by cancer patients.[14] In a study with 60 women diagnosed with uterine cancer, Ahlberg and colleagues[15] found significant correlations between general fatigue and anxiety and also between general fatigue and depression. In fact, depression explained 44% of the variance in general fatigue.

Anxiety can be defined as an unpleasant subjective experience associated with the perception of a real or imagined threat and is a common symptom in connection with cancer. Cancer diagnosis and its treatments often are associated with negative side effects, such as increased anxiety;[16-18] however, anxiety after cancer diagnosis is not necessarily abnormal. Anxiety may not present a problem, or may even be a constructive part of dealing with problems.[19] An assessment of the level of anxiety in cancer patient populations is important because abnormal anxiety is disruptive[20] and amenable to pharmacologic and psychologic treatment.[21]

ETIOLOGY AND RISK FACTORS

Researchers who have attempted to determine whether female cancer patients are at greater risk for anxiety and/or depression have mostly been unsuccessful. One study found that women had higher levels of anxiety when compared to men in a study of 178 patients with various cancer diagnoses (lymphoma, renal cell carcinoma, malignant melanoma).[22] The information presented in this section speaks to the etiology and risk factors for anxiety and depression in cancer patients. Most studies discussed had primarily female participants; departures from gender-based predictions are noted.

Internal and External Factors

Studies have found that several internal and external factors contribute to the experiences of psychologic distress in cancer patients. Internal factors include sociodemographic characteristics such as age and education level, and disease-related factors such as stage, functional status, and physical distress such as pain and dyspnea. Coping responses and personality characteristics (pessimism, optimism) are additional internal factors that contribute to cancer patients' psychologic distress. External factors include treatment-related factors, social support systems, and experiences with health care providers.

Sociodemographic Characteristics

Sociodemographic characteristics such as younger age and low educational level have been associated with psychologic distress in cancer patients. Thewes and colleagues[23] found in a qualitative study with women with breast cancer that being under the age of 50 greatly increased reports of depression compared to older women. These findings were supported in a study with women with metastatic disease in Australia. Kissane and colleagues[24] found younger women (under 50 years of age) with metastatic breast disease were significantly more depressed than women without metastatic disease or older women with metastatic disease. Educational level was found to be a significant predictor of psychologic distress. In a study with 212 patients with non–small cell lung cancer 1 year after curative resection, educational level below junior high school was a significant predictor of depression.[25]

Disease-related Factors

Disease-related factors such as advanced disease stage, poor functional status, and physical distress from pain and dyspnea have been associated with psychologic distress in cancer patients. Stage of illness is different from the length of diagnosis with cancer. Newly diagnosed patients often express more anxiety and depression than those who have been diagnosed for a longer time. Stage of illness, indicating degree of metastasis, is associated with higher levels of anxiety and depression across cancer types. The most common studies of cancer in women have been conducted with breast cancer. These studies have consistently shown a strong association between advanced stage of illness and increased levels of depression and anxiety.[26,27] Functional status before and following cancer diagnosis have been found to be predictors of psychologic distress in cancer patients. Specifically, poorer functional status is associated with higher levels of depression and anxiety in cancer patients.[28,29]

Physical Symptoms

Physical symptoms, specifically pain and dyspnea, have been associated with increased psychologic distress in cancer patients. The relationship between pain and depression is a complex one. Some scientists hypothesize that pain results in higher depression levels, while others think that depression increases pain levels. A study with 121 hospitalized cancer patients found those with depression reported higher levels of pain, insomnia, anorexia, and fatigue than cancer patients who were not depressed.[30] Patients with uncontrolled pain were found to report significantly higher levels of depression and anxiety than those without pain.[27,31,32] Patients with dyspnea were more likely to report higher levels of depression and anxiety than those with fewer respiratory symptoms.[33] Depression adds significantly to the burden of illness experienced by cancer patients. Depression may also result in physical symptoms becoming resistant to conventional treatments, with improvement seen only when depression is appropriately treated.[27,31]

Treatment-related Factors

Treatment-related factors, chemotherapy, surgery, and radiation therapy have been significantly associated with psychologic distress.[34-37] For example, chemotherapy, although essential, often challenges the patient and family with several adverse side effects. These side effects can control the patient's life. Fatigue severely disrupts the individual's ability to carry out activities of daily living.[38,39] Nausea and vomiting prevent adequate nutrition.[40] Dyspnea is a frightful experience for both the family and patient. The sensation of "not being able to catch one's breath" or "air hunger" is very distressing for both the patient and family.[41] Mucositis, sexual dysfunction, alopecia, pain, and anemia are a few more common symptoms related to chemotherapy that can influence patients' quality of life and cause psychologic distress. The focus of this chapter is not to review the symptoms commonly seen as a result of cancer therapies, only to raise the awareness that these symptoms can contribute to psychologic distress in cancer patients.

Coping

Coping responses and lack of social support have been associated with psychologic distress in cancer patients. Coping responses are broadly defined in many studies. A study conducted by Akechi and colleagues[42] with 148 postoperative ambulatory breast cancer patients in Japan identified low fighting spirit, high fatalism, and high helplessness/hopelessness as significantly correlated with increased symptoms of depression and anxiety. These findings support those from other studies of the relationship between psychologic distress and coping that have found that the most beneficial response is fighting spirit and the most deleterious response may be helplessness/ hopelessness.[26,43,44]

Similarly, fatalism, avoidance, and hopelessness were found to be significant predictors of depression in Grassi and colleagues[45] study with Mediterranean cancer patients. Furthermore, some studies have revealed that the coping response may affect the patient's physical outcomes. A follow-up study of breast cancer patients revealed that those who responded to cancer with fighting spirit were more likely to be alive and free of recurrence at 15-year follow-up than those who responded with helplessness/hopelessness.[46] These findings suggest that coping response may play a significant role in psychologic distress outcomes.

Social Support

Social support may be an important factor in how well patients adapt to their cancer experience. Social support has been found to be beneficial in helping individuals adjust to stressful situations, including medical illness, and researchers have found that perceived social support moderates the negative effects of stressful life events.[44,47] Several years have been dedicated to exploring the relationships between social support and overall health and well-being; however, relatively little is known about this relationship within the context of the cancer experience. One study conducted with cancer patients undergoing surgery revealed that patients with very high levels of social support had less psychologic distress.[44] Others have found that high social support was associated with better emotional adjustment and better mood.[48] The benefits of social support have also been documented in patients with head and neck cancers.[49] Burgess and colleagues[4] found in a 5-year observational cohort study that a "lack of an intimate confiding relationship" was a significant predictor of long-term depression and anxiety in cancer patients.

Personality Characteristics

Personality characteristics influence how an individual will view the diagnosis of cancer: is the cancer a threat to be feared (pessimism) or a challenge to be overcome (optimism)? Pessimism was the strongest predictor of anxiety and depression 1 year following cancer surgery.[50] Optimists and pessimists differed not only in regard to coping styles, but also in regard to predictors of depression and anxiety. Optimists experiencing anxiety at the time of diagnosis had about a 6-times higher risk of experiencing anxiety 1 year later, compared to optimists without preoperative anxiety. For pessimists, the more pessimistic one was about one's overall future, the higher the risk for developing anxiety 1 year after surgery. Pessimists who used helpless/hopeless coping style when receiving a diagnosis of cancer had 3 times the risk for experiencing depression than pessimists who did not.

PATIENT AND PROVIDER INTERACTIONS

The quality of the interactions between cancer patients and their health care providers has been a strong predictor of psychologic distress. Specifically the experience of hearing "bad news" appears to have an effect on the patient's overall experience. Negative experiences during all stages of treatment were found to be associated with high anxiety and depression scores.[51] A cancer diagnosis confronts a patient with a completely new world of medical terminology, different diagnostic and therapeutic procedures, and emotional, cognitive, and behavioral reactions, as well as reactions of significant others. The patient meets a multitude of new people such as nurses, doctors, and therapists, who can influence the experience to be more positive or more negative.

Much effort focuses on studying the impact on patients' psychologic reaction of breaking bad news.[52] Attempts have also been made to assess patients' opinions and perceptions about the process of breaking bad news. Girgis and colleagues,[53] for example, found that patients and doctors agree only minimally over the importance of the order of the different steps and principles defined as the "breaking bad news" guidelines. The medical system comprises not only dimensions of treatment, but to a great extent the social contacts a patient makes with the medical and health care staff during cancer treatment. These contacts can be an important source of support for coping with the illness, or they can act as an additional stressor.

The ultimate goal of cancer treatment, second to cure, is quality of life. Studies using formal assessments of quality of life have confirmed an association between depression, anxiety, and impaired quality of life.[28,54,55] Smith, Gomm, and Dickens[56] examined the association between depression and various dimensions of quality of life. They confirmed that pain, anxiety, and depression were associated with impaired quality of life in a study with 65 palliative care cancer patients. Anxiety and depression contributed independently toward global health status, emotional and cognitive functioning, and fatigue. Anxiety further contributed significantly towards poor social functioning, and increased nausea and vomiting.

PREVENTION RELATING SPECIFICALLY TO WOMEN

It may be an unrealistic goal to attempt to prevent *all* anxiety and depression in cancer patients. Conversely, a "realistic" goal is to decrease the intensity of and the negative outcomes from anxiety and depression symptoms. The next section discusses ways to detect, assess, and treat anxiety and depression in cancer patients.

TREATMENT AND SYMPTOM MANAGEMENT

Anxiety and depression can mimic physical symptoms of cancer treatments, and consequently emotional distress may not be detected. This is important to recognize, since depression has been significantly correlated with increased mortality in cancer patients. Hjerl and colleagues[57] used survival analysis of data from three central registers and found that breast cancer patients with depression had a modestly but significantly higher risk of mortality depending on stage of cancer and time of depression. Of the 20,593 cases reviewed 5,648 patients died from natural causes. Preoperative depression was associated with a significantly higher relative rate of mortality for late-stage breast cancer patients. The same trend was seen for early-stage breast cancer patients, although it was not significant. For early-stage patients, postoperative depression was a significantly higher relative risk for mortality. The same effect was not seen in the late-stage patients. Watson and colleagues[58] found depression to significantly contribute to increased mortality rates in a study with 578 early-stage breast cancer patients.

Assessment and Detection

In order to treat depression and anxiety the clinician must first be able to detect and assess these complex symptoms. Patients may present verbal and nonverbal cues of their distress, or they may somaticize and appear for treatment with physical complaints. This last presentation may be the most challenging for clinicians. Each of these presentations will be discussed, followed by suggestions for techniques that can be used by clinicians to detect and assess anxiety and depression in cancer patients.

Patients experiencing emotional distress are likely to provide verbal cues or report symptoms of psychologic nature in primary care consultations[59] (e.g., "I'm feeling really upset about my diagnosis."). In contrast, cancer patients tend not to disclose psychologic distress, and therefore verbal cues are likely to be indirect (e.g., "I guess a lot of people feel down when they get cancer."). Patients with higher levels of emotional distress are more likely to mention psychologic symptoms, signal emotional needs, and request information during a medical consultation.[60,61] Some patients may not be this direct; however, nonverbal behavior often conveys more information than verbal behavior in the communication process.[62] Nonverbal behaviors that suggest possible psychologic morbidity include postural or movement cues, such as dejected pose or excessive or lack of movement, and vocal cues, such as an unmodulated or distressed tone.[60,63]

Patients who are first seen with physical symptoms are less likely to have their depression recognized, especially if psychologic symptoms are mentioned late in the consultation or not at all.[64] This could potentially result from patients' somaticizing or normalizing their feelings of depression.[64] Patients may first be seen with gastrointestinal problems, chronic pain, or fatigue.[61,65] Oncologists expect to observe and treat these symptoms in their patients and, in the absence of other indications of distress, may not suspect an underlying emotional cause. Sayar and colleagues[65] found that 75% of patients who have clinically significant anxiety or depression manifest somatic symptoms, and that accurate recognition of psychologic distress becomes less likely with increasing somatization.

Establishing Rapport

Given these challenges presented by patients, what is a clinician to do? Clinicians must elicit feelings and emotions from their patients. Rapport between the patient and the clinician is essential for effective communication; it requires clinicians to be interested in the feelings and concerns of their patients and to generate an atmosphere in which patients feel comfortable enough to disclose feelings and concerns. This process involves active listening and the identification of verbal and nonverbal cues. If clinicians are not familiar with these techniques, they may unintentionally create barriers to communication. In addition, patients may also conceal their emotions or block discussions of this nature for a variety of reasons, such as attitudes toward the clinician's role and toward their condition, and differences in willingness to disclose emotional concerns.

Patient Attitudes

Patients' attitudes about the clinician's role can affect the amount of information they disclose about psychosocial issues. Patients perceive their doctors to be too busy to be burdened with this type of information.[60,63] Cape[66,67] interviewed patients experiencing high levels of psychologic distress, and found that almost half of them did not disclose their symptoms because they felt embarrassed or hesitant to trouble the physician with their problems, while almost 20% felt deterred by the behavior of the doctor.

Patients' attitudes towards their own condition can also influence their willingness to disclose information. Data suggest that patients may perceive that their fears and concerns are silly or unreasonable, or that their symptoms are a predictable result of their illness, and therefore they do not disclose them to their doctor. Patients may also be embarrassed about discussing psychosocial issues because they feel it reflects badly on their coping abilities.[60,63]

Differences in patients' willingness to disclose emotional concerns may be related to demographic factors; however, these associations are not consistent. Studies of the effect of age,[68] gender[20,69-71] and ethnicity[72] have failed to determine systematic differences. However the relationship between educational level and communication style appears more consistent. Patients with higher levels of education are more likely to request information and provide evidence of emotional needs.[20] Because of the high level of contradictory evidence, demographic characteristics are not reliable indicators of distress or psychologic morbidity.

INTERVENTION TECHNIQUES

Techniques such as active listening, using open questions and emotional words, responding appropriately to patients' emotional cues, and a patient-centered consulting style can assist in detection of depression and anxiety in patients. Screening tools for psychologic distress and patient question prompt sheets administered before the consultation can also be useful.

Active Listening

Active listening is perhaps the most important technique of identifying cues and distress in cancer patients. Active listening involves attending to and observing verbal and nonverbal behaviors, and understanding them in the context of the patient's life and circumstances.[60] Special emphasis on attention to nonverbal communication increases detection of cues and distress. Active listening involves using eye contact, having an attentive posture, and facilitating the patient's disclosure through behaviors such as nodding and making noises of agreement or encouragement. The patient is aware of whether or not they are being listened to, and are more likely to disclose information if the listener is conveying empathy and interest both verbally and nonverbally. A brief summary of what the person has conveyed at the end of her statement confirms that the listener has accurately heard and understood, and permits the speaker to correct any misconceptions. Active listening requires an objective state of mind and genuine interest in the concerns of the patient, and thereby leads to the ability to detect cues that may convey information about the patient's state.[17,60]

Patient-centered consulting is where the needs and wants of the patient are put first, dealing with the patient holistically rather than specifically with her illness. This style involves listening and allowing the patient to explain her issues and expectations, and can also involve shared decision making.[73,74] Thus the patient is involved in making treatment decisions, and her true needs are addressed. This style of consultation is preferred by the majority of patients[75] and is conducive to more effective communication when compared with clinician-centered consultations, where the clinician makes the agenda.

Alternative Treatments

Alternative treatments that have been tried to reduce anxiety and depression in cancer patients include progressive muscle relaxation, guided imagery, relaxation training, and support groups. Progressive muscle relaxation and guided imagery techniques have been used for several years in nursing and the medical management of patients with cancer. These techniques have been found useful in treating cancer pain;[76,77] for relieving the adverse side effects of chemotherapy, such as nausea and vomiting, and for promoting improved quality of life.[78]

Sloman[77] reported significant improvement in depression and quality of life following progressive muscle relaxation and guided imagery with 56 advanced-stage cancer patients. Women diagnosed with cancer who participated in a study conducted by Alder and Bitzer[51] most frequently expressed a need for relaxation training. Over one quarter of the women expressed a need for additional counseling for body image changes and sexuality, creative therapy, and group therapy that focuses on anxiety reduction and coping strategies in general. Only 35% of the women did not want to take part in any psycho-oncology treatments. Further analysis revealed that these women who requested no additional treatment reported significantly lower anxiety and depression scores than those who requested more treatments.

SPECIAL CONSIDERATIONS

Elderly

More rigorous cancer treatment, often centered today in outpatient facilities, requires a higher level of patient participation and responsibility. There is usually more frank disclosure of diagnosis, prognosis, and treatment options by physicians than in the past. Patients and families appear more interested in treatment issues and quality of life, both during and after treatment. Since many patients are surviving longer today, there are more delayed effects of treatment. Consequently, clinical management has been challenged to include the emotional, physical, and behavioral consequences of rigorous treatment regimens on quality of life, in addition to dealing with issues of death, dying, and biologic survival.

Even with tremendous improvement in screening techniques and treatment, a cancer diagnosis may shatter the dream of a dignified old age for elderly patients who grew up in an era where the word "cancer" was unmentionable. For these people, cancer means hopelessness, pain, fear, and death. A cancer diagnosis and its treatment often produce psychologic stresses resulting from actual symptoms of the disease as well as the patient's and family's perceptions of the disease and its stigma. Patient fears include worries about death, dependency, disfigurement, disability, and sexual dysfunction, disruption of relationships, and finally discomfort or pain in later stages of illness. Concerns related to cancer have particular meaning for aging individuals who undergo these situations in the context of retirement, widowhood, other medical disabilities, and other losses. Similar to younger patients, the elderly patient's ability to manage these stresses depends on disease characteristics (such as site, symptoms, treatments), prior level of adjustment to medical illnesses, cultural and religious attitudes, the presence of supportive others, previous experiences with cancer, and the patient's personality and coping styles.

Depression in the elderly may mask, amplify, or be the hallmark of physical disabilities and illness. Symptoms often tend to improve as physical status improves. Somatic complaints are often more common defining symptoms of depression in the elderly than in younger patients. Physiologic changes seen with depression in the elderly include fatigue, poor appetite, and decreased motivation. It is important to remember that major depression is not a normal part of aging.

Depressed mood and sadness can be appropriate responses to cancer, but when the patient's normal depressed mood is severe and accompanied by hopelessness, despondence, guilty feelings, and suicidal thoughts it can be considered major depression, and the patient should be referred for treatment.

Risk factors for depression in elderly cancer patients include loss of spouse, functional disability, inadequacy of emotional support, uncontrolled pain, poor physical condition, advanced illness, previous history of depression, other life stresses or losses, family history of depression or suicide, and the patient taking medications known to cause depression. Increasing disability and deterioration in health are strong predictors of depression.[79] Higher levels of symptom severity, lower levels of prior physical functioning, and greater physical functioning deficits have predicted higher levels of depression.[80]

Depression in older cancer patients is optimally managed using a combination of supportive psychotherapy and cognitive-behavioral techniques, as well as antidepressant medications if needed. Psychotherapeutic treatment is directed at helping the patient adapt to the stresses he/she is undergoing, and to help strengthen his/her coping abilities.

The level of distress that a person experiences, the inability to carry out daily activities, and the response to psychotherapeutic interventions determine when a psychotropic medication is needed.[81,82] Some clinicians are willing to start antidepressant medication in cancer patients sooner than in the general population because of the desire to offer some relief to the patient. The general rule of thumb for dosing antidepressants in elderly cancer patients is "Start low and go slow." It is important to educate patients about the therapeutic response time of these medications. It can take at least 2 weeks and possibly up to 5 to 6 weeks for most antidepressants to work. If there is no response or insufficient response by this time, the dose may be increased as indicated and tolerated. If patients are not aware of this time frame, they may become prematurely noncompliant with the drug.

The prevalence of anxiety in the elderly cancer patient is similar to what is seen with younger patients. The challenges for clinicians come with determining the etiology of anxiety seen in this medically complex population. Anxiety may be a sign of pain, respiratory distress, sepsis, endocrine abnormalities, hypoglycemia, hypercalcemia, or hormone-secreting tumors.[81,82] Aside from these physiologic symptoms, pharmacologic treatments may result in anxiety (e.g., steroids). Regardless of the cause, uncontrolled anxiety is detrimental to the patient and family and requires intervention. Once it is determined that the patient's anxiety is not the result of a physiologic condition and/or pharmacologic treatment, elderly patients with anxiety may benefit from cognitive-behavioral interventions (reframing, relaxation training, mediation, etc). There are several pharmacologic therapies that may also be helpful (e.g., benzodiazepines); however, they should be used with caution with elderly clients.[81,82]

IMPLICATIONS

Practice Implications

It is evident that cancer patients experience symptoms of depression and anxiety, and that it often goes unrecognized by the health care team. Given the severity of the negative outcomes associated with untreated anxiety and depression in cancer patients, it is essential that these symptoms be assessed in every client at every visit. Use of active listening techniques and client-centered consultation will assist in eliciting emotional thoughts and feelings from these clients; however, it is not sufficient to just detect the symptom. The first choice for treatment is often pharmacologic; however, clinicians must include in their repertoire of treatments cognitive-behavioral therapies for the treatment of anxiety and depression.

Pharmacologically treating the symptom without determining the cause (e.g., fear of chemotherapy, sexual dysfunction, disfigurement) does not help the patient in the long run. It must be acknowledged that many clinical sites are overburdened and have neither the time nor the expertise to provide cognitive-behavioral therapies for clients and their families; however, assessing for anxiety and depression and providing referrals for treatment is manageable even in the busiest of offices.

Education Implications

Similar to the recommendations for clinical practice, new clinicians need to be educated to detect, assess, and treat psychologic distress in their clients. Education regarding active listening techniques and client-centered consultations must be incorporated into all levels of nursing education. Often the focus on pathology and pharmacology take precedence over the human side of nursing. Holistic treatment of cancer patients includes genuine caring for their psychologic as well as their physiologic state.

Research Implications

The body of research assessing anxiety and depression in cancer patients goes back several decades. Therefore it seems paradoxical that more research would be called for; nevertheless, more research is needed. Specifically, research in populations of female patients with cancers other than breast cancer is needed. These studies are indicated to determine if the factors contributing to anxiety and depression in women with other cancers are the same or different from those in breast cancer populations. Similarly, intervention and survival studies are needed in other cancer populations. This is not to say that breast cancer is unimportant, only that women also suffer from cancers other than breast cancer and those populations warrant similar attention from the research community.

REFERENCES

1. Massie MJ: Prevalence of depression in patients with cancer, *J Natl Cancer Inst Monogr* 32:57-71, 2004.
2. Sharpe M and others: Major depression in outpatients attending a regional cancer center: screening and unmet treatment needs, *Br J Cancer* 90:314-320, 2004.
3. Spiegel D, Giese-Davis J: Depression and cancer: mechanisms and disease progression, *Biol Psychiatry* 54:269-282, 2003.
4. Burgess C and others: Depression and anxiety in women with early breast cancer: five year observational cohort study, *BMJ* 330:702-706, 2005.
5. Bodurka-Bevers D and others: Depression, anxiety, and quality of life in patients with epithelial ovarian cancer, *Gynecol Oncol* 78: 302-308, 2000.
6. Berard RM: Depression and anxiety in oncology: the psychiatrist's perspective, *J Clin Psychiatry* 62(Suppl 8): 58-61, 2001.
7. Sanson-Fisher R and others: The unmet supportive care needs of patients with cancer, *Cancer* 88:226-237, 2000.
8. Chochinov, HM: Depression in cancer patients, *Lancet Oncol* 2:499-405, 2001.
9. Zabora J and others: The prevalence of psychological distress by cancer site, *Psychooncology* 10:19-28, 2001.
10. Girgis A, Burton L: Cancer patients' supportive care needs: strategies for assessment and intervention, *NSW Public Health Bull* 12:269-272, 2001.
11. Fallowfield L and others: Psychiatric morbidity and its recognition by doctors in patients with cancer, *Br J Cancer* 84:1011-1015, 2001.
12. Passik SD and others: Oncology staff recognition of depressive symptoms on videotaped interviews of depressed cancer patients: implications for designing a training program, *J Pain Symptom Manage* 19:329-338, 2000.
13. Ozalp G and others: Preoperative emotional states inpatients with breast cancer and postoperative pain, *ACTA Anaesthesiol Sand* 47:26-29, 2003.
14. Badger TA, Braden CJ, Mishel MH: Depression burden, self-help interventions, and side effect experience in women receiving treatment for breast cancer, *Oncol Nurs Forum* 28:567-574, 2001.
15. Ahlberg K and others: Fatigue, psychological distress, coping and quality of life in patients with uterine cancer, *J Adv Nurs* 45:205-213, 2004.
16. Fulton C: Patients with metastatic breast cancer: their physical and psychological rehabilitation needs, *Int J Rehabil Res* 22:291-301, 1999.
17. Newell SA, Sanson-Fisher RW, Savolainen NJ: Systematic review of psychological therapies for cancer patients: overview and recommendations for future research, *J Natl Cancer Inst* 17:558-584, 2002.
18. Payne DK and others: Screening for anxiety and depression in women with breast cancer: Psychiatry and medical oncology gear up for managed care, *Psychosom* 40:64-69, 1999.
19. Golden-Kreutz DM, Andersen BL: Depressive symptoms after breast cancer surgery: relationships with global, cancer-related, and life event stress, *Psychooncology* 13:211-220, 2004.
20. Sherbourn CD, Dwight-Johnson M, Klap R: Psychological distress, unmet need, and barriers to mental health care for women, *Womens Health Issues* 11:231-243, 2001.
21. Sheard T, Maguire P: The effect of psychological interventions on anxiety and depression in cancer patients: results of two meta-analyses, *Br J Cancer* 80:1770-1780, 1999.
22. Stark D and others: Anxiety disorders in cancer patients: their nature, associations, and relation to quality of life, *J Clin Oncol* 20:3137-3148, 2002.
23. Thewes B and others: The psychosocial needs of breast cancer survivors; a qualitative study of the shared and unique needs of younger versus older survivors, *Psychooncology* 13:177-189, 2004.
24. Kissane DW and others: Psychiatric disorder in women with early stage and advanced breast cancer: A comparative analysis, *Austr NZJ Psychiatry* 38:320-326, 2004.

25. Uchitomi Y and others: Depression and psychological distress in patients during the year after curative resection of non-small-cell lung cancer, *J Clin Oncol* 21:69-77, 2003.
26. Kungaya A and others: Prevalence, predictive factors, and screening for psychologic distress in patients with newly diagnosed head and neck cancer, *Cancer* 88:2817-2823, 2000.
27. Lloyd-Williams M, Dennis M, Taylor F: A prospective study to determine the association between physical symptoms and depression in patients with advanced cancer, *Palliat Med* 18:558-563, 2004.
28. Stommel M and others: A longitudinal analysis of the course of depressive symptomatology in geriatric patients with cancer of the breast, colon, lung or prostate, *Health Psychol* 23:564-573, 2004.
29. Prieto JM and others: Patient-rated emotional and physical functioning among hematologic cancer patients during hospitalization for stem-cell transplantation, *Bone Marrow Transplant* 35:307-314, 2005.
30. Chen M-L, Chang H-K: Physical symptom profiles of depressed and nondepressed patients with cancer, *Palliat Med* 18:712-718, 2004.
31. Bair MJ, Robinson RL, Eckert GJ, et al: Impact of pain on depression treatment response in primary care, *Psychosom Med* 66:17-22, 2004.
32. Miaskowski C: Gender differences in pain, fatigue, and depression in patients with cancer, *J Natl Cancer Inst Monogr* 32:139-143, 2004.
33. Hopwood P, Stephens RJ: Depression in patients with lung cancer: prevalence and risk factors derived from quality-of-life data, *J Clin Oncol* 18:893-903, 2000.
34. Ahles TA and others: Neuropsychologic impact of standard-dose systemic chemotherapy in long-term survivors of breast cancer and lymphoma, *J Clin Oncol* 20:485-493, 2002.
35. Dodd MJ and others: A comparison of the affective state and quality of life of chemotherapy patients who do and do not develop chemotherapy-induced oral mucositis, *J Pain Symptom Manage* 21:498-505, 2001.
36. Farrell C and others: Identifying the concerns of women undergoing chemotherapy, *Patient Educ Couns* 56:72-77, 2005.
37. Stiegelis HE, Ranchor AV, Sanderman R: Psychological functioning in cancer patients treated with radiotherapy, *Patient Educ Couns* 52:131-141, 2004.
38. Curt GA and others: Impact of cancer-related fatigue on the lives of patients: new findings from the fatigue coalition, *Oncologist* 5:353-360, 2000.
39. Portenoy RK: Cancer-related fatigue: an immense problem, *Oncologist* 5:350-352, 2000.
40. Francoeur RB: The relationship of cancer symptom clusters to depressive affect in the initial phase of palliative radiation, *J Pain Symptom Manage* 29:130-155, 2005.
41. Chiu T-Y and others: Dyspnea and its correlates in Taiwanese patients with terminal cancer, *J Pain Symptom Manage* 28:123-132, 2004.
42. Akechi T and others: Biomedical and psychosocial determinants of psychiatric morbidity among postoperative ambulatory breast cancer patients, *Breast Cancer Res Treat* 65:195-202, 2001.
43. Akechi T and others: Major depression, adjustment disorders and post-traumatic stress disorder in terminally ill cancer patients: associated and predictive factors, *J Clin Oncol* 22:1957-1965, 2004.
44. Chan CW and others: Social support and coping in Chinese patients undergoing cancer surgery, *Cancer Nurs* 27:230-236, 2004.
45. Grassi L and others: Psychosocial morbidity and its correlates in cancer patients of the Mediterranean area: findings for the Southern European Psycho-Oncology Study, *J Affect Disord* 83:243-248, 2004.
46. Greer S and others: Psychological response to breast cancer and 15 year outcome, *Lancet* 355:49-50, 1990.
47. Han WT and others: Breast cancer and problems with medical interactions: Relationships with traumatic stress, emotional self-efficacy, and social support, *Psychooncology* 14:318-330, 2004.
48. Heinonen H and others: Quality of life and factors related to perceived satisfaction with quality of life after allogeneic bone marrow transplantation, *Ann Hematol* 80:137-143, 2001.
49. De Leeuw J and others: Negative and positive influences of social support on depression in patients with head and neck cancer: a prospective study, *Psychooncology* 9:20-28, 2000.
50. Schou I and others: Pessimism as a predictor of emotional morbidity on year following breast cancer surgery, *Psychooncology* 13:309-320, 2004.
51. Alder J, Bitzer J: Retrospective evaluation of the treatment for breast cancer: how does the patient's personal experience of the treatment affect later adjustment to the illness? *Arch Womens Mental Health* 6:91-97, 2003.
52. Dickson D and others: Health professionals' perceptions of breaking bad news, *Int J Health Care Qual Assur Inc Ledersh Health Serv* 15:324-336, 2002.
53. Girgis A, Sanson-Fisher RW, Schofield MJ: Is there consensus between breast cancer patients and providers on guidelines for breaking bad news? *Behav Med* 25:69-77, 1999.
54. Bang SM and others: Changes in quality of life during palliative chemotherapy for solid cancers, *Support Care Cancer* 13:515-521, 2005.
55. Kohda R and others: Prospective studies on mental status and quality of life inpatients with head and neck cancer treated by radiation, *Psychooncology* 14:331-336, 2005.
56. Smith EM, Gomm SA, Dickens CM: Assessing the independent contribution to quality of life from anxiety and depression in patients with advanced cancer, *Palliat Med* 17:509-513, 2003.
57. Hjerl K and others: Depression as a prognostic factor for breast cancer mortality, *Psychosom* 44:24-30, 2003.
58. Watson M and others: Influence of psychological response on survival in breast cancer: population-based cohort study, *Lancet* 354:1331-1336, 1999.
59. Del Piccolo L and others: Differences in verbal behaviors of patients with and without emotional distress during primary care consultations, *Psychol Med* 30:629-643, 2000.
60. Ryan H and others: How to recognize and manage psychological distress in cancer patients, *Eur J Cancer Care* 14:7-15, 2005.
61. Kirmayer LJ and others: Explaining medically unexplained symptoms, *Can J Psychiatry* 49:663-672, 2004.
62. Egan G: *The Skilled Helper: A Problem-Management Approach to Helping,* ed 5, Pacific Grove, CA, 1994, Brooks/Cole.
63. Street RL Jr, Millay B: Analyzing patient participation in medical encounters, *Health Commun* 13:61-73, 2001.

64. Kessler D and others: Cross sectional study of symptoms attribution and recognition of depression and anxiety in primary care, *BMJ* 318:436-440, 1999.
65. Sayar K, Kirmayer LJ, Taillefer SS: Predictors of somatic symptoms in depressive disorder, *Gen Hosp Psychiatry* 25: 108-114, 2003.
66. Cape, J: Consultation length, patient-estimated consultation length, and satisfaction with consultation, *Br J Gen Pract* 52:1004-1006, 2002.
67. Cape J: How general practice patients with emotional problems presenting with somatic or psychological symptoms explain their improvement, *Br J Genl Pract* 51: 724-729, 2001.
68. O'Connor DW, Rosewarne R, Bruce A: Depression in primary care 1: elderly patients' disclosure of depressive symptoms to their doctors, *Int Psychogeriatr* 13:359-365, 2001.
69. Butow PN and others: Oncologists' reactions to cancer patients' verbal cues, *Psychooncology* 11:47-58, 2002.
70. Street RL Jr: Gender differences in health care provider-patient communication: are they due to style, stereotypes, or accommodation? *Patient Educ Couns* 48:201-206, 2002.
71. Emslie C and others: Gender differences in mental health: evidence from three organizations, *Soc Sci Med* 54: 621-624, 2002.
72. Harris PA: The impact of age, gender, race, and ethnicity on the diagnosis and treatment of depression, Manage Care Pharm 10(2 Suppl):S2-S7, 2004.
73. Lewin SA and others: Interventions for providers to promote a patient-centered approach in clinical consultations, *Cochrane Database of Syst Rev* 4:CD003267, 2001.
74. Price J, Leaver L: Beginning treatment [clinical review: ABC of psychological medicine], *BMJ* 325:33-35, 2002.
75. Dowsett SM and others: Communication styles in the cancer consultation: preferences for a patient-centered approach, *Psychooncology* 9:147-156, 2000.
76. Astin JA: Mind-body therapies for management of pain, *Clin J Pain,* 20:27-32, 2004.
77. Sloman R: Relaxation and imagery for anxiety and depression control in community patients with advanced cancer, *Cancer Nurs* 25:432-435, 2002.
78. Deng G, Cassileth BR, Yeng KS: Complementary therapies for cancer-related symptoms, *J Support Oncol* 2:419-426, 2004.
79. Hybels CF, Blazer, DG: Epidemiology of late-life mental disorders, *Clin Geriatr Med* 19:663-696, 2003.
80. Kurtz ME and others: Physical functioning and depression among older persons with cancer, *Cancer Pract* 9:11-18, 2001.
81. Roth A, Modi R: Psychiatric issues in older cancer patients, *Crit Rev Oncol Hematol* 48:185-197, 2003.
82. Winell J, Roth AJ: Depression in cancer patients, *Oncology,* 18:1554-1560, 2004.

CHAPTER

16 Body Image and Sexual Functioning

Judith A. Shell

INTRODUCTION

Women commonly associate energy and productivity with strength and femininity, which promote the feeling that they are worthwhile members of society. Likewise, in the American culture the sense of being desirable and capable of bonding or connecting sexually is also extremely important. Often, this is equated with a sense of adequacy as a woman. In fact, if she feels sexually inadequate, it may be a reason for a woman to feel like an inadequate person in most respects. Logically, such an analogy is ridiculous, but our emotions are usually not logical.

If cancer enters a woman's life and creates weakness and debilitation, she may believe that she has become worthless and that sexual expression and activity that she shared with her partner may have to end.[1] The couple may feel cheated, not only because they realize that life as they knew it has changed, but they also may believe in the general myth that everyone else is already "having more sex than we are." Michael and colleagues explain that "America has a message about sex, and that message is none too subtle. Anyone who watches a movie, reads a magazine, or turns on the television has seen it. It says that almost everyone but you is having endless, fascinating, varied sex. But we have found the public image of sex in America bears virtually no relationship to the truth. The public image consists of myths, and they are not harmless, for they elicit at best unrealistic and at worst, dangerous misconceptions of what people do sexually. The resulting false expectations can badly affect self-esteem, marriages, relationships, even physical health."[2] Fortunately, the diagnosis of cancer does not preclude a person's being sexual, but the patient and her partner will undoubtedly require reassurance and inspiration to devote many of their resources to retain an intimate relationship.

There are at present an estimated 9.2 million cancer survivors, and anywhere from 10% to 90% of them have reported some manifestation of sexual problems during and/or after their treatment, depending on diagnosis, sex, and type of treatment.[3] Consequently, it comes as no surprise that recognition of psychosexual aspects of cancer care has become more evident in the literature and journal articles have increased from 50 in 1960 to over 1,000 publications in 2001.[4]

Much of the research regarding sexual function in female cancer survivors has revolved around treatments for breast and gynecologic cancers.[3,5-10] However, other research has recently looked at sexual function specifically related to women and the effects from bone marrow transplant and genitourinary, head and neck, and lung cancers.[11-14]

While sexual happiness is not only a question of anatomy or endocrinology in the woman, it is important to briefly review some aspects of her human sexual response. The body's vasocongestive-neuromuscular response is mediated through the autonomic nervous system, and there can be impairment of the mechanism that underlies vasocongestion as a result of pelvic or vaginal irradiation or from the loss of estrogenic hormones.[15,16] Even though there may be a delay in physiologic response, sexual function is usually not completely destroyed. Several sources, however, report there is a definite impact on sexual function with the advent of these treatments. Lamb and colleagues all state that sexual activity and satisfaction was decreased in women who were treated for gynecologic cancers as evidenced by lack of desire and decreased frequency of intercourse, orgasm, and feelings of enjoyment.[10,17,18] Corney and colleagues assessed 105 women following radical pelvic surgery and revealed that after 6 months, 66% had sexual problems, of which lack of desire was the most common.[19] Of the women, 50% said that they felt their relationship had deteriorated, although only 16% thought their marriage had gotten worse. There were also psychogenic factors, which included concerns over loss of fertility, depression, and anxiety about desirability as a sexual partner. On a positive note, the presence of a stable relationship before diagnosis seemed to enhance coping.[19]

Even when women experience surgical changes of their anatomy such as removal of the vagina or clitoris, they are often able to learn to have a good sexual response through stimulation of other erogenous areas with proper and appropriately timed rehabilitation. Increasing the sensitivity in the thigh and breast area or stimulation of the anus, the ostia of an ileostomy or colostomy, or scar tissue in the area of the vulva, or even finding a heightened enjoyment in bringing one's partner to orgasm through mutual masturbation can enhance and provide for a satisfactory sexual response.[20]

Some of the most important elements in sexual rehabilitation relative to any type of cancer are a partner who has an understanding of the patient's treatment, an uninterrupted interest in pleasure with her, and an open, honest method of communication. John Rowland put it best when he said that "Couples that can redefine intimacy and nurturance in broader than purely sexual terms can successfully adapt to losses in the sexual component of their relationship. This redefinition includes valuing a mutually caring companionate relationship in other dimensions, with shared interests and pleasurable activities."[21] This chapter will explore the professional's responsibility to address sexuality with their female clients, site-specific physical and psychosocial aspects, the assessment of sexual function, and interventions relative to the sexual rehabilitation of women who have experienced cancer and the ramifications of its treatments.

PROFESSIONAL RESPONSIBILITY TO DISCUSS SEXUALITY

Routine care of oncology survivors should include discussion of sexual function, which is a vital element of quality of life. The integration of education and appropriate intervention can be fostered through communication between patient, partner, and health care team regardless of age, marital status, or sexual orientation. Although attitude has improved and providers are more liberal and aware of the importance of human sexuality, Brunner and Boyd note that professionals are still not adequately addressing sexuality issues.[22] Consequently, several changes must be made to promote sexuality assessment and counseling (Box 16-1).

To normalize the patient and partner's sexual concerns and increase their comfort, it is appropriate to address sexual function before, during, and after cancer treatment. An intimate relationship can be a solace and an affirmation of life for those women who have or wish to have a partner. For those women who either have no partner or who simply have decided that sexual activity is no longer an important aspect of their lives, this too is a normal, healthy choice. However, such women will most likely continue to see themselves as sexual beings with worries about their femininity.

It is also necessary to remember that not all women have partners of the opposite sex: providers should not make the inaccurate assumption that all women are in heterosexual relationships. This can be detrimental to both the lesbian patient and her partner. Fields and Scout cite a lesbian woman

Box 16-1 Changes Needed To Promote Assessment & Counseling

Knowledge of the extent of sexual problems generated by cancer
- Increased appreciation of how significant the nurses' efforts may be to augment quality of life for patients & partners.

Increased comfort related to the discussion of sexual issues with patients and partners
- Practice in the development of skills to consult and talk with patients and partners
- Awareness of the normal sexual concerns related to cancer and its treatment
- Increase the ability to either initiate conversation, or facilitate the patient's initiation of the conversation

Knowledge of resources and referrals are available for support

who had had her first Pap smear at age 42 because of "multiple bad experiences with doctors…the cost to her was a large ulcerated cervical tumor and a diagnosis of cervical cancer."[23] One study reported that over 25% of lesbians who "came out" to their physicians felt their health care was negatively affected.[24] In addition, researchers hypothesize that because of studies that profile lesbian behavioral risk factors (higher rates of smoking, alcohol consumption, and obesity, and nulliparity), lesbians and women who partner with women may receive a lesser standard of care and thus may be at increased risk for the development of cancer.[25] Once cancer has occurred, if a woman's partner is excluded from the treatment process as a result of provider ignorance, she may have greater difficulty with decision making, and the discomfited couple may show little or no affection toward each other during office visits or hospitalizations. Whether a couple is gay or heterosexual, they are usually nervous and worried about each other and want to be protective during their cancer experience; all providers must acknowledge this supportive relationship.

Women who experience cancer in the later years of life have some special issues. They have often lost friends, family, and their spouse or partner, which causes them to think more about their own mortality. Women must adjust to the social stigma of being "old" and to several physical irritations like the pain of arthritis, decreased eyesight and hearing, and gravity's pull on face, bosom, and buttocks. The preconceived notions about older women have changed somewhat, though, because of the "baby boomers" and their resistance to growing old as evidenced by botox, liposuction and face lifts, running marathons, and staying sexually active.[26]

Along with a new cancer diagnosis, an older woman may be dealing with retirement and reduced income, the death of her spouse or partner, a decrease in physical strength and general health, and the challenge of establishing a satisfactory living arrangement either with a child or perhaps in an assisted living facility. A chronic or recurrent cancer may compound her problems, especially if multimodal therapy is necessary. These tasks may preempt the energy usually available for interest in sex and an intimate relationship. Because a woman's sexuality and sense of femininity remain throughout the life cycle and are integral to her self-esteem, it is important that nurses remain aware of life stage reactions that are important factors in sexual rehabilitation.

FACTORS THAT AFFECT THE SEXUAL FUNCTION OF WOMEN WITH CANCER

Site-Specific Factors Related to Surgery

Bladder Cancer

Bladder cancer occurs primarily in older women, and the incidence increases with age. If tumors are superficial and noninvasive, cystectomy is not necessary and they are usually treated with bacillus Calmette-Guérin (BCG).[18] The instillation of BCG through repeated cystoscopies can be uncomfortable and cause urethral irritation, even though surgery has been avoided.[18] Intercourse may be painful, desire for sexual activity inhibited, and the woman's partner may be concerned about becoming "contaminated" during intercourse and avoid her altogether.

Cystectomy remains the treatment of choice with or without radiation therapy if the bladder tumor is invasive, and this entails removal of the urethra, the uterus, the cervix, the ovaries, and the anterior wall of the vagina.[27,28] There will be a continent urinary reservoir that needs to be catheterized frequently, or a urostomy stoma will be placed. Body image is often negatively affected and problems with sexual desire, and function can be similar to those who have stoma placement because of colon cancer. However, women tend to be more independent than men in the care of their stomas.[28] Gallo-Silver explains that women can still have a positive sexual experience with their partners even after radical cystectomy: "Although Helen did not want to experiment with vaginal penetration, she and Max enjoyed physical intimacy by using a side by side position in which Max approached her lubricated inner thighs from behind her. This position also protected and avoided the ostomy site."[29] Women who do wish to resume sexual relations with vaginal penetration may wish to use vaginal hormone cream, vaginal dilatation (see the later discussion on site-specific factors related to radiation therapy), and/or Kegel exercises (tensing and relaxing of the muscles in the pubic area), which promote more comfortable intercourse.[10]

Breast Cancer

American culture has used the female breast to symbolize various concepts and to exploit symbolic meanings, and as an agent of cultural presumption, the female breast represents femininity and sexuality. However, clarification is needed to remind us that breasts are not primarily sexual organs, but may have some secondary effects on a woman's sexual function.

Continued improvements in the treatment for breast cancer have resulted in less radical surgery, although all treatment is accompanied by some risk to self-image and sexual function since it may entail not only surgery, but a combination including chemotherapy, radiation, and hormonal therapies.[30] Initially, it was believed that breast-conserving surgery would have less impact on sexual function than mastectomy; however, several studies have reported little to no difference in overall sexual functioning following the two treatments.[9,31-35]

Wilmoth and Ross described the responses of 105 women in an exploratory study who explained how their sexuality had changed since being diagnosed with breast cancer.[33] Content-analytic methods identified four themes: physical sexual functioning, relationship quality, psychologic self, and self as female. Qualitative and quantitative data revealed that there was no significant difference in sexual functioning in women who were treated with either mastectomy or lumpectomy. However, there is some advantage for breast conservation related to body image, pleasure and frequency of breast caressing, comfort with nudity, and frequency of intercourse.[22,32,34] Women who have had either type of treatment complain that they were not prepared for the lack of sensation in the breast/breast area after surgery, and they found that this was distressing and detrimental to sexual arousal.[33] Several studies found that type of surgery did not have as much impact on sexual function as did the administration of chemotherapy in addition to the surgery.[32-37]

One other concern related to surgery for breast cancer is the age of the woman. Fifty women (28 premenopausal and 22 postmenopausal) who had undergone surgery for breast cancer participated in a study that assessed the reaction to illness and scarring and marital satisfaction, and what impact these factors had on the patient's ability to resume an enjoyable sexual life after surgery and radiation therapy.[37] The data revealed that for younger women, adjustment to illness and the required treatment and adequate sexual function seemed to depend on how well the marital relationship functioned. For postmenopausal women, the illness adjustments depended on an extended network of emotional support, and surprisingly marital contentment and agency did not affect sexual function. However, the ability of all couples to communicate their intimate and often fearful feelings fostered the resumption of a satisfying sexual intimacy.[37]

Colorectal Cancer

The mainstay of treatment for colorectal cancer continues to be surgery, with or without chemotherapy.[31] Although much is known about how these surgical procedures affect the sexual function of men, there is a flagrant lack of studies related to sexual function in women who have been treated for colorectal neoplasms.[17,18] Abdominoperineal resection can include hysterectomy, excision of the posterior vaginal wall, and pelvic lymphadenectomy, which can disturb sympathetic nerves and affect vaginal lubrication, resulting in uncomfortable intercourse. Other physical effects may involve genital numbness, removal of the rectum, and the formation of a stoma.[38-40] Turnbull reports, "Dyspareunia can result if the back wall of the vagina is removed. Even if the vagina is not surgically damaged, the absence of the rectum removes the cushioning behind the rear wall of the vagina and can result in pain with thrusting during intercourse. In addition, bands of scar tissue from the surgery can develop around the vagina, causing narrowing."[38] If the rectum must be removed, it is recommended that the woman abstain from intercourse to avoid the potential for infection and to promote tissue healing.[39] Lamb reports that women may not only experience genital numbness and vaginal dryness, but they may also have a diminished sexual libido.[10] If ovaries and uterus must be removed, women endure a surgically-induced menopause and are no longer able to have children.

If a woman must undergo the placement of a stoma, there is enormous distress along with problems adjusting to a changed body image, and sexual behavior may be negatively affected.[40] Several "normal" responses to ostomy surgery may occur regardless of the type (colostomy or ileostomy) or where the stoma is placed (Box 16-2). Shame and embarrassment often accompany the overwhelmed feeling of the loss of the bodily control so painstakingly secured as a child. Also, since many women equate physical beauty with sexual attraction, a new stoma could make it awkward and difficult to feel alluring to a potential lover. Now, even the smallest negative reaction can create a sense of being unacceptable, and she may decide to withdraw from all social interaction and potential relationships. Sprangers and colleagues found that sexual functioning in female stoma patients was consistently more impaired than that of women with intact sphincters, and they reported limitations in their level of social functioning, with increased levels of psychologic distress.[41]

There may also be problems with partner acceptance of ostomy disfigurement—viewing the stoma at an early stage helps to desensitize both patient and partner—and both partners may have difficulty with feelings of sexual adequacy,

Box 16-2 NORMAL PSYCHOSOCIAL RESPONSES TO OSTOMY SURGERY

Anxiety about cancer-related surgery; death and dying
Overwhelming sense of loss of control related to bowel elimination
The perception of being mutilated or violated
Hopelessness at the first sight of the stoma
Feeling fragile and damaged
Feeling like an invalid
Being depressed, which in turn causes decreased libido
An unexpected increase in fatigue and weakness
Revulsion by an external pouching system for stool
Apprehension and embarrassment about accidents, odor, noise, leakage, and staining
A conscious obsession about cleanliness
An excessive emotional investment in the stoma

desirability, and feeling lovable. Lesbian partners will have similar concerns and should be encouraged to discuss their feelings and anxieties regarding how the stoma will affect their relationship.[42] Spouses/partners often fear they will hurt the stoma. Northouse and colleagues found that spouses of patients with colon cancer judged the diagnosis more negatively than did the patients.[43] In one survey of people with colon cancer 50 years and older, 8% were divorced and 63% of those divorced said the separation occurred after their surgery, and they believed that the surgery was responsible for the divorce.[44]

Gynecologic Cancers

Disclosure of low levels of sexual satisfaction from women with gynecologic (GYN) cancer and their partners is not uncommon.[10,46] GYN surgery can alter self-image, endocrine status, and the anatomy of these women, as evidenced by a decrease in sexual desire and increased discomfort during intercourse; however, they often remain sexually active.[47] Many women fear that they will "grow old" faster, loose their libido completely, or simply feel empty because they no longer have the ability to become pregnant. On the other hand, while some women have lost the ability to have multiple orgasms after hysterectomy, others actually have an increased sense of sexual enjoyment *because* they can no longer get pregnant.[48]

Hysterectomy is one of the most common treatment procedures for GYN cancers (cervix, endometrium, and/or ovaries), and may create devastating sequelae if the woman has been used to experiencing uterine contractions during orgasm. Orgasm may be less exciting and pleasurable after surgery if she no longer has these contractions. In radical hysterectomy, the uterus, cervix, and a portion of the vaginal vault (upper third to half) is removed. Scarring, nerve damage, or venous damage may affect vaginal expansion, engorgement and lubrication, which may affect sexual enjoyment; penile thrusting may also be painful.[10,17,31,47] Another annoying problem may be the need for a long-term indwelling urinary catheter that stays in place after surgery until the bladder begins to function again. If bladder function is delayed and the catheter stays in place, after the woman is able to resume intercourse, she may need to alter positions for intercourse and/or tape up the catheter over the abdomen.[10,20]

Other surgical procedures such as oophorectomy may be performed as part of a radical hysterectomy for invasive cervical cancer, but is not usually suggested unless the woman is over 40 years old.[31] If oophorectomy is necessary, it will create a surgical menopause in younger women, and estrogen replacement therapy can begin if there is no contraindication.[31] Without ovarian hormones, thinning of the vaginal wall and vaginal dryness will occur and adversely affect sexuality and decrease sexual response; this is true in both benign and malignant disease.[22]

Simple vulvectomy entails only removal of the labia majora and minora, but in radical vulvectomy the vulva, the clitoris, and femoral and inguinal lymph nodes, and occasionally the distal urethra, are all removed.[17] There is loss of erogenous tissue, and introital stenosis may also result. It is often difficult to resume vaginal intercourse for several reasons including perineal numbness, the formation of scar tissue as healing takes place, some measure of urinary incontinence, and occasional edema of the perineum and lower extremities. Partners may be fearful to attempt sexual stimulation, and surgical ramifications, due to a change in physical appearance and in sensation, are often difficult to accept.[17,20] Foreplay may now need to include stimulation in other erogenous zones such as the earlobes, breasts, fingers, toes, and inner thighs. A pilot survey study to evaluate sexual dysfunction after vulvectomy elicited the agreement of 47 women to participate, and 41 of them returned the survey.[49] Results indicated that regardless of the extent of surgery or type of vulvectomy, women experienced significant sexual dysfunction. Other risk factors for dysfunction included age, depression, worsening performance status as measured by the Gynecologic Oncology Group (GOG), and preoperative hypoactive sexual dysfunction.

Finally, pelvic exenteration is the most devastating GYN surgery, since it involves not only the removal of the vagina, the uterus, the ovaries, and the urethra, but also the bladder and the rectum wherein a colostomy and ileal conduit must be created.[18] Obviously, a woman's sense of self-esteem, body image and sexual function will be oppressively affected. Lamb indicates that although there may be a decrease in sexual activity and satisfaction initially, this may also depend on the couple's previous sexual practice, and their desire and determination to resume sexual activity.[10]

Site-specific Factors Related to Systemic Chemotherapy

Hematologic Cancers

A multitude of studies have been done relative to female sexuality as it is affected by particular diseases such as breast and gynecologic cancers; however, there is a paucity of work accomplished in cancers not typically associated with sexuality such as hematologic, lung, and head and neck cancers. Although a diagnosis of leukemia or lymphoma does not denote the need for surgery, some type of biopsy is invariably needed to establish a diagnosis. The leukemias and lymphomas can strike at any age. In the Hodgkin's lymphoma population, one report acknowledged various psychosocial problems including separation or divorce, and 21% had high levels of psychologic distress.[50] Sexual issues are demonstrated by decreased interest in sexual intimacy, painful intercourse, and a poor self-image. In a leukemia and non-Hodgkin's lymphoma cancer survivor group, it was learned that both groups had serious marital problems, and 33% of the leukemia population thought their divorce or separation was owing to the disease itself.[50] Again, a decreased interest in sexual activity and painful intercourse for women occurred for both groups, as they did in the Hodgkin's patient group.

Chemotherapy is the mainstay of treatment for leukemia and lymphoma and may be given in high doses along with blood or bone marrow transplantation (BMT) to rescue the patient. Chemotherapy, even if given in normal doses, can cause adverse affects on ovarian function such as the destruction of ova and follicles, which leads to a perimenopausal or menopausal state along with fertility modifications.[10,17,40,51]

Amenorrhea, hot flashes, vaginal dryness, skin changes, and anovulatory cycles are the result. Loss of sexual desire can follow, and of course, this decreased desire for sexual intimacy can also be attributed to increased weakness and fatigue, intermittent nausea and vomiting, possible diarrhea or constipation, and low blood counts.[17,20] In 2 to 3 weeks, alopecia will also begin, which will most likely be destructive to self-image and the sense of femininity even though the nurse may have compassionately explained that there is a variety of attractive wigs and creative headwear available. Hair loss in itself has been shown to alter body image and self-esteem.[52] No woman is ever ready for hair loss.

With BMT, sexual difficulties may follow that are not reversible. Syrjala and others reported that 67% of women reported sexual dysfunctions for 3 years after treatment with BMT.[11] Other investigators have reported rates of sexual function difficulties between 25% and 44% in quality of life outcome studies across genders for up to 18 years after transplant.[53,54] Changes in hormone levels may cause disruption in the sexual response cycle (desire, arousal, excitement, or orgasmic phase). Tierney explains, "Social factors may contribute to sexual dissatisfaction in transplant recipients. In the context of sexuality, the most important social relationship is that of the intimate partner. Variables influencing this relationship include partner uncertainty and anxiety, difficult communicating, and role shifting within the couple during treatment and recovery."[55] During an illness crisis such as this, the sexual partner is often the caregiver, and this can have an untoward effect on the couple relationship because of role changes and intensified dependence on the caregiver. After experiencing the distinct lack of privacy and ability to be intimate that results from prolonged treatment and hospitalization, reestablishing an intimate relationship can be difficult at best.

Lung Cancer

Of the many women faced with cancer each year, those with the diagnosis of lung cancer are among the most common. Treatment depends heavily on chemotherapy, since advanced disease at the time of diagnosis often requires it be primarily palliative. Radiation therapy is often added, and surgery is occasionally performed when the disease is diagnosed early. Lifestyle adjustments will be required because of psychosocial and emotional distress, the possible spread of the malignancy, and an uncertain prognosis.[56] Chemotherapy treatments can be devastating especially if the patient begins treatment in an incapacitated state. A woman's personhood and femininity may be threatened as a result of changes in role function such as the inability to work or be a mom, a deflated body image from an altered appearance, fatigue from disease or treatment, and the loss of physical ability to function sexually. Fatigue may be increased, as well, by nausea and vomiting and increased shortness of breath due to tumor or low hemoglobin. These intermittent symptoms are not only troublesome but can cause depression and the lack of sexual desire; the woman may even choose to withdraw from intimacy, affection, and physical closeness.[14,56]

Sarna explored the impact of lung cancer on the lives of 69 women and revealed that fatigue, pain, and insomnia were the three most distressing symptoms, and these symptoms most likely affected their "poor outlook."[14,57] Sarna stated, "Increased symptom distress in lung cancer has been associated with greater awareness of dying and with a decline in positive attitude."[14] Women with lung cancer experienced more disturbance in their quality of life as compared with women with other cancers. If their disease recurred, they had greater marital dysfunction. A decrease in sexual activity was reported by 38% of the women: they did not feel sexually attractive, and/or they were no longer interested in engaging in sex.[57] It is suggested that this may not only be due to the disease process, but also to the fact that a woman may be affected by her inability to care for family and other home-making responsibilities.[57]

Other studies have been done relative to quality of life issues, but they include both men and women. Ginsberg and colleagues examined psychiatric illness and psychosocial concerns in 52 lung cancer patients, 75% male and 25% female.[58] Only *one* of 20 outcome measures related to sexuality, and that was "loss of libido." These patients often experienced symptoms of potential psychiatric significance and psychosocial concern. Loss of libido was acknowledged by 48%, and this was severe in 27%.

One study has been completed in a lung cancer population currently under treatment, with sexuality as the primary focus. Shell reported on 59 lung cancer patients (27 were female) in a 4-month longitudinal study.[59] Sexual function included sexual cognition/fantasy, sexual arousal, sexual behavior/experiences, orgasm, and drive and relationship. Results indicated that sexual function worsened with treatment over time; other variables that affected sexual function were age, gender, and mood status; women had more dysfunction.[59]

Head and Neck Cancer

Ofman notes that there is little research in the cancer population with tumors that do not affect the "sexual" organs directly, and head and neck cancer is no exception.[18] This cancer can impose a particularly severe challenge physically and emotionally.[13,60,61] With today's emphasis on youth and beauty, these women will most likely feel grossly unattractive, have difficulties with body image, and will encounter insecurities with simple tasks like talking and eating and, in particular, breathing.[20,62] Consequently, needs for things such as closeness, touching, and intimate sexual pleasures may receive little attention, and a woman's partner may be repulsed by her inability to talk or by the sight and smell if the disease has progressed to the later stages. Women may be embarrassed by the need to use an electronic device to speak because of the masculine sound it produces. If a tracheostomy is placed, it is accompanied by a hissing sound, which often elicits fear of suffocation during sexual intercourse. Alcohol and smoking history may also be contributing factors to sexual dysfunction that have predated development of the cancer.[17]

In a study of 36 head and neck cancer patients who had received treatment for more than a year, it was learned that 75% rated their sexual relationship as "somewhat" to "very important" and 50%

reported problems with their sexuality.[63] Since head and neck cancer may also be treated with surgery, either before or after chemotherapy, rehabilitation due to cosmetic and functional impairments will have a definite effect on body image, particularly in women. Katz and others concluded in a study with 82 ambulatory patients at least 6 months past treatment that women had higher levels of depression and lower life happiness, and those with greater disfigurement suffered more depression.[13] Those at greater risk for psychosocial dysfunction had lower levels of social support and underwent more face-disfiguring treatment. Clearly, treatment with radiation therapy, chemotherapy, and even surgery for head and neck cancer does not have a direct impact on the sexual organs, but it does indirectly affect the sexual response cycle: desire, arousal, excitement, and orgasm.[17]

TREATMENT EFFECTS SECONDARY TO RADIATION THERAPY

Radiation Therapy Effects to the Upper Body

Severe problems can arise because of radiation to the head and neck area; they can manifest themselves as xerostomia and problems with chewing, swallowing, and talking. Pain is often part of this symptom cluster, and all must be well controlled to promote quality of life, especially where intimacy is concerned.[64] One of the author's patients complained that one of her "favorite parts of intimacy was having oral sex with her husband, and now she couldn't enjoy this with him because she had no saliva." The artificial salivas were not acceptable to her during sex, and this frustrated both her and her partner. Taste and the ability to swallow may also indirectly affect sexuality: if a woman will not eat and loses weight, a poor body image may be the result and sexual self-esteem may be damaged. Radiation therapy can cause changes in the skin that are very noticeable such as redness and peeling in the treatment area on the face, neck, chest, or back. As a result, a woman can become self-conscious and embarrassed. If soreness and pain is a problem, sexual intimacy may again be deterred.

Monga and colleagues conducted a study with 55 head and neck cancer patients, of whom only one subject was a woman. However, the results are notable.[60] A majority reported arousal problems, 58% had orgasmic problems and/or did not participate in sexual intercourse; however, 85% did have an interest in sex and 49% were satisfied with current sexual function.

Another troublesome side effect from radiation therapy can be the cough that results from treatment to the chest for lung and esophageal cancers and the lymphomas. Sexual desire may have to be deferred because of a poorly controlled cough that often leads to shortness of breath and fatigue. It may be necessary to give attention to sexual closeness rather than to focus on intercourse.

Radiation Therapy Effects to the Lower Body

Women with colorectal and GYN cancers most often receive radiation therapy to the lower body. It is important that women and their partners are aware of the progressive anatomic changes that can take place and the difficulty this can cause in sexual function. Some of the more immediate and troublesome side effects are nausea and vomiting, abdominal cramping and diarrhea, dysuria and cystitis, and vaginal bleeding.[64] Some of the long-term direct effects of radiation will include vaginal stenosis, fibrosis, vaginal shortening and narrowing, rectovaginal or vesicovaginal fistulas, and gastrointestinal dysfunction.[30] Of women younger than 40 years of age who undergo radiation, more than 95% experience termination of menses after a cumulative radiation dose of 500 to 1000 cGy; and a cumulative radiation dose of 375 cGy may induce amenorrhea in women who are older than 40 years of age.[17] In premenopausal women, if the ovaries are within the radiation field they will experience menopausal symptoms that include hot flashes, loss of libido, decreased vaginal lubrication, and vaginal thinning due to cessation of estradiol and progesterone production.[17,65] Ofman explains that more radiation than surgical patients report "diminished sexual functioning, with severe dyspareunia, postcoital bleeding, and pain on penetration."[18] However, in one study only 22%

of 107 women with a partner expressed dissatisfaction with their sexual lives after radiation treatment.[66]

To decrease the impact that radiation therapy has on the vagina, women are encouraged to remain sexually active for as long as it is comfortable and to return to activity as soon as any discomfort has resolved.[65] If she is not sexually active, a woman must use a vaginal dilator with lubricant for at least 3 years to ensure vaginal patency and to maintain the ability of the radiation oncologist to monitor for possible recurrent cancer.[20]

TREATMENT EFFECTS SECONDARY TO HORMONE THERAPY

Women with newly diagnosed as well as advanced breast cancer are often treated with hormone therapy; this treatment began in the 1970s with tamoxifen.[67] At present, various therapy options are available depending on a woman's menopausal and estrogen/progesterone status. These hormones include fulvestrant, anastrozole, exemestane, toremifene, letrozole, and tamoxifen, and all of them can cause sexual side effects, especially hot flashes. Vaginal dryness and discharge, vaginitis, weight gain, and loss of libido are other sexual concerns that plague women taking hormone therapy.[68] The study done by Mortimer and colleagues with 57 breast cancer patients who were treated with tamoxifen revealed that all of the women suffered from hot flashes, and tamoxifen was also associated with dyspareunia.[69] These women reported a significant incidence of "negative feelings" during intercourse ($P = 0.02$), although the frequency of having sex corresponded to the desire for sex.[69]

Counseling for these women to relieve and manage the aforementioned effects is imperative. In particular, conversation is needed regarding the controversy related to the use of local estrogen to relieve vaginal irritations. One choice advocated by Versea and Rosenzweig is the estradiol vaginal ring, which is placed in the vagina by a gynecologist every 3 months to help relieve dysuria and vaginal dryness.[68] Clearly these women will have an increased body image and sense of self-esteem if they are able to continue to be sexually active with their partners, and the bonus is that they can do so without discomfort.

THE IMPACT OF CANCER ON THE PSYCHOSEXUAL FEMININE SELF

Death is often the first fear to invade a woman's spiritual environment when a diagnosis of cancer is given. The possibility of metastasis or an uncertain prognosis, the loss of personal control, changes in role function, and a negative body image or altered sense of self-esteem can also affect a woman's sense of femininity and can create untold stress.[20] Nishimoto says, "The cancer experience and treatment radically change what was normal in a patient's life and normalization is not static, but a process that occurs as a person incorporates the cancer experience into his or her life and then adapts to the changes that have occurred."[40] A patient may ask herself whether she will be able to function like "normal people do." She may feel shame and self-disgust due to physical damage or disability from the disease, and may deny her own sexual desires because she thinks that "sick" people aren't supposed to be sexual and that she should feel lucky to be alive. Fear of abandonment may be enhanced if she is unable or has a lack of desire to experience sexual intimacy or to satisfy her partner.

The patient and her partner may deny themselves the therapeutic comfort that intimate and sexual contact provides during this frightening and powerless time if they have no information to correct distorted views and myths. It is often a healthy sexual and/or intimate relationship that enables the woman to actually feel "alive" while traveling along this devastating journey.[20] The literature is encouraging in that it demonstrates that after a cancer diagnosis, a woman's partner does tend to be steadfast and to remain in the relationship if the relationship has been strong and supportive through the years.[23,70] Fortunately, a person's sexuality does not cease to exist with the diagnosis of cancer, although couples may require inspiration and reassurance to retain their intimacy.

ASSESSMENT OF SEXUAL FUNCTION

Discomfort with the topic of sexuality, lack of time and education, and the fear of being intrusive are among the reasons why the health professional tends to shy away from the issue of sexuality, all the more so when a patient is single, widowed, lesbian, very young, or old.[71] Nurses may decide that since the patient has remained silent or voiced no questions, she has no interest in her sexual function. Normally, she feels grateful to have survived the diagnosis and treatment trajectory and may think that her sexual concerns are insignificant, especially if these haven't been addressed at any point in time by the nurse or physician.

As soon as time permits, a sexual assessment should be completed, preferably along with the nursing history and physical (see Table 16-1). Because time is usually limited, a few brief questions may be asked that will inform the clinician whether or not there are immediate concerns (Box 16-3). An in-depth assessment will, of course, provide more extensive information; the Activity, Libido/desire, Arousal/orgasm, Resolution, Medical history (ALARM) method can guide the nurse in this endeavor (Box 16-4).

Nurses and physicians should be cautious about becoming too ardent in their effort to alleviate the sexual side effects of cancer and its treatment. While it is important to assess and address the issue, if the patient does not want to discuss her sexuality, this wish should also be respected. The clinician can take comfort in knowing, nonetheless, that the patient was afforded the opportunity, and that she knows that this subject is one that will be discussed if she chooses to do so at a later date. Patients will have varied emotional and verbal responses when

Table **16-1** Sexual Assessment Components[18,20,40]

Component	Process
Privacy	Do not discuss when making rounds or if roommate is present; move to another room or private area if possible.
Confidentiality	Usual practice is to meet with the patient first, then include the partner with permission. This decreases anxiety.
Obtain sexual history early	Ascertain sexual function before disease occurred; the psychologic status of the patient; the relationship with and attitude of his sexual partner.
Avoid overreaction	Listen attentively with genuine interest; this conveys acceptance.
Move from less sensitive (general) questions to more sensitive (specific) issues	Introduce concept during other informational/educational conversation.
Determine patient goals	Clear and detailed information assists in patient/partner decisions and helps to anticipate problems.
Realize when a problem is too complex	Refer patient to a sex therapist, preferably one who is Assoc. of Sex, Education, Counseling, and Therapy (ASSECT)–certified.

Box 16-3 Brief Assessment Questions

- Has having cancer (or its treatment) interfered with your being a father (partner, husband)?
- Has your cancer (or its treatment) changed the way you see yourself as a man?
- Has your cancer (or its treatment) caused any change in your sexual functioning (sex life)?
- Do you expect your sexual functioning (sex life) to be changed in any way after you leave the hospital (after treatment is finished)?

From McPhetridge L: Nursing history: one means to personalize care, *Am J Nurs* 68:73, 1968.

Box 16-4 ALARM Assessment Method[80]

A = **A**ctivity: frequency of sexual activity
L = **L**ibido/desire: changes in desire or interest in sexual activity
A = **A**rousal/orgasm: changes in ability to get an erection, ability to ejaculate with sexual excitement
R = **R**esolution: changes in sense of release of tension or sexual contentment after intercourse
M = **M**edical history: description of history relative to disruption of sexual activity

pondering sexuality changes due to their cancer. And, discussion about this most intimate aspect of their lives should be perceived as an opportunity rather than an annoyance or embarrassment.

There are several research assessment instruments that can be adapted to the clinical setting, and the information gathered can be quantitatively analyzed.[22,71,72] The Derogatis Interview for Sexual Functioning (DISF), which also has a self-report component, is a tool that measures the quality of sexual function in five sections (sexual cognition/fantasy, sexual arousal, sexual behavior/experiences, orgasm, and drive and relationship).[73] The DISF parallels the sexual response cycle, it has a female and male version, and it takes less than 15 minutes to complete. Studies regarding the sexual function of patients with head and neck, prostate, and lung cancer have used this brief instrument.[61,74]

INTERVENTIONS RELATED TO SEXUAL DYSFUNCTION

Once the clinician has determined the patient's desire to learn, her present level of knowledge, and her social and sexual value systems, it is essential to educate the patient and her partner about the sexual ramifications of treatment and potential forms of sexual expression that they may find acceptable. Varied expressions of affection and love (e.g., holding, touching, caressing, kissing, fondling) are reassuring behaviors. Rather than dwelling on what is missing, encourage patients and their partners to focus on their positive attributes and the methods of expression still available to them during recovery and in survivorship. Cancer and its therapies can impede many facets of sexual expression, but many other characteristics remain intact like the simple pleasure of being close and of receiving comfort from a loving partner. An excellent resource for the woman with cancer and her partner, written by Schover and published by the American Cancer Society, is available free of charge.[75] Schover and colleagues have also written an in-depth account for the professional of the female sexual response during the cancer experience.[16]

Sexual happiness may be achieved by the integration of emotional needs and physical needs. Many interventions may be suggested and employed by the clinician so that the patient and her partner are well informed and have permission to be as physical as they wish to be together (Box 16-5). Further emotional support may be

Box 16-5 General Interventions to Fulfill Physical and Emotional Needs[20]

ALWAYS PRACTICE SAFE SEX

BREAST CANCER

1. If mastectomy has occurred and she feels self conscious showing her partner her surgical scar, it is advocated that the couple both takes their clothes off, put robes on, and then stand in front of a mirror *together* and disrobe. This prevents the woman from feeling totally vulnerable because both of them have their clothes removed.
2. She can camouflage the wound (whether mastectomy or lumpectomy and radiation) by wearing a camisole or fancy short nightgown, which also enhances femininity.
3. The couple may wish to try other positions for intercourse that do not enhance a direct view of the treated breast. A side-lying or rear-entry position is recommended.
4. She may wish to make love by candlelight or to replace a white light bulb with a red one to enhance the ambiance.
5. Many women derive great pleasure from manipulation, touching, or sucking on the breast. Inform her that she will not cause a cancer in the other breast while enjoying this kind of stimulation. If the breast is reconstructed, it is important that she know there will be little to no sensation in this breast.

COLORECTAL CANCERS

Hints for Women

1. Encourage the use of personal lubricants for vaginal dryness (e.g., Astroglide, Slippery Stuff, KY jelly) found in most grocery and drug stores. Replens can be used as a moisturizer daily.
2. Hormone creams or vaginal suppositories (Vagifem, not absorbed systemically) may also be prescribed for dryness.
3. Encourage her to experiment with "teddies," fancy night-wear, crotch-less panties or something with a snap crotch or a cut-out crotch.
4. The patient may not come to orgasm the first time she has sexual intercourse after surgery. Explain that this is normal and not to worry about it.

If a Stoma is in Place

1. The focus should be on feelings and not on the pouch!
2. The pouch should be emptied and secured and reinforced with paper tape around the edges. Use a "lock-ring" mechanism for security if a two-piece system is in place.
3. Gassy foods such as cabbage, sodas, beer, beans, and chili should be avoided.
4. If a urostomy is in place, foods that cause strong odor in the urine like asparagus should be avoided.
5. Encourage the use of deodorizers: one for the pouch (Banish) and perhaps a pill or liquid taken by mouth (e.g., Breath-Assure, Bean-O, Devrom).
6. Pouch covers can be obtained that are not transparent. A "passion pouch" can be used during sex. These are smaller, closed-end, disposable pouches that are shorter and less bulky than standard drainable pouches. Many brands are available.
7. In the "woman on top" position, the bottom of the pouch can be tucked into a belt or held out of the way with a cloth cover.
8. The side-lying position works best on the stoma side because the pouch will fall away and not come between the woman and her partner

Continued

Box 16-5 General Interventions to Fulfill Physical and Emotional Needs[20]—cont'd

GYNECOLOGIC CANCERS

1. Sexual intercourse should not be resumed until 6 to 8 weeks after gynecologic surgery (hysterectomy, vulvectomy, pelvic exenteration). This waiting time will promote healing, and rehabilitation may be needed if reconstruction of the vagina was needed or a neovagina has been created.
2. Alternatives to intercourse must be provided and encouraged even if intercourse is possible. These include nudity and cuddling with general pleasuring, autoeroticism and mutual masturbation, oral-genital stimulation, anal loveplay, and fantasy with DVD or videos. The Kāma Sũtra created by the Sinclair Intimacy Institute is a good choice; it can be contacted online at www.BetterSex.com.
3. Vaginal estrogen products, which decrease dryness and irritability, are an option, and several are on the market such as Estrace (a vaginal cream), Vagifem tablets, and the Estring. The tablets and Estring incur the least systemic absorption.
4. Kegel exercises (tensing and relaxing the pelvic muscles) will help to relieve tension, increase elasticity, reduce urinary incontinence, and decrease dyspareunia.
5. During sexual activity, the hips may be elevated to improve stimulation. If rear entry is preferred, the thighs may be adducted and lubricated to emulate a deeper vaginal barrel. More control is afforded in the female superior position, but it may not be as comfortable.

If radiation has been administered to the pelvis, the following interventions may be helpful:

1. Encourage the woman to continue intercourse during treatment until it becomes uncomfortable and resume when the vagina is healed. This helps prevent adhesions and shortening of the vagina.
2. If the woman does not have a partner, she should be encouraged to use a dilator (they come in sizes from extra-small to large) on a daily basis. It should also be used during the period in which the woman cannot tolerate intercourse. Sensitivity must be used when explaining dilator use.
3. A water-soluble lubricant must be used for intercourse or when using a dilator, since the ability of the vagina to lubricate will be damaged from the radiation. A lubricant can be applied either privately or as part of foreplay. Lubricants include Astroglide, Slippery-Stuff, KY jelly products, and others. They are obtained at any local drugstore or supermarket. Replens is another commercially available vaginal moisturizer; it can be applied on a daily basis and is useful especially in women who have had total body radiation.

HEAD AND NECK CANCER

1. Before sexual activity, tracheostomies should be cleaned and shielded with a cover obtained from Byram Health Care Center, Inc., Greenwich, CT, 800-354-4054. Women may also wish to wear some kind of fancy high neckwear.
2. Sugarless mints help to freshen breath and artificial salivas (Moi-Stir, Xerolube) will lubricate a dry mouth.
3. Because of a decreased sense of smell resulting from radiation treatments, fragrance may not be appreciated, but candles, scented or not, will still enhance ambience.
4. Partners may be fearful of smothering her or obstructing her air supply, so various positions may need to be tried (see Schover LR: *Sexuality and cancer: For the woman who has cancer and her partner,* Atlanta, GA, 2001, American Cancer Society).
5. If her larynx has been removed, heavy breathing will sound different and a sexy voice will be absent. If she must use an artificial larynx, her voice will sound rather masculine and distract from her sense of femininity.

Continued

Box 16-5 GENERAL INTERVENTIONS TO FULFILL PHYSICAL AND EMOTIONAL NEEDS[20]—CONT'D

HEMATOLOGIC MALIGNANCIES

1. Patients with neutropenia or thrombocytopenia should be cautioned against oral, vaginal, and anal manipulation. Suggest "nonperformance" activities like a warm bubble bath with candlelight, romantic music, and some wine (in plastic glasses).
2. Avoid heavy meals and alcohol.
3. Plan a sexual interlude after antiemetics have taken effect.
4. To decrease fatigue, a supine or side-lying position for intercourse uses less energy. A nap may also be helpful.
5. Emphasize the importance of contraception during chemotherapy; encourage sperm banking before chemotherapy begins, or within the first 10-14 days.[78,79] If quality or quantity of preserved sperm is too low for intrauterine insemination, in vitro fertilization or intracytoplasmic sperm injection (ICSI) may be used. ICSI is a new technique whereby a single sperm is isolated and injected into the egg, which is cultured until an embryo develops, and then transferred to the uterus.[78]

LUNG CANCER

1. Experience sexual closeness that does not necessarily lead to intercourse, which may exacerbate fatigue and dyspnea. These precious moments allow the patient to feel "alive," especially when she is not being treated like an invalid.
2. Nonperformance closeness and touching, like soft caressing or light massage with oils or creams is sensual and helps reduce discomfort.
3. To conserve energy, partners can be sexual with mutual masturbation and watching erotic videos.
4. To prevent bronchospasm, decrease or eliminate environmental irritants like perfumes, colognes, and hairsprays.
5. Avoid long, slow kisses on the mouth because patients can become fearful of not getting enough oxygen.
6. To reduce exertion during sexual activity, encourage the use of a waterbed; movement is created without effort.

EMOTIONAL INTIMACY

1. Focus on the development of increased intimacy in the relationship rather than simply thinking about sex. Remember that intimacy and affection whet the appetite for lovemaking.
2. Encourage communication between partners about their day, their jobs, the relationship, and their feelings. A relationship is no place for the "strong, silent" type.
3. Encourage development of a high degree of comfort with sensuality. Too often the value of sensual touching gets replaced with a fixed focus on sexuality.
4. Encourage patients to hold realistic expectations of themselves and their mate about sexual performance. Discard the false expectation that in a good relationship, sexual desire will always be as strong as it was in the beginning.
5. Time for fun and companionship with a partner should be planned. Time should be carved out in schedules to play together and to laugh, travel, listen to music, go for walks, communicate, and be emotionally available.

Colorectal information data from Turnbull G: Intimacy, sexuality and an ostomy, patient education booklet, Irvine, CA, 2001, United Ostomy Association.

offered by the nurse, or the patient and her partner may be better served by a referral to a therapist who specializes in dealing with cancer patients and/or sexuality issues. If couples can appreciate and enjoy each other and share in each other's companionship during this wearisome experience, a stronger emotional bond may be enhanced or created.

SUMMARY

Feelings of femininity and normal sexual function will be interrupted by specific physiologic and psychologic changes depending on the cancer site, type of cancer, and treatment employed. At present, the professional literature focuses on the incidence and prevalence of sexual dysfunction and does little to promote or propagate sexual function with good, evidence-based intervention research. More randomized controlled studies are needed to provide information as to what education is needed and when. However, even before those studies are accomplished, it is imperative to provide information to patients and partners before treatment begins, as well as during treatment and after it has finished. Then, psychosexual side effects may be diminished or prevented altogether. Women are not only interested in broad-spectrum quality of life, they also with to safeguard and protect their sexual quality of life.

Tiefer notes that women can experience sexual and erotic pleasures irrespective of whether they have a partner or have the full use of their bodies.[76] Although changes in health and circumstances may challenge traditional notions of sexuality and sexual pleasure, they do not preclude other rich and satisfying avenues to the expression and experiencing of women's sexual desires and energy. That part of the self that is women's "erotic life force" can still be a powerful source of pleasure and enjoyment.

REFERENCES

1. Shell JA: Do you like the things that life is showing you? The sensitive self-image of the person with cancer, *Oncol Nurs Forum* 22:907, 1995.
2. Michael R and others: *Sex in America,* Boston, 1994, Little Brown.
3. Syrjala K and others: Sexual function measurement and outcomes in cancer survivors and matched controls, *J Sex Research* 37:213, 2000.
4. Jeffry D: Overview: cancer survivorship and sexual function, *J Sex Educat Therapy* 26:170, 2001.
5. Anderson BL: Predicting sexual and psychologic morbidity and improving the quality of life for women with gynecologic cancer, *Cancer* 71:1678, 1993.
6. Bergmark K and others: Vaginal changes and sexuality in women with a history of cervical cancer, *New Engl J Med* 340:1383, 1999.
7. Bines J, Oleske DM, Cobleigh MA: Ovarian function in pre-menopausal women treated with adjuvant chemotherapy for breast cancer, *J Clin Oncol* 14:1718, 1996.
8. Ganz PA: Sexual functioning after breast cancer: a conceptual framework for future studies, *Ann Oncol* 8:105, 1997.
9. Gantz PA and others: Life after breast cancer: understanding women's health-related quality of life and sexual functioning, *J Clin Oncol* 16:501, 1998.
10. Lamb MA: Effects of cancer on the sexuality and fertility of women, *Semin Oncol Nurs* 11:120, 1995.
11. Syrjala KL and others: Prevalence and predictors of sexual dysfunction in long-term survivors of marrow transplantation, *J Clin Oncol* 16:3148, 1998.
12. Schover LR, von Eschenbach AC: Sexual function and female radical cystectomy: a case series, *J Urol* 134:465, 1985.
13. Katz MR and others: Psychosocial adjustment in head and neck cancer: the impact of disfigurement, gender, and social support, *Head Neck* 25:103, 2003.
14. Sarna L: Correlates of symptom distress in women with lung cancer, *Cancer Pract* 1:21, 1993.
15. Masters W, Johnson V, Kolodny R: *Heterosexuality,* New York, 1994, Harper Perennial.
16. Schover L, Montague D, Lakin M: Sexual problems. In DeVita VT, Hellman S, Rosenberg SA, editors: *Cancer: principles and practices of oncology,* ed. 5, Philadelphia, 1997, Lippincott-Raven.
17. Monga U: Sexuality in cancer patients, *Arch Phys Med Rehab* 9:417, 1995.
18. Ofman US: Disorders of sexuality and reproduction. In Berger A, Portenoy RK, Weissman, DE, editors: *Principles and practice of supportive oncology,* Philadelphia, 1998, Lippincott Williams & Wilkins.
19. Corney RH And others: Psychosexual dysfunction in women with gynecological cancer following radical pelvic surgery, *Br J Obstet Gynecol* 100:73, 1993.
20. Shell JA: Impact of cancer on sexuality. In Otto S, editor: *Oncology nursing,* ed. 4, St. Louis, 2001, Mosby.
21. Rowland J: In sickness and in health: the impact of illness on couples' relationships, *J Marital Fam Therapy* 20:327, 1994.
22. Brunner DW, Boyd CP: Assessing sexuality, *Cancer Nurs* 22:440, 1999.
23. Fields B, Scout: Addressing the needs of lesbian patients, *J Sex Educ Therapy* 26:182, 2001.
24. Lehmann J, Lehmann C, Kelly P: Development and health care needs of lesbians, *J Womens Health* 7:379, 1998.
25. Institute of Medicine: *Lesbian health: current assessment and directions for the future,* Washington, DC, 2000, National Academy Press.
26. National Council on Aging: *Healthy sexuality and vital aging,* Washington, DC, 1998, Author.

27. Little FA, Howard GC: Sexual function following radial radiotherapy for bladder cancer, *Radiother Oncol* 49:157, 1998.
28. Ofman US: *Preservation of function in genitourinary cancers: psychosexual and psychosocial issues,* New York, 1995, Marcel Dekker.
29. Gallo-Silver L: The sexual rehabilitation of persons with cancer, *Cancer Pract* 8:10, 2000.
30. Schover LR: Sexuality and body image in younger women with breast cancer, *Monogr Natl Cancer Instit* 16:177, 1994.
31. Wilmoth MC, Bruner DW: Integrating sexuality into cancer nursing practice. In Hubbard SM, Goodman M, Knobf, MT editors: *Oncol Nurs Updates* 19:10, 2002.
32. Wilmoth MC, Townsend, JA: A comparison of the effects of lumpectomy versus mastectomy on sexual behaviors, *Cancer Pract* 3:279, 1995.
33. Wilmoth MC, Ross JA: Women's perception: breast cancer treatments and sexuality, *Cancer Pract* 5:353, 1997.
34. Schover L and others: Comparison of partial mastectomy with breast reconstruction on psychosocial adjustment, body image, and sexuality, *Cancer* 75:54, 1995.
35. Carlsson M, Hamrin E: Psychological and psychosocial aspects of breast cancer and breast cancer treatment: a literature review, *Cancer Nurs* 17:418, 1994.
36. Young-McCaughan S: Sexual functioning in women with breast cancer after treatment with adjuvant therapy, *Cancer Nurs* 19:308, 1996.
37. Ghizzani A and others: The evaluation of some factors influencing the sexual life of women affected by breast cancer, *J Sex Marital Ther* 21:57, 1995.
38. Turnbull GB: *Intimacy, sexuality, and an ostomy,* Irvine, CA, 2001, United Ostomy Association.
39. Sprunk E, Alteneder RR: The impact of an ostomy on sexuality, *Clin J Oncol Nurs* 4:85, 2000.
40. Nishimoto PW: Sex and sexuality in the cancer patient, Nurse Pract Forum 6:221, 1995.
41. Sprangers MA and others: Quality of life in colorectal cancer: Stoma vs. nonstoma patients, Dis Colon Rectum 38:361, 1995.
42. Caldwell K: Homosexuality: a neglected issue in stoma care, *Br J Nurs* 4:1009, 1995.
43. Northouse LL and others: The concerns of patients and spouses after the diagnosis of colon cancer: a qualitative analysis, *J Wound Ostomy Continence Nurs* 26(1): 8-17, 1999.
44. Mihalopoulos NG and others: The psychologic impact of ostomy surgery on persons 50 years of age and older, *JWOCN* 21:149, 1994.
45. Zacharias DR, Gilg CA, Foxall MJ: Quality of life and coping in patients with gynecological cancer and their spouses, *Oncol Nurs Forum* 21:1699, 1994.
46. Wilmoth MC, Spinelli A: Sexual implications of gynecologic cancer treatments, *J Obstet Gynecol Nurs* 29:413, 2000.
47. Lefkowitz GK, McCullough AR: Influence of abdominal, pelvic, and genital surgery on sexual function in women, *J Sex Educ Ther* 25:45, 2000.
48. Darling CA, McKoy-Smith YM: Understanding hysterectomies: sexual satisfaction and quality of life, *J Sex Res* 30:324, 1993.
49. Green MS and others: Sexual dysfunction following vulvectomy, *Gynecol Oncol,* 77:73, 2000.
50. Kattlove H, Winn R.J: Ongoing care of patients after primary treatment for their cancer, *Cancer J Clin* 53:172, 2003.
51. Otto SE: Chemotherapy. In Otto S, editor: *Oncology nursing,* St. Louis, 2001, Mosby.
52. Burt K: The effects of cancer on body image and sexuality, *Nurs Times* 91:36, 1995.
53. Bush NE and others: Quality of life of 125 adults surviving 6-18 years after bone marrow transplantation, *Soc Sci Med* 40:479, 1995.
54. Marks DI and others: A prospective study of the effects of high-dose chemotherapy and bone marrow transplantation on sexual function in the first year after transplant, *Bone Marrow Transplant* 19:819, 1997.
55. Tierney DK: Sexuality following hematopoietic cell transplantation, *Clin J Oncol Nurs* 8:43, 2004.
56. Sarna L: Women with lung cancer: impact on quality of life, *Qual Life Res* 2:13, 1993.
57. Sarna L: Functional status in women with lung cancer, *Cancer Nurs* 17:87, 1994.
58. Ginsberg M and others: Psychiatric illness and psychosocial concerns of patients with newly diagnosed lung cancer, *CMAJ* 5:701, 1995.
59. Shell JA: *The longitudinal effects of cancer treatment on sexuality in individuals with lung cancer,* Unpublished doctoral dissertation, East Lansing MI, 2002, Michigan State University.
60. Monga U and others: Sexuality in head and neck cancer patients, *Arch Physical Med Rehab* 78:298, 1997.
61. Gritz ER and others: First year after head and neck cancer: quality of life, *J Clin Oncol* 17:352, 1999.
62. Dropkin, MJ: Body image and quality of life after head and neck cancer surgery, *Cancer Pract* 7:309, 1999.
63. Siston AK and others: Sexual functioning and head and neck cancer, *J Psychosoc Oncol* 15:107, 1997.
64. Iwamoto R: Radiation therapy. In Otto S, editor: *Oncology nursing,* ed. 4, St. Louis, 2001, Mosby.
65. Ezzell P: Managing the effects of gynecologic cancer treatment on quality of life and sexuality, *Soc Gynecol Nurs Oncol* 8:23, 1999.
66. Thranov I, Klee M: Sexuality among gynecological cancer patients—a cross-sectional study, *Gynecol Oncol* 52:14, 1994.
67. Powles TJ: Efficacy of tamoxifen as treatment of breast cancer, *Semin Oncol* 24(Suppl. 1):S148, 1997.
68. Versea L, Rosenzweig M: Hormonal therapy for breast cancer: focus on fulvestrant, *Clin J Oncol Nurs* 7:307, 2003.
69. Mortimer JE and others: Effect of tamoxifen on sexual functioning in patients with breast cancer, *J Clin Oncol* 17:1488, 1999.
70. McDaniel SH, Hepworth J, Doherty WJ: *Medical family therapy: a biopsychosocial approach to families with health problems,* New York, 1992, Basic Books.
71. Shell JA: Evidence-based practice for symptom management in adults with cancer: sexual dysfunction, *Oncol Nurs Forum* 29:53, 2002.
72. Barton D, Wilwerding MB, Carpenter L, Loprinzi, C: Libido as part of sexuality in female cancer survivors, *Oncol Nurs Forum* 31:599, 2004.
73. Derogatis LR: *The DISF/DISF-SR manual,* Baltimore, 1987,Clinical Psychometric Research.
74. Zinreich E and others: Pre- and post-treatment evaluation of sexual function in patients with adenocarcinoma of the prostate, *Intl J Radiat Oncol Biol Phys* 19:729, 1990.

75. Schover LR: *Sexuality and cancer: For the woman who has cancer and her partner*, Atlanta, GA, 2001, American Cancer Society.
76. Tiefer L: Towards a feminist sex therapy, *Women Therapy* [Special Issue: Sexualities], 19:53, 1996.
77. McPhetridge L: Nursing history: one means to personalize care, *Am J Nurs* 68:73, 1968.
78. Hershlag A, Schuster M: Return of fertility after autologous stem cell transplantation, *Fertility and Sterility* 77: 419, 2002.
79. Meirow D, Nugent D: The effects of radiotherapy and chemotherapy on female reproduction, *Human Reproduction Update* 7:535, 2001.
80. Anderson BL: How cancer affects sexual functioning, *Oncology* 4:81-94, 1990.

CHAPTER

17 Fatigue

Rita Musanti

"For the one who is tired, the feelings experienced are the fatigue."
—Howard Bartley and Eloise Chutes: "Fatigue and Impairment in Man," 1947

INTRODUCTION

Fatigue is a common human experience of interest to many disciplines because, when present, it has the potential to decrease functional performance and affect human safety and quality of life. *Cancer-related fatigue* (CRF) is a term that identifies the fatigue that is experienced by cancer patients. It has unique characteristics that distinguish it from other fatigue states.

Cancer-related fatigue is reported as the most prevalent complaint of cancer patients, with reported incidence rates ranging from 4% to 91%.[1] CRF can occur at any time during the cancer experience; that is, as a presenting sign, during treatment, during times of survivorship and remission, and in the palliative care setting. CRF is implicated as a cause of distress and suffering in cancer patients and is considered a significant contributor to decreased quality of life in these patients. A growing body of literature related to CRF has developed since the 1970s attesting to the desire by health care professionals to gain an understanding of CRF and to find ways to minimize its effect on the cancer patient.

CANCER-RELATED FATIGUE AND WOMEN

Cancer-related fatigue is not sex-specific, but the impact of this sensation on women is profound. Across the life span, women fill vital roles in the family, the work force, and in the communities in which they live. From the time of diagnosis through survivorship, the presence of CRF has the potential to affect the developmental tasks associated with a woman's stage in life. Improvements in early detection and treatment of cancer, and the successful management of dose-limiting toxicities of cancer therapeutics, have changed the landscape of cancer survivorship. Current treatments for women diagnosed with early-stage breast, cervical, uterine, and colon cancer offer the possibility of long-term survivorship. Unfortunately, high rates of mortality and morbidity still exist for ovarian and lung cancer, since screening and early detection methods for these cancers are lacking.[4] Increasing survival from cancer is certainly welcome, but survivorship is not without problems for some women. Residual treatment effects, such as persistent CRF, are present for years after treatment is competed.[5] Understanding CRF in women is important because it is common, distressing, debilitating, and frequently persistent.

CANCER-RELATED FATIGUE AND DEVELOPMENTAL STAGE

Of all women diagnosed with cancer, approximately 30% will be diagnosed with breast cancer, 20% with gynecologic cancers, 18% with digestive system cancers, 12% with lung cancer, and the remainder of women with other types of tumors.[6] Most women will be diagnosed after the age of 50. In terms of assessing women for CRF, a clinician must take into account the age of the woman, family and occupational roles, and other developmental, contextual matters.

Several approaches have been taken with respect to developmental life span theory. On the one hand, theories divide adulthood into progressive stages based on chronologic age.[7] Specific goals or tasks are assigned to each stage. Adult tasks are focused on forming intimate relationships, generativity, and self-understanding.[8] An alternative approach is to view the adult life span trajectory based on important events such as marriage, childbearing, educational and career milestones, and caregiver responsibilities. In the latter view, developmental stage tasks in midlife are not so much dictated by age as by societal and cultural norms. The women's movement over the last 30 years has resulted in more career and family planning options for women. For example, women may choose to pursue educational or career goals first and delay marriage and childbearing until their late 30s and early 40s; or they may choose the opposite sequence and establish a family first and then proceed with career development.

All developmental life span theories, in essence, propose that women continue to evolve over their lifetimes, and that at any given time there are external and internal circumstances that influence behavior and reactions to subjective states such as CRF. The circumstances are variable and are not dictated by a women's age anymore. Therefore, when evaluating a subjective symptom such as CRF, the context of a woman's life must be taken into consideration. The impact of CRF on Erikson's developmental stages is presented in Table 17-1. Even though stages are age-defined, they are a useful framework when combined with the knowledge of specific life span events pertinent to the individual.

CLASSIFICATION OF FATIGUE

Cancer-related fatigue is a subjective state that may be acute or chronic, and that involves both the peripheral and central neuromuscular system.

Subjective vs. Objective Fatigue

Initially considered and measured as an objective state, fatigue is now considered by widespread agreement to be a subjective phenomenon that is best measured by self-report.[1,9,10] It is important to recognize that objective measures of behavior such as work output and functional performance should not be considered surrogate measures of fatigue. These measures are undoubtedly useful in the assessment of quality of life. However, to maintain conceptual clarity about fatigue, the point must be made that although these objective measures may be influenced by the perceived state of fatigue, they are not a true measure of fatigue.

Acute or Chronic Fatigue

Acute fatigue is fatigue that is of short duration and is usually relieved by rest. It is considered protective because it prompts the cessation of activity before injury occurs. It is usually experienced after prolonged physical or mental exertion. Chronic fatigue is of longer duration and is not relieved by rest or sleep; it is unpredictable in pattern, is distressful, and impairs function. It is considered pathologic. Examples include the fatigue associated with disease states such as chronic fatigue syndrome, muscular sclerosis, posttraumatic stress syndrome, Lyme disease, rheumatoid arthritis, and cancer.

Peripheral or Central Fatigue

The distinction between central and peripheral fatigue points to the conceptualization of fatigue

Table 17-1 Impact of Cancer-Related Fatigue on Developmental Stages in Adult Women

Developmental Stage Age Groups	Life Span Development Tasks[54]	Influential Cancers by Developmental Stage	Potential Impact of Cancer-Related Fatigue by Developmental Stage
Young adult women (ages 18-28)	**Intimacy vs. isolation** (ages 19-25): Identity is established and intimacy is established with another adult. **Generativity vs. stagnation** (ages 26-40): Individuals aim to produce, to contribute to society, to create a legacy; can be achieved through childrearing or personal achievement.	Cervical, rarely breast	CRF may interfere with role function in the family; dependence on others may cause developmental delay in separation from parents in younger women; social development may be impeded or delayed; educational and career goals may not be realized or need adjustment.
Women in their 30s (ages 29-39)	**Generativity vs. stagnation**	Cervical, breast	Women may be affected as younger or midlife women are; effect will depend on life events pertinent to the individual
Midlife women (ages 40-55)	**Ego integrity vs. despair** (age 41 and beyond): Acceptance of self; previous stages must have been successfully experienced and achieved.	Cervical, breast, uterine	Emotional response to sudden, premature treatment-induced menopause may exacerbate symptom of CRF. Altered role function and loss of independence, temporary or permanent, may lead to redefining of a woman's family, career, and social roles and capabilities. Deconditioning related to CRF can accelerate and/or exacerbate age-related or hormonally-induced changes in physical state such as fitness level, bone density, body composition, and risk for other chronic diseases.
Later adulthood (ages 56-75)	**Ego integrity vs. despair**	Cervical, breast, ovarian, uterine, colon, lung, lymphoma	Lesser impact on occupational role and may not be considered as distressful to women when compared to younger age group, however, impact must be assessed individually. Deconditioning-related impairment in physical and social functioning may be significant and lead to loss of independence, and loss of treatment options if disease recurs. Elder caregiver and grandparenting roles may be affected.
Older women (beyond age 75)	**Ego integrity vs. despair**	Cervical, ovarian, uterine, colon, lung, lymphoma	Deconditioning may be profound leading to greater dependence on others, despair, and safety issues for both patient and caregiver.

as a phenomenon of the neuromuscular system. Centrally-mediated fatigue implies that the fatigue sensation emanates by means of inhibition of motor neuron activation at the level of the cerebral cortex.[11] Medications such as the opioids induce fatigue through action on the central nervous system.

Peripheral fatigue is produced by means of events that occur distal to the central nervous system at the neuromuscular level. Peripheral fatigue has been demonstrated in both in vitro and in vivo studies of muscle contractile force and is attributed to neuromuscular transmission failure at the level of the neuromuscular synapse.[11,12]

DEFINITION OF CANCER-RELATED FATIGUE

Earlier fatigue research performed in numerous disciplines laid the groundwork upon which oncology researchers built their own investigations into the phenomenon that has become known as *cancer-related fatigue.*

A definition commonly cited for cancer-related fatigue is the National Comprehensive Cancer Network definition, which states the following: "Cancer-related fatigue is a persistent, subjective sense of tiredness related to cancer or cancer treatment that interferes with usual functioning."[13]

"Usual functioning" assumes functioning in the cognitive, physical, and psychosocial domains of the individual. The persistent characterization of fatigue in this definition refers to the chronic nature of fatigue, as described earlier. It does not refer to the specific pattern of presentation; that is, continuous or intermittent, or sudden or insidious onset.

Individuals interpret the meaning of this phenomenon and report it using words such as the following: inability to think, lack of concentration or diminished ability to do computations, memory impairment, tiredness, weakness, lack of energy, exhausted, lack of motivation, inability to carry out role functions at home or work, irritability, and emotional lability.

Pathogenesis and Models of Cancer-Related Fatigue

The etiology of CRF is not known. However, research shows that CRF is an abstract construct with factors in the cognitive, physiologic, and psychosocial domains of individual functioning. A unifying or common pathway to the sensation of CRF has not been elucidated. Animal models are sometimes useful in researching mechanistic pathways but the use of animal models to glean physiologic and behavioral data relevant to CRF is limited by the subjective nature of fatigue.[14] Animal studies use activity level as a surrogate for fatigue. Whether in animal models or in clinical trials, using activity as a surrogate for fatigue incorrectly assumes that fatigue and activity level are situated inversely along the same behavioral continuum.[15] This thinking ignores the voluntary dimension of fatigue. The presence of energy cannot be excluded just because fatigue is present. Patients will frequently comment on how they felt incredibly fatigued but "pushed through" to maintain their activities of daily living. Compare this with other causes of decreased activity, such as anemia or neuromuscular impairment, where voluntarily pushing through is not possible.

Several pathogenic models of CRF have been proposed. These models are based on identified factors within the physiologic, psychosocial, cognitive, and contextual domains of CRF. Commonly cited factors associated with CRF are presented in Box 17-1.

The multiplicity of factors that contribute to CRF is illustrated in Piper's fatigue framework (Figure 17-1).[16] Some models focus primarily on only one domain, such as the cognitive domain in the attentional fatigue model.[17] The physical domain is favored in the deconditioning and energy system dysfunction that is at the core of Winningham's psychobiologic-entrophy model.[18] Others have proposed that CRF is the product of an uncontrolled stress response.[19] Clearly, CRF fatigue is a broad construct comprised of a complex interplay of factors within the physiologic, psychologic, and cognitive domains of the individual.

A unique characteristic of the Piper model is that it encompasses patterning of the contributing

Box 17-1 Factors Associated with Cancer-Related Fatigue

PHYSIOLOGIC

Cancer-Related
- Abnormalities of energy metabolism
- Decreased availability of metabolic substrates
- Abnormal cytokine production
- Neurophysiologic changes of skeletal muscles
- Chronic stress response
- Hormonal changes

Treatment-Related
- Surgery
- Chemotherapy
- Radiotherapy
- Biologic response modifiers
- Hormonal therapy

Concomitant Disease States
- Anemia
- Infections
- Lung disease
- Liver disease
- Renal disease
- Malnutrition
- Neuromuscular dysfunction
- Dehydration or electrolyte imbalances
- Thyroid disease

Sleep Disorders

Immobility or Lack of Exercise

Pain or Other Symptoms

Medications

PSYCHOSOCIAL

Anxiety Disorders

Depressive Disorders

factors. The fluctuation in pattern and intensity of CRF-related factors translates into a potential change in the perception of fatigue by the individual. In addition to the variable nature of these factors is the value assigned to that variable by the individual. For example, chemotherapy treatments contribute to CRF. During treatment, varying agents and administration schedules result in different fatigue patterns.[20] A chemotherapy agent that is delivered once every 3 weeks may result in fatigue for a couple of days after the therapy. This is followed by a 2-week hiatus from the fatigue. In contrast, weekly chemotherapy administration can result in a more cumulative, daily fatigue. The former scenario may be mildly problematic to a patient who must continue to work during treatment (her job holds high value) but it is doable; she may choose to schedule her chemotherapy on a Friday so that she has the weekend to recover. However, in this same patient the second scenario may mean that she cannot continue working. This pattern of fatigue is more pervasive and debilitating and carries the potential to cause significant distress in the individual. Although somewhat simplistic, this example is illustrative of how the complex interplay of factors related to CRF is filtered through the value system of the individual.

FACTORS ASSOCIATED WITH CANCER-RELATED FATIGUE

Physiologic Factors

Abnormalities of Energy Metabolism

Energy metabolism encompasses virtually every system in the body. Lack of appetite, malnutrition, and inadequate caloric intact are all related to CRF. Hwang found a lack of appetite to be an independent predictor of fatigue in mixed cancer patients.[21] Attesting to the multiplicity of factors usually present in the setting of CRF, pain, dyspnea, feeling drowsy, feeling sad, feeling irritable, and use of analgesics were also noted to be predictors of CRF.

Energy metabolism is also affected by the transport of oxygen through the pulmonary system to the neuromuscular system via the hematologic and cardiorespiratory systems. Anemia is a well-known correlate of fatigue and one that is frequently amenable to treatment.[22,23] Anemia is a significant dose-limiting toxicity in women receiving carboplatin or cisplatin chemotherapy for gynecologic cancers. Anthracyclines, a mainstay of breast cancer treatment, expose women to the risk of cardiotoxicity with cumulative dosing. When cardiotoxicity occurs, the resultant decrease in cardiac ejection fraction impairs the ability of the

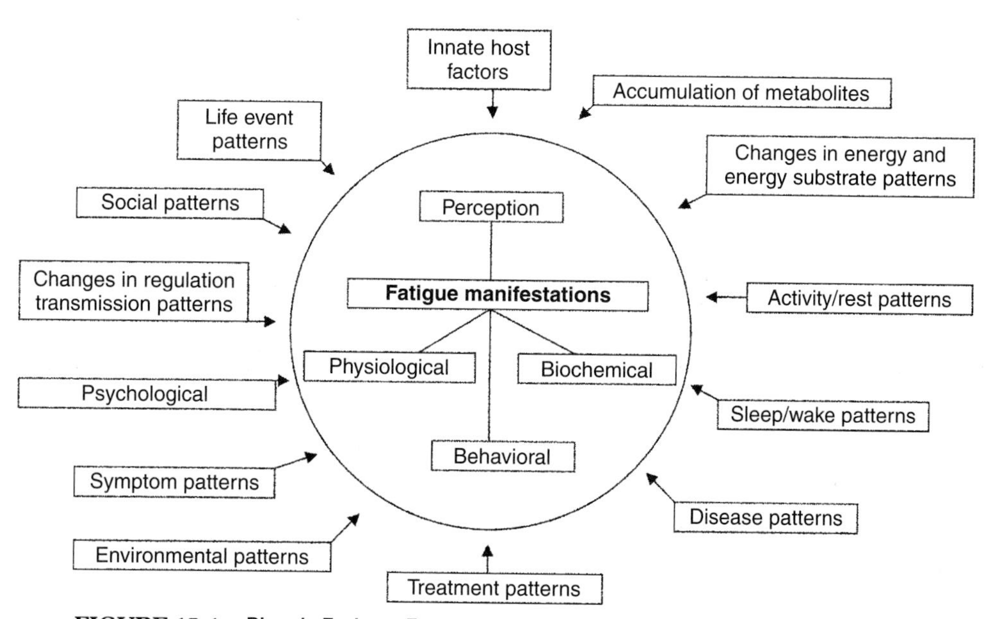

FIGURE 17-1 Piper's Fatigue Framework. (From Piper B, Lindsey A, Dodd M: Fatigue mechanisms in cancer patients: developing nursing theory, *Oncol Nurs Forum,* 14(6):17-23, 1987.)

heart to provide oxygen and nutrients to the working muscle and adequately remove metabolic wastes. The consequences are limited tolerance to physical activity, the potential for fatigue, and deconditioning. Combining poor baseline physical fitness with either anemia or cardiotoxicity can result in further deconditioning and initiation of the downward spiral of deconditioning and CRF.[18,22]

Deconditioning brings with it decreases in capacity as well as prolongation of recovery. When this condition is related to cachexia, a cytokine-driven abnormality of metabolism, the dramatic increase in whole-body protein turnover and abnormal substrate utilization leads to muscle wasting and fatigue states.[14]

Dysregulation of cytokine function has been associated with CRF.[24-26] Interleukin-1 (IL-1), interleukin-6 (IL-6), erythropoeitin, and tumor necrosis factor-α (TNF-α) dysregulation includes endogenous production by the tumor cells and inappropriate inhibitory or stimulatory control. Cytokines influence cellular signal transduction pathways. These pathways transmit signals in a stepwise manner, facilitating sequential reactions within the cell. Cytokine dysregulation provides the tumor cells with growth factors, induces immune dysfunction, and can produce symptoms such as fever, night sweats, weight loss, cachexia, anemia, and fatigue.

Attentional Fatigue

Attentional fatigue and cognitive dysfunction are frequently described by patients and commonly referred to as "chemo brain."[27] It is a phenomena that Cimprich originally described as a decreased capacity for maintaining thoughts, and an increased susceptibility to distraction and impulsivity.[17] The characterization of this attentional deficit is very similar to that described as attention deficit disorder, or ADD. *ADD* is defined as a dysfunction of the frontal lobe in areas responsible for executive functioning; it is presumed to be caused by neurotransmitter dysfunction. Wefel and colleagues used a prospective, longitudinal design to study cognitive function in breast cancer patients undergoing chemotherapy.[28] Although the sample size was small (n = 18), findings in this study confirmed a decline in frontal lobe functioning in 61% of the women. Women recovered functioning as they moved away from treatment, but not all returned to their baseline functioning level. This is a significant finding when one considers the impact such losses can have on occupational, family, and social functioning. More research is necessary in this area, specifically related to the identification of risk factors and interventions to prevent or remedy this effect if it occurs.

Psychologic Factors

Emotional distress and symptom distress are frequently reported by cancer patients. Depression, anxiety, and concurrent symptoms such as pain, nausea, vomiting, and insomnia correlate with CRF.[29-31] Emotional and symptom distress impacts negatively on coping skills and can easily exacerbate feelings of fatigue.[29] From a clinical standpoint it is challenging to determine which came first—the emotional distress or fatigue. In some cases, feeling sad and irritable are predictive signs of fatigue.[21] This is not a surprising finding when one consider how closely linked psychologic factors and mood disorders are with fatigue. It is for this reason that mood disorders must always be considered when assessing CRF.

Contextual Factors

Patterns of CRF can be described for contextual variables such as treatment modality and administration schedule.[20,23] Contextual variables that influence the perception of CRF include surgery, radiation therapy, chemotherapy, short- and long-term survivorship, and the presence and patterns of comorbid conditions.

CANCER-RELATED FATIGUE SYNDROME

The complexity of CRF is evident. In the absence of a satisfactory definition of fatigue and with the etiology of CRF still elusive, some researchers proposed that CRF should be approached as a syndrome.[32] A syndrome occurs when some predetermined arrangement of criteria are met. Box 17-2 lists the criteria accepted by the

Box 17-2 ICD-10 Cancer-Related Fatigue Criteria[55]

The following symptoms have been present every day or nearly every day during the same 2-week period in the past month:

1. Significant fatigue, diminished energy, or increased need to rest, disproportionate to any recent change in activity level; plus 5 or more of the following:
    1. Complaints of generalized weakness, limb heaviness
    2. Diminished concentration or attention
    3. Decreased motivation or interest to engage in usual activities
    4. Insomnia or hypersomnia
    5. Experience of sleep as unrefreshing or nonrestorative
    6. Perceived need to struggle to overcome inactivity
    7. Marked emotional reactivity (e.g., sadness, frustration, or irritability) to feeling fatigued
    8. Difficulty completing daily tasks attributed to feeling fatigued
    9. Perceived problems with short-term memory
    10. Postexertional fatigue lasting several hours
2. The symptoms cause clinically significant distress or impairment in social, occupational, or other important areas of functioning.
3. There is evidence from the history, physical examination, or laboratory findings that the symptoms are a consequence of cancer or cancer therapy.
4. The symptoms are not primarily a consequence of comorbid psychiatric disorders such as major depression, somatization disorder, somatoform disorder, or delirium.

International Classification of Diseases (ICD-10). The similarity of these criteria to those of a depression disorder dictates ruling out depression before these criteria can be applied to an individual experiencing a fatigue state.

Studies that have evaluated the syndrome approach to CRF identification have shown that the criteria are able to discriminate severe fatigue from mild or moderate fatigue but are not able to discriminate between mild and moderate levels.[33] In addition, because CRF must be present every day for a 2-week period, alternative CRF pattern presentations may be minimized or missed completely.

This CRF syndrome approach requires further testing for validity and reliability in identifying patients with all intensities of CRF. As currently proposed it has limited utility in identifying CRF in individuals who experience low to moderate CRF or who have fluctuations or intermittent patterns of CRF. In addition, the overlap in the criteria with symptoms of depressive disorder makes it harder to distinguish a CRF from a depressive disorder diagnosis.

Measurement of Cancer-Related Fatigue

It is generally agreed that CRF is most appropriately measured subjectively by self-report.[2,33] There are several self-report measurement tools available. The choice of CRF instrument is based on the purpose of the measurement. The measurement tool should be short and easy to complete to minimize the burden on the patient.

A primary consideration is whether or not the instrument measures fatigue unidimensionally or multidimensionally. Although limited by the fact that they measure only one dimension of fatigue, the unidimensional scales are useful to rapidly determine if fatigue is present. This is most useful in screening for fatigue, although these scales have been used extensively in fatigue research. The most common unidimensional scales seen in the literature include the Profile of Mood States—Fatigue (POMS-F)[34], the FACT-F (Functional Assessment of Cancer Therapy—Fatigue),[35] the VAS and the Brief Fatigue Inventory (BFI).[36] The multidimensional fatigue scales are intended to render more information about the patient's fatigue experience. Examples of these instruments include the Revised Piper Fatigue Scale,[37] the Revised Schwartz Cancer Fatigue Scale (SCFS-6),[38] and the Multidimensional Fatigue Symptom Inventory (MFSI).[39]

A secondary consideration is the time reference of the measurement. Fatigue patterns vary greatly and are dependent on an interplay of contributing factors. Querying the patient over the wrong time period may result in clinically significant fatigue going undetected. Selected unidimensional and multidimensional CRF measurement instruments are presented in Table 17-2. These instruments range from those that detect only the presence or absence of fatigue to those that recall the presence of fatigue over the prior week. Patterns may not be easily elicited. A patient diary is useful in detecting patterns of fatigue. An example of a fatigue diary is presented in Figure 17-2. Richardson suggests the use of a patient diary in order to document fatigue patterns and assist patients in identifying associated factors and behaviors that may both contribute to and help ameliorate the CRF.[40,41] Diaries may aid a clinician during the more detailed assessment of fatigue and could potentially prove an efficient way to garner detailed information about the patient's fatigue in a short time. Provided the patient completed the diary in real time, this method is more reliable than patient recall of the fatigue experience.

Assessment of Cancer-Related Fatigue

Management of patients with CRF requires first that fatigued patients be identified, and then that these patients be assessed for contributing factors, that appropriate interventions be prescribed, and that patients be reevaluated at pertinent intervals. The long-held assumption that CRF is an inevitable consequence of having cancer has resulted in patients quietly suffering with their fatigue. Over the last 10 years, educational initiatives aimed at increasing patient and professional awareness about CRF have been instituted by cancer care organizations such as the Oncology Nursing Society and the American Cancer Society. Awareness is

Table 17-2 CANCER-RELATED FATIGUE MEASUREMENT INSTRUMENTS

Instrument	Dimension	Description	Reference Period	Comments	Utility
Unidimensional – Global Fatigue Score					
VISUAL-ANALOG FATIGUE SCALE (VAS-F)	Fatigue intensity	One item; 0-10 scale; 0 = no fatigue, 10 = worst fatigue	Present	Reported breakpoints include 0-3, mild fatigue; 4-6, moderate fatigue; 7-10, severe fatigue	Screening
PROFILE OF MOOD STATES (POMS-F)	Fatigue intensity; includes only psychologic aspects	7 items; 5-point Likert scale: 0 = not at all, 4 = extremely	Over the past week	Fatigue-inertia subscale of the Profile of Mood States Questionnaire; widely used in the cancer population; frequently used to validate other instruments; valid and reliable. Good test–retest reliability	Screening and outcome measure
FUNCTIONAL ASSESSMENT OF CANCER THERAPY—FATIGUE (FACT-F)	Fatigue intensity; includes psychologic and physical aspects	13 items; 5-point Likert scale; 0 = not at all, 4 = very much so	Over the past week	Part of the larger FACT Quality of Life questionnaire; may be administered as a subscale; valid and reliable in the cancer population; good test–retest reliability	Screening (subscale only) and outcome measure
BRIEF FATIGUE INVENTORY (BFI)	Fatigue intensity and interference; includes both physical and psychologic aspects	9 items; 11-point Likert; 0 = no fatigue or no interference, 10 = as bad as you can imagine or complete interference	Present level, worst, and usual level over last 24 hours; past week	Fatigue-only questionnaire; valid and reliable measure of fatigue; can best discriminate between severe fatigue (score 7 and above) and not-severe (score below 7). Test–retest reliability not evaluated	Screening

Continued

Table 17-2 CANCER-RELATED FATIGUE MEASUREMENT INSTRUMENTS—CONT'D

Instrument	Dimension	Description	Reference Period	Comments	Utility
	Multidimensional Fatigue Measurement Instruments—Subscale Plus Global Fatigue Score				
PIPER FATIGUE SCALE	Behavioral/ severity, affective meaning, sensory, and cognitive/mood	27 items 22 use an 11-point Likert scale; 5 are open-ended qualitative questions	Present	Valid and reliable in women; internal reliability of subscales established; good test–retest reliability	Screening and outcome of multiple fatigue dimensions
MULTIDIMENSIONAL FATIGUE SYMPTOM INVENTORY-SHORT FORM (MFSI-SF)	General fatigue, physical fatigue, emotional fatigue, mental fatigue, and vigor	30 items; 5-point Likert scale; 0 = not at all and 4 = extremely	Over the last 7 days	Valid and reliable, 5-factor model recently supported in male and female cancer patients receiving chemotherapy; good test–retest reliability	Screening and outcome measures of multiple dimensions of fatigue
THE SCHWARTZ CANCER FATIGUE SCALE (SCFS-6)	Physical and perceptual dimensions	6 items; 1-5 rating scale; 1 = not at all, and 5 = extremely	Over the past 2-3 days	Valid and reliable in experimental conditions	Screening; needs further psychometric testing in clinical populations

Daily Fatigue Diary

1. Did you feel fatigued today: ______Yes ______No

If yes please answer the questions below. . If no there is no need to complete the diary today.

2. To what extent did you experience fatigue today?

0 1 2 3 4 5 6 7 8 9 10
No Fatigue — Worst Fatigue

3. To what degree did your fatigue cause you distress today?

0 1 2 3 4 5 6 7 8 9 10
No Distress — Worst Distress

4. To what degree did the fatigue interfere with your ability to carry out your daily activities and chores?

0 1 2 3 4 5 6 7 8 9 10
No Interference — Complete Interference

5. To what degree did the fatigue interfere with your ability to do the things that you enjoy?

0 1 2 3 4 5 6 7 8 9 10
No Interference — Complete Interference

6. Please mark the time of the day which indicate when you felt fatigued. You may indicate more than one time.

____ early morning ______late morning ____early afternoon ____late afternoon

____early evening ____late evening

7. Did you perform any actions you hoped would relieve your fatigue?
_____**Yes** ____**No**

If you answered yes please indicate what action you took and level of relief you felt.

Action Taken	Relief Obtained		
	Complete	Partial Relief	No Relief at All

8. Did you experience any other symptoms or problems today? Please list these symptoms or problems.

____
____
____
____

FIGURE 17-2 Cancer-Related Fatigue Daily Diary. (Adapted from Richardson A: The health diary: an examination of its use as a data collection method, *J Adv Nurs* 19:782-791, 1994.)

still limited, and health care providers still fail to suggest interventions. This is presumably because of a lack of knowledge regarding assessment and interventional strategies on the part of health care providers.[42,43]

A systematic assessment approach is necessary to identify patients experiencing CRF. There is currently only one organization that provides definitive practice guidelines for the management of CRF. The National Comprehensive Cancer Network (NCCN) has published guidelines that provide clinicians with CRF standards of care as well as screening and treatment algorithms. They were originally developed by a panel of CRF experts and are now updated on a yearly basis.[44] The guideline assumes that fatigue is assessed at each patient visit. Screening for fatigue is done by using a severity scale of 0-10. The time frame reference is "since the last visit." A fatigue severity level of 1-3 (mild) prompts patient education about fatigue, and a severity level equal to or greater than 4 prompts further assessment. Assessment, intervention, and evaluation strategies are outlined for patients undergoing active treatment, in posttreatment follow-up, and at end of life. The practice guidelines for primary evaluation are shown in Figure 17-3.

One can see by looking at the guideline that the comprehensive assessment of fatigue is time-consuming. This poses a challenge to busy health care providers, who have little time during any given visit to address all patients' needs. In general, systematic screening for fatigue is not done at each visit in most cancer care institutions. It is this author's contention that the complexity of CRF, along with a lack of knowledge regarding helpful interventions and the time pressures during clinic visits, leads to some issues taking priority over others. All too frequently, fatigue falls to the bottom of the list. In addition, patients do not want to appear to complain, and they are concerned that if fatigue is mentioned it will be treated with yet another medication; thus they are hesitant to bring the problem up during the visit.[43]

A recent study of women undergoing treatment for gynecologic cancers by Donovan and others bears this out.[45] These women reported that they believed their fatigue was related to their cancer and chemotherapy, that it was not controllable, and that it was severe and distressing. Even so, they did not bring it to the attention of their health care provider. Health care providers, in turn, did not offer remedial interventions, thus potentially reinforcing the patients' perception that CRF is uncontrollable. Interestingly, 7% of the women in this study attributed their fatigue to some other variable. The literature notes that in many instances, neither the patient nor the clinician mentions fatigue during the visit for reasons previously discussed. Knowing that this is the case strongly argues for the systematic screening of fatigue in patients at each visit. A fatigue assessment form similar to the one presented in Figure 17-4 can prompt and guide clinicians to put the NCCN guidelines into effect.

A CRF score of 4 or greater prompts a standard symptom assessment. Potential contributing factors are also assessed. If a factor is found to be present, it is considered a possible contributor and handled accordingly. The fatigue assessment form provides clinicians with a framework from which to assess fatigue and can thus guide interventions. The back of the form may be used to list potential interventional strategies. The form serves to reinforce health care provider education about CRF and should minimize the perception that health care providers have that there are no interventions to use against CRF. The clinician may be referred to other guidelines such as pain or anemia management guidelines, or referral numbers may be listed for services such as sleep or pulmonary specialists. Suggested handouts can be listed, making it easier for the clinician to access or suggest materials for his or her patients.

One element of assessment that is particularly important is the temporal nature of fatigue. Because fatigue is a dynamic state, assessment must take into account patient-specific patterning. A patient-completed diary has been used successfully to record this information.[41] Delineating fatigue patterns, especially during treatment, not only facilitates improved symptom management, but gives patients a sense of control at a time that is laden with a sense of helplessness and lack of control.

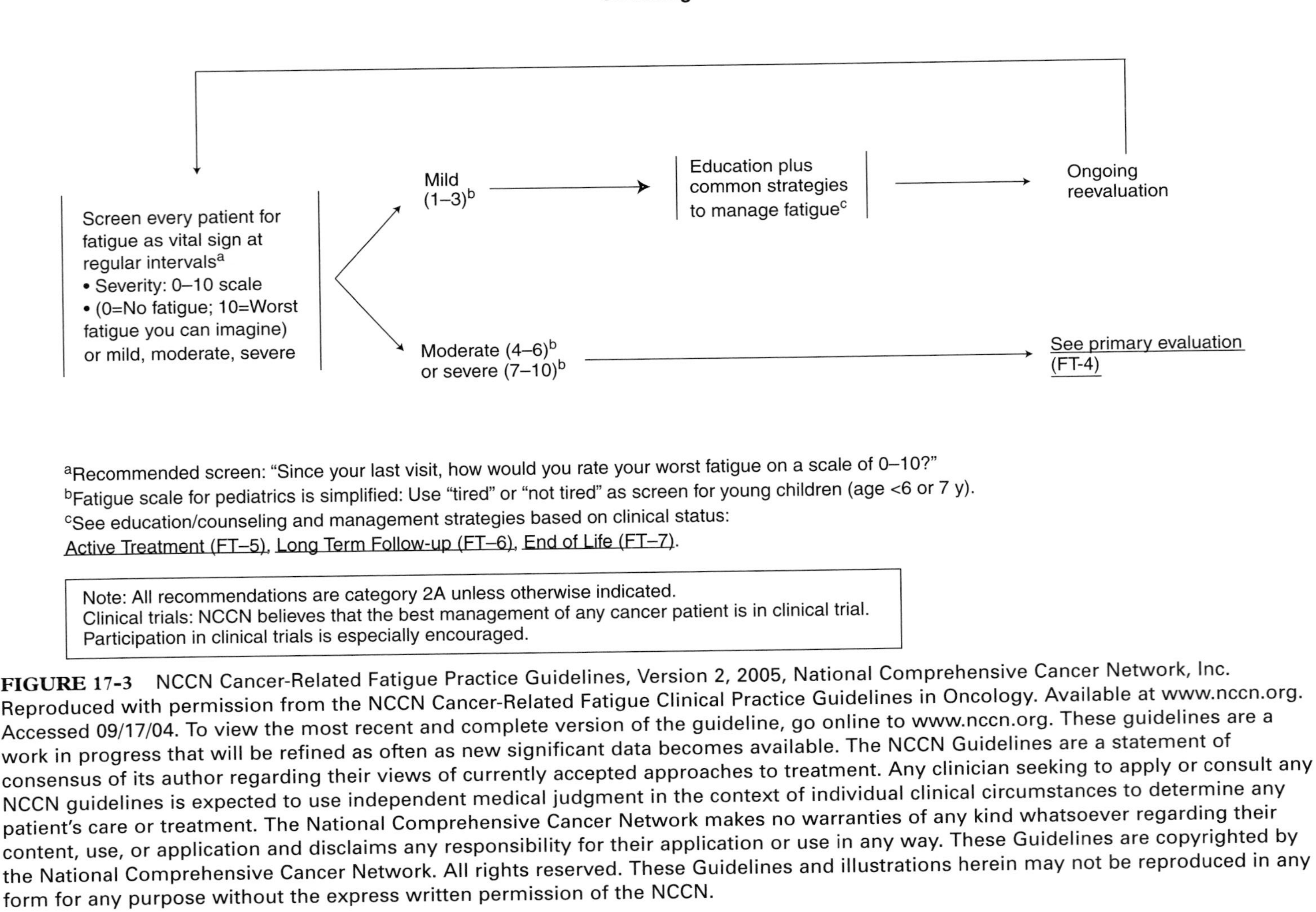

FIGURE 17-3 NCCN Cancer-Related Fatigue Practice Guidelines, Version 2, 2005, National Comprehensive Cancer Network, Inc. Reproduced with permission from the NCCN Cancer-Related Fatigue Clinical Practice Guidelines in Oncology. Available at www.nccn.org. Accessed 09/17/04. To view the most recent and complete version of the guideline, go online to www.nccn.org. These guidelines are a work in progress that will be refined as often as new significant data becomes available. The NCCN Guidelines are a statement of consensus of its author regarding their views of currently accepted approaches to treatment. Any clinician seeking to apply or consult any NCCN guidelines is expected to use independent medical judgment in the context of individual clinical circumstances to determine any patient's care or treatment. The National Comprehensive Cancer Network makes no warranties of any kind whatsoever regarding their content, use, or application and disclaims any responsibility for their application or use in any way. These Guidelines are copyrighted by the National Comprehensive Cancer Network. All rights reserved. These Guidelines and illustrations herein may not be reproduced in any form for any purpose without the express written permission of the NCCN.

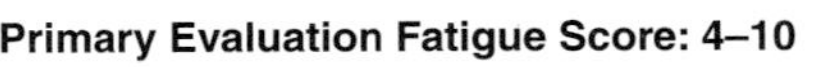

Primary Evaluation Fatigue Score: 4–10

Focused history
- Disease status and treatment
  - ▶ Rule out recurrence or progression
  - ▶ Current medications/medication changes
- Review of systems
- In-depth fatigue assessment
  - ▶ On-set, pattern, duration
  - ▶ Change over time
  - ▶ Associated or alleviating factors
  - ▶ Interference with function

Assessment of treatable contributing factors:
- Pain
- Emotional distress
  - ▶ Depression
  - ▶ Anxiety
- Sleep disturbance
- Anemia
- Nutrition assessment
  - ▶ Weight/caloric intake changes
  - ▶ Fluid electrolyte imbalance: sodium, potassium, calcium, magnesium
- Activity level
  - ▶ Decreased activity
  - ▶ Decreased physical fitness
- Comorbidities
  - ▶ Infection
  - ▶ Cardiac dysfunction
  - ▶ Pulmonary dysfunction
  - ▶ Renal dysfunction
  - ▶ Hepatic dysfunction
  - ▶ Neurologic dysfunction
  - ▶ Endocrine dysfunction (hypothyroidism)

→ Treatable contributing factors →
- No other factors →
- Pain: See NCCN Cancer Pain Guideline →
- Emotional distress: See NCCN Distress Management Guideline →
- Anemia: See NCCN Cancer and Treatment-Related Anemia Guideline →
- Sleep disturance →
- Nutrition evaluation/medical interventions →
- Activity level →
- Comorbidities →

Patient Clinical Status
- Active treatment → See Interventions (FT–5)
- Follow-up, no active treatment (except hormonal therapy) → See Interventions (FT–6)
- End of life → See Interventions (FT–7)

Note: All recommendations are category 2A unless otherwise indicated.
Clinical trials: NCCN believes that the best management of any cancer patient is in a clinical trial. Participation in clinical trials is especially encouraged.

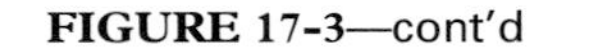

FIGURE 17-3—cont'd

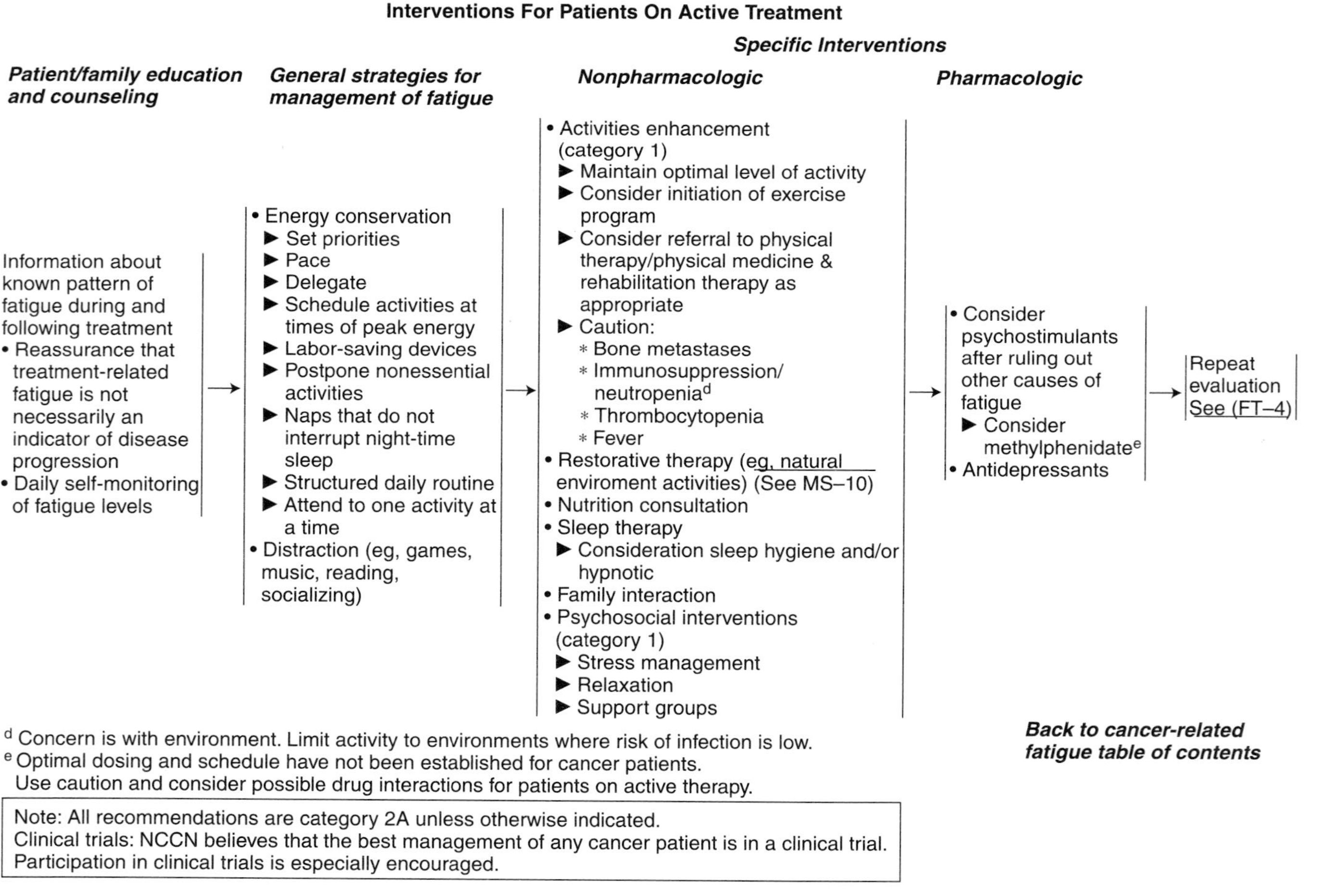

FIGURE 17-3—cont'd

Initial/Interim Fatigue Screening and Assessment Tool

Patient's Name_______________ **Date**_______________
Diagnosis:_______________ **Physician**_______________

On a scale of 0-10, zero being no fatigue at all and 10 being the most fatigue, what number best describes fatigue that you have experienced over the past week, including today?

0 1 2 3 4 5 6 7 8 9 10

If score is 4 or greater than notify clinician.

Assessment

Quality (use patient's own words)_______________

Onset, pattern, duration_______________

Relieving factors_______________

Aggravating factors_______________

Does fatigue interfere with daily activities _______yes _______no
(Consider life-span concerns)_______________

Assess for the presence of the following contributing factors:

	Yes[a]	No	Maybe[a]		Yes[a]	No	Maybe[a]
Pain rating				Infection			
Emotional distress				Cardiac dysfunction			
Sleep disturbance				Pulmonary dysfunction			
Anemia				Renal dysfunction			
Hypothyroidism				Neurological dysfunction			
Nutritional Alteration				Endocrine dysfunction			
Activity level change				Hepatic dysfunction			
Medications				Increased tumor burden			

[a]If yes or maybe is checked further assessment of this condition is required.

Plan (see back of form for resources): 1.Consider for fatigue or exercise clinical trial:_____2. Other_______________

Signature: _______________ Date: _______________

Suggestions for Interventions

Pain rating : Complete Pain Assessment Form
Emotional distress: Social Work Consult
Sleep disturbance: Refer to Sleep Disorder Center, (XXX_XXX_XXXX); Pamplets/Patient Ed materials: Resource and Learning Center
Anemia : Treat as per Anemia Guidelines
Hypothyroidism: Obtain serum TSH
Nutritional Alteration: Dietary Consult
Activity level change: Encourage Physical Activity, Learning and Resource Center, PT or Exercise Intervention.
Medications: Multi-disciplinary consult with Pharmacy
Infection: Evaluate and treat appropriately.
Cardiac dysfunction: Evaluate and refer if necessary.
Pulmonary dysfunction: Evaluate and refer if necessary.
Renal dysfunction: Evaluate and refer if necessary.
Neurological dysfunction: Evaluate and refer if necessary.
Endocrine dysfunction: Evaluate and refer if necessary.
Hepatic dysfunction: Evaluate and refer if necessary.
Suspected increase tumor burden: Restage.

FIGURE 17-4 Cancer-Related Fatigue Assessment Tool. (Adapted from Fatigue Assessment Form: Cancer Institute of New Jersey Comprehensive Cancer Center.)

Management of Cancer-Related Fatigue

Research to date has not revealed a common pathway in which all the contributing factors converge and result in CRF. Theoretically, if this were the case, this pathway could be targeted in some way and CRF could potentially be relieved with one intervention. Given what is known today, the most effective strategy to manage CRF is to use a comprehensive assessment that identifies the contributing factors followed by appropriate intervention and follow-up evaluation.

TREATING UNDERLYING CAUSES OF FATIGUE

Anemia

Anemia is a known cause of CRF, and once identified by a proper work-up it can usually be successfully treated. Transfusion with packed red blood cells provides quick, effective relief of symptomatic anemia. Supplemental iron to replace depleted stores, and/or recombinant human erythropoietin, provides ongoing stimulation and the raw materials to boost red blood cell production. Erythropoietin has been shown to be useful in treating therapy-induced anemias and decreases the chance of having to receive a RBC transfusion, and it improves self-reported functional status and QOL.[42,46]

Current clinical guidelines published by the American Society of Clinical Oncologists (ASCO) and the NCCN recommend treatment if the hemoglobin level falls below 10 or 11 g/dl respectively.[47,48] ASCO recommends using clinical judgment when deciding to treat patients whose hemoglobin is between 10 and 12 g/dl. Erythropoietin is withheld when the hemoglobin level reaches 12 g/dl. It is imperative that reevaluation of the hemoglobin response be incorporated into the treatment plan at no less than once per month. Pretreatment evaluation and periodic monitoring of iron, total iron binding capacity (TIBC), transferrin saturation, or ferritin levels are also recommended. If an increase in hemoglobin response is not achieved at the recommended starting dose, the dose is titrated up and response is assessed over the next 4 to 8 weeks. Once an adequate response is obtained (i.e., hemoglobin level around 12 g/dl) the dose of erythropoietin can be titrated to maintain a hemoglobin level of greater than 10 g/dl. Both triweekly and weekly doses have been found to be effective. A longer-acting erythropoietin stimulation medication, darbopoeitin, is now available and undergoing clinical trials to ascertain its optimal dosing schedule to treat chemotherapy-induced anemia.

Depression

Patients with depression may be treated with antidepressants and/or be offered opportunities for psychosocial support, either through referral to a mental health professional for individual counseling or to a cancer support group. Psychosocial support can include stress management techniques, relaxation techniques, and attendance at support groups.

Alterations in Activity and Rest Pattern

Patient education about activity and rest patterns should include strategies for energy conservation, exercise, and sleep patterns. A patient diary or journal in which a patient monitors fatigue, sleep, rest, activity, and other symptoms has been successfully used to teach patients energy conservation techniques.[49] The diary provided the basis for analyzing the patterns of activity, rest, and fatigue so patients could be taught to plan and carry out activities while keeping fatigue to a minimum. Energy-conserving activities include setting priorities, pacing activities, delegation of tasks to others, performing important or high energy–requiring activities at time of peak energy and minimal fatigue, balancing activity with rest periods or naps, and not doing unnecessary activities.

The clinician should address the issue of sleep disorders. The use of sleep medication should be considered, when indicated, for insomnia. A sleep protocol consisting of routine bedtime activities and timing is considered an important first step in preparing the body for sleep.[50] In addition, a block of night time sleep is preferential to intermittent sleep with daytime napping. These naps should be limited to no longer than 15 to 20 minutes. Long periods of daytime inactivity and napping can contribute to overall physical deconditioning, which increases fatigue. Patients whose sleep is seriously impaired should be referred to a specialist on sleep disorders.

Exercise is one of the few evidence-based interventions against CRF. In addition to decreasing fatigue, it is instrumental in guarding against deconditioning, improving mood, and improving sleep quality. The reader is referred to the chapter on exercise.

Multiple Symptom Management

Symptom clustering is a new term that refers to the well-known phenomenon of more than one symptom occurring simultaneously. In patients with lung cancer, symptoms of weight loss, dyspnea, and fatigue are often seen together; in patients with breast cancer, symptoms of weight gain, fatigue, depression, and anxiety have been noted to occur together in survivors; in women with advanced cancers, pain, fatigue, and depression are commonly seen concurrently. Fatigue is often associated with other symptoms, and symptom distress has been frequently found to correlate with fatigue. The challenge of multiple symptom management lies in a comprehensive assessment of the patient and the subsequent attention to all symptoms. It is plausible that with further research into symptom clusters, one will be able to identify sentinel symptoms. The appearance of these symptoms is a harbinger of what may follow. Theoretically appropriate treatment of these symptoms will pave the way for minimizing additional symptoms. For example, uncontrolled pain will undoubtedly lead to sleep impairment and fatigue if left unchecked. In providing proper pain management at the onset, the impairment of sleep and the emergence of fatigue are less likely.

Nutrition

The reader is referred to Chapter 18 "Nutrition" for specifics related to proper nutrition. Inappropriate caloric or nutrient consumption, poor hydration, and vitamin deficiencies can jeopardize the efficiency of metabolic systems and affect energy levels. Many patients have misconceptions about diet, and a referral to a dietician can help dispel myths and assist in patient education.

Patient Education

Patient education is vital to the management of CRF. Behavioral strategies such as those just discussed involve educating the patient about activity, nutrition, exercise, mental health, and other symptoms. Women need to be encouraged to report their symptoms to their health care providers and not minimize the impact that symptoms such as CRF have on their quality of life. In addition, health care providers can prescribe and educate regarding preventive and management measures. It is important for health care providers to stay abreast of new developments so that as interventions are uncovered these can be passed on to patients.

Pharmacologic Agents

The psychostimulants methylphenidate and dextroamphetamine are prescribed to ameliorate CRF.[51] Methylphenidate relieves fatigue, improves appetite, and decreases anxiety, depression, nausea, pain, and drowsiness when self-administered in patients with advanced cancer.[52] The psychostimulants enhance alertness and attention. They are short-acting and so can be useful for daytime administration that doesn't interfere with the sleep cycle. Patients must be educated that these medications, when taken in the evening, have the potential to interfere with sleep and that this should be avoided. Appetite suppression is a side effect of these medications and may be problematic for some patients. Interestingly, the drug methylphenidate is the mainstay of the treatment of attention-deficit hyperactivity disorder (ADHD). No studies to date have examined the effectiveness in treating the attention deficit identified in cancer patients. Modafinil is a newer central nervous stimulant medication that has not been studied in the cancer population but that could potentially offer benefit.

In the palliative care setting, glucocorticoids are prescribed for fatigue. These steroid medications also cause an increase in feelings of general well-being in most patients and increases appetite.

Long-term use is not recommended because of undesirable side effects such as propensity to infection, myopathy, and adrenal insufficiency.

Antidepressant medications have been considered as a treatment of CRF, based on the theory that CRF is centrally mediated and because of its close association to depression. Alteration in brain 5-hydroxytryptamine (5-HT) in chronic fatigue syndrome led researchers to hypothesize that perhaps a similar mechanism was operative in CRF during treatment and that fatigue and depression shared a common pathway involving serotonin.[53] Although the selective serotonin reuptake inhibitors have not yet been proven effective in combating CRF, these medications are still valuable in the treatment of depression in cancer patients.

SUMMARY

Cancer-related fatigue is a prevalent symptom experienced by women cancer patients. It has a profound impact on quality of life. It is often underreported, and there remains a general contention among health care providers and patients alike that little can be done to ameliorate this symptom. However, there is evidence that psychosocial support and exercise interventions effectively reduce CRF. It is imperative that further research continue in the area of CRF. Relieving this symptom will not only decrease suffering but will allow women to engage more fully in the things they choose to do.

REFERENCES

1. Agency for Healthcare Research and Quality: *Management of cancer symptoms: pain, depression, and fatigue*, Rockville, Maryland, 2002.
2. Ferrell BR and others: Quality of life in breast cancer, *Cancer Pract*, 4:331, 1996.
3. Bower JE and others: Fatigue in breast cancer survivors: occurrence, correlates, and impact on quality of life, *J Clin Oncol* 18:743, 2000.
4. Jemal A and others: Cancer statistics, *Cancer J Clin* 55:10, 2005.
5. Andrykowski MA, Curran SL, Lightner R: Off-treatment fatigue in breast cancer survivors: A controlled comparison, *J Behav Med* 21:1, 1998.
6. American Cancer Society: *Cancer facts and figures*, Atlanta, Ga., 2005, The Society. Available online at www.cancer.org.
7. Erickson JM: Fatigue in adolescents with cancer: a review of the literature, *Clin J Oncol Nurs* 8:139, 2004.
8. Staudinger UB, Bluck S: A view on midlife development from life-span theory. In Lachman M, editor: *Handbook of midlife development*, New York, 2001, John Wiley & Sons.
9. Ferrell BR and others: Quality of life in breast cancer survivors: implications for developing support services, *Oncol Nurs Forum* 25:887, 1998.
10. Pearce S, Richardson A: Fatigue in cancer: a phenomenological perspective, *Eur J Cancer Care* 5:111, 1996.
11. Gardiner P: *Neuromuscular aspects of physical activity*, Champaign, Il, 2001, Human Kinetics.
12. Cairns S and others: Evaluation of models used to study neuromuscular fatigue, *Exercise Sport Sci Rev* 33:9, 2005.
13. Mock V and others: *NCCN practice guidelines for cancer-related fatigue*, National Comprehensive Cancer Network, 2004. On the Web at www.nccn.org/professionals/physician_gls/f_guidelines.asp.
14. Stasi R and others: Cancer-related fatigue: Evolving concepts in evaluation and treatment, *Cancer* 98:1786, 2003.
15. Nail LM: Fatigue in patients with cancer, *Oncol Nurs Forum* 29:537, 2002.
16. Piper B, Lindsey A, Dodd M: Fatigue mechanisms in cancer patients: developing nursing theory, *Oncol Nurs Forum* 14:17, 1987.
17. Cimprich B: Development of an intervention to restore attention in cancer patients, *Cancer Nurs* 16:83, 1993.
18. Winningham ML, Barton-Burke M: *Fatigue in cancer: a multidimensional approach*, Sudbury, Mass., 2000, Jones and Bartlett.
19. Aistars J: Fatigue in the cancer patient: a conceptual approach to a clinical problem, *Oncol Nurs Forum* 14:25, 1987.
20. Richardson A, Ream E: The experience of fatigue and other symptoms in patients receiving chemotherapy, *Eur J Cancer Care* 5:24, 1996.
21. Hwang SS and others: Multidimensional independent predictors of cancer-related fatigue, *J Pain Symptom Manage* 26:604, 2003.
22. Cella D: The effects of anemia and anemia treatment on the quality of life of people with cancer, *Oncology* 16:125, 2002.
23. Payne JK: The trajectory of fatigue in adult patients with breast and ovarian cancer receiving chemotherapy, *Oncol Nurs Forum* 29:1334, 2002.
24. Kurzrock R: The role of cytokines in cancer-related fatigue, *Cancer* 92:1684, 2001.
25. Bower JE and others: Fatigue and proinflammatory cytokine activity in breast cancer survivors, *Psychosom Med* 64:604, 2002.
26. St.Pierre B, Kasper C, Lindsey, A: Fatigue mechanisms in patients with cancer: effects of tumor necrosis factor and exercise on skeletal muscle, *Oncol Nurs Forum* 19:419, 1992.
27. Wefel JS and others: "Chemobrain" in breast carcinoma? A prologue, *Cancer* 101:466, 2004.
28. Wefel JS and others: The cognitive sequelae of standard-dose adjuvant chemotherapy in women with breast carcinoma: results of a prospective, randomized, longitudinal trial, *Cancer* 100:2292, 2004.
29. Ahlberg K and others: Fatigue, psychological distress, coping and quality of life in patients with uterine cancer, *J Adv Nurs* 45:205, 2004.

30. Berger AM and others: Adherence, sleep, and fatigue outcomes after adjuvant breast cancer chemotherapy: results of a feasibility intervention study, *Oncol Nurs Forum* 30:513, 2003.
31. Redeker NS, Lev EL, Ruggiero J: Insomnia, fatigue, anxiety, depression, and quality of life of cancer patients undergoing chemotherapy, *Sch Inq Nurs Pract* 14:275, 2000.
32. Cella D and others: Progress toward guidelines for the management of fatigue, *Oncology* 12:369, 1998.
33. Cella D and others: Cancer-related fatigue: prevalence of proposed diagnostic criteria in a United States sample of cancer survivors, *J Clin Oncol* 19:3385, 2001.
34. Mcnair D and others: *Manual for the profile of mood states,* San Diego, California, 1971, Educational and Industrial Testing Service.
35. Cella D: The functional assessment of cancer therapy-anemia (fact-an) scale: a new tool for the assessment of outcomes in cancer anemia and fatigue, *Semin Hematol* 34:13, 1997.
36. Mendoza T and others: The rapid assessment of fatigue severity in cancer patients: use of the brief fatigue inventory, *Cancer* 85:1186, 1999.
37. Piper BF and others: The revised Piper Fatigue Scale: psychometric evaluation in women with breast cancer, *Oncol Nurs Forum* 25:677, 1998.
38. Schwartz AL: The Schwartz cancer fatigue scale: testing reliability and validity, *Oncol Nurs Forum* 25:711, 1998.
39. Stein KD and others: Further validation of the multidimensional fatigue symptom inventory-short form, *J Pain Symptom Manage* 27:14, 2004.
40. Richardson A: Measuring fatigue in patients with cancer, *Support Care Cancer* 6:94, 1998.
41. Richardson A: The health diary: an examination of its use as a data collection method, *J Adv Nurs* 19:782, 1994.
42. Passik SD: Impediments and solutions to improving the management of cancer-related fatigue, *J Natl Cancer Inst Monogr* 136, 2004.
43. Passik SD and others: Patient-related barriers to fatigue communication: initial validation of the fatigue management barriers questionnaire, *J Pain Symptom Manage* 24:481, 2002.
44. Mock V and others: Cancer-related fatigue, 2004. Available online at www.nccn.org.
45. Donovan HS, Ward S: Representations of fatigue in women receiving chemotherapy for gynecologic cancers, *Oncol Nurs Forum* 32:113, 2005.
46. Glaspy J and others: Impact of therapy with epoetin alfa on clinical outcomes in patients with nonmyeloid malignancies during cancer chemotherapy in community oncology practice, Procrit study group, *J Clin Oncol* 15:1218, 1997.
47. Rizzo D and others: Use of epoetin in patients with cancer, www.asco.org. 2002.
48. Sabbatini P: Cancer and treatment-related anemia, 2004. Available online at www.nccn.org.
49. Barsevick AM and others: A randomized clinical trial of energy conservation for patients with cancer-related fatigue, *Cancer* 100:1302, 2004.
50. Berger AM and others: Feasibilty of a sleep intervention during adjuvant breast cancer chemotherapy, *Oncol Nurs Forum* 29:1431, 2002.
51. Burks TF: New agents for the treatment of cancer-related fatigue, *Cancer* 92:1714, 2001.
52. Bruera E and others: Patient-controlled methylphenidate for the management of fatigue in patients with advanced cancer: a preliminary report, *J Clin Oncol* 21:4439, 2003.
53. Morrow GR and others: Differential effects of paroxetine on fatigue and depression: a randomized, double-blind trial from the University of Rochester cancer center community clinical oncology program, *J Clin Oncol* 21:4635, 2003.
54. Erikson EH: *Childhood and society,* 1963, New York, Norton.
55. International Classification of Diseases, Tenth Revision, Clinical Modification (ICD-10-CM), National Center for Health Statistics, Bethesda, Maryland, 1998, National Institutes of Health, National Cancer Institute.

CHAPTER

18 Nutrition

Maureen B. Huhmann

MALNUTRITION IN CANCER

Malnutrition is an important issue in the treatment of cancer patients. The term "malnutrition" applies to both underweight and overweight populations. Malnutrition is defined as "any disorder of nutrition status including disorders resulting from deficiency of nutrient intake, impaired nutrient metabolism, or overnutrition."[1] Malnutrition has many undesired consequences on both the patient and treatment outcome.[2,3]

The term *nutritional status* is often poorly defined. Although no single index can accurately indicate poor nutritional status,[4] weight and weight history are the parameters most commonly used.[5] This method has limitations. Weight alone does not indicate the nature and extent of tissue loss in patients with cachexia.[6] It also does not indicate specific metabolic or biochemical nutritional issues.

Nutritional status has been linked to clinical outcome.[3,7] Malnutrition has been correlated with decreased response to cancer therapy,[2] decreased survival,[3] and decreased quality of life.[3,8] Malnutrition can also affect surgical outcomes and complications rates.[9-12]

CHANGES IN METABOLISM IN CANCER

The malnutrition that occurs in cancer is often due to changes in metabolism caused by the cancer itself or the treatment. Energy, carbohydrate, protein, and fat metabolism can be affected.

The impact of cancer on basal energy expenditure is variable. Cancer patients may have reduced, normal, or increased energy expenditure.[13,14] This variability is caused by individual responses to the tumor, body composition, and tumor type and stage.[15] In addition, byproducts of the tumor can affect metabolism.[16] Because of this variability it is hard to predict energy requirements for cancer patients.

Glucose intolerance and abnormal insulin response have been frequently observed in patients with cancer-induced weight loss.[14] It is hypothesized that this occurs as a result of insulin resistance or decreased pancreatic function.[17] Tumors use glucose to produce large amounts of lactate, which is converted back into glucose through gluconeogenesis in the liver. This use and recycling of glucose is called the Cori cycle.[18] This process is inefficient and requires adenosine triphosphate (ATP), or energy. This increase in ATP use contributes to hypermetabolism and further weight loss.

Loss of adipose, or fat, tissue is a common feature in weight-losing cancer patients. Lipolysis, or the breakdown of fat, and turnover of glycerol and fatty acids are increased in cancer patients. Supplemental glucose provided through infusion does not prevent or reverse this problem.[19] Lipid-mobilizing factor (LMF), a tumor byproduct, may be responsible for this increased lipolysis. LMF seems to act directly on adipocytes, causing a release of free fatty acids and glycerol.[18]

Muscle wasting contributes to the fatigue, weakness, asthenia, and respiratory complications observed in patients with advanced cancer.[20] Muscle wasting is a consequence of protein degradation occurring to provide amino acids for gluconeogenesis.[18] In normal patients these amino acids would be spared, but this protective mechanism is defective in weight-losing cancer patients. Whole body protein turnover is normal or increased because of increases in liver protein synthesis, also called the *acute phase response.*[18] Supplementation of protein does not seem to affect this turnover.[21,22] The tumor byproduct proteolysis-inducing factor (PIF) has been implicated in the increased turnover of body protein stores. PIF appears to induce protein degradation and inhibit protein synthesis.[23] A loss of 30% of body weight has been correlated with a loss of 75% of skeletal muscle mass due to protein degradation.[13]

TREATMENT-INDUCED WEIGHT GAIN

Although once thought to be impossible in cancer patients, weight gain can occur during cancer treatment. Weight gain has been reported in 50% to 96% of breast cancer patients receiving adjuvant cancer treatment.[24] A significant number gain more than 20 pounds.[24,25] Weight gain has also been observed in prostate cancer patients who receive androgen deprivation therapy.[26] The weight is gained in the form of sarcopenic obesity, or weight gain in the absence of lean tissue gain.[25] Weight gain may be related to an increase in food intake to manage symptoms or anxiety, decreased physical activity, and modification of metabolic rate.[24] Weight gain and overweight have been associated with increased risk of cancer recurrence and mortality in breast cancer survivors.[27] Current interventions in breast cancer to decrease weight gain include calorie restriction and exercise training.[25]

CANCER-INDUCED WEIGHT LOSS

The prevalence of weight loss in oncology patients ranges from 31% to 100% depending upon tumor site, stage, and treatment.[3,28-31] Minimal weight loss, in the range of 5%, is associated with increased mortality and poor prognosis.[3] Multiple factors contribute to the weight loss observed in cancer patients.[9-12] Some of the causes of weight loss[9,11,12] are presented in Box 18-1. Patients who experience gastrointestinal (GI) symptoms such as nausea, vomiting, diarrhea, and constipation, and oral symptoms such as xerostomia and mucositis, may experience weight loss early in the course of cancer.[5] Fatigue and psychologic symptoms such as depression and anxiety also influence weight loss.[11] The presence of weight loss itself is a constant reminder of disease that interferes with patient quality of life.[32]

Loss of body weight by patients with solid tumors is attributed to losses of fat, water, and fat free mass (FFM); there is little loss of protein in patients with solid tumors.[33-37] Patients with lung, GI, and head and neck tumors experience not only weight loss that is greater than 10%, but also loss of both muscle and fat. Individuals with GI malignancies seem to experience the largest decreases (more than 50%) in muscle mass and protein content, as well as 30% to 40% loss in body fat. However, even in severe wasting, patients retain some body fat. Visceral mass is also preserved to an extent, and skeletal muscle loss is the primary form of lean body mass loss.[38]

Box 18-1 Causes of Weight Loss in Cancer Patients[9,11,12]

Physiologic abnormalities associated with the tumor:
- Malabsorption
- Obstruction
- Diarrhea
- Vomiting

Host response to the tumor
- Anorexia
- Altered metabolism

Side effects of anti-cancer treatment
- Mucositis
- Radiation enteritis
- Xerostomia

Nutritional decline is often accepted as part of the cancer course and its treatment. Each anticancer treatment modality, surgery, chemotherapy, and radiation therapy presents risks to patients' nutritional integrity.

Surgery causes metabolic stress, which can lead to hypermetabolism. This hypermetabolism contributes to muscle and fat breakdown leading to postoperative weight loss.[39] Decreased dietary intake secondary to diet restriction and poor appetite further contribute to this weight loss.[11] Surgical resection that results in a change in anatomy of the GI tract may present mechanical barriers to food ingestion. Colon resections can lead to diarrhea, malabsorption, and dehydration. Pancreatic surgery can affect pancreatic enzyme and insulin production and secretion, leading to metabolic consequences.[11]

Chemotherapy is highly toxic to rapidly dividing cells such as those that line the GI tract.[11] Side effects related to chemotherapy administration vary greatly. These drugs may impair food intake directly by way of stomatoxic reactions such as mucositis, diarrhea, and vomiting, or indirectly by way of fatigue, pain, food aversions, and taste changes. Nausea and vomiting are among the most distressing side effects associated with chemotherapy.[11] Symptoms can occur before treatment, during treatment, or 1 to 2 weeks later and can last from several hours to days.[11]

Similar to chemotherapy, radiation therapy is most toxic to cells with a high turnover rate.[11] Radiation to any portion of the GI tract can cause extreme susceptibility to malnutrition. Greater that 70% of patients who receive radiation to the pelvic area experience acute inflammatory intestinal changes that cause diarrhea, abdominal pain, and nausea.[40] In some patients, this develops into chronic radiation enteritis, necessitating lifelong medicating and changes in diet. Treatment-related side effects of radiation to the head and neck such as mucositis, xerostomia, taste change, and dysphagia peak two thirds of the way through treatment and can become permanent.[41] Radiation therapy in the area of the thyroid gland can cause permanent thyroid damage, leading to changes in metabolism.[42]

Cancer Cachexia Syndrome

Cancer cachexia syndrome (CCS) refers to the characteristic wasting seen in cancer patients. Symptoms associated with CCS include weight loss, anorexia (loss of appetite), fatigue, early satiety, and asthenia.[14] CCS is a complex metabolic state that leads to depletion of energy and muscle stores. Unlike in starvation, patients experiencing CCS lose both adipose and skeletal muscle mass, while preserving visceral muscle mass and increasing hepatic mass.[43] Also unlike starvation, the weight loss associated with CCS cannot be reversed with increases in nutrient provision.[44] In the presence of CCS, weight loss will continue despite increased administration of nutrients.[43] This is most dramatically illustrated in cachectic patients receiving enteral feedings, in whom caloric intake can be increased with little patient burden. Studies in these patients have indicated no benefit of increased caloric intake on weight, survival, or quality of life (QOL).[14] Appetite stimulants are not effective in the treatment of CCS for this reason. The most effective treatment of CCS is the treatment of the underlying disease with the appropriate anticancer therapy.[43]

Although there is no universally accepted model that adequately explains the etiology of CCS in all patients,[45] CCS is blamed in part on changes in cytokine and hormone levels. Proinflammatory cytokines such as tumor necrosis factor (TNF), interferon-γ (IFN-γ), and interleukins 1 and 6 (IL-1 and IL-6) are considered important mediators of CCS. In addition, tumor byproducts such as PIF, LMF, and mitochondria-uncoupling proteins (UCP) 1, 2, and 3 exhibit specific effects on nutrient metabolism.[16]

IMPACT OF CANCER ON BODY COMPOSITION

Body composition is a breakdown for descriptive purposes of the body makeup into the compartments of the body. These compartments can be described several ways and on several levels. At the most basic level the body can be divided into fat mass and lean body mass (LBM). However, body composition is frequently described in more detail. Body compartments commonly described include body cell mass (BCM), extracellular fluids (ECF), fat mass, bone, and collagen. Descriptions of these compartments[46,47] and the impact of cancer[36-38,48] on them are presented in Table 18-1.

BCM and body fat are commonly decreased in cancer patients. The decreased BCM and accompanying expansion of ECF creates a different extracellular-intracellular water ratio specific to cachexia.[48] Malnourished cancer patients may experience a 41% decrease in BCM and a 25% increase in ECF.[47] Patients with solid tumors can lose as much as 1.34 kg of fat-free mass (FFM) in 4 weeks.[49] However, a degree of body fat remains even in patients with severe weight loss.

Changes in body composition affect symptom control and complication rates. Patients with GI malignancies experience increasing rates of severe complications associated with surgical intervention and decreasing LBM.[50] Decreases in fat mass after gastric resection were associated with increased GI symptoms and diarrhea.[51] Increased incidence of nutritional symptoms is correlated with decreases in QOL.

NUTRITION AND QUALITY OF LIFE

Health-related QOL refers to the physical, psychologic, and social domains of health that are influenced by an individual's experiences, beliefs, expectations, and perceptions. Aggressive cancer treatments influence the social, psychologic, and emotional aspects of patients' lives.[52]

The presence of malnutrition can affect a patient's QOL. Difficulty with eating because of the side effects of treatment or disease may cause patients to pass up social interactions with family and friends. This in turn leads to further depression of appetite.[53,54] Poorer overall QOL has been observed in patients experiencing symptoms that have an impact on socializing such as mouth pain, hoarseness, and unclear speech.[54]

A relationship has been established between weight loss and QOL in oncology patients. Most studies of nutrition and QOL have been limited to exploration of the impact of aggressive medical nutrition therapy, such as total parenteral nutrition, on QOL.[53] To date, there is little information correlating changes in specific body compartments to QOL. Preliminary research relating to the use

Table **18-1** IMPACT OF CANCER ON BODY COMPARTMENTS

Body Compartment	Description	Impact of Cancer
Body cell mass (BCM)	Metabolically active, oxygen-requiring, carbon dioxide–producing, glucose burning cellular mass[46] Includes skeletal muscle, tissue, organs, glands, bone marrow, and lymphatic system[46]	Decreased skeletal muscle[36,37] Visceral mass preserved[38]
Extracellular mass (ECM)	Nonmetabolically active components of fat-free mass (FFM) located outside the cellular compartment[47]	Decreased[36,37]
Extracellular fluid (ECF)	95% water and found in vascular, lymphatic, and interstitial spaces Approximately 22%-28% of body weight is ECF.[46]	Increased[48]
Fat mass	Should contribute 12%-25% of body composition, increased in obesity Comprised of stored lipid, adipocytes, and extracellular water (ECW)[46]	May be increased in breast and prostate cancer Decreased in CCS[36,37]

CCS, cancer cachexia syndrome.

of oxandrolone, an anabolic steroid, indicate that increases in BCM are associated with improved QOL and Eastern Cooperative Oncology Group (ECOG) performance scores in head and neck and lung cancer patients.[55] However, there has been little quantification of the impact of loss of LBM on QOL.

Nutritional Screening

Effective management of nutritional issues requires early intervention. Nutritional screening provides the vehicle to facilitate the early recognition of malnutrition. The purpose of screening is to quickly identify individuals at nutritional risk.[56] To create a clear picture of the patient's nutritional status, objective and subjective data are incorporated into the nutritional screening. Height, weight, weight change, primary diagnosis, disease stage, and the presence of comorbidities are objective measures commonly included in nutritional screening tools.[1] Individual objective measures alone, such as a laboratory value or current weight, are not specific enough to indicate nutritional risk,[4] so multiple objective measures are combined with subjective measures related to nutrition.[56] To facilitate routine screening of all patients, nutritional screening tools should be easy to use, cost-effective, valid, reliable, and sensitive.[1] The American Society for Parenteral and Enteral Nutrition (ASPEN) and the American Dietetic Association (ADA) recommend that all patients receive nutritional screening as a component of their initial evaluation.[1,56]

Several nutritional screening tools have been used in cancer settings to identify those patients who are at greatest risk to develop nutritional problems. The Patient-Generated Subjective Global Assessment (PG-SGA) and the Mini Nutritional Assessment (MNA) are commonly used in the outpatient oncology setting. Many acute care facilities have designed facility-specific screening forms to be completed by the nursing staff upon admission. These acute care forms commonly combine nutrition with other disciplines.

The PG-SGA[57] (Figure 18-1) is a modification of an earlier screening tool called the Subjective Global Assessment (SGA).[58] Faith Ottery, a surgical oncologist, understood the impact of malnutrition on morbidity and mortality in cancer patients, so she designed the PG-SGA specifically for the oncology population. The PG-SGA is divided into two sections: a patient-completed section and a section completed by the health care professional. Patients provide data regarding weight history, symptoms, dietary intake, and activity level. Health care professionals evaluate metabolic demand, disease in relation to nutritional requirements, and perform a physical assessment. The nursing staff, a nurse practitioner, a registered dietitian, or a physician can complete this section. The Oncology Practice Group of the American Dietetic Association created a video instructional tool to train and assist practitioners in using the PG-SGA.[59] A numeric score is calculated by adding the points obtained in sections one and two. Figure 18-2 describes how the sections of the PG-SGA are tabulated to arrive at this score. A SGA score of mild, moderate, or severe malnutrition is assigned based on this overall assessment. The numeric scores can be used as a triage system to initiate intervention and guide follow-up.[60,61] The PG-SGA numeric score, when repeated at subsequent time points, is useful in illustrating small improvements or deteriorations in nutritional status.[62]

The Nestle Mini Nutritional Assessment (MNA) (Figure 18-3) is nutritional screening tool commonly used in the elderly population. The 18-item MNA was developed by Guigoz with the Nestle Nutritional Corporation.[63] The MNA is comprised of two main components, screening and assessment. The six-item screening takes approximately 3 minutes to complete and includes questions related to decline in food intake, weight loss, mobility, stress, and body mass index (BMI). The health care practitioner is directed to complete the assessment section of the MNA if the screening provided a score of 11 or less.[63] The assessment component includes specific medical history and eating habits as well as some anthropometric measurements. A total score of less than 17 points signifies protein energy malnutrition (PEM); a score of 17-23.5 indicates risk for malnutrition.[63,64]

Worksheets for PG-SGA Scoring

© FD Ottery, 2001

Boxes 1-4 of the PG-SGA are designed to be completed by the patient. The PG-SGA numerical score is determined using 1) the parenthetical points noted in boxes 1-4 and 2) the worksheets below for items not marked with parenthetical points. Scores for boxes 1 and 3 are additive within each box and scores for boxes 2 and 4 are based on the highest scored item checked off by the patient.

Worksheet 1 - Scoring Weight (Wt) Loss

To determine score, use 1 month weight data if available. Use 6 month data only if there is no 1 month weight data. Use points below to score weight change and add one extra point if patient has lost weight during the past 2 weeks. Enter total point score in Box 1 of the PG-SGA.

Wt loss in 1 month	Points	Wt loss in 6 months
10% or greater	4	20% or greater
5-9.9%	3	10 -19.9%
3-4.9%	2	6 - 9.9%
2-2.9%	1	2 - 5.9%
0-1.9%	0	0 - 1.9%

Score for Worksheet 1 ☐
Record in Box 1

Worksheet 2 - Scoring Criteria for Condition

Score is derived by adding 1 point for each of the conditions listed below that pertain to the patient.

Category	Points
Cancer	1
AIDS	1
Pulmonary or cardiac cachexia	1
Presence of decubitus, open wound, or fistula	1
Presence of trauma	1
Age greater than 65 years	1

Score for Worksheet 2 = ☐
Record in Box B

Worksheet 3 - Scoring Metabolic Stress

Score for metabolic stress is determined by a number of variables known to increase protein & calorie needs. The score is additive so that a patient who has a fever of > 102 degrees (3 points) and is on 10 mg of prednisone chronically (2 points) would have an additive score for this section of 5 points.

Stress	none (0)	low (1)	moderate (2)	high (3)
Fever	no fever	>99 and <101	≥101 and <102	≥102
Fever duration	no fever	<72 hrs	72 hrs	> 72 hrs
Corticosteroids	no corticosteroids	low dose (<10mg prednisone equivalents/day)	moderate dose (≥10 and <30mg prednisone equivalents/day)	high dose steroids (≥30mg prednisone equivalents/day)

Score for Worksheet 3 = ☐
Record in Box C

Worksheet 4 - Physical Examination

Physical exam includes a subjective evaluation of 3 aspects of body composition: fat, muscle, & fluid status. Since this is subjective, each aspect of the exam is rated for degree of deficit. Muscle deficit impacts point score more than fat deficit. Definition of categories: 0 = no deficit, 1+ = mild deficit, 2+ = moderate deficit, 3+ = severe deficit. Rating of deficit in these categories are *not* additive but are used to clinically assess the degree of deficit (or presence of excess fluid).

Fat Stores:				
orbital fat pads	0	1+	2+	3+
triceps skin fold	0	1+	2+	3+
fat overlying lower ribs	0	1+	2+	3+
Global fat deficit rating	**0**	**1+**	**2+**	**3+**
Muscle Status:				
temples (temporalis muscle)	0	1+	2+	3+
clavicles (pectoralis & deltoids)	0	1+	2+	3+
shoulders (deltoids)	0	1+	2+	3+
interosseous muscles	0	1+	2+	3+
scapula (latissimus dorsi, trapezius, deltoids)	0	1+	2+	3+
thigh (quadriceps)	0	1+	2+	3+
calf (gastrocnemius)	0	1+	2+	3+
Global muscle status rating	**0**	**1+**	**2+**	**3+**

Fluid Status:				
ankle edema	0	1+	2+	3+
sacral edema	0	1+	2+	3+
ascites	0	1+	2+	3+
Global fluid status rating	**0**	**1+**	**2+**	**3+**

Point score for the physical exam is determined by the overall subjective rating of total body deficit.

No deficit	score = 0 points
Mild deficit	score = 1 point
Moderate deficit	score = 2 points
Severe deficit	score = 3 points

Score for Worksheet 4 = ☐
Record in Box D

Worksheet 5 - PG-SGA Global Assessment Categories

Category	**Stage A** Well-nourished	**Stage B** Moderately malnourished or suspected malnutrition	**Stage C** Severely malnourished
Weight	No wt loss **OR** Recent non-fluid wt gain	~5% wt loss within 1 month (or 10% in 6 months) **OR** No wt stabilization or wt gain (i.e., continued wt loss)	> 5% wt loss in 1 month (or >10% in 6 months) **OR** No wt stabilization or wt gain (i.e., continued wt loss)
Nutrient Intake	No deficit **OR** Significant recent improvement	Definite decrease in intake	Severe deficit in intake
Nutrition Impact Symptoms	None **OR** Significant recent improvement allowing adequate intake	Presence of nutrition impact symptoms (Box 3 of PG-SGA)	Presence of nutrition impact symptoms (Box 3 of PG-SGA)
Functioning	No deficit **OR** Significant recent improvement	Moderate functional deficit **OR** Recent deterioration	Severe functional deficit **OR** recent significant deterioration
Physical Exam	No deficit **OR** Chronic deficit but with recent clinical improvement	Evidence of mild to moderate loss of SQ fat &/or muscle mass &/or muscle tone on palpation	Obvious signs of malnutrition (e.g., severe loss of SQ tissues, possible edema)

Global PG-SGA rating (A, B, or C) = ☐

FIGURE 18-1 The Patient-Generated Subjective Global Assessment (PG-SGA). (Copyright Faith Ottery 2004.)

Scored Patient-Generated Subjective Global Assessment (PG-SGA)

Patient ID Information

History **(Boxes 1-4 are designed to be completed by the patient.)**

1. Weight *(See Worksheet 1)*

In summary of my current and recent weight:

I currently weigh about _______ pounds
I am about _________ feet _________ tall

One month ago I weighed about _________ pounds
Six months ago I weighed about _________ pounds

During the past two weeks my weight has:
☐ decreased (1) ☐ not changed (0) ☐ increased (0)

Box 1 ☐

2. Food Intake: As compared to my normal intake, I would rate my food intake during the past month as:
- ☐ unchanged (0)
- ☐ more than usual (0)
- ☐ less than usual (1)

I am now taking:
- ☐ *normal food* but less than normal amount (1)
- ☐ little solid food (2)
- ☐ only liquids (3)
- ☐ only nutritonal supplements (3)
- ☐ very little of anything (4)
- ☐ only tube feedings or only nutrition by vein (0)

Box 2 ☐

3. Symptoms: I have had the following problems that have kept me from eating enough during the past two weeks (check all that apply):
- ☐ no problems eating (0)
- ☐ no appetite, just did not feel like eating (3)
- ☐ nausea (1)
- ☐ vomiting (3)
- ☐ constipation (1)
- ☐ diarrhea (3)
- ☐ mouth sores (2)
- ☐ dry mouth (1)
- ☐ things taste funny or have no taste (1)
- ☐ smells bother me (1)
- ☐ problems swallowing (2)
- ☐ feel full quickly (1)
- ☐ pain; where? (3) _________
- ☐ fatigue (1)
- ☐ other** (1) ____________________

** Examples: depression, money, or dental problems

Box 3 ☐

4. Activities and Function: Over the past month, I would generally rate my activity as:
- ☐ normal with no limitations (0)
- ☐ not my normal self, but able to be up and about with fairly normal activities (1)
- ☐ not feeling up to most things, but in bed or chair less than half the day (2)
- ☐ able to do little activity and spend most of the day in bed or chair (3)
- ☐ pretty much bedridden, rarely out of bed (3)

Box 4 ☐

Additive Score of the Boxes 1-4 ☐ **A**

The remainder of this form will be completed by your doctor, nurse, or therapist. Thank you.

5. Disease and its relation to nutritional requirements *(See Worksheet 2)*

All relevant diagnoses (specify) ____________________________

Primary disease stage (circle if known or appropriate) I II III IV Other ____________

Age ________

Numerical score from Worksheet 2 ☐ **B**

6. Metabolic Demand *(See Worksheet 3)*

Numerical score from Worksheet 3 ☐ **C**

Numerical score from Worksheet 4 ☐ **D**

7. Physical *(See Worksheet 4)*

Global Assessment *(See Worksheet 5)*
- ☐ Well-nourished or anabolic (SGA-A)
- ☐ Moderate or suspected malnutrition (SGA-B)
- ☐ Severely malnourished (SGA-C)

Total PG-SGA score
(Total numerical score of A+B+C+D above) ☐
(See triage recommendations below)

Clinician Signature ______________________ RD RN PA MD DO Other ___ Date ________

Nutritional Triage Recommendations: Additive score is used to define specific nutritional interventions including patient & family education, symptom management including pharmacologic intervention, and appropriate nutrient intervention (food, nutritional supplements, enteral, or parenteral triage). First line nutrition intervention includes optimal symptom management.

0-1 No intervention required at this time. Re-assessment on routine and regular basis during treatment.
2-3 Patient & family education by dietitian, nurse, or other clinician with pharmacologic intervention as indicated by symptom survey (Box 3) and laboratory values as appropriate.
4-8 Requires intervention by dietitian, in conjunction with nurse or physician as indicated by symptoms survey (Box 3).
≥9 Indicates a critical need for improved symptom management and/or nutrient intervention options.

 email: fdottery@savientpharma.com or noatpres1@aol.com

FIGURE 18-2 The Patient-Generated Subjective Global Assessment (PG-SGA) Worksheet. This form directs clinicians as to how to score the PG-SGA. The numeric score is obtained by adding the subscores of each section. The SGA score is designated by the clinician. (Copyright Faith Ottery 2004.)

NESTLÉ NUTRITION SERVICES

Nestlé

Mini Nutritional Assessment MNA®

Last name: First name: Sex: Date:

Age: Weight, kg: Height, cm: I.D. Number:

Complete the screen by filling in the boxes with the appropriate numbers.
Add the numbers for the screen. If score is 11 or less, continue with the assessment to gain a Malnutrition Indicator Score.

Screening

A Has food intake declined over the past 3 months due to loss of appetite, digestive problems, chewing or swallowing difficulties?
- 0 = severe loss of appetite
- 1 = moderate loss of appetite
- 2 = no loss of appetite ☐

B Weight loss during the last 3 months
- 0 = weight loss greater than 3 kg (6.6 lbs)
- 1 = does not know
- 2 = weight loss between 1 and 3 kg (2.2 and 6.6 lbs)
- 3 = no weight loss ☐

C Mobility
- 0 = bed or chair bound
- 1 = able to get out of bed/chair but does not go out
- 2 = goes out ☐

D Has suffered psychological stress or acute disease in the past 3 months
- 0 = yes   2 = no ☐

E Neuropsychological problems
- 0 = severe dementia or depression
- 1 = mild dementia
- 2 = no psychological problems ☐

F Body Mass Index (BMI) (weight in kg) / (height in m)^2
- 0 = BMI less than 19
- 1 = BMI 19 to less than 21
- 2 = BMI 21 to less than 23
- 3 = BMI 23 or greater ☐

Screening score (subtotal max. 14 points) ☐ ☐

12 points or greater Normal – not at risk – no need to complete assessment
11 points or below Possible malnutrition – continue assessment

Assessment

G Lives independently (not in a nursing home or hospital)
- 0 = no   1 = yes ☐

H Takes more than 3 prescription drugs per day
- 0 = yes   1 = no ☐

I Pressure sores or skin ulcers
- 0 = yes   1 = no ☐

Ref.: Guigoz Y, Vellas B and Garry PJ. 1994. Mini Nutritional Assessment: A practical assessment tool for grading the nutritional state of elderly patients. *Facts and Research in Gerontology.* Supplement #2:15-59.
Rubenstein LZ, Harker J, Guigoz Y and Vellas B. Comprehensive Geriatric Assessment (CGA) and the MNA: An Overview of CGA, Nutritional Assessment, and Development of a Shortened Version of the MNA. In: "Mini Nutritional Assessment (MNA): Research and Practice in the Elderly". Vellas B, Garry PJ and Guigoz Y, editors. Nestlé Nutrition Workshop Series. Clinical & Performance Programme, vol. 1. Karger, Bâle, in press.

J How many full meals does the patient eat daily?
- 0 = 1 meal
- 1 = 2 meals
- 2 = 3 meals ☐

K Selected consumption markers for protein intake
- At least one serving of dairy products (milk, cheese, yogurt) per day? yes ☐ no ☐
- Two or more servings of legumes or eggs per week? yes ☐ no ☐
- Meat, fish or poultry every day yes ☐ no ☐

0.0 = if 0 or 1 yes
0.5 = if 2 yes
1.0 = if 3 yes ☐.☐

L Consumes two or more servings of fruits or vegetables per day?
- 0 = no   1 = yes ☐

M How much fluid (water, juice, coffee, tea, milk...) is consumed per day?
- 0.0 = less than 3 cups
- 0.5 = 3 to 5 cups
- 1.0 = more than 5 cups ☐.☐

N Mode of feeding
- 0 = unable to eat without assistance
- 1 = self-fed with some difficulty
- 2 = self-fed without any problem ☐

O Self view of nutritional status
- 0 = views self as being malnourished
- 1 = is uncertain of nutritional state
- 2 = views self as having no nutritional problem ☐

P In comparison with other people of the same age, how does the patient consider his/her health status?
- 0.0 = not as good
- 0.5 = does not know
- 1.0 = as good
- 2.0 = better ☐.☐

Q Mid-arm circumference (MAC) in cm
- 0.0 = MAC less than 21
- 0.5 = MAC 21 to 22
- 1.0 = MAC 22 or greater ☐.☐

R Calf circumference (CC) in cm
- 0 = CC less than 31   1 = CC 31 or greater ☐

Assessment (max. 16 points) ☐ ☐.☐

Screening score ☐ ☐

Total Assessment (max. 30 points) ☐ ☐.☐

Malnutrition Indicator Score

17 to 23.5 points at risk of malnutrition ☐
Less than 17 points malnourished ☐

FIGURE 18-3 The Mini Nutritional Assessment. The Mini Nutritional Assessment has been validated in the elderly oncology population. This tool is commonly used in the outpatient setting. (From Nestle Nutrition Services, available online at www.mna-elderly.com/navigation_frames/clinicalpractice/navigation-clinicalpractice-frame-mnaforms.htm.)

The Malnutrition Screening Tool (MST), although not commonly used in the US, is a short nutritional screening tool. This three-item tool uses data on weight history and appetite to predict nutritional risk The MST, developed by Maree Ferguson, has been validated in both acute care patients[65] and oncology patients receiving radiation therapy.[66]

Anthropometric Measures

The term *anthropometric* refers to comparative measurements of the human body. Body parameters such as weight, height, and BMI are commonly used to assess nutritional status. Other anthropometric measurements less commonly used in routine practice include waist and hip circumference and skinfold measurements. Each of these measures provides valuable information about the individual's body composition, but they also have limitations. For example, skinfold measurements are associated with a high degree of error, and they can put the patient to significant inconvenience, so they are rarely used in clinical practice.

Weight should be obtained from a calibrated scale at each patient visit, or as determined by the facility. Weight information should be gathered in several ways. Usual body weight (UBW) refers to the patient's last stable weight. Data regarding the timeline for last stable weight should also be collected. Ideal body weight (IBW) describes the reference weight considered to be optimal for the patient; this can be obtained from reference tables. Actual body weight (ABW) is a measure of the current weight of the patient. ABW should be compared to UBW and IBW. The change in a patient's weight over time is an inexpensive and relatively accurate tool for predicting nutritional status. Table 18-2 illustrates ways of categorizing the severity of weight loss and malnutrition according to amount of weight lost.[67]

BMI defines weight in relation to height. It is commonly used to describe the degree of adiposity and disease risk.[68] Table 18-3 defines weight by BMI score.[68] BMI can be calculated or obtained from a BMI chart (Figure 18-4). BMI alone is not a perfect predictor of overweight or obesity. Its use is limited in the elderly because it underestimates body fat in those who have lost muscle mass.[68] When evaluating muscular individuals such as body builders, or patients with large amounts of edema or ascites, clinical judgment must be used because these physiologic states may lead to false overestimation of the degree of fatness.[69]

In research settings, more detailed measures of specific body compartments are employed. The most reliable method of body composition measurement is cadaver dissection; however, this is not an option for living patients.[50] Other

Table **18-2** DEGREES OF MALNUTRITION AS DETERMINED BY WEIGHT[66]

Percent Weight Lost	Weight Measurement Used	Period of Time	Categorization of Weight Loss/Malnutrition
5%	ABW	1-3 months	Severe weight loss
>5%	ABW	1 month	Severe weight loss
7.5%	ABW	3-6 months	Significant weight loss
>7.5%	ABW	3 months	Severe weight loss
10%	ABW	6 or more months	Significant weight loss
>10%	ABW	6 months	Severe weight loss
10%-15%	UBW		Mild malnutrition
16%-25%	UBW		Moderate malnutrition
>25%	UBW		Severe malnutrition

ABW, Actual body weight; *UBW,* usual body weight.

Table **18-3** CATEGORIZATION OF BODY MASS INDEX[68]

Weight Status	BMI Score
Underweight	Below 18.5
Normal	18.5-24.9
Overweight	25.0-29.9
Obesity	30.0-39.9
Extreme Obesity	40.0 or more

methods used by research teams include hydrodensitometry, isotope dilution, total body potassium, neutron activation, air-displacement plethysmography, dual x-ray absorptiometry (DXA), and bioelectrical impedance (BIA).[34,37,70-75] Most methods require significant effort on the part of the subject. Laboratory methods such as isotope dilution, total body potassium, and underwater weighing are expensive and not suitable for routine use.

Health care professionals in routine practice are becoming more interested in obtaining measures and tracking changes in body composition. Outpatient cancer centers are beginning to use BIA technology to obtain regular measurements of LBM and fat mass. BIA is based on the principle that the body is a biologic circuit, and a fixed low-voltage high-frequency current introduced into the human body would be conducted almost completely through the electrolyte component of FFM. It is assumed that the total conductive volume of the body is equivalent to total body water (TBW).[72,76] A small electrical current, which the patient cannot sense physically, is measured for resistance as it travels through the body. The measured resistance is approximately equivalent to that of muscle tissue. The electric current typically used with single-frequency BIA (SFBIA) is 50 kHz, the characteristic frequency for skeletal muscle tissue.[72,74] Using values of TBW derived from BIA, one can then estimate FFM and body fat by means of prediction equations.[74]

BIA is inexpensive, can be performed without specific operator skills, and imposes no burden on the subject.[50,76,77] It relies on various assumptions that vary in validity depending upon the individual. Potential factors that could influence measurements include level of hydration, posture, environmental and skin temperatures, age, sex, and athletic status.[72] BIA appears to systematically overestimate TBW in underweight patients (BMI <19.6) by 5% when a prediction model for normal weight subjects is used.[76] The increase in hydration associated with cancer cachexia would lead to underestimation of fat.[34,78] However, the interference of many of these factors with accuracy of measurements can be avoided with proper measurement technique and the use of appropriate prediction equations.

It is important to remember that prediction of body composition using any of the experimental methods is most accurate and provides the best picture of change when carried out with serial measurements over time. A single measurement at any time provides little useful data. The change in measurement over time is indicative of changes in nutritional status.

Nutritional Assessment

Once malnutrition or the risk of malnutrition has been identified, the next step is systematic nutritional assessment and creating a plan of care. Nutritional assessment differs from nutritional screening in that it is a thorough evaluation which assimilates data obtained from the medical history, dietary history, physical examination, anthropometric measurements, and laboratory data.[56] The nutritional assessment integrates the review of body composition with data on disease and clinical status to evaluate impact on metabolism and nutrient need.[1] In addition, appraisal of disease- and treatment-related symptoms is necessary to plan nutritional interventions. This process leads to the identification and diagnosis of nutritional issues. This nutritional diagnosis includes the problem, etiology, and signs and symptoms, which in turn directs the nutritional intervention.[79] The nutritional assessment is usually completed by a registered dietitian (RD) or nutrition professional, however

Body Mass Index Table

	Normal						Overweight					Obese									
BMI	19	20	21	22	23	24	25	26	27	28	29	30	31	32	33	34	35	36	37	38	39
Height (inches)	Body Weight (pounds)																				
58	91	96	100	105	110	115	119	124	129	134	138	143	148	153	158	162	167	172	177	181	186
59	94	99	104	109	114	119	124	128	133	138	143	148	153	158	163	168	173	178	183	188	193
60	97	102	107	112	118	123	128	133	138	143	148	153	158	163	168	174	179	184	189	194	199
61	100	106	111	116	122	127	132	137	143	148	153	158	164	169	174	180	185	190	195	201	206
62	104	109	115	120	126	131	136	142	147	153	158	164	169	175	180	186	191	196	202	207	213
63	107	113	118	124	130	135	141	146	152	158	163	169	175	180	186	191	197	203	208	214	220
64	110	116	122	128	134	140	145	151	157	163	169	174	180	186	192	197	204	209	215	221	227
65	114	120	126	132	138	144	150	156	162	168	174	180	186	192	198	204	210	216	222	228	234
66	118	124	130	136	142	148	155	161	167	173	179	186	192	198	204	210	216	223	229	235	241
67	121	127	134	140	146	153	159	166	172	178	185	191	198	204	211	217	223	230	236	242	249
68	125	131	138	144	151	158	164	171	177	184	190	197	203	210	216	223	230	236	243	249	256
69	128	135	142	149	155	162	169	176	182	189	196	203	209	216	223	230	236	243	250	257	263
70	132	139	146	153	160	167	174	181	188	195	202	209	216	222	229	236	243	250	257	264	271
71	136	143	150	157	165	172	179	186	193	200	208	215	222	229	236	243	250	257	265	272	279
72	140	147	154	162	169	177	184	191	199	206	213	221	228	235	242	250	258	265	272	279	287
73	144	151	159	166	174	182	189	197	204	212	219	227	235	242	250	257	265	272	280	288	295
74	148	155	163	171	179	186	194	202	210	218	225	233	241	249	256	264	272	280	287	295	303
75	152	160	168	176	184	192	200	208	216	224	232	240	248	256	264	272	279	287	295	303	311
76	156	164	172	180	189	197	205	213	221	230	238	246	254	263	271	279	287	295	304	312	320

	Extreme Obesity														
BMI	40	41	42	43	44	45	46	47	48	49	50	51	52	53	54
Height (inches)	Body Weight (pounds)														
58	191	196	201	205	210	215	220	224	229	234	239	244	248	253	258
59	198	203	208	212	217	222	227	232	237	242	247	252	257	262	267
60	204	209	215	220	225	230	235	240	245	250	255	261	266	271	276
61	211	217	222	227	232	238	243	248	254	259	264	269	275	280	285
62	218	224	229	235	240	246	251	256	262	267	273	278	284	289	295
63	225	231	237	242	248	254	259	265	270	278	282	287	293	299	304
64	232	238	244	250	256	262	267	273	279	285	291	296	302	308	314
65	240	246	252	258	264	270	276	282	288	294	300	306	312	318	324
66	247	253	260	266	272	278	284	291	297	303	309	315	322	328	334
67	255	261	268	274	280	287	293	299	306	312	319	325	331	338	344
68	262	269	276	282	289	295	302	308	315	322	328	335	341	348	354
69	270	277	284	291	297	304	311	318	324	331	338	345	351	358	365
70	278	285	292	299	306	313	320	327	334	341	348	355	362	369	376
71	286	293	301	308	315	322	329	338	343	351	358	365	372	379	386
72	294	302	309	316	324	331	338	346	353	361	368	375	383	390	397
73	302	310	318	325	333	340	348	355	363	371	378	386	393	401	408
74	311	319	326	334	342	350	358	365	373	381	389	396	404	412	420
75	319	327	335	343	351	359	367	375	383	391	399	407	415	423	431
76	328	336	344	353	361	369	377	385	394	402	410	418	426	435	443

Source: Adapted from *Clinical Guidelines on the Identification, Evaluation, and Treatment of Overweight and Obesity in Adults: The Evidence Report.*

FIGURE 18-4 Body Mass Index Chart. The BMI is used to categorize weight by height. The categories of weight are commonly used to classify disease risk. (Adapted from Clinical guidelines on the identification, evaluation, and treatment of overweight and obesity in adults: The Evidentiary Report, National Heart Lung Blood Institute, 1998.)

other members of the health care team can complete it as well. The PG-SGA and the MNA have been designed so that they can be used as nutritional screening or assessment tools.[11,63]

Nutritional Intervention

Nutritional intervention refers to the specific activities required to address and correct the nutritional diagnosis.[79] The nutritional intervention is selected, planned, and implemented with the intent of improving nutritional status.[79] Planning of the nutritional intervention requires the input of all disciplines involved in patient care. Attention must be given to the causes of weight loss or weight gain. Box 18-2 presents some of the factors to be considered;[15,56] with these kept in mind, the patient should remain at the center of the intervention and paramount importance be placed on patient preferences.[80]

The goals of the intervention must be documented and reevaluated frequently.[79] The intervention must be individualized to the patient, and consideration should be given to patient comfort and wishes.[60,79] Although there are variations between and among patients, common nutritional goals include symptom management, weight maintenance, and preservation of functional status.[60] Attaining these goals may require modified diets, the addition of oral nutritional supplements, or the initiation of enteral or parenteral nutrition. Figure 18-5 presents an algorithm for the treatment of cancer-induced weight loss. These modifications to dietary intake can be costly, and flexibility is required on the part of the individual designing the intervention with respect to specific formulas and administration. The services of financial planners and social workers are very beneficial in this situation.

Role of the Registered Dietitian

A registered dietitian (RD) is an individual who has completed the minimum of a baccalaureate degree; completed an accredited, organized preprofessional experience or internship; passed the registration examination for dietitians; and accrued 75 hours of approved continuing professional education every 5 years.[81] The nutritional care provided by a RD is called medical nutrition therapy (MNT). MNT is described as nutritional assessment, intervention, and follow-up by a RD or nutrition professional to manage disease.[79] The proper educational background equips the RD to deal with complex nutritional issues that arise in the course of cancer treatment. Resources such as the American Dietetic Association's Medical Nutrition Therapy Protocols, published in 1998, provide guidelines for the MNT on working with cancer patients receiving chemotherapy and radiation. These protocols were published to define the detailed care provided by dietitians and the expected outcomes of MNT in the oncology setting.[82]

Role of the Multidisciplinary Team

Very few cancer centers employ an RD to provide MNT.[83,84] The nurse commonly has the most direct patient contact in institutions providing care for cancer patients. It would seem logical that the nurse would perform the nutritional screening and assessment. It has been suggested that the nurse's role as a patient advocate and expert clinician makes the oncology nurse ideal to contribute to a comprehensive nutritional assessment.[83] In fact, many acute care facilities use data collected in the initial nursing screening to identify patients at nutritional risk. The complete care of the oncology patient should include the input of many disciplines.[50] Providing nutritional

Box 18-2 Considerations in Designing Nutrition Interventions[15,56]

- Food and nutrient intake patterns
- Psychologic factors
- Social factors
- Physical conditions
- Abnormal laboratory values
- Medication use
- Presence of a functional gastrointestinal tract
- Type of anticancer therapy
- Quality of life
- Performance status
- Prognosis
- Cost effectiveness

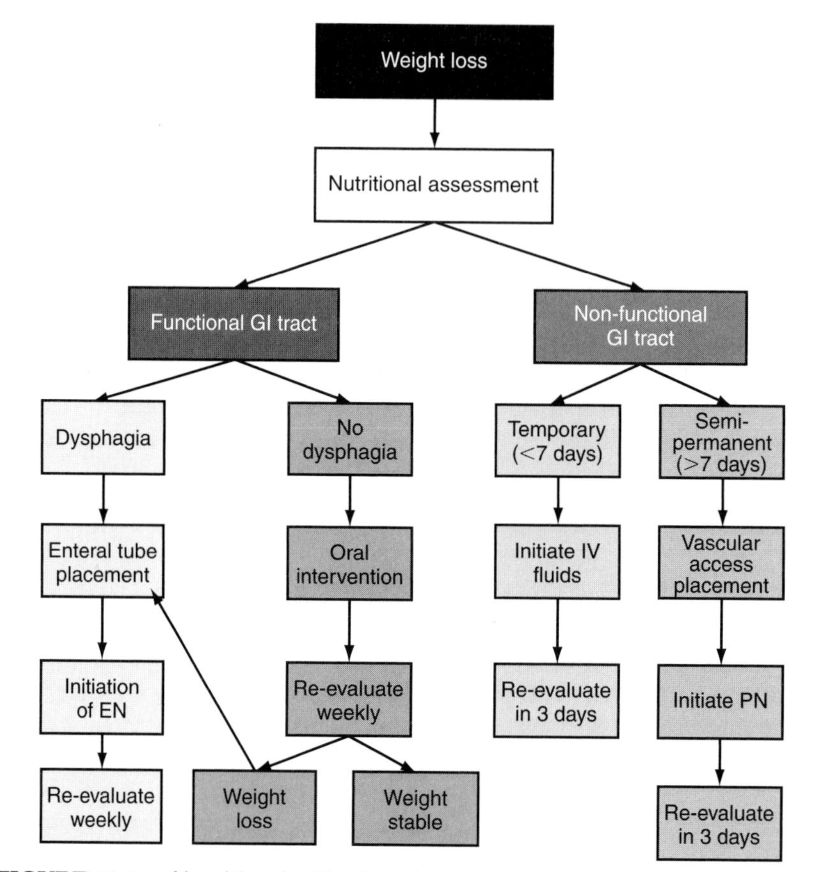

FIGURE 18-5 Algorithm for Nutrition Intervention in Cancer-Induced Weight Loss. The presence or absence of a functional GI tract should direct the intervention in patients with cancer-induced weight loss. Although these are general recommendations, interventions should be individualized.

care is a multidisciplinary activity that includes the physician, nurse, pharmacist, dietitian, psychologist, social worker, and physical therapist.[83]

The Joint Commission on Accreditation of Healthcare Organizations (JCAHO) requires the assessment of nutritional status and education regarding nutritional interventions when warranted by the disease state.[85] In the acute setting this function must be provided by nutrition professionals, but JCAHO has made no designation of responsibility in the ambulatory setting. Trained personnel of any discipline can use standardized nutritional assessment tools, such as the PG-SGA and MNA. If necessary, the RD can be consulted to assist at this point with specific nutritional intervention and follow-up, via referral by the primary health care providers.[86]

Nutritional Approaches to Symptom Management

Many symptoms and side effects commonly occur in cancer patients. Food and eating problems experienced during chemotherapy are perceived by patients as highly stressful.[54] Nutrition-related symptoms have been implicated in exacerbating patients' weight loss.[80] These symptoms must be aggressively managed to minimize this effect.[47] Table 18-4 presents approaches to some of the common side effects experienced by cancer patients.[87]

Table **18-4** SYMPTOM-RELATED NUTRITIONAL INTERVENTIONS

Symptom	Intervention
Taste changes	Eat tart foods Use flavorful seasonings Use plastic utensils and dishes Marinate foods
Xerostomia	Drink fluids with meals Moisten and/or puree foods Use oral moistening mouthwash/gel Drink papaya juice Avoid the following: • Caffeine • Alcohol • Commercial mouthwashes
Stomatitis/ mucositis	Avoid the following: • Acidic foods • Spicy foods • Rough food • Salty foods Eat bland, soft foods that are easy to swallow Cook food (especially vegetables) until it is soft and tender Cut food into small pieces, or puree food in blender Mix food with broth, gravies, or sauces to make it easier to swallow Eat capsaicin candy
Diarrhea	Adopt BRAT diet (banana, rice, applesauce, toast) Initially keep diet low-fiber → slowly increase soluble fiber Avoid the following: • High-fat foods • Caffeine • Alcohol • Tobacco • Strong spices Temporarily avoid milk products (with the exception of yogurt) Increase fluid intake (include juice and broth in this recommendation)
Dumping syndrome	Eat small, frequent meals (every 2 hours) Increase protein and fat content of meals Drink fluids between meals Limit intake of simple carbohydrates
Constipation	Gradually increase total fiber Drink 8 to 10 glasses of fluid daily Drink 4 to 8 ounces of prune juice once or twice a day Increase physical activity Use (progressively as need) a fiber supplement → stool softener → laxative
Nausea	Drink fluids between meals Avoid the following: • Foods with strong odors • High fat foods • Strong spices Cold foods may be better tolerated
Vomiting	Progress from NPO → Clear Liquid → Full Liquid → Soft Maintain fluid intake (include juice and broth in this recommendation)
Early satiety	Limit excessive intake of fat and fiber Small, frequent meals (every 2 hours) Increase protein and carbohydrate content of meals Fluids between meals

NPO, nothing by mouth.
From Huhmann MB, Cunningham RS: Importance of nutritional screening in the treatment of cancer related weight loss, *Lancet Oncol*, 6, p. 338, 2005.

Specialized Nutrition Support

The term *specialized nutrition support* (SNS) refers to the use of parenteral nutrition (PN) or enteral nutrition (EN) in the treatment or prevention of malnutrition. SNS is considered an invasive and aggressive nutritional approach. There are risks and benefits associated with the use of both EN and PN. Some of the risks and benefits of SNS[1] are described in Table 18-5. Because of these risks, the use of SNS in cancer patients is a highly debated topic. Both EN and PN have been associated with improved nitrogen balance and weight gain; however, PN produces weight gain more consistently.[28] Unfortunately this weight gain appears to be in the form of fat.[28] Unlike in other disease states, SNS does not appear to have an effect on serum proteins when administered for 7 days or more.[1]

ASPEN and the American Gastroenterological Association have both published guidelines for the use of SNS in cancer patients.[1,88] These guidelines highlight the lack of benefit associated with the use of SNS in large subgroups of the oncology population and reinforce the need for ample consideration when contemplating the use of SNS.

Enteral Nutrition

EN refers to the provision of nutrition by means of the introduction of liquid nutritional supplements into the GI tract. EN can be broken into two categories: oral EN and EN tube feeding.[89] Oral EN is consumed via the mouth, and EN tube feeding is provided via a delivery system directly into the GI tract.[89] Common access sites to the GI tract include gastrostomy and jejunostomy tubes. EN is contraindicated in patients without a functioning GI tract, those experiencing severe bleeding, diarrhea, or intractable vomiting, or those with a fistula or with a poor prognosis.[1]

There are several methods of EN tube feeding administration. EN tube feeding administration can be facilitated through a programmable pump, syringe, or gravity drip bag.[90] The administration schedule and dosing will dictate the equipment required. Hospitalized patients commonly receive continuous feedings using an enteral feeding pump. Continuous feedings are provided throughout the day at a specific rate for a specified period of time. These feedings can be provided with a gravity drip bag or programmable pump. Gravity drip bags allow for a limited level of control over the drip. Flow control is adjusted manually with a dial on the tubing. Programmable pumps allow for a controlled amount and timing of feeding. Bolus feedings are administered with a syringe. The bolus method is more commonly used in the outpatient setting. Bolus feedings are limited in the volume that can be administered at one time, but the use of bolus feedings allows for less of a patient

Table **18-5** RISKS AND BENEFITS OF SPECIALIZED NUTRITION SUPPORT[1]

Enteral Nutrition		Parenteral Nutrition	
Benefits	Risks	Benefits	Risks
Prevention of bacterial translocation	Intolerance	Consistently causes weight gain	Venous thrombosis
Prevention of mucosal atrophy	Obstruction	Increases body fat	Metabolic abnormalities
Provision of glutamine	Tube dislocation	Improves nitrogen balance	Infections
Provision of fiber (short chain fatty acids)		Little effect on lean body mass	
Usually causes weight gain			
Improves nitrogen balance			

burden and more freedom with timing of administration, and negates the need to carry a pump or gravity bag.

EN has received somewhat less criticism than PN. It has been suggested that intestinal integrity deteriorates in the absence of nutrient provision directly into the GI tract.[90] Therefore EN is the preferred method of feeding. EN is also less expensive than PN.[91] The use of perioperative EN has been associated with a reduction in the number of complications, earlier return of bowel function,[92,93] decreased incidence of infection,[94] and shorter postoperative stay.[93] Metabolically, EN is associated with improved protein balance[95] and reduced incidence of hypoglycemia and electrolyte abnormalities.[91]

Parenteral Nutrition

PN refers to the administration of nutrients intravenously, bypassing the GI tract. PN is contraindicated in the following situations: in patients with a functional GI tract and those who will require support for less than 5 days; where there is lack of vascular access, hemodynamic instability, or profound metabolic or electrolyte disturbance; and in patients with a poor prognosis.[1] According to ASPEN recommendations, PN provided adjuvantly to chemotherapy or radiation therapy provides no additional benefit and increases risk of complications.[1] PN should only be considered in patients predicted to be unable to ingest or absorb nutrients for a period greater than 5 to 10 days. A life expectancy of less than 40 to 60 days is a contraindication to PN. The only intravenous (IV) intervention recommended for these patients is IV fluids administration.[1]

The benefits of using PN in cancer are highly debated. Early studies indicating benefit have been criticized for inclusion of multiple tumor groups and stages, inconsistent provision of calories and protein, and suboptimal sample sizes.[87] Recent studies indicate a lack of benefit, an increased incidence of infection, and no increase in survival.[93,96] Concerns have been raised regarding the possibility of "feeding the tumor" with PN administration. Recent research has indicated that although glucose uptake is higher in malignant cells, uptake was not increased with the provision of glucose-based PN.[97]

Benefits of PN observed in postoperative patients when compared to EN are decreased incidence of GI symptoms such as diarrhea and distention.[91,93] This finding has been contradicted in several recent studies in which EN was carefully initiated and carried out in a controlled manner.[98,99] PN seems to provide no benefit when supplied adjuvantly during chemotherapy,[100-102] except in stem cell transplantation (SCT).[103-105] PN reduces length of stay[103-105] and may prevent weight loss associated with SCT.[106]

Immunonutrition

Immunonutrition is a relatively new field of nutrition in which nutrients are provided with the intent of "boosting" immunity.[107] Nutrients currently under investigation for their benefits in the oncology population include glutamine (GLN), arginine (ARG), omega-3 fatty acids (ω-3 FAs), and combinations of all three. One of the most well-researched immune-enhancing formulas, Impact, Novartis Nutrition, contains ARG, ω-3 FAs, and ribonucleic acid (RNA).

GLN is an amino acid. It is considered the primary fuel for enterocytes in the intestine. GLN has been investigated for the treatment of several treatment-induced side effects such as mucositis, diarrhea, neuropathy, and hepatic venoocclusive disease.[108] GLN is unstable in liquid form, so it is often provided as a dipeptide in PN or added as a powder to enteral formulas. PN supplemented with GLN has been associated with improved nitrogen balance[109] and improved neutrophil count.[110] SCT recipients receiving enteral GLN experienced decreased length of stay and decreased need for PN.[105,111]

A limited number of studies have examined ARG supplementation in the absence of other immunonutrients. These studies indicate improvement in morbidity and length of stay with enteral ARG adminstration[112] and enhanced immune response with parenteral ARG administration.[113] ARG is most commonly investigated with other immunonutrients. The results of these studies suggest improvement in nutrition and immune parameters and incidence of infections.[114,115] Immunonutrient formulas highest in ARG content are associated with the lowest incidence of infectious complications in patients after surgery.[116]

ω-3 FAs are essential fatty acids that must be obtained from the diet. They are important in prostaglandin synthesis and are hypothesized to have the ability to modulate the inflammatory response.[117] The possible impact on the inflammatory response has led to the study of ω-3 FAs in the treatment of cachexia. Research exploring the use of ω-3 FAs in cancer patients has used several forms of the lipid. The early studies of ω-3 FAs used fish oil pills, which were poorly tolerated because of GI side effects.[118] More recently ω-3 FAs have been added to PN and EN. Parenterally-administered ω-3 FAs are associated with improvements in markers of inflammation and in levels of cytokines such as TNF.[119] Enteral administration of ω-3 FAs has been associated with weight stabilization and gain in weight-losing cancer patients.[120-122] Improvements have also been observed in nutritional status, performance status, and QOL in patients receiving enteral ω-3 FAs.[123]

NUTRITION IN END OF LIFE CARE

The preparation and provision of food symbolizes love and care to many individuals.[124] Cancer patients with advanced disease and no further treatment options, and their families, view nutritional support as life-sustaining and may use this to assert some control in their final days.[124] Patient and family members may request EN or PN when a cancer patient is eating poorly. These questions should be addressed thoughtfully and carefully on an individual basis.[125] Discussion should include the benefits and risks of employing these measures.

Loss of appetite and poor oral intake are common in terminally ill patients. This does not reduce the quality of life. In advanced oncology patients, hunger is rare and transient.[126] Most terminally patients do not experience hunger; thirst is more common.[127,128] Dehydration causes ketosis, hemoconcentration, and hyperosmolality, which leads to azotemia, hypernatremia, and hypercalcemia.[124,128] This combination produces a physiologic adaptation that sedates the person.[128-130]

The ethics of end of life care is an issue for all members of the health care team. All health care professionals are ethically bound to respect the life as well as the comfort of the patient. Nutrition is no exception. The ADA recommends that the primary goals of palliative health care is to minimize human suffering by reducing the intensity of disturbing symptoms.[129]

The ADA further recommends that the health care team develop clinical and ethical criteria for the nutrition and hydration of persons through the life span. The multidisciplinary team must work collaboratively to make recommendations regarding nutrition, hydration, and feeding on an individual-case basis.[129] Box 18-3 presents considerations to keep in mind when designing nutritional care plans for patients at end of life. The most important concept is that the decision should center on the patient.[129,130]

Commonly, persons with advanced cancers who express a consistent and strong desire to die meet the criteria for clinical depression.[131] This desire for death has been correlated with ratings of pain and low family support; however, the most significant correlation has been made with

Box **18-3** Consideration in Palliative Nutrition at End of Life[128]

- Patient preferences guide the decision making process.
- When the patients preference is not known—a substitute decision maker is guided by the best interests of the patient.
- Informed and shared decision making is the best ethical practice.
- All stakeholders are encouraged to collaborate in the decision making process.

depression.[131] It has been recommended that patients with the desire to die should be carefully assessed and provided with treatment for depression.[126,131] When dealing with an incompetent patient, the clinician should strongly encourage input from all family members, and if no surrogate is available, team members should agree before withdrawing nutritional support.[126]

The ADA recommends, "When in doubt, feed." However, feeding should be stopped based on the expression of patient wishes, if feeding is contraindicated medically, if the patient is diagnosed as persistently vegetative, or if the team has evidence of the patient's wish to stop nutrition and hydration.[129] It is important to remember, "Nutrition support treats malnutrition, but not the underlying pathology."[132]

NUTRITIONAL FOLLOW-UP AND REASSESSMENT

Nutritional monitoring and evaluation is a vital step in the nutritional care of patients. Desired outcomes and goals must be selected and tracked to measure the effectiveness of the nutritional care plan. The purpose of this monitoring is to determine if progress has been made.[79] If goals are not met, the plan must be reevaluated and revised to be more aggressive.[133] An effective nutritional care plan evolves and includes persistent follow-up, revision of interventions, and reevaluation of goals.

NUTRITION AND CANCER PREVENTION

A popular topic at any time is cancer prevention. The field of cancer prevention has grown tremendously in the last 20 years. The use of food and food derivatives, or nutraceuticals, for the prevention of cancer is gaining more research attention.

Obesity, sedentary lifestyle, and alcohol and tobacco use have been implicated as probable cancer promoters. Specific foods have also been suggested to have cancer-promoting activity such as dietary fat, charbroiled meats, and pickled foods. However, some of these associations are still considered controversial.

The process of carcinogenesis occurs over decades.[134] All of the steps and pathways leading to a cancer diagnosis have not been identified. It is difficult to identify single foods or food groups as cancer-causing or cancer-preventing because of the amount and type of research required to substantiate such a claim. The majority of research on which such claims are based is epidemiologic. These studies require participants to complete surveys to assess current or past dietary intake. There are many limitations associated with this method, most important of which is the inability of most people to accurately recall their intake. This method also does not account for exposure to nondietary carcinogens.[135] Case control studies are able to control for more factors, but are expensive to conduct for short periods of time, let alone over an entire lifetime. Animal studies are helpful in testing theories; however, the extrapolation to humans is not always exact. For this reason, it is important to review the research regarding cancer prevention claims. As a rule, the claims made regarding groups of foods are more reliable than those regarding individual foods.[135]

In acknowledging the confusion regarding cancer prevention, the American Cancer Society has published guidelines for cancer prevention[135] (Box 18-4). These evidence-based guidelines are intended to provide general guidance to the public. They do not provide specific interventions because of limited applicability to the entire population. The American Cancer Society and the American Institute for Cancer Research developed supplemental educational materials to address more specific aspects of cancer prevention. These materials are available free to patients via the Internet.

SUMMARY

In summary, nutrition has a vital role in care of women with cancer. Malnutrition has an impact on quality of life throughout the cancer continuum from prevention through treatment,

Box 18-4 American Cancer Society Guidelines for Cancer Prevention[136]

Eat a variety of healthful foods, with an emphasis on plant sources:
- Eat 5 or more servings of a variety of fruits and vegetables.
- Choose whole grains in preference to processed grains.
- Limit consumption of red meats, especially those high in fat and those that are processed.
- Choose foods that help maintain a healthful weight.

Adopt a physically active lifestyle:
- Adults: engage in moderate activity for 30 minutes or more, 5 or more days per week.
- Children and adolescents: moderate-vigorous activity for 45 minutes or more, 5 or more days per week.

Maintain a healthful weight throughout life:
- Balance caloric intake with physical activity.
- Lose weight if you are currently overweight or obese.

Limit alcohol intake.

Do not use tobacco in any form.

survivorship, and end of life. The registered dietitian is an important resource for the patient, the family, and the oncology team.

REFERENCES

1. American Society for Parenteral and Enteral Nutrition Board of Directors: Guidelines for the use of parenteral and enteral nutrition in adult and pediatric patients, *JPEN J Parenter Enteral Nutr* 26(1 Suppl):1-138SA, 2002.
2. Murry DJ, Riva L, Poplack DG: Impact of nutrition on pharmacokinetics of anti-neoplastic agents, *Int J Cancer Suppl* 11:48-51, 1998.
3. Dewys WD and others: Prognostic effect of weight loss prior to chemotherapy in cancer patients. Eastern Cooperative Oncology Group, *Am J Med* 69(4):491-497, 1980.
4. Sarhill N and others: Evaluation of nutritional status in advanced metastatic cancer, *Support Care Cancer* 11(10):652-659, 2003.
5. Bloch A, Charuhas P: Cancer and cancer therapy. In Gottschlich M, editor: *The science and practice of nutrition support*, Dubuque, 2001, Kendall Hunt.
6. Wigmore SJ and others: Changes in nutritional status associated with unresectable pancreatic cancer, *Br J Cancer* 75(1):106-109, 1997.
7. Cunningham RS, Bell R: Nutrition in cancer: an overview, *Semin Oncol Nurs* 16(2):90-98, 2000.
8. Hammerlid E and others: Malnutrition and food intake in relation to quality of life in head and neck cancer patients, *Head Neck* 20(6):540-548, 1998.
9. McCallum PD, Polisena, CG, editors: *The clinical guide to oncology nutrition*, Chicago, 2000, American Dietetic Association.
10. Rivadeneira DE and others: Nutritional support of the cancer patient, *CA Cancer J Clin* 48(2):69-80, 1998.
11. Capra S, Ferguson M, Ried K: Cancer: impact of nutrition intervention outcome—nutrition issues for patients, *Nutrition* 17(9):769-772, 2001.
12. Parnes HL, Aisner J: Protein calorie malnutrition and cancer therapy, *Drug Saf* 7(6):404-416, 1992.
13. Tisdale MJ: Pathogenesis of cancer cachexia, *J Support Oncol* 1(3):159-168, 2003.
14. Barber M: The pathophysiology and treatment of cancer cachexia, *Nutr Clin Pract* 17(4):203-209, 2002.
15. Martin C: Calorie, protein, fluid and micronutrient requirements. In McCallum P, Polisena C, editors: *The clinical guide to oncology nutrition*, Chicago, 2000, American Dietetic Association.
16. Tisdale MJ: Tumor-host interactions, *J Cell Biochem* 93(5):871-877, 2004.
17. Nebeling L: Changes in carbohydrate, protein, and fat metabolism in cancer. In McCallum P, Polisena C, editors: *The clinical guide to oncology nutrition*, Chicago, 2000, American Dietetic Association.
18. Inui A: Cancer anorexia-cachexia syndrome: current issues in research and management, *CA Cancer J Clin* 52(2):72-91, 2002.
19. Shaw JH, Wolfe RR: Fatty acid and glycerol kinetics in septic patients and in patients with gastrointestinal cancer. The response to glucose infusion and parenteral feeding, *Ann Surg* 205(4):368-376, 1987.
20. Ravasco P and others: Nutritional deterioration in cancer: the role of disease and diet, *Clin Oncol (R Coll Radiol)* 15(8):443-450, 2003.
21. Jeevanandam M and others: Effect of total parenteral nutrition on whole body protein kinetics in cachectic patients with benign or malignant disease, *JPEN J Parenter Enteral Nutr* 12(3):229-236, 1988.
22. Norton JA, Stein TP, Brennan MF: Whole body protein synthesis and turnover in normal man and malnourished patients with and without known cancer, *Ann Surg* 194(2):123-128, 1981.
23. Tisdale MJ: Metabolic abnormalities in cachexia and anorexia, *Nutrition* 16(10):1013-1014, 2000.
24. Costa LJ, Varella PC, del Giglio A: Weight changes during chemotherapy for breast cancer, *Sao Paulo Med J* 120(4): 113-117, 2002.
25. Demark-Wahnefried W and others: Changes in weight, body composition, and factors influencing energy balance among premenopausal breast cancer patients receiving adjuvant chemotherapy, *J Clin Oncol* 19(9): 2381-2389, 2001.

26. Holzbeierlein JM, Castle E, Thrasher JB: Complications of androgen deprivation therapy: prevention and treatment, *Oncology (Huntingt)* 18(3):303-309; discussion 310, 315, 319-321, 2004.
27. Ingram CDR, Brown JKPFR: Patterns of weight and body composition change in premenopausal women with early stage breast cancer: has weight gain been overestimated? *Cancer Nurs* 27(6):483-490, 2004.
28. Bozzetti F: Rationale and indications for preoperative feeding of malnourished surgical cancer patients, *Nutrition* 18(11-12):953-959, 2002.
29. Linn BS, Robinson DS, Klimas NG: Effects of age and nutritional status on surgical outcomes in head and neck cancer, *Ann Surg* 207(3):267-273, 1988.
30. Nguyen TV, Yueh B: Weight loss predicts mortality after recurrent oral cavity and oropharyngeal carcinomas, *Cancer* 95(3):553-562, 2002.
31. Haugstvedt TK and others: Factors related to and consequences of weight loss in patients with stomach cancer. The Norwegian Multicenter experience. Norwegian Stomach Cancer Trial, *Cancer* 67(3):722-729, 1991.
32. Ovesen L and others: Effect of dietary counseling on food intake, body weight, response rate, survival, and quality of life in cancer patients undergoing chemotherapy: a prospective, randomized study, *J Clin Oncol* 11(10): 2043-2049, 1993.
33. Cohn S, Sawitsky A, Vartsky D: In vivo quantification of body nitrogen and body composition in cancer patients and cancer nutrition studies, *Nutr Cancer* 2: 67-71, 1980.
34. Cohn S, Ellis K, Vartsky D: Comparison of methods of estimating body fat in normal subjects and cancer patients, *Am J Clin Nutr* 34:2839-2347, 1981.
35. Cohn S, Gartenhaus W, Sawitsky A: Compartmental body composition of cancer patients by measurement of total body nitrogen, potassium, and water, *Metabolism* 30:222-229, 1981.
36. Cohn S, Gartenhaus W, Vartsky D: Body composition and dietary intake in neoplastic disease, *Am J Clin Nutr* 34(10):1997-2004, 1981.
37 Cohn S, Vaswani A, Vartsky D: In vivo quantification of body nitrogen for nutritional assessment, *Am J Clin Nutr* 35(5 suppl):1186-1191, 1982.
38. Marian M: Cancer cachexia: Prevalence, mechanisms, and interventions, *Support Line* 20:3-12, 1998.
39. Bosaeus I and others: Dietary intake and resting energy expenditure in relation to weight loss in unselected cancer patients, *Int J Cancer* 93(3):380-383, 2001.
40. McGough C and others: Role of nutritional intervention in patients treated with radiotherapy for pelvic malignancy, *Br J Cancer* 90(12):2278-2287, 2004.
41. Isenring EA, Capra S, Bauer JD: Nutrition intervention is beneficial in oncology outpatients receiving radiotherapy to the gastrointestinal or head and neck area, *Br J Cancer* 91(3):447-452, 2004.
42. Jereczek-Fossa BA and others: Radiotherapy-induced thyroid disorders, *Cancer Treat Rev* 30(4):369-384, 2004.
43. Tisdale MJ: Cachexia in cancer patients, *Nat Rev Cancer* 2(11):862-871, 2002.
44. MacDonald N and others: Understanding and managing cancer cachexia, *J Am Coll Surg* 197(1):143-161, 2003.
45. Lind D, Souba W, Copeland E: Weight loss and cachexia. In Abeloff M and others, editors: *Clinical oncology*, New York, 1995, Churchill Livingstone.
46. Classroom N: Body composition evaluation using single frequency tetrapolar bioelectrical impedance analysis (BIA). *Nutrition Classroom*, 2001, retrieved 3/2/01 from www.nutritionclassroom.com/CLASS/BIA/body_compartments.htm.
47. Shizgal HM: Body composition of patients with malnutrition and cancer. Summary of methods of assessment, *Cancer* 55(1 Suppl):250-253, 1985.
48. Giacosa A and others: Food intake and body composition in cancer cachexia, *Nutr Cancer* 12(1):s20-23, 1996.
49. May P and others: Reversal of cancer related wasting using oral supplementation with a combination of B-hydroxy-B-methylbutyrate, arginine, and glutamine, *Am J Surg* 183:471-479, 2002.
50. Fritz T and others: The predictive role of bioelectrical impedance analysis (BIA) in postoperative complications in cancer patients, *Eur J Surg Oncol* 16:326-331, 1990.
51. Liedman B and others: Symptom control may improve food intake, body composition, and aspects of quality of life after gastrectomy in cancer patients, *Dig Dis Sci* 46(12):2673-2680, 2001.
52. Speca M and others: Patients evaluate a quality of life scale: whose life is it anyway? *Cancer Pract* 2(5):365-370, 1994.
53 Small W and others: Quality of life and nutrition in the patient with cancer, *Oncology Issues* Integrating nutrition into your cancer program:13-4, 2002.
54. McGrath P: Reflections on nutritional issues associated with cancer therapy, *Cancer Pract* 10(2):94-101, 2002.
55. Tchekmedyian S and others: Ongoing placebo-controlled study of oxandrolone in cancer-related weight loss, *Int J Radiat Oncol Biol Phys* 57(2 Suppl):S283-S284, 2003.
56. Council on Practice (COP) Quality Management Committee: Identifying patients at risk: ADA's definitions for nutrition screening and nutrition assessment, *J Am Diet Assoc* 94(8):838-839, 1994.
57. Ottery FD: Definition of standardized nutritional assessment and interventional pathways in oncology, *Nutrition* 12(1 Suppl):S15-S19, 1996.
58. Detsky AS and others: What is subjective global assessment of nutritional status? *JPEN J Parenter Enteral Nutr* 11(1):8-13, 1987.
59. Oncology Nutrition Practice Group: *Patient generated subjective global assessment video* [Video]. Chicago, 2001, American Dietetic Association.
60. Luthringer S, Kulakowski K: Medical nutrition therapy protocols. In McCallum P, Polisena C, editors: *The clinical guide to oncology nutrition*, Chicago, 2000, American Dietetic Association.
61. Ottery F, Bender F, Kasenic S: The design and implementation of a model nutritional oncology clinic, *Oncology Issues* Integrating nutrition into your cancer program: 2-6, 2002.
62. Ferguson M: Patient-generated subjective global assessment, *Oncology (Huntingt)* 17(2 Suppl 2):13-14, 2003.
63. Guigoz Y, Vellas B, Garry PJ: Assessing the nutritional status of the elderly: the Mini Nutritional Assessment as part of the geriatric evaluation, *Nutr Rev* 54(1 Pt 2): S59-S65, 1996.
64. Guigoz Y, Vellas B: The Mini Nutritional Assessment (MNA) for grading the nutritional state of elderly

patients: presentation of the MNA, history and validation, *Nestle Nutr Workshop Ser Clin Perform Programme* 1:3-11, 1999.

65. Ferguson M and others: Development of a valid and reliable malnutrition screening tool for adult acute hospital patients, *Nutrition* 15(6):458-464, 1999.
66. Ferguson ML and others: Validation of a malnutrition screening tool for patients receiving radiotherapy, *Australas Radiol* 43(3):325-327, 1999.
67. Blackburn GL and others: Nutritional and metabolic assessment of the hospitalized patient, *JPEN J Parenter Enteral Nutr* 1(1):11-22, 1977.
68. National Heart Lung and Blood Institute: Part 1 assessing your risk. *National Institutes of Health,* retrieved 1/25/05 from www.nhlbi.nih.gov/health/public/heart/obesity/lose_wt/risk.htm.
69. Expert Panel on the Identification Evaluation, and Treatment of Overweight and Obesity in Adults: *The practical guide identification, evaluation, and treatment of overweight and obesity in adults,* Bethesda, Md., 2000, National Institutes of Health.
70. Ali PA and others: Body composition measurements using DXA and other techniques in tamoxifen-treated patients, *Appl Radiat Isot* 49(5-6):643-645, 1998.
71. Beddoe A, Graham G: Clinical measurement of body composition using in-vivo neutron activation analysis, *JPEN J Parenter Enteral Nutr* 9(4):504-520, 1985.
72. Hills A, Byrne N: Bioelectrical impedance and body composition assessment, *Malaysian Journal of Nutrition* 4:107-112, 1998.
73. Lukaski HC: Methods for the assessment of human body composition: traditional and new, *Am J Clin Nutr* 46(4): 537-556, 1987.
74. NIH Technology Assessment Program: *bioelectrical impedance analysis in body composition measurement,* Bethesda, 1994, National Institutes of Health.
75. Smith MR and others: Measurement of body fat by dual-energy x-ray absorptiometry and bioimpedance analysis in men with prostate cancer, *Nutrition* 18(7-8):574-577, 2002.
76. Simons J and others: The use of bioelectrical impedance analysis to predict total body water in patients with cancer cachexia, *American J Clin Nutr* 61:741-745, 1995.
77. Toso S and others: Bioimpedance vector pattern in cancer patients without disease versus locally advanced or disseminated disease, *Nutr Cancer* 19(6):510-514, 2003.
78. McMillan D and others: Lean body mass changes in cancer patients with weight loss., *Clin Nutr* 19(6):403-406, 2000.
79. Lacey K, Pritchett E: Nutrition care process and model: ADA adopts road map to quality care and outcomes management, *J Am Diet Assoc* 103(8):1061-1072, 2003.
80. Ottery FD: Supportive nutrition to prevent cachexia and improve quality of life, *Semin Oncol* 22(2 Suppl 3): 98-111, 1995.
81. Commission on Dietetics Registration: Who is a registered dietitian? *Commission on Dietetics Registration,* retrieved 1/25/05 from www.cdrnet.org/certifications/rddtr/rddefinition.htm.
82. Johnson E, Inman-Felton A: Overview of the medical nutrition therapy protocols. In Gilbreath J and others, editors: *Medical nutrition therapy across the continuum of care,* Chicago, 1998, American Dietetic Association.
83. McMahon K, Brown JK: Nutritional screening and assessment, *Semin Oncol Nurs* 16(2):106-112, 2000.
84. Tesauro GM, Rowland JH, Lustig C: Survivorship resources for post-treatment cancer survivors, *Cancer Pract* 10(6):277-283, 2002.
85. Joint Commission on the Accreditation of Hospitals Organization: Crosswalk of 2002-2003 Standards for Ambulatory Care to 2004 Provision of Care, Treatment, and Services Standards for Ambulatory Care. *Joint Commission on Accreditation of Healthcare Organizations,* retrieved 1/3/05 from www.jcaho.org/accredited+organizations/ambulatory+care/standards/new+standards/pc_xwalk_amb.pdf.
86. Groenwald S: Continuity of care: nursing challenges, *CancerSource,* retrieved 1/3/05 from www. cancer-sourcern.com/search/getcontent.cfm?DiseaseID=21&Contentid=16722.
87. Huhmann MB, Cunningham RS: Identification and nutritional treatment of cancer related weight loss, *Lancet Oncology,* in press, 2005.
88. American Gastroenterological Association: American Gastroenterological Association medical position statement: parenteral nutrition, *Gastroenterology* 121(4): 966-969, 2001.
89. Murphy L, Mirtallo J, Bradsher K: A.S.P.EN. Communicates with Medicare chief regarding enteral nutrition definition. *American Society for Parenteral and Enteral Nutrition,* retrieved 1/26/05 from www. nutritioncare. org/news/HFCA514.html.
90. American Gastroenterological Association: American Gastroenterological Association medical position statement: guidelines for the use of enteral nutrition, *Gastroenterology* 108(4):1280-1281, 1995.
91. Braga M and others: Early postoperative enteral nutrition improves gut oxygenation and reduces costs compared with total parenteral nutrition, *Crit Care Med* 29(2):242-248, 2001.
92. Jiang XH, Li N, Li JS: Intestinal permeability in patients after surgical trauma and effect of enteral nutrition versus parenteral nutrition, *World J Gastroenterol* 9(8):1878-1880, 2003.
93. Bozzetti F and others: Postoperative enteral versus parenteral nutrition in malnourished patients with gastrointestinal cancer: a randomised multicentre trial, *Lancet* 358(9292):1487-1492, 2001.
94. Braunschweig CL and others: Enteral compared with parenteral nutrition: a meta-analysis, *Am J Clin Nutr* 74(4):534-542, 2001.
95. Harrison LE and others: Early postoperative enteral nutrition improves peripheral protein kinetics in upper gastrointestinal cancer patients undergoing complete resection: a randomized trial, *JPEN J Parenter Enteral Nutr* 21(4):202-207, 1997.
96. Koretz RL, Lipman TO, Klein S: AGA technical review on parenteral nutrition, *Gastroenterology* 121(4):970-1001, 2001.
97. Bozzetti F and others: Glucose-based total parenteral nutrition does not stimulate glucose uptake by humans' tumours, *Clin Nutr* 23(3):417-421, 2004.
98. Aiko S and others: Beneficial effects of immediate enteral nutrition after esophageal cancer surgery, *Surg Today* 31(11):971-978, 2001.

99. Page RD and others: Intravenous hydration versus naso-jejunal enteral feeding after esophagectomy: a randomised study, *Eur J Cardiothorac Surg* 22(5):666-672, 2002.
100. De Cicco M and others: Parenteral nutrition in cancer patients receiving chemotherapy: effects on toxicity and nutritional status, *JPEN J Parenter Enteral Nutr* 17(6):513-518, 1993.
101. Tandon SP and others: Nutritional support as an adjunct therapy of advanced cancer patients, *Indian J Med Res* 80:180-188, 1984.
102. Valdivieso M and others: Long-term effects of intravenous hyperalimentation administered during intensive chemotherapy for small cell bronchogenic carcinoma, *Cancer* 59(2):362-369, 1987.
103. Weisdorf SA and others: Positive effect of prophylactic total parenteral nutrition on long-term outcome of bone marrow transplantation, *Transplantation* 43(6):833-838, 1987.
104. Szeluga DJ and others: Nutritional support of bone marrow transplant recipients: a prospective, randomized clinical trial comparing total parenteral nutrition to an enteral feeding program, *Cancer Res* 47(12):3309-3316, 1987.
105. Schloerb PR, Amare M: Total parenteral nutrition with glutamine in bone marrow transplantation and other clinical applications (a randomized, double-blind study), *JPEN J Parenter Enteral Nutr* 17(5):407-413, 1993.
106. Roberts S and others: Total parenteral nutrition vs oral diet in autologous hematopoietic cell transplant recipients, *Bone Marrow Transplant* 32(7):715-721, 2003.
107. Macfie J: European round table: the use of immuno-nutrients in the critically ill, *Clin Nutr* 23(6):1426-1429, 2004.
108. Savarese DM and others: Prevention of chemotherapy and radiation toxicity with glutamine, *Cancer Treat Rev* 29(6):501-513, 2003.
109. Morlion BJ and others: Total parenteral nutrition with glutamine dipeptide after major abdominal surgery: a randomized, double-blind, controlled study, *Ann Surg* 227(2):302-308, 1998.
110. Scheid C and others: Randomized, double-blind, controlled study of glycyl-glutamine-dipeptide in the parenteral nutrition of patients with acute leukemia undergoing intensive chemotherapy, *Nutrition* 20(3): 249-254, 2004.
111. Coghlin-Dickson TM and others: Effect of oral glutamine supplementation during bone marrow transplantation, *JPEN J Parenter Enteral Nutr* 24(2):61-66, 2000.
112. de Luis DA and others: Randomized clinical trial with an enteral arginine-enhanced formula in early postsurgical head and neck cancer patients, *Eur J Clin Nutr* 58(11): 1505-1508, 2004.
113. Song JX and others: Effect of parenteral nutrition with L-arginine supplementation on postoperative immune function in patients with colorectal cancer, *Di Yi Jun Yi Da Xue Xue Bao* 22(6):545-547, 2002.
114. Daly JM and others: Enteral nutrition with supplemental arginine, RNA, and omega-3 fatty acids in patients after operation: immunologic, metabolic, and clinical outcome, *Surgery* 112(1):56-67, 1992.
115. Braga M and others: Gut function and immune and inflammatory responses in patients perioperatively fed with supplemented enteral formulas, *Arch Surg* 131(12): 1257-1264, 1996.
116. Heyland DK and others: Should immunonutrition become routine in critically ill patients? A systematic review of the evidence, *JAMA* 286(8):944-953, 2001.
117. Jho DH and others: Role of omega-3 fatty acid supplementation in inflammation and malignancy, *Integr Cancer Ther* 3(2):98-111, 2004.
118. Burns CP and others: Phase II study of high-dose fish oil capsules for patients with cancer-related cachexia, *Cancer* 101(2):370-378, 2004.
119. Wachtler P and others: Influence of a total parenteral nutrition enriched with omega-3 fatty acids on leukotriene synthesis of peripheral leukocytes and systemic cytokine levels in patients with major surgery, *J Trauma* 42(2):191-198, 1997.
120. Jatoi A and others: An eicosapentaenoic acid supplement versus megestrol acetate versus both for patients with cancer-associated wasting: a North Central Cancer Treatment Group and National Cancer Institute of Canada collaborative effort, *J Clin Oncol* 22(12):2469-2476, 2004.
121. Moses AW and others: Reduced total energy expenditure and physical activity in cachectic patients with pancreatic cancer can be modulated by an energy and protein dense oral supplement enriched with n-3 fatty acids, *Br J Cancer* 90(5):996-1002, 2004.
122. Fearon K and others: An energy and protein dense, high omega 3 fatty acid oral supplement promotes weight gain in cancer cachexia, *Eur J Cancer* 37(Supp 6): S27-S28, 2001.
123. Bauer JD, Capra S: Nutrition intervention improves outcomes in patients with cancer cachexia receiving chemotherapy-a pilot study, retrieved from www.springerlink.com/(533ngd45rvi1u555rhkuhsaw)/app/home/contribution.asp?referrer=parent&backto=issue,11,11;journal,9,76;linkingpublicationresults, 1:101182,1.
124. Schwarte A: Ethical decisions regarding nutrition and the terminally ill, *Gastroenterol Nurs* 24(1):29-33, 2001.
125. Whitworth MK and others: Doctor, does this mean I'm going to starve to death? *J Clin Oncol* 22(1):199-201, 2004.
126. Quill TE, Byock IR: Responding to intractable terminal suffering: the role of terminal sedation and voluntary refusal of food and fluids. ACP-ASIM End-of-Life Care Consensus Panel. American College of Physicians-American Society of Internal Medicine, *Ann Intern Med* 132(5):408-414, 2000.
127. McCann R: Lack of evidence about tube feeding—food for thought, *JAMA* 282(14):1380-1381, 1999.
128. McCann RM, Hall WJ, Groth-Juncker A: Comfort care for terminally ill patients. The appropriate use of nutrition and hydration, *JAMA* 272(16):1263-1266, 1994.
129. Maillet JO, Potter RL, Heller L: Position of the American Dietetic Association: ethical and legal issues in nutrition, hydration, and feeding, *J Am Diet Assoc* 102(5):716-726, 2002.
130. Dorner B and others: The "to feed or not to feed" dilemma, *J Am Diet Assoc* 97(10 Suppl 2):S172-S176, 1997.

131. Chochinov HM and others: Desire for death in the terminally ill, *Am J Psychiatry* 152(8):1185-1191, 1995.
132. MacFie J: Ethical and legal considerations in the provision of nutritional support to the perioperative patient, *Curr Opin Clin Nutr Metab Care* 3(1):23-29, 2000.
133. Capra S and others: Nutritional therapy for cancer induced weight loss, *Nutr Clin Pract* 17(4):210-213, 2002.
134. O'Shaughnessy JA and others: Treatment and prevention of intraepithelial neoplasia: an important target for accelerated new agent development, *Clin Cancer Res* 8(2):314-346, 2002.
135. August D: Nutritional care of cancer patients. In Norton J and others, editors: *Surgery: basic science and clinical evidence,* ed 1, New York, 2000, Springer-Verlag.
136. Byers T, Nestle M, McTiernan A, et al. American Cancer Society guidelines on nutrition and physical activity for cancer prevention: Reducing the risk of cancer with healthy food choices and physical activity. *CA Cancer J Clin* 52(2):92-119, 2002.

UNIT IV

Maintaining Health After Cancer

CHAPTER

19 Sleep and Wakefulness

Ann M. Berger

INTRODUCTION

Healthy adults awaken from sleep feeling rested and ready to perform their daily activities. They remain alert and have energy throughout the day. When a pattern of deprived sleeping time or disrupted sleep occurs in adults, there are adverse physical, cognitive, emotional, and social consequences. Impaired total sleep time has been linked to impaired alertness,[1] performance, and memory[2] and an increased risk of car accidents due to sleepiness,[3] a reduced pain threshold,[4] and a resistance to insulin.[5] Women at all stages of cancer often experience problems falling asleep and staying asleep and report that they awaken feeling fatigued and unmotivated to perform their daily activities.[6-16] Patterns of deprived sleeping time or disrupted sleep develop more frequently in women with cancer than they do in healthy women.[17] Health care team members in primary care and oncology settings must systematically screen all patients and make referrals to sleep specialists for disturbances in sleep and wakefulness. Teaching women in all settings of the importance of adequate sleep must become an integral part of the instructions regarding the maintenance of physical and mental health. Advancing knowledge through research regarding the role of sleep in prevention and control of cancer will move the science forward in the most expedient fashion. These efforts are important, because sleep disturbances and the consequences of fatigue and daytime sleepiness can influence quality of life (QOL).[18,19] The cost of cancer in the US is estimated to be over $180 billion/year, and these costs are not limited to treatment but also include lost productivity and poor health status secondary to treatment and its side effects, including disturbances in sleep and wakefulness.[19]

OVERVIEW

This chapter will focus on maintaining health by assisting women with cancer to get the sleep their bodies need during each 24-hour circadian cycle. When sleep needs are met, women are more likely to wake up feeling refreshed and be able to function optimally during the day. After reading this chapter, it is hoped that the reader will have more knowledge on the role of sleep in maintaining health and be able to integrate procedures to screen, assess, and treat disturbances in sleep and wakefulness in women, particularly those with cancer. In recent years, there have been excellent book chapters on sleep[20] and its measurement,[21] and key articles focusing on sleep and cancer.[15,17,19,22-24] This chapter will focus on synthesizing the information on this topic. Readers are referred to these sentinel publications to gain further knowledge and appreciation for the scope of the problem and the need for the health care system to incorporate assessment and treatment of disturbances in sleep and daytime wakefulness into each patient encounter.

Leading types of cancer in women include breast cancer, followed by lung, colon, and gynecologic cancers.[25] The majority of research thus far regarding sleep in women with cancer has been conducted in breast cancer, with minimal research conducted in women with lung and colon cancer despite the prevalence of these cancers.[19] Studies that have examined sleep in lung and colon cancer patients have usually included mixed samples of both men and women. There have been very few studies of sleep in women with gynecologic cancers.[19] Further study of sleep in women with common cancer diagnoses is needed.

PROCESSES THAT REGULATE SLEEP

Sleep is recognized as an active process that is regulated by multiple behavioral, neuroendocrine, and central nervous system factors. When sleep is insufficient or of poor quality, a variety of adverse effects have been shown to occur.[24] A recent study's findings suggest that chronic insomnia negatively affects host immune defenses.[26] Despite advances in the understanding of sleep, dissemination of knowledge to health care professionals hasn't kept pace. Therefore, not surprisingly, the sleep problems of patients frequently go unaddressed.[27] Many patients do not discuss sleep problems with health care providers because their concerns have been dismissed in the past. To improve clinical outcomes, health care providers need to recognize and respond to the sleep and wakefulness concerns of patients in primary care and oncology settings.

Sleep disorders include a group of problems that are characterized by insomnia, abnormal movements, behaviors or sensations during sleep, or excessive daytime sleepiness.[24] Very broadly, sleep disorders fall into the following primary groups: insomnia, sleep related breathing disorders, hypersomnias of central origin, circadian rhythm sleep disorders, parasomnias, sleep-related movement disorders, isolated symptoms, apparently normal variants and unresolved issues, and other sleep disorders.[28] There is no current or proposed disorder that is specific to sleep in the context of cancer.

Homeostasis has been defined as the coordinated physiologic processes that maintain most of the steady states in the organism.[29] Homeostatic processes that regulate activity, nutrition, stress, and sleep play vital roles in maintaining health and preventing the initiation and promotion of cancer. The two-process model of sleep regulation provides the framework for understanding the mechanisms that play vital roles in the initiation and maintenance of regular sleep patterns.[30,31] The model is based on the interaction of two key processes, the homeostatic process S and the circadian process C. The level of the sleep/wake–dependent process S rises during waking and declines during sleep. It can be referred to as the "sleep pressure" that humans feel when they remain awake for increasing number of hours each day. Process C, or the circadian component, is independent of sleep and waking. It can be described as the endogenous circadian pacemaker located in the suprachismatic nuclei (SCN) of the brain that cycles approximately every 24 hours. Its role is to modulate two thresholds that make humans feel sleepy in the evening and ready to rise in the morning. Sleep homeostasis refers to the sleep/wake–dependent aspect of sleep regulation that adjusts sleep propensity in response to prior deprivation or excessive sleep.[32]

A "sleep debt" that results from a poor night's sleep can't be accumulated over several days but must be restored within the next 24-hour cycle by homeostatic mechanisms. The two-process model has also been successful in predicting alertness and sleepiness. The strength of the S and C processes has been examined in healthy, young subjects. The extent of circadian rhythm alterations with cancer has varied in animal models according to tumor type, growth rate, and level of differentiation.[33] In mice, disruption of circadian rhythms was associated with tumor growth acceleration of two types of malignant tumors (osteosarcoma or pancreatic adenocarcinoma), suggesting that the host circadian clock may plan a key role in endogenous control of tumor progression.[34] The circadian rhythms in women with cancer is a promising area for future research.

Rapid eye movement (REM) sleep and non-REM (NREM) are the two major sleep states. The alternation of REM and NREM sleep constitutes the sleep cycle. NREM sleep is more prevalent in the first part of the night and contains more deep sleep. During the night, NREM sleep becomes progressively lighter, and REM sleep becomes more frequent. Each REM cycle follows an NREM cycle and increases in length and intensity during the second half of the night, as shown in Figure 19-1.[35] Knowledge of the sleep cycle is fundamental to understanding sleep in health and illness. Sleep intensity is reflected by the extent of slow waves in the sleep electroencephalogram (EEG), and these slow, or delta, waves appear to play an important role in perceptions of restorative sleep.

Circadian rhythms of most human bodily functions, including physiologic, biochemical, and behavioral, are generated and maintained by the biologic clock. Examples of these functions include the hormones melatonin, cortisol, prolactin, and growth hormone. Core body temperature, task performance, blood pressure, triacyglycerol activity, and sleep-wakefulness are other processes regulated by the biologic clock.[36] In health, these rhythms are carefully regulated to maintain internal stability that complements the organism's needs and to increase its chances of survival. Maintenance of robust circadian rhythms of sleeping and waking are a vital component of healthy adaptation throughout the life cycle.

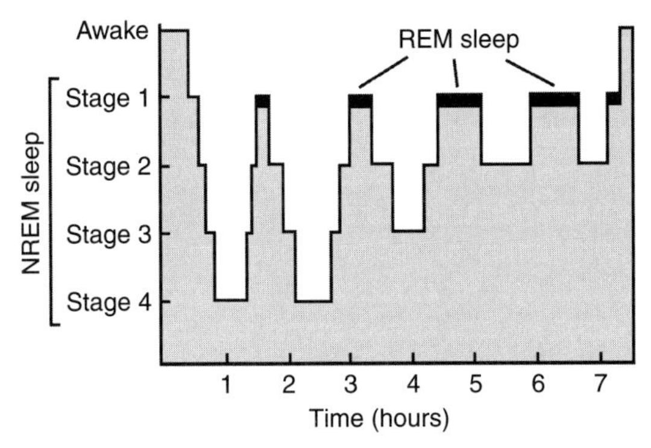

FIGURE 19-1 REM sleep cycles. (From Scammel TE: The regulations of sleep and circadian rhythms. *Sleep Medicine Alert* (8), p. 2, National Sleep Foundation, 2004.)

A metaanalysis of age-related changes in initiation and maintenance of sleep found that waking frequency and duration increased with age. A limitation of studies included in the metaanalysis was that few studied women.[37] Shift workers provide us with evidence that attempts to sleep at inappropriate phases of the circadian cycle will usually result in shorter sleep episodes and more awakenings.[38] Health consequences of working and sleeping out of phase with the innate biologic clock, as observed in shift workers, include increased rates of gastrointestinal, cardiovascular, and hormonal disturbances[39] and increased risk of colorectal[40] and breast cancer.[41] These same consequences may result when individuals, including patients with cancer, adopt unhealthy sleep/wake patterns or experience inflammatory responses that result in chronic sleep deprivation and disruption. Interventions aimed at entraining the circadian clock and increasing sleep pressure may assist in reducing impaired sleep. This is a particularly timely topic since recent advances in cancer diagnosis and treatment have resulted in increased numbers of cancer survivors (currently over 9 million persons, including over 2.5 million with breast cancer).[42]

A conceptual framework of insomnia for primary care practitioners, known as the 3P model, focuses on predisposing, precipitating, and perpetuating factors that influence sleep.[43] These factors interfere with the homeostatic processes that regulate sleep in health. Predisposing traits within the individual that create vulnerability to sleep disturbance are associated with measures of heightened arousal. The hypothalamic-pituitary-adrenal (HPA) axis response to stress in some persons is easily and frequently evoked, producing chronic hyperarousal. Precipitating factors are events, outside the individual, that trigger insomnia. If coping capacity is insufficient or the presenting problem persists, acute insomnia may progress into chronic insomnia.

Women are known to report insomnia more frequently than men.[44] Perpetuating factors include behaviors and attitudes that develop during acute insomnia that lead to persistent sleeping problems. These maladaptive patterns are often not assessed in clinical practice, even though they offer a therapeutic target that can be addressed and successfully treated.[43] In primary care patients, predisposing factors for insomnia may include past history of poor sleep related to poor sleep hygiene or lifestyle factors, or having been diagnosed with one of the common sleep disorders such as sleep apnea, narcolepsy, or restless leg syndrome.[19] Precipitating factors may include stressful life events. Common perpetuating factors include spending more time in bed and taking long naps. Figure 19-2 shows a schematic depiction of insomnia in an at-risk hyperaroused person, triggered by a precipitating event and then perpetuated by adoption of maladaptive practices and attitudes that exceeds the insomnia threshold.[43]

The Conceptual Model of Impaired Sleep, developed by Lee and colleagues,[20] suggests that impaired sleep may be due to either sleep deprivation, conceptualized as an inadequate amount of sleep that is often due to a lifestyle or developmental issue, and/or sleep disruption resulting from fragmented sleep due to one or more health-related issues (Figure 19-3). Sleep deprivation is prevalent in today's 24/7 society.[36]

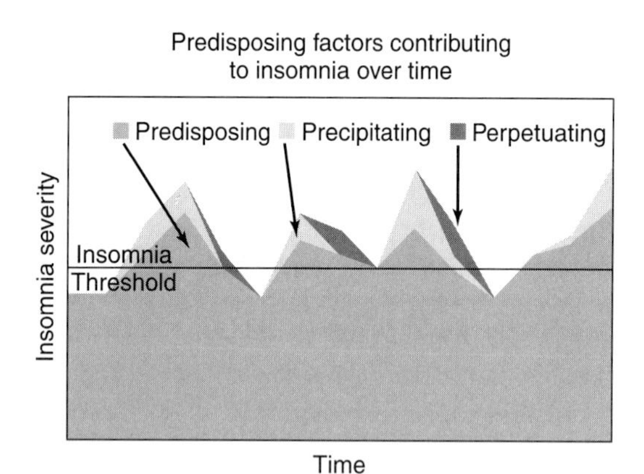

FIGURE 19-2 Process model. (From Spielman AJ, Glovinsky PB: A conceptual framework of insomnia for primary care practitioners. *Sleep Medicine Alert 9*(1), National Sleep Foundation, 2004.)

The major risk factor for impaired sleep among healthy adults is a stressful lifestyle, which heightens the classic stress response, the HPA axis response, and alertness. The prevalence of disrupted sleep in healthy women varies in relationship to menstrual cycles, pregnancy, motherhood, and the menopausal trajectory—all times of high prevalence for sleep disruption.[45,46] Female sex has been identified as a factor that doubles the risk of insomnia.[19,47] Increased fragmentation of sleep occurs with aging, especially when a woman has comorbid diseases that disrupt sleep or has adopted poor health habits over the long term. Older women are more likely to complain of sleep difficulties,[48] even though men have more objective changes in sleep architecture. Increased frequency of primary sleep disorders also occurs with aging. The most prevalent specific cause of fragmented sleep in adult women is sleep-disordered breathing; its incidence ranges from 5% to 20% of women between 30 and 60 years of age.[49] Restless leg syndrome and periodic limb movement disorder also interfere with sleep in approximately 1% to 10% of persons from different ethnic backgrounds and with anemia,[50] and increases with aging in women.[51] Disturbances in sleep and daytime wakefulness are often perceived as symptoms secondary to depressive or anxiety disorders that will resolve with time and are often ignored or minimized in clinical practice, despite their link to chronic insomnia.[52]

Lee's model identifies the adverse health outcomes that result from impaired sleep and divides them into physiologic, cognitive/behavioral, emotional, and social categories (Figure 19-3).[20] Impaired functioning in all dimensions creates significant reduction in QOL and puts the person at risk for increased morbidity and mortality. Prevention of these adverse outcomes is important for women both before and after a diagnosis of cancer. A chronic inflammatory process involving the T cell compartment has been linked to persistent fatigue in breast cancer survivors.[53]

Comparison of the two-process model, the 3P model, and the Conceptual Model of Impaired Sleep provides scientifically sound knowledge for

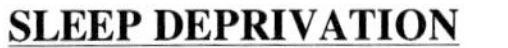
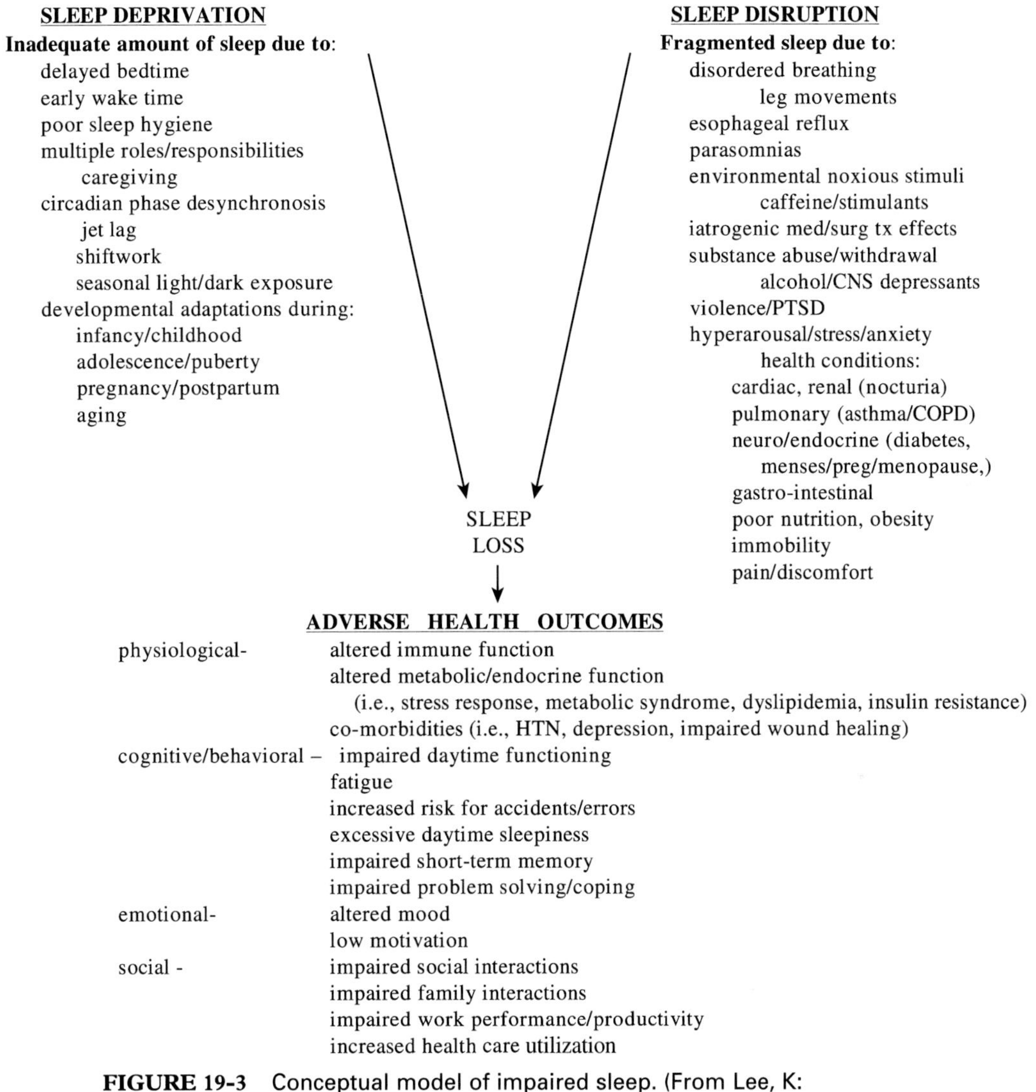

FIGURE 19-3 Conceptual model of impaired sleep. (From Lee, K: Pathophysiological phenomena in nursing. Saunders, St. Louis, 2003.)

understanding the homeostatic process, the factors that positively and negatively influence sleep, and the adverse outcomes of impaired sleep. Healthy sleep is important for maintaining optimal health and immune function to prevent the initiation and promotion of cancer. When predisposing, precipitating, and/or perpetuating factors are activated and/or normal amplitudes of circadian rhythms are lost, sleep deprivation or disruption occurs that may result in adverse health outcomes. There are gaps in what is known about sleep in women who are healthy and those with cancer. As understanding of sleep advances, health care professionals must integrate this knowledge into prevention and patient care delivery in primary and oncology clinical settings.

INSOMNIA

Insomnia is defined as a heterogeneous complaint that may involve difficulty in falling to sleep, trouble staying asleep with prolonged nocturnal awakenings, and/or early morning awakenings with an inability to resume sleep that is associated with daytime dysfunction.[28] Insomnia is a very common complaint in patients with cancer;[54] in fact, it is the most prevalent cause of impaired sleep in women with breast cancer.[16] Studies conducted among heterogeneous samples of both male and female cancer patients suggest that between 30% and 50% of newly diagnosed or recently treated cancer patients report difficulties with sleep, a finding that confirms insomnia's frequent presence.[15] In addition, 23% to 44% of breast cancer survivors (2 to 6 years after diagnosis) report difficulties with sleep; a finding that denotes insomnia's chronic nature in a subset of women.[16]

Potential etiologic factors for insomnia are multifactorial because of the fact that cancer is not a single event but rather a succession of severe stressors. When patients are diagnosed and undergo cancer treatment, numerous stimuli increase the risk for varying durations of insomnia; transient (less than 1 month), acute (more than 1 but less than 6 months), and/or chronic insomnia (more than 6 months).[16] These factors fall into several categories: demographic, lifestyle, psychologic, disease-related, and treatment-related.[24] Demographic factors include older age, female sex, and Caucasian race.[55] Lifestyle factors, such as daytime napping patterns and excessive environmental stimulation, contribute to sleep disturbances.[22] Sleep patterns are influenced by ongoing concerns and worries about the disease. Anxiety and depression are common and believed to affect sleep in patients with cancer, but it is not clear if these relationships begin at the time of, or after, cancer has been found.[24]

Disease-related factors that may influence sleep include pain and other symptoms, changes in activity/rest patterns, and altered hormone and cytokine production. The estrogen deficiency produced by chemotherapy and hormonal treatments given for many cancers may result in premature menopause or aggravated menopausal symptoms that interfere with sleep.[56,57] Most troubling are the vasomotor symptoms of hot flashes and sweating that are reported during cancer chemotherapy[58] and by at least half of the women taking tamoxifen and that usually persist for a considerable portion of the 5-year period of administration.[59-61]

The circadian rhythm of hot flashes has been shown to be different in women with breast cancer as compared to healthy norms, suggesting that an alteration of the circadian process may play a role in the quality of night sleep.[62] A need to void, pain, and coughing or snoring were the three most frequent reasons for disturbed sleep given by breast cancer patients in a study where menopausal symptoms were not discussed.[63] Factors that may contribute to sleep disorders in various types and stages of cancer must be identified. Cancer survivors who chronically experience symptoms are at increased risk for perpetuating disturbances in sleep and wakefulness. Mechanisms to explain how menopausal symptoms, pain, mood, activity, inflammation, and clusters of symptoms affect sleep have to be clarified. Clusters of symptoms can have adverse effects on patient outcomes and may have a synergistic effect as a predictor of patient morbidity.[64]

Biologic processes that are involved in circadian processes may be affected by inadequate sleep and result in blunted or erratic rhythms of cortisol, melatonin, and other substances.[65] In addition, cancer cells alter the production of cytokines, including interleukin 1, and may be related to daytime sleepiness and longer sleep times.[66] A combination of animal and human research suggests that several cancer-related symptoms may involve the actions of pro-inflammatory cytokines.[19,67] Daytime melatonin assay levels changed during the course of chemotherapy treatment in one study. Additional work regarding the relationship between melatonin patterns, fatigue and sleep is needed.[68,69] Further understanding of the interaction between biologic and cancer disease processes is needed so that interventions can be developed that positively influence patient outcomes.

PREVALENCE OF SLEEP PROBLEMS IN PATIENTS WITH CANCER

The prevalence of sleep problems in cancer patients is difficult to determine because of the various methods used in epidemiologic studies. The estimated prevalence of insomnia is about 20% in the general population,[70] but it has not yet been determined if disturbances in sleep are more prevalent in certain groups of cancer patients.[22] Although disturbances in sleep and wakefulness in women with cancer have received little attention from researchers, estimates are that 30% to 40% of these women experience these symptoms.[44] A range of 30% to 88% of women with breast cancer has been reported.[17] A prevalence of 54% to 68% of male and female patients with a variety of cancer diagnoses report "feeling drowsy" during the day.[17] Only a few studies have measured sleep objectively with actigraphy or polysomnography to determine prevalence.[22] Two descriptive studies reported that 43% to 44% of hospitalized cancer patients had prescriptions for hypnotics.[71,72]

A review of studies conducted between 1977 and 1999[15] on the prevalence of insomnia in cancer patients determined that most samples included both men and women and mixed cancer sites and stages. Samples that included only women reported the prevalence of insomnia to be between 23% and 44%.[73-75] Another study compared men and women with lung or breast cancer with age- and sex-matched healthy controls and healthy insomniacs. Lung cancer patients slept as poorly as insomniacs but underreported their sleep difficulties. No breakdown based on sex was provided.[76] No studies were found that described the prevalence of sleep disturbances in women with colorectal cancer. In studies of lung cancer or colon cancer, samples have been too small to examine sex differences.

Approximately 30% of women undergoing radiation therapy for cervical cancer (n = 31) or uterine cancer (n = 19) had problems either with failing asleep or waking up during the night at the initiation of therapy. Sleep problems peaked at 60% of women during the fourth or fifth week of radiation and continued to be the second most problematic symptom (after fatigue) when treatments were completed.[77] Sleep quality and immune functioning were studied in 91 women with abnormal Papanicolaou smears who had cervical biopsies to determine if cancer was present. Those who self-reported getting adequate sleep had significantly more T helper cells and B cells, and fewer T suppressor cells.[78] This study must be repeated before results can be conclusive. A link between chronic primary insomnia and reduced immune function of CD3+, CD4+, CD8+, and CD16+/CD56+ has been reported, but more research is needed to determine the finding's clinical significance, particularly in the context of women with cancer.[26]

Sleep has been studied in a few other cancer diagnoses, usually with mixed samples (male and female). A sample of 72 men and 72 women with melanoma were studied 3 months after surgery and again at 7 and 13 months.[79] Although men had a significantly greater thickness of melanoma lesion (and therefore a poorer prognosis) compared to women, significantly more sleep problems and lower sleep quality were reported by the women. A mixed sample of 91 patients who were at least 6 months post–bone marrow transplant (mean of 40 months) and 73 patients who were at least 6 months post–chemotherapy (mean of 39 months) were examined in relationship to fatigue and sleep. The most interesting finding was that fatigue was related to changes in sleep patterns rather than duration of sleep, a finding supported by other studies.[80,81] Persistent sleep problems are more common in persons who undergo bone marrow transplantation who are over 40 years of age at the time of the transplant, women, and those who received total body irradiation before the transplant.[82] In samples that include several types of cancer and treatment modalities, younger patients were more likely to report insomnia.[44]

Very little research has focused on sleep in the late or terminal phases of cancer.[19] The prevalence of sleep problems in women with metastatic breast cancer who were receiving palliative chemotherapy to reduce pain was 68% at baseline. Insomnia improved for 55%, remained the same for 28%, and became worse for 17% during chemotherapy.[83] The prevalence of one or more types of sleep disturbance was 63% in another sample of women with metastatic breast cancer, with 37% having used sleeping pills within the last month. Greater pain and depression were associated with problems falling and staying asleep.[14] Salivary cortisol samples were collected 4 times each day for 3 days to assess circadian rhythm amplitude as a predictor of 7-year survival rates in metastatic breast cancer patients.[84] Flat or dampened amplitudes in cortisol rhythm were associated with fewer natural killer (NK) cells and suppressed NK activity and with more self-reported night awakenings. The few studies that have examined the role of circadian rhythms in cancer treatment outcomes suggest that prognosis and QOL may be more positive for those who maintain robust circadian rhythms and regular sleep/wake patterns of activity.[19] Linking immune function with cancer morbidity and mortality is a promising area for future study and will support the importance of obtaining quality sleep to preserve immunity and health.

The largest study to date, conducted to determine prevalence and nature of sleep disturbances in persons with cancer by use of self-report, was recently reported.[44] Most of the entire mixed sample (n = 982) had more than one type of insomnia, with maintenance insomnia the most common type (76%) with several awakenings during the night. The sample also reported trouble falling asleep (44%), being awake for a long time (35%), and waking up too early in the morning (33%). The prevalence of insomnia was 37.8% in breast, 29.4% in gynecologic, and 30.5% in all cancer patients, with men reporting fewer problems than women. The reasons for the insomnia include pain or discomfort, concerns about family and finances, and physical effects of the cancer itself. Odds of insomnia were increased if the patient's spirits were down or if patients had concerns, restlessness in their legs, or used sleeping pills—findings that are similar to the general population. Those patients who had received radiation to the head were more likely to report excessive sleepiness and sleeping more than usual. Patients who reported being overly fatigued were 2.5 times more likely to also report insomnia. The contribution of insomnia to cancer-related fatigue has been largely overlooked, and this warrants further investigation. The actigraphic recordings of number of awakenings/night and/or the number of minutes awake after sleep onset have been found to be excessive in several samples of women with early-stage breast cancer and correlated with higher fatigue.[6-8,85,86] Figure 19-4 illustrates the ability of actigraphs to objectively capture the number and length of night awakenings in a more rigorous manner than by sleep diaries to assist in clarifying the relationship between sleep, activity, and fatigue.[6]

The onset of sleep-wake disturbances occurs before diagnosis in a subset of patients and prevalence increases after the diagnosis. Three hundred women (mean time since diagnosis of 48.6 months) who had been treated with radiation therapy for nonmetastatic breast cancer completed an investigator-developed insomnia screening questionnaire.[15] Those who reported sleep difficulties were then interviewed by phone to further evaluate the specifics of their symptoms. Current sleep difficulties were reported by 145 (48%) and 83 (28%) were currently using hypnotics. When combined, 51% (n = 154) of the total sample was considered to display insomnia symptoms. Using the same criteria, 15% (n = 45) of the entire sample reported a past history of sleep difficulties. Of those with current symptoms of insomnia, 33% (n = 45) felt their sleep difficulties followed the diagnosis of cancer and the remaining 91 patients (67%) reported that sleep disturbance was a preexisting condition. Most of those who reported that their sleep difficulties began after diagnosis reported that the problems began within 6 months after diagnosis (76%, n = 25), and about one half of them (51%, n = 13) estimated that insomnia began within the first month after diagnosis. The most frequent reason that was identified for their difficulties was stress

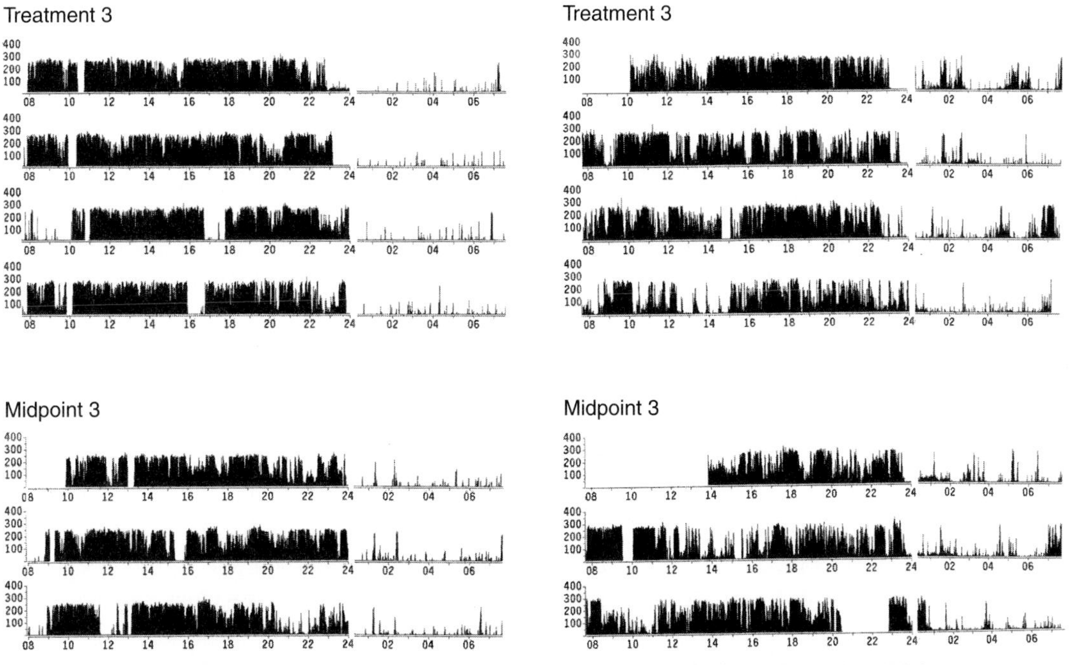

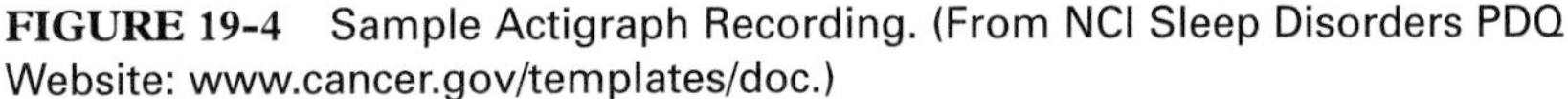
FIGURE 19-4 Sample Actigraph Recording. (From NCI Sleep Disorders PDQ Website: www.cancer.gov/templates/doc.)

or worry associated with cancer. There was a fourfold increased risk of sleep problems after diagnosis in highly educated women living alone. This study's findings indicate that breast cancer may aggravate occasional or mild preexisting sleep disturbances in vulnerable individuals and result in chronic and severe sleep onset and maintenance disturbances. In order to reduce the likelihood of progressive sleep disturbances, targeted treatment has to be proactively offered before the problem becomes chronic.

Chronic Insomnia in Patients with Cancer

It is currently believed that chronic insomnia is more likely to be present among individuals who are initially more vulnerable to this condition as a result of a hyperarousability trait. The individual's response to the initial acute insomnia is thought to determine in large part whether the sleep problems persist or not. According to a cognitive-behavioral conceptualization of insomnia, maladaptive sleep habits and dysfunctional beliefs about sleep play key roles in maintenance of insomnia. Both of these factors then work to increase physiologic, cognitive, and emotional arousal as well as performance anxiety regarding sleep, which are not congruent with the relaxation state required for sleep.[47,87]

To further compound the problem, individuals with chronic insomnia often develop sleep habits such as napping more during the day, spending more time in bed, and having irregular sleep/wake schedules. Although they may be helpful in acute insomnia, these perpetuating habits desynchronize the sleep-wake cycle and weaken the association between the bedroom cues and sleep.[47,87] Patients with cancer frequently adopt these maladaptive sleep behaviors when they are encouraged to take it easy and to rest.[86,88] Faulty ideas and attitudes about sleep also may contribute to sleep maintenance problems over time.[47] These misconceptions about sleep can be summarized as the following: unrealistic expectations about sleep requirements, inaccurate appraisals of difficulty sleeping, misattributions regarding daytime impairments, and inaccurate conceptions about the causes of insomnia. Cancer patients often report dysfunctional ideas about the relationship between sleep and cancer that may contribute to the development of sleep problems.[15] They also report that the frequency and intensity of and the distress from other symptoms interferes with their sleep.[89] Research in this area is needed that better delineates the role of each of these potential etiologic factors in chronic insomnia in women with cancer and women who are caregivers to patients with cancer.[90]

Measurement of Sleep in Patients with Cancer

Little is known about sleep quality in patients with cancer. A limitation of studies has been a lack of consensus among researchers studying sleep in cancer patients about which sleep variables to examine and on preferred instruments to measure variables of interest. Sleep quality can be measured by several methods: self-report (questionnaire, diary), behavioral (observation, actigraphy), and physiologic (polysomnography). Despite attempts, no single item tool of global sleep quality has established reliability and validity for use with cancer patients.[91] No multicomponent tool has consistently been used in studies conducted thus far. Variables most consistently examined include latency, the number and length of awakenings, total sleep time, daytime naps, daytime sleepiness, quality of perceived sleep, and sleep efficiency. Detailed information regarding measuring oncology nursing–sensitive patient outcomes of sleep and wakefulness in patients with cancer has been recently made available on the Oncology Nursing Society (ONS) website.[92]

Descriptions of the self-reported sleep and wakefulness tools and their psychometric properties when used in patients with cancer are shown in Tables 19-1 and 19-2.[23] Actigraphy and polysomnography also have established reliability and validity for use with patients with cancer. They have been used to deepen the understanding of relationships between activity, rest, and sleep, and fatigue. Guidelines for the use of actigraphy in research and practice were recently published,[93] and consistent use of these guidelines will aid in comparison of findings across studies. The American Association of Sleep Medicine guideline, "Practice parameters for the evaluation of chronic insomnia,"[94] provides major recommendations for the evaluation and diagnosis of chronic insomnia without comorbid diseases. Researchers are encouraged to overcome past measurement limitations by considering consistent adoption of instruments with established reliability and validity for use in patients with cancer.

Evidence Relating to Treatment and Interventions

During the last 20 years, there has been increasing recognition that psychologic and behavioral factors play an important role in insomnia. More than a dozen nonpharmacologic interventions have been developed; about one half of these have received adequate empirical evaluation of their clinical efficacy. A metaanalysis reported that stimulus control, sleep restriction, sleep hygiene counseling, and relaxation therapy interventions have been shown to produce reliable and durable improvements in sleep patterns in about 60% to 80% of patients with primary and chronic insomnia.[95] Both sleep induction and sleep maintenance were significantly improved; stimulus control and sleep restriction were the most effective single-therapy procedures and were well maintained at a 6-month follow-up.

Examples of cognitive-behavioral therapies that have been tested to promote quality sleep include stimulus control, sleep restriction, paradoxical intention, sleep hygiene, cognitive restructuring, relaxation therapy, phototherapy, and exercise.[23] Two excellent textbooks[47,96] and one edited journal issue[97] are essential reading for the clinician who is involved in the assessment and treatment of insomnia. These resources contain detailed information about several cognitive-behavioral therapies. Appendices in both books and the ONS website also provide helpful information for the clinician.

Table 19-1 SELF-REPORT TOOLS FROM EVIDENCE-BASED OUTCOMES—ONS

Name of Tool	Author/Year	Domains or Factors	# of items	Scaling	Scoring	Language
Insomnia Severity Index (ISI)	Bastien, Vallieres, and Morin, 2001; Savard, Savard, and Ivers, 2004	Focus is on daytime symptoms: insomnia severity, sleep worry, functional impairment, social concern, and sleep satisfaction Used to compare medication vs. cognitive-behavioral treatments of insomnia	7	5-point scale items;	7-35	English French
Pittsburgh Sleep Quality Index (PSQI)	Buysse and others, 1989; Beck and others, 2004	Global score of sleep quality	19 basic, 5 roommate -rated	Mixed format	Complex Global score plus 7 subscales, range is 0-21 Subscales: sleep quality, sleep latency, sleep duration, habitual sleep efficiency, sleep disturbance, use of sleeping medication, daytime functioning	Widely translated

Continued

Table 19-1 Self-Report Tools from Evidence-Based Outcomes—ONS—cont'd

Name of Tool	Author/Year	Domains or Factors	# of items	Scaling	Scoring	Language
Morin's Sleep Diary	Morin, 1993; Morin and Espie, 2003; Berger and others, 2002 and 2003	Sleep parameters	10	Mixed format	Reports napping, sleep, use of aids/alcohol, morning refreshment, and sleep restedness (important component in the behavioral evaluation of sleep)	English French
Epworth Sleepiness Scale	Johns, 1991; Johns, 1992	Tendency to doze in particular situations; daytime sleepiness	8	4-point sscale	0-24	English German Italian Chinese English
Structured Interview for Sleep Disorders (DSMIII-R) (SIS-D)	Schramm and others, 1993	Structured clinical interview: semistructured section plus structured section (sleep disorder symptoms)	Interview	Interview	Interview	Widely translated

Table 19-2 PSYCHOMETRIC PROPERTIES OF TOOLS THAT HAVE BEEN USED IN STUDIES WITH PATIENTS WITH CANCER AND CAREGIVERS

Name of Tool	Populations	Reliability and Validity	Sensitivity	Clinical Utility	Comment
Insomnia Severity Index (ISI)	1. 145 patients evaluated for insomnia in a sleep disorders clinic in Study 1; 78 older patients with insomnia for Study 2 (Bastien and others, 2001) 2. 1670 cancer patients (Savard and others, 2004)	*Reliability* 1. Internal consistency Chronbach's alpha coefficient in insomnia patients = 0.74 (Bastien, 2001); coefficient in cancer patients = 0.90 overall and item-total correlations ranging from 0.65 to 0.78 (Savard, 2004) 2. Test-retest reliability R = 0.83 at 1 month; 0.77 at 2 months; and 0.73 at 3 months (Savard, 2004) *Validity* 1. Convergent validity with different indices derived from self-reports of sleep (r = 0.32-0.91, all $p < 0.05$) (Bastien, 2001). Items correlate significantly with items of sleep diary, but correlations between ISI and polysomnogram are weaker (Savard, 2004). 2. Factor analysis found 2 factors (severity and impact of the sleep difficulties (Savard, 2004).	Change scores demonstrated a significant relationship between sleep efficiency scores and ISI scores (Savard, 2004). Clinical cut-off score associated with optimal sensitivity and specificity to detect change.	Focus on daytime symptoms of insomnia; brief screening or outcome measure in treatment of insomnia only (Bastien, 2001)	Past week Has been used to compare medications vs. cognitive-behavioral treatment of insomnia

Continued

Table **19-2** Psychometric Properties of Tools That Have Been Used in Studies with Patients with Cancer and Caregivers—cont'd

Name of Tool	Populations	Reliability and Validity	Sensitivity	Clinical Utility	Comment
Pittsburgh Sleep Quality Index (PSQI)	Adult patients with cancer: Study 1 and 249 cases in Study 2 (Beck, 2004) 2. 25 women with breast cancer (Berger, 2002) 3. 21 women with breast cancer (Berger, 2003) 4. 102 women with breast cancer (Carpenter, 1998) 5. 47 caregivers of patients with advanced-stage cancer (Carter, 2002) 6. 51 caregivers of patients with advanced-stage cancer (Carter, 2000) 7. 15 cancer patients, 52 healthy adults (Owen, 1999)	*Reliability* 1. Internal consistency: coefficient for global sleep quality index (GSQI) in cancer patients and caregivers = 0.77-0.81 (Beck and others, 2004; Berger, 2002; Berger, 2003; Carpenter, 1998; Carter, 2000; Carter, 2002). Chronbach's alpha coefficient for GSQI in cancer patients and controls = 0.75 (Fortner, 2002). Internal consistency among health and chronically ill persons and caregivers = 0.83-0.89 (Buysse and others, 1989) 2. Test-retest: r = 0.85 Internal consistency among healthy and chronically ill persons and caregivers = 0.83-0.89 (Buysse and others, 1989)	Tests support internal consistency reliability and construct validity. Global score of 5 was shown to differentiate good from poor sleepers without cancer.	Scoring rather cumbersome; otherwise appropriate in adults Integrates nocturnal and daytime assessments; a score of 8 and above is identified as the cut-off score in patients with cancer (Carpenter, 1998); above 5 in healthy adults (Buysse and others, 1989)	1-month recall Most widely used tool throughout sleep studies

	8. 72 breast cancer patients (19 precancer treatment, 29 receiving treatment, and 23 posttreatment), and 50 female medical patients being seen for physical exams) (Fortner, 2002) 9. Healthy adults (Buysse, 1989)	*Validity* Validity examined by comparing PSQI estimates of sleep variables with those obtained by PSG from healthy adults. There were no significant differences in sleep latency; but subjects tended to overestimate sleep duration and efficiency ($p<0.001$). (Buysse, 1989)			
Sleep Diary	Adult patients with cancer; 1. 12 women with breast cancer (Morin diary) (Berger, 2000); 2. 10 patients with chronic insomnia and nonmetastatic breast cancer post	*Reliability and Validity* Reliability and validity of diaries is a major concern. Some studies have reported high reliability of diary versus observation; others have reported items ranges of 0.38-0.62 for coefficients of stability. Reliable for most patients (Lashley, 2004).	Sensitive to day-to-day or night-to-night fluctuations in sleep and naps	Easy to complete; scoring rather cumbersome and time-consuming	Last day and night; inexpensive, may be burdensome; can be used to show adherence to therapy

Continued

Table 19-2 Psychometric Properties of Tools That Have Been Used in Studies with Patients with Cancer and Caregivers—cont'd

Name of Tool	Populations	Reliability and Validity	Sensitivity	Clinical Utility	Comment
Epworth Sleepiness Scale (ESS)	1. 180 adults (30 normal men and women and 150 with a range of sleep disorders (Johns, 1991) 2. 87 healthy medical students for test-retest reliability; 104 medical students and 15 patients with sleep disorders for factor analysis (Johns, 1992) 3. Adult patients with cancer: 13 prescreened men (60-76 years old) with prostate cancer 1-2 weeks before radiation therapy (RT), at the end of 8 weeks of RT, and at 5-6 weeks after completing RT (Monga and others, 1997) 4. 36 veterans with localized prostate cancer before, during, and after RT (Monga and others, 1999) 5. Miletin and Hanly, 2003	*Reliability* Internal consistency: Cronbach's alpha coefficient = 0.88 (Johns, 1992); No report (Monga, 1997; Monga, 1999) Test-retest reliability = 0.82 (Johns, 1992) *Validity* Factor analysis: only one factor (Johns, 1992) ESS distinguished between those with and those without excessive daytime sleepiness; is a valid measure of sleep propensity in adults. ESS scores were correlated with sleep latency measured during the multiple sleep latency test and during overnight PSG (Johns, 1991) 4. To summarize: There is little data to support ESS as a measure of daytime sleepiness or sleep propensity, perhaps owing to a lack of consensus over the definition of the concept.	Total ESS scores significantly distinguished normal subjects from patients in various sleep diagnostic groups. In sleep apnea, ESS scores were correlated with the respiratory disturbance index and the minimum SaO_2 (Johns, 1991). Sensitive to treatment for sleep apnea (Johns, 1992)	Simple test to measure general level of sleepiness; preferred over multiple sleep latency test (MSLT), which takes all day for the subject and the polysomnographer. Quick and easy to use and score	Past week Important to assess daytime consequences of poor sleep

Nonpharmacologic intervention studies that address disturbances in sleep and wakefulness in women with cancer are found in Table 19-3.[23] A search (Medline, PubMed, Cumulative Index to Nursing and Allied Health Literature, and PsychLit) was conducted to identify all intervention studies that examined the effect of a cognitive and/or behavioral intervention on sleep disturbance or sleep quality in women with cancer. Only 6 studies were found that met the criteria, although 19 studies were found as of January 2005 that have tested interventions in patients with mixed samples, stages and types of cancer.[23] The interventions used combinations of cognitive and/or behavioral techniques.[7,8,98-101] All studies reported improvement or stability of some sleep parameters. Most of the interventions were conducted in three to eight sessions; the individualized sleep promotion plan was both revised and reinforced every 21 to 30 days.[7,8]

Although these first attempts at intervening to promote quality sleep in women with cancer include some positive findings, the quality of the evidence on the effects of these interventions for sleep was not strong. Only one study used a randomized controlled trial (RCT) design,[98] one used a quasi-experimental design,[100] and none of the studies had sample sizes greater than 100 participants, which has been identified as a criterion for the strongest level of evidence.[102] The use of combinations of intervention strategies makes it difficult to specify the essential elements that accounted for the success of a given intervention. Future studies will have to carefully examine these issues before conclusions can be drawn about the most effective interventions to improve sleep in cancer patients.

No guidelines have been developed for the screening, diagnosis, or management of disturbances in sleep and wakefulness specifically for patients with cancer. The National Comprehensive Cancer Network (NCCN)[103] has been very active during the last 5 years in developing evidence-based clinical practice guidelines in oncology for numerous types of cancer and supportive care needs. A review of the website[103] reveals an extensive list of guidelines for symptoms frequently experienced by patients with cancer, but none are found for disturbances in sleep and wakefulness. Nor are any of the existing guidelines are written in a gender-specific manner.

No guidelines at the National Guideline Clearinghouse[104] are found that are specific to disturbances in sleep and wakefulness in patients with cancer. General practice parameters are available from this website for several sleep-related issues, including but not limited to the following: use of polysomnography to evaluate insomnia, use of light therapy, nonpharmacologic treatment of chronic insomnia, as well as treatment of sleep apnea, narcolepsy, restless legs syndrome, and periodic limb movement disorder. The guideline, "Practice parameters for the nonpharmacologic treatment of chronic insomnia"[105] ranks stimulus control as Level II evidence and progressive muscle relaxation, paradoxical intention, biofeedback, and sleep restriction as Levels II-III evidence; and multicomponent behavioral therapy as Levels II, III, and V. Insufficient evidence was available for sleep hygiene education, imagery training, and cognitive therapy to be recommended as a single therapy.

No report of a metaanalysis of interventions for disturbed sleep and cancer is available, but currently published comparative reviews and metaanalyses on management of insomnia in non–cancer populations can be found at the Cochrane Library website.[106] These include reviews of bright light therapy,[107] physical exercise[108] and cognitive-behavioral interventions in non–cancer populations.[95,109,110] These resources may be of assistance to researchers who are developing interventions to treat cancer patients with chronic insomnia. While the cognitive-behavioral interventions may appear promising for use in patients with cancer, it is important to emphasize that they have not been tested in this unique population. These interventions will require pilot and larger studies to test their effects in this more complex situation, where homeostasis may be much more difficult to achieve because of the cancer process–related immunologic and inflammatory changes. Interventions will have to

Table 19-3 Nonpharmacologic Interventions in Cancer Patients[7,8,98-100,115]

Author, Date	Interventions tested/compared	Design	Sample	Outcomes
(Berger, and others, 2002)	Individualized sleep promotion plan • Sleep hygiene • Relaxation therapy • Stimulus control • Sleep restriction 1 2-hr session; 4 15-min problem-solving sessions; 3 30-min revision sessions	1-group pretest/ post-test design	25 breast cancer patients	• Moderate to high adherence (46%-80%) with components of sleep plan • Sleep latency, efficiency, total rest, and rating of awakening were stable • Time awake after sleep onset and night-time awakenings exceeded desired levels • Conclusion: intervention feasible, adherence improved over time, most sleep/wake patterns consistent with normal values
(Berger and others, 2003)	Individualized sleep promotion plan • Sleep hygiene • Relaxation therapy • Stimulus control • Sleep restriction 1 2-hr session; 4 15-min problem-solving sessions; 3 30-min revision sessions	1-group pretest/ post-test design	21 breast cancer patients	• Adherence to intervention high except stimulus control • Sleep latency remained stable • Sleep efficiency ranged from 82%-92% • Total rest ranged from 7-8 hr per night • Night awakenings ranged from 10-11 per night • Daytime naps ranged from 10-15 min in length • Fatigue was 2.9-3.5 on 10-point scale
(Fobair and others, 2002)	Supportive-expressive group therapy discussion of the following: • Problem of new diagnosis • Coping with illness, treatment, mood changes • Self-efficacy • Improving relationships • Managing pain, sleep, body image, sexuality	1-group pretest/ post-test design	20 lesbians diagnosed with early-stage breast cancer within past 12 months	• Improved sleep, less pain • Decreased emotional distress, intrusiveness, and avoidance • Improved coping • Reduced social support • Trend toward more family cohesiveness and expressiveness • No change in body image, sexuality, or attitude toward health care providers

(Mock and others, 1997)	Individualized, self-paced, home-based walking exercise program: • 20- to 30-min walk • 5-min cool-down • 4-5 sessions/week for 6 weeks	Quasi-experimental 2-group design, alternate assignment to groups	46 breast cancer patients receiving radiotherapy Groups: Exercise: n = 22; Usual care: n = 24	Exercise group reported the following: • Improved physical functioning • Reduced symptom intensity (fatigue, anxiety, and difficulty sleeping)
(Quesnel and others, 2003)	Multimodal cognitive-behavioral therapy for insomnia Components: • Stimulus control • Sleep restriction • Coping strategies for fatigue • Reframing maladaptive cognitions • Sleep hygiene 8 sessions	1-group multiple baseline A-B experimental design	10 patients with chronic insomnia and nonmetastatic breast cancer who had completed chemotherapy and radiation therapy	• Daily variability in sleep decreased after initiation of the intervention. • Significant improvement in sleep efficiency and total wake time • Significant improvements in mood, general and physical fatigue, and global and cognitive dimensions of quality of life.
(Shapiro and others, 2003)	Mindfulness-based stress reduction (MBSR): • Sitting meditation • Body scan • Hatha yoga (stretches and postures) 6 sessions and 1-day silent retreat	Randomized controlled trial	63 women with breast cancer Groups: • MBSR: n = 31 • Control: n = 32	• Both MBSR and free-choice groups had significant improvement in sleep quality. • Neither group had improvement in sleep efficiency. • MBSR group members who practiced more improved more on sleep measure associated with distress.

Min, Minute(s); *hr*, hour(s).

be tested in individuals with various types and stages of disease while also controlling for age, sex, and menopausal status.

A helpful source for clinicians to learn more about sleep disorders in general, and more specifically in cancer patients, can be found at the National Cancer Institute website.[111] This PDQ version for health professionals provides basic information on sleep disturbances in cancer patients, suggestions for assessment, non-pharmacologic, and pharmacologic management, and special considerations. Links to additional PDQ summaries, such as information on complementary and alternative medicine, are also included.

Pharmacologic management of sleep disturbances in patients with cancer begins with identifying the medications the patient is receiving for the treatment of cancer and the accompanying side effects, to determine if they play a role in the development of insomnia. Use of central nervous system stimulants, sedatives, and hypnotics, as well as of chemotherapy agents, anticonvulsants, beta blockers, and thyroid preparations can result in insomnia and should be reduced or discontinued if possible if it is suspected to be contributing to sleep problems.[111] Use and withdrawal from some of the most commonly prescribed hypnotics can interfere with sleep and result in irritability, nervousness, apathy, and decreased daytime alertness. Behavioral techniques may be preferred by both patients and clinicians because of concerns related to polypharmacy.

When sleep disturbances are not resolved after attempting nonpharmacologic interventions, the short-term (7 to 10 days) use of pharmacologic agents to promote sleep may be helpful. Long-term use is discouraged, since these drugs can interfere with natural sleep patterns and result in tolerance, dependence, and drug hangover.[111] Medications commonly used to promote sleep in persons with cancer are displayed in Table 19-4.[111] Only a few studies have examined use of pharmaceuticals to improve sleep in women with cancer, usually an attempt to treat hot flashes. One recent study reported that the antidepressant paroxetine was helpful for hot flashes and related symptoms of fatigue, sleep disturbance, and depression in women treated with breast cancer chemotherapy.[112] Future studies are recommended that attempt to balance the use of pharmaceuticals for symptom control with the need for restorative sleep.

Special considerations are the final component of the Sleep Disorders PDQ.[111] These special considerations include dealing with sleep in these patients: the patient with pain, the older patient, and the patient with sleep apnea following mandibulectomy. These may be helpful resources for clinicians caring for women with these special issues.

Researchers have only recently begun to test interventions to reduce disturbances in sleep and wakefulness in women with cancer. There is a critical need for development and testing of strategies likely to improve sleep and daytime wakefulness in these patients. If pilot studies demonstrate an effect, controlled studies are needed to more fully evaluate the efficacy of the interventions. A critical component of these intervention studies will be the selection of reliable, valid, and conceptually sound instruments. Standard assessment methods to document outcomes, and criteria to define successful outcomes in the treatment of disturbances in sleep and wakefulness are needed to move the science forward in the most effective manner. Finally, a consensus is needed on what the clinically relevant outcomes are for interventions to improve sleep and wakefulness. Outcomes will have to include multidimensional functioning and QOL.

IMPLICATIONS FOR PRACTICE, EDUCATION, AND RESEARCH

Implications for practice include a recommendation to screen for disturbances in sleep and wakefulness in all women with cancer at each care encounter. The Clinical Sleep Screen instrument is recommended.[23] This tool can be used to screen and refer selected patients to an accredited sleep disorders clinic for diagnostic evaluation of a treatable sleep disorder. This screen can be as brief

Table 19-4 MEDICATIONS COMMONLY USED TO PROMOTE SLEEP

Drug Category	Medication	Hypnotic Dose (route)	Onset (duration of action)
Benzodiazepines	diazepam (Valium)	5-10 mg (capsule, tablet)	30-60 min (6-8 hr)
	temazepam (Restoril)	15-30 mg (capsule)	60 min, minimum (6-8 hr)
	triazolam (Halcion)	0.125-0.5 mg (tablet)	30 min (peaks 1-1.5 hr)
	clonazepam (Klonopin)	0.5-2.0 mg (tablet)	30-60 min (8-12 hr)
Tricyclic antidepressants	doxepin (Sinequan)	10-150 mg	30 min
	amitriptyline (Elavil)	10-300 mg	30 min
	nortriptyline (Pamelor)	10-50 mg	30 min
Chloral derivatives	chloral hydrate	0.5-1.0 g (capsule, syrup, suppository)	30-60 min (4-8 hr)
Second-generation antidepressants	trazodone (Desyrel)	25-150 mg	30 min
	nefazadone (Serzone)	50-100 mg	30 min
	mirtazapine (Remeron)	15-60 mg	30 min
Antihistamines	diphenhydramine (Benadryl)	25-100 mg (tablet, capsule, syrup)	10-30 min (4-6 hr)
	hydroxyzine (Vistaril, Atarax)	10-100 mg (tablet, capsule, syrup)	15-30 min (4-6 hr)
Neuroleptics	thioridazine (Mellaril)	10-50 mg	30-60 min
	chlorpromazine (Thorazine)	10-50 mg	30-60 min
Other	zolpidem tartrate (Ambien)	5-20 mg	30 min (4-6 hr)
	zaleplon (Sonata)	10-20 mg	30 min (4-6 hr)

Min, Minute(s); *hr,* hour(s).

as asking four essential questions. An evidence-based patient education teaching sheet that includes key information regarding the techniques of stimulus control, sleep restriction, sleep hygiene, and relaxation strategies should be made available to all women in conjunction with the initial screening.

Disturbances in sleep and wakefulness are often ignored or underappreciated by both the health care team members and women with cancer in comparison to other symptoms that accompany the disease and its treatment. The Clinical Sleep Screen is recommended to be used consistently in conjunction with assessment of these other symptoms to identify and treat clusters of symptoms.

Clinicians will need staff development programs to assist them in learning how to teach women about the restorative function of sleep and how sleep disturbances can influence QOL, fatigue, and daytime sleepiness.[89] Clinicians also must discuss with women the possible drug-drug interactions that can occur when over-the-counter and herbal sleep aids are combined with chemotherapy and supportive therapy prescription drugs. Emphasis must be placed on the importance of obtaining approval of the health care team before taking over-the-counter and herbal products.

Sleep deprivation can be reduced by the adoption of good sleep hygiene practices and regular bedtimes and wake times. Clinicians can also assist women to recognize predisposing, precipitating, and perpetuating risk factors for insomnia such as a history of prior sleep problems, presence of pain, anxiety, or depression, younger age, and being single. They can teach women basic relaxation training exercises and promote low- to moderate-intensity aerobic exercise programs and adequate treatment of other symptoms, using nonpharmacologic interventions when possible to avoid drug-drug interactions. Group cognitive-behavioral therapy to assist with coping with the diagnosis of cancer and to assist in side effects management can also be encouraged. Another intervention is to help women distinguish between fatigue and daytime sleepiness. Women commonly develop a pattern of taking long daytime naps when they feel fatigued, whereas adoption of low-intensity restorative activities may be more helpful. When sleepiness occurs related to a sleep debt from disrupted sleep the previous night, short naps (30 to 45 minutes) should be taken as early in the day as possible and at least 4 hours before bedtime, if needed.

Implications for nursing education are many. Nursing education has not generally included knowledge about sleep and circadian rhythms in undergraduate curriculum content. This is despite the fact that considerable emphasis has been given to physical activity, nutrition, and stress management as key components related to human health and wellness. A nursing task force, including members of the Association of Professional Sleep Societies, has developed educational competencies for sleep and chronobiology.[113] The undergraduate objectives are organized into learning objectives, suggested clinical experiences, suggested clinical competency objectives, and clinical evaluation possibilities that can be integrated into medical-surgical and psychiatric nursing courses. In addition, graduate-level learning objectives for clinical nurse specialist and primary care roles are developed. These learning activities will prepare advanced practice nurses to work as a member of an interdisciplinary team at an accredited sleep disorders center or in a general practice setting. This content can also be used to organize staff development offerings for clinical nurses, advanced practice clinical nurses, nursing educators, and researchers.

Implications for research are broad. Disturbances of sleep and wakefulness in all types and stages of cancer in women is an understudied area. There is a need for descriptive studies regarding sleep in women with the most prevalent cancers (breast, lung, colon, and gynecologic). Breast cancer is the only type of cancer in which several descriptive studies have been conducted. However, various investigator-developed measures limit the generalizability of the findings. There are gaps in knowledge regarding the clusters of symptoms most commonly associated with disturbances in sleep in various stages and types of cancer. More about the relationships between the quality or quantity of sleep and the sleep/wake circadian rhythm cycle must be understood. Studies that identify the factors that predict and influence the frequency and intensity of and distress from sleep disturbances in women with cancer will also advance the science to the development of targeted interventions to improve QOL during treatment and survivorship. Box 19-1 lists several key focal areas for future research studies, but is not intended to be comprehensive.

Box 19-1 Focus Areas for Future Research Studies

- Identify sleep patterns of women with the most common cancers (breast, gastrointestinal, lung, gynecologic) at baseline, during various single or multimodal therapies, and following completion of therapy.
- Identify sleep patterns of women with the most common cancers at various stages of disease (prediagnosis, at diagnosis, initial treatment survivors, treatment for metastatic disease, end of life).
- Identify sleep patterns of various age groups of females (pediatric, adolescent, young adult, middle-aged adult, older adult) during and following therapy.
- Identify symptoms that cluster with disturbances in sleep and wakefulness in women. Identify effects of individual and clusters on multidimensional functioning and quality of life.
- Identify a core battery of standardized instruments to document disturbances in sleep and wakefulness in women with cancer.
- Test interventions designed to promote and maintain restorative sleep, functioning, and quality of life in women with cancer and women who are caregivers of patients with cancer.

Identification of important predictor variables will assist in development of interventions to reduce the prevalence of disturbed sleep in women with cancer. Several possible predictor variables to consider testing include the following: anxiety, depression, psychologic distress, history of sleep disturbances, abuse (physical/verbal), or use of hypnotics, pain, low functional status at baseline or during treatment, advanced cancer, the presence of hot flashes, and other symptoms.

Evidence-based interventions to treat disturbances in sleep and wakefulness in women with cancer will have to be designed to bring about successful treatment outcomes as measured by variables that reflect difficulty falling asleep, staying asleep, early morning awakenings, and daytime functioning. These include variables to quantify early morning awakenings, daytime sleepiness, multidimensional functioning, and the use of sleeping medications. It will be important to include key outcome variables that are influenced by sleep disturbances, such as measures of daytime functioning, psychologic symptoms, and QOL.[114] Outcomes may include feelings of rest on awakening, midday energy/fatigue, mood, anxiety, depression, cognitive functioning, serotonin and melatonin neuropeptide hormone levels, performance/functional status, use of prescription drugs for sleep, morbidity (i.e., rates of infection, use of sick days if employed, depression, chronic insomnia, cancer recurrence), and mortality.

A final area for research is the development of accepted criteria to define a successful outcome in the treatment of insomnia. This is an area that is also being recognized and addressed by the larger sleep science community.[114] It has been recommended that success be measured not just by improvements in sleep, but also by improvement in daytime functioning, fatigue, mood, and QOL.

REFERENCES

1. Rosenthal L and others: Level of sleepiness and total sleep time following various time in bed conditions, *Sleep* 16:226-232, 1993.
2. Drake CL and others: Effects of rapid versus slow accumulation of eight hours of sleep loss, *Psychophysiology* 38:979-989, 2001.
3. Roth T, Ancoli-Israel S: Daytime consequences and correlates of insomnia in the United States: results of the 1991 National Sleep Foundation Survey, 2, *Sleep* 22(Suppl 2):S354-S358, 1999.
4. Roehrs TA and others: Pain threshold and sleep loss, *Sleep* 26(Suppl):A196, 2003 (abstract).
5. Spiegel K, Leproult R, VanCauter E: Impact of sleep debt on metabolic and endocrine function, *Lancet* 354: 1435-1439, 1999.
6. Berger AM, Farr L: The influence of daytime inactivity and nighttime restlessness on cancer-related fatigue, *Oncol Nurs Forum* 26(10):1663-1671, 1999.
7. Berger AM and others: Feasibility of a sleep intervention during adjuvant breast cancer chemotherapy, *Oncol Nurs Forum* 29(10):1431-1441, 2002.
8. Berger AM and others: Adherence, sleep, and fatigue outcomes after adjuvant breast cancer chemotherapy: results of a feasibility intervention study, *Oncol Nurs Forum* 30(3):513-522, 2003.
9. Carpenter JS and others: Hot flashes and related outcomes in breast cancer survivors and matched comparison women, *Oncol Nurs Forum* 29(3):E16-25, 2002.
10. Carpenter JS and others: Sleep, fatigue, and depressive symptoms in breast cancer survivors and matched healthy women experiencing hot flashes, *Oncol Nurs Forum* 31(3):591-598, 2004.
11. Cimprich B: Pretreatment symptom distress in women newly diagnosed with breast cancer, *Cancer Nurs* 22(3):185-194, quiz 195, 1999.
12. Dow KH and others: An evaluation of the quality of life among long-term survivors of breast cancer, *Breast Cancer Res Treat* 39:261-273, 1996.
13. Dow KH: Seventh National Conference on Cancer Nursing Research keynote address: challenges and opportunities in cancer survivorship research, *Oncol Nurs Forum* 30(3):455-469, 2003.
14. Koopman C and others: Sleep disturbances in women with metastatic breast cancer, *Breast J* 8(6):362-370, 2002.
15. Savard J, Morin CM: Insomnia in the context of cancer: a review of a neglected problem, *J Clin Oncol* 19(3): 895-908, 2001.
16. Savard J and others: Prevalence, clinical characteristics, and risk factors for insomnia in the context of breast cancer, *Sleep* 24(5):583-590, 2001.
17. Clark J and others: Sleep-wake disturbances in people with cancer part II: evaluating the evidence for clinical decision making, *Oncol Nurs Forum* 31(4):747-771, 2004.
18. Bardwell WA and others: Health-related quality of life in women previously treated for early-stage breast cancer, *Psychooncology* 13(9):595-604, 2004.
19. Lee K and others: Impaired sleep and rhythms in persons with cancer, *Sleep Med Rev* 8(3):199-212, 2004.
20. Lee KA: Impaired sleep. In Carrieri-Kohlman V, editor: *Pathophysiological phenomena in nursing*, ed 3, Philadelphia, 2003, Saunders.
21. Lashley F: Measuring sleep. In Frank-Stromborg M, Olsen S, eds: Instruments for clinical health care research, ed 3, Boston, 2004, Jones and Bartlett.
22. Ancoli-Israel S, Moore PJ, Jones V: The relationship between fatigue and sleep in cancer patients: a review, *Eur J Cancer Care (Engl)* 10(4):245-255, 2001.

23. Berger A and others: Sleep/wake disturbances in people with cancer and their caregivers: state of the science, Oncol Nurs Forum, 32 E98-E126. Retrieved 11/3/05 from www.ons.org/publications/journals/ONF/volume32/issue6/32061097.asp
24. Vena C and others: Sleep-wake disturbances in people with cancer part I: an overview of sleep, sleep regulation, and effects of disease and treatment, *Oncol Nurs Forum* 31(4):735-746, 2004.
25. American Cancer Society: *Cancer facts and figures 2004*, Atlanta, Ga., 2004, The Society.
26. Savard J and others: Chronic insomnia and immune functioning, *Psychosom Med* 65(2):211-221, 2003.
27. Dement WC: History of sleep physiology and medicine. In Kryger MH, Roth T, Dement, WC, editor: *Principles and practice of sleep medicine*, ed 3, Philadelphia, 2000, Saunders.
28. American Academy of Sleep Medicine: *The international classification of sleep disorders*, ed 2, Westchester, Il., 2005, The Academy.
29. Cannon WB: *The wisdom of the body*, New York, 1939, WW Norton.
30. Achermann P: The two-process model of sleep regulation revisited, *Aviat Space Environ Med* 75:A37-A43, 2004.
31. Borbely A: A two-process model of sleep regulation, *Human Neurobiol* 1:195-204, 1982.
32. Borbely A: Sleep circadian rhythm versus recovery process. In Koukkou M, Lehmann D, Angst J, editors: *Functional states of the brain, their determinants*, Amsterdam, 1980, Elsevier.
33. Mormont MC, Levi F: Circadian-system alterations during cancer processes: a review, *Int J Cancer* 70(2): 241-247, 1997.
34. Filipski E and others: Host circadian clock as a control point in tumor progression, *J Natl Cancer Inst* 94(9): 690-697, 2002.
35. Scammell T: The regulation of sleep and circadian rhythms, *Sleep Medicine Alerts* 8(1):1-6, 2004.
36. Rajaratnam S, Arendt J: Health in a 24-h society, *Lancet* 358:999-1005, 2001.
37. Floyd JA and others: Age-related changes in initiation and maintenance of sleep: a meta-analysis, *Res Nurs Health* 23(2):106-117, 2000.
38. Dijk DJ and others: Aging and the circadian and homeostatic regulation of human sleep during forced desynchrony of rest, melatonin and temperature rhythms, *J Physiol* 516:611-627, 1999.
39. Garbarino S and others: Sleepiness and sleep disorders in shift workers: a study on a group of Italian police officers, *Sleep* 25(6):648-653, 2002.
40. Schernhammer ES and others: Night-shift work and risk of colorectal cancer in the nurses' health study, *J Natl Cancer Inst* 95(11):825-828, 2003.
41. Schernhammer ES and others: Rotating night shifts and risk of breast cancer in women participating in the nurses' health study, *J Natl Cancer Inst* 93(20):1563-1568, 2001.
42. American Cancer Society: *Cancer facts and figures 2005*, Atlanta, Ga., on the Web at www.cancer.org/docroot/STT/content/STT_1x_Cancer_Facts_Figures_2005.asp, accessed January 10, 2005.
43. Spielman AJ, Glovinsky P: A conceptual framework of insomnia for primary care practitioners: predisposing, precipitating and perpetuating factors, *Sleep Medicine Alerts* 9(1):1-6, 2004.
44. Davidson JR and others: Sleep disturbance in cancer patients, *Soc Sci Med* 54(9):1309-1321, 2002.
45. Lee KA, Zaffke ME, McEnany G: Parity and sleep patterns during and after pregnancy, *Obstet Gynecol* 95:14-18, 2000.
46. Lee KA, Taylor, DL: Is there a generic midlife woman? The health and symptom experience of midlife women, *Menopause* 3:154-164, 1996.
47. Morin CM, Espie CA: *Insomnia*, Boston, 2003, Plenum.
48. Ancoli-Israel S, Roth T: Characteristics of insomnia in the United States: results of the 1991 National Sleep Foundation Survey. I, *Sleep* 22(Suppl 2):S347-S353, 1999.
49. Lindberg E, Gislason T: Epidemiology of sleep-related obstructive breathing, *Sleep Med Rev* 4:411-433, 2000.
50. Rama AN, Kushida C: Restless legs syndrome and periodic limb movement disorder, *Med Clin North Am* 88:653-667, 2004.
51. Moline M, Broch L, Zak R: Sleep in women across the life cycle from adulthood through menopause, *Med Clin North Am* 88:705-736, 2004.
52. Zammit GK and others: Quality of life in people with insomnia, *Sleep* 22:S379-S385, 1999.
53. Bower JE and others: T-cell homeostasis in breast cancer survivors with persistent fatigue, *J Natl Cancer Inst* 95(15):1165-1168, 2003.
54. Hu DS, Silberfarb PM: Management of sleep problems in cancer patients, *Oncology (Huntingt)* 5(9):23-27; discussion 28, 1991.
55. Bliwise DL: Normal again. In Kryger MH, Roth T, Dement WC, editors: *Principles and practice of sleep medicine*, Philadelphia, 2000, Saunders.
56. Knobf MT: Natural menopause and ovarian toxicity associated with breast cancer therapy, *Oncol Nurs Forum* 25(9):1519-1530, quiz 1531-1532, 1998.
57. Savard J and others: The association between nocturnal hot flashes and sleep in breast cancer survivors, *J Pain Symptom Manage* 27(6):513-522, 2004.
58. Broeckel JA and others: Characteristics and correlates of fatigue after adjuvant chemotherapy for breast cancer, *J Clin Oncol* 16(5):1689-1696, 1998.
59. Carpenter JS and others: Hot flashes in postmenopausal women treated for breast cancer: Prevalence, severity, correlates, management, and relation to quality of life, *Cancer* 82:1682-1691, 1998.
60. Carpenter JS, Andrykowski MA: Menopausal symptoms in breast cancer survivors, *Oncol Nurs Forum* 26: 1311-1317, 1999.
61. Love RR and others: Symptoms associated with tamoxifen treatment in post-menopausal women, *Arch Intern Med* 151:1842-1847, 1991.
62. Carpenter JS and others: Circadian rhythm of objectively recorded hot flashes in postmenopausal breast cancer survivors, *Menopause* 8(3):181-188, 2001.
63. Fortner BV and others: Sleep and quality of life in breast cancer patients, *J Pain Symptom Manage* 24(5):471-480, 2002.
64. Dodd MJ, Miaskowski C, Paul SM: Symptom clusters and their effect on the functional status of patients with cancer, *Oncol Nurs Forum* 28(3):465-470, 2001.

65. Spiegel K, Leproult R, Van Cauter E: Impact of sleep debt on physiological rhythms, *Rev Neurol (Paris)* 159(11 Suppl):6S11-20, 2003.
66. Krueger JM, Karnovsky, ML: Sleep as a neuroimmune phenomenon: a brief historical perspective, *Adv Neuroimmunol* 5:5-12, 1995.
67. Cleeland CC and others: Are the symptoms of cancer and cancer treatment due to a shared biologic mechanism? *Cancer* 97(11):2919-2925, 2003.
68. Payne JK: The trajectory of fatigue in adult patients with breast and ovarian cancer receiving chemotherapy, *Oncol Nurs Forum* 29(9):1334-1340, 2002.
69. Payne JK: A neuroendocrine-based regulatory fatigue model, *Biol Res Nurs* 6(2):141-150, 2004.
70. Ohayon MM, Caulet M, Lemoine P: Comorbidity of mental and insomnia disorders in the general population, *Cancer Psychiatr* 39(4):185-197, 1998.
71. Derogatis LR: A survey of psychotropic drug prescriptions in an oncology population, *Cancer* 44:1919-1929, 1979.
72. Stiefel FC, Kornblith AB, Holland JC: Changes in the prescription patterns of psychotropic drugs for cancer patients during a 10-year period, *Cancer* 65:1048-1053, 1990.
73. Couzi RJ, Helzlsouer KJ, Fetting JH: Prevalence of menopausal symptoms among women with a history of breast cancer and attitudes toward estrogen replacement therapy, *J Clin Oncol* 13:2737-2744, 1995.
74. Lindley C and others: Quality of life and preferences for treatment following systemic adjuvant therapy for early-stage breast cancer, *J Clin Oncol* 16:1380-1387, 1998.
75. Sarna L: Correlates of symptom distress in women with lung cancer, *Cancer Pract* 1:21-28, 1993.
76. Silberfarb PM: Assessment of sleep in patients with lung cancer and breast cancer, *J Clin Oncol* 11(5):997-1004, 1993.
77. Christman NJ, Oakley MG, Cronin SN: Developing and using preparatory information for women undergoing radiation therapy for cervical or uterine cancer, *Oncol Nurs Forum* 28:93-98, 2001.
78. Savard J, Miller and others: Association between subjective sleep quality and depression on immunocompetence in low-income women at risk for cervical cancer, *Psychosom Med* 61:496-507, 1999.
79. Brandberg Y and others: Psychological reactions in patients with malignant melanoma, *Eur J Cancer* 2:157-162, 1995.
80. Smets EM and others: Fatigue and radiotherapy: (A) experience in patients undergoing treatment, *Br J Cancer* 78:899-906, 1998.
81. Smets EM and others: Fatigue and radiotherapy: (B) experience with patients 9 months following treatment, *Br J Cancer* 78:907-912, 1998.
82. Andrykowski MA and others: Energy level and sleep quality following bone marrow transplantation, *Bone Marrow Transpl* 20(8):669-679, 1997.
83. Geels P and others: Palliative effect of chemotherapy: objective tumor response is associated with symptom improvement in patients with metastatic breast cancer, *J Clin Oncol* 12:2396-2405, 2000.
84. Sephton SE and others: Diurnal cortisol rhythm as a predictor of breast cancer survival, *J Natl Cancer Inst* 92:994-1000, 2000.
85. Berger AM: Patterns of fatigue and activity and rest during adjuvant breast cancer chemotherapy, *Oncol Nurs Forum* 25(1):51-62, 1998.
86. Berger AM, Higginbotham P: Correlates of fatigue during and following adjuvant breast cancer chemotherapy: a pilot study, *Oncol Nurs Forum* 27(9):1443-1448, 2000.
87. Morin C: *Insomnia*, New York, 1993, The Guilford Press.
88. Richardson A, Ream E: Self-care behaviours initiated by chemotherapy patients in response to fatigue, *Int J Nurs Stud* 34:35-43, 1997.
89. Byar K and others: Impact of adjuvant breast cancer chemotherapy on fatigue, other symptom and quality of life, *Oncol Nurs Forum*, in press.
90. Carter PA: Caregivers' descriptions of sleep changes and depressive symptoms, *Oncol Nurs Forum* 29(9): 1277-1283, 2002.
91. Passik SD and others: An unsuccessful attempt to develop a single-item screen for insomnia in cancer patients, *J Pain Symptom Manage* 25(3):284-287, 2003.
92. Oncology Nursing Society: Evidence-based practice resource area. Nursing-sensitive patient outcomes, retrieved 7/18/05 from http://ons.opcontent.ons.org/toolkits/evidence/clinicaloutcomes.html.
93. Littner M and others: Practice parameters for the role of actigraphy in the study of sleep and circadian rhythms: an update for 2002, *Sleep* 26(3):337-341, 2003.
94. American Academy of Sleep Medicine: Practice parameters for the evaluation of chronic insomnia, *Sleep* 23(2):237-241, 2000.
95. Morin CM, Culbert JP, Schwartz SM: Nonpharmacological interventions for insomnia: a meta-analysis of treatment efficacy, *Am J Psychiatr* 151(8):1172-1180, 1994.
96. Szuba MP, Kloss JE, Dinges DF: *Insomnia Principles and Management*, New York, 2003, Cambridge University Press.
97. Lee-Chiong TL: Sleep and sleep disorders: an overview. *Med Clin North Am* 88:xi-xiv, 2004.
98. Shapiro SL and others: The efficacy of mindfulness-based stress reduction in the treatment of sleep disturbance in women with breast cancer: an exploratory study, *J Psychosom Res* 54(1):85-91, 2003.
99. Fobair P and others: Psychosocial intervention for lesbians with primary breast cancer, *Psychooncology* 11(5):427-438, 2002.
100. Mock V and others: Effects of exercise on fatigue, physical functioning, and emotional distress during radiation therapy for breast cancer, *Oncol Nurs Forum* 24(6): 991-1000, 1997.
101. Quesnel C and others: Efficacy of cognitive-behavioral therapy for insomnia in women treated for nonmetastatic breast cancer, *J Consult Clin Psychol* 71(1):189-200, 2003.
102. Ropka ME, Spencer-Cisek P: PRISM: Priority Symptom Management Project phase I: assessment, *Oncol Nurs Forum* 28(10):1585-1594, 2001.
103. National Comprehensive Cancer Network: Guidelines for Supportive Care, retrieved 7/18/05 from www.nccn.org/professionals/physician_gls/f_guidelines.asp?button=I+Agree#care.
104. National Guideline Clearinghouse: On the Web at www.guidelines.gov. Accessed July 18, 2005.
105. American Academy of Sleep Medicine: Practice parameters for the nonpharmacologic treatment of chronic insomnia, *Sleep* 22(8):1128-1133, 1999.

106. Cochrane Library: Main index of Cochrane Reviews, available on the Web at www.cochrane.org/reviews/mainindex.html, accessed July, 18, 2005.
107. Montgomery P, Dennis J: Bright light therapy for sleep problems in adults aged 60+, *Cochrane Database Syst Rev* (2):CD003403, 2002.
108. Montgomery P, Dennis J: Physical exercise for sleep problems in adults aged 60+, *Cochrane Database Syst Rev* (4):CD003404, 2002.
109. Montgomery P, Dennis J: Cognitive behavioural interventions for sleep problems in adults aged 60+, *Cochrane Database Syst Rev* (1):CD003161, 2003.
110. Murtagh DR, Greenwood KM: Identifying effective psychological treatments for insomnia: a meta-analysis, *J Consult Clin Psychol* 63(1):79-89, 1995.
111. National Cancer Institute: Sleep disorders PDQ®. On the Web at www.cancer.gov. Accessed July 18, 2005.
112. Weitzner MA and others: A pilot trial of paroxetine for the treatment of hot flashes and associated symptoms in women with breast cancer, *J Pain Symptom Manage* 23(4):337-345, 2002.
113. Lee KA and others: Sleep and chronobiology: recommendations for nursing education, *Nurs Outlook* 52(3):126-133, 2004.
114. Morin CM: Measuring outcomes in randomized clinical trials of insomnia treatments, *Sleep Med Rev* 7(3):263-279, 2003.
115. Quesnel, C and others: Efficacy of cognitive-behavioral therapy for insomnia in women treated for nonmetastatic breast cancer, *J Consulting Clin Psychol* 71(1):189-200, 2003.

CHAPTER

20 Physical Activity in Women Cancer Survivors

Kerry S. Courneya, Kristin L. Campbell, Margaret L. McNeely, and Kristina H. Karvinen

The purpose of this chapter is to provide an overview of the role that physical activity can play in improving and maintaining health in women cancer survivors. It begins by defining physical activity and exercise-related terms. Then, a detailed review is presented of exercise studies that have focused exclusively on women cancer survivors, as well as a more basic review of studies that included women cancer survivors. After noting that none of the mixed-sex studies analyzed the data separately for women, an ancillary analysis from one of the author's trials on colorectal cancer survivors is discussed. This analysis showed that women colorectal cancer survivors may respond differently to an exercise intervention than men. This is followed by a summary of the general literature about the effects of exercise on outcomes particularly important to women cancer survivors that have not been adequately addressed in the cancer studies (e.g., menopausal symptoms, osteoporosis, lymphedema, body image). After that, the authors review the prevalence and determinants of exercise in women cancer survivors and ways to promote exercise in this population. Finally, future research directions and clinical guidelines for women cancer survivors are discussed.

Acknowledgement: Kerry S. Courneya, PhD, is supported by the Canada Research Chairs Program and a Research Team Grant from the National Cancer Institute of Canada with funds from the Canadian Cancer Society and the Sociobehavioral Cancer Research Network. Kristin L. Campbell, MSc, Margaret L. McNeely, MSc, and Kristina H. Karvinen, MA are supported by Health Research Studentships from the Alberta Heritage Foundation for Medical Research.

DEFINITIONS OF PHYSICAL ACTIVITY AND RELATED TERMS

Bouchard and Shephard[1] have provided definitions of *physical activity* and its related terms. These researchers define physical activity as any bodily movement produced by the skeletal muscles that results in a substantial increase in energy expenditure over resting levels. They define *leisure-time physical activity* as physical activity undertaken during discretionary time with an element of personal choice. This form of physical activity is often contrasted with *occupational* and *household physical activity. Exercise* is defined as a subset of leisure-time physical activity that is usually performed on a repeated basis over an extended period of time with the intention of improving fitness, performance, or health. An exercise training prescription usually includes activity mode or type (e.g., walking, swimming), volume (i.e., frequency, intensity, and duration), progression and/or periodization (i.e., variation over time), and context (i.e., physical and social environment). *Physical fitness* is defined as the ability to perform muscular work satisfactorily and commonly includes the components of body composition, cardiorespiratory fitness, muscular fitness, flexibility, and agility/balance.

EXERCISE RESEARCH IN WOMEN CANCER SURVIVORS

The authors conducted a systematic literature search in December 2004 using the CD-ROM databases Medline, Embase, Cinahl, Psychlit, Pedro, Cochrane databases, Dissertation Abstracts, and Sport Discus. Key words that related to cancer (i.e., cancer, oncology, tumor, neoplasm, carcinoma), the postdiagnosis time period (i.e., rehabilitation, therapy, adjuvant therapy, treatment, intervention, palliation), and exercise (i.e., exercise, physical activity, physical therapy, sport, weight training) were combined and searched. Relevant articles were then hand-searched for further pertinent references. To be included in the review, a study had to (a) focus exclusively on women cancer survivors, (b) report a randomized controlled trial, and (c) examine aerobic or resistance exercise. Ten studies focus exclusively on women cancer survivors.[2-11] The details of these studies are reported in Table 20-1 and a brief summary of the studies is provided here.

STUDIES FOCUSING EXCLUSIVELY ON WOMEN CANCER SURVIVORS

All 10 studies were conducted in breast cancer survivors and were restricted to women without metastatic disease (i.e., stages 0/I-III). The sample sizes of these studies ranged from 14 to 123, but most were small, with six studies having sample size less than 30. Six of 10 studies examined exercise interventions **during** adjuvant cancer therapy, with the types of adjuvant therapies being mixed. One study examined exercise during chemotherapy, one study focused on radiation therapy, one included participants receiving chemotherapy or hormonal therapy, two studies included participants receiving chemotherapy or radiation therapy, and one study included participants receiving chemotherapy, radiation therapy, or hormonal therapy.

Six studies tested supervised exercise interventions, three tested home-based (self-directed) exercise interventions, and one study included both supervised and home-based exercise groups. There was considerable variation in the prescribed exercise interventions. The chosen types of exercise were aerobic for four studies, aerobic interval training for one study, combined aerobic and resistance exercise for two studies, and tai chi chuan for one study. Walking was the mode of exercise for five of the aerobic studies, two studies used stationary cycle ergometers, one study used an arm ergometer, and one study varied the mode of exercise. The frequency of exercise sessions ranged from 2 to 6 times per week. The length of the interventions ranged from 6 to 26 weeks and the duration of each exercise session ranged from 10 to 60 minutes. The intensity of the prescribed exercise protocols varied, but most studies prescribed moderate-intensity exercise based on heart rate. Adherence to the exercise intervention was reported in six studies and ranged from approximately 70% to 98%.

The studies examined a wide range of biopsychosocial outcomes. The most commonly reported outcome was cardiopulmonary fitness. Nine of the 10 trials included a measure of cardiopulmonary fitness, and most reported a statistically significant and clinically meaningful change in fitness. Quality of life (QOL) was reported in four studies, and the results showed support for the benefits of exercise after cancer treatment, but there was insufficient evidence to support the benefits of exercise during treatment. Nevertheless, statistically and clinically significant improvements in physical functioning and/or physical well-being components of QOL were reported during treatment.

The effect of exercise on fatigue was also evaluated in four studies. Evidence suggests that exercise is beneficial in improving fatigue after cancer treatment but has more mixed results during treatment. Nevertheless, exercise appears to be beneficial in attenuating symptoms of fatigue for women who are able to adhere to an exercise program. Three studies monitored for changes in body weight and/or body mass index. Though reductions in body weight occurred as a result of the exercise intervention, the findings were not statistically or clinically significant. It is not known, however, if positive changes in body

Table 20-1 Characteristics of Exercise Studies in Women with Breast Cancer

Study	Participants	Intervention/Comparison	Outcomes	Results
Campbell 2004 United Kingdom	19 women aged 47.5 (±8) years with early-stage breast cancer undergoing adjuvant radiation therapy or chemotherapy. All subjects had previous breast surgery but no other cancer treatments.	**Supervised exercise vs. usual care** Exercise subjects participated in a mixed aerobic and resistance exercise (varied mode) program 2x per week for 12 weeks. The exercise intensity was 60%-75% of heart rate maximum. Each session was 10-20 minutes.	Quality of life: satisfaction with life scale, FACT-G, FACT-B Cardiopulmonary fitness: 12-minute walk test Fatigue: Piper Fatigue Scale	Significant improvements in 12-minute walk test and quality of life (FACT-G) in favor of exercise group
Courneya 2003 Canada	53 postmenopausal women aged 59 (± 6) years with Stages I-IIIa breast cancer 1 year after treatment. All subjects had previous breast surgery with or without radiation therapy/chemotherapy/hormonal therapy.	**Supervised exercise vs. control** Exercise subjects participated in an aerobic exercise program on an upright or recumbent cycle ergometer 3x per week for 15 weeks. The exercise intensity corresponded to approximately 70%-75% of maximum oxygen consumption. Exercise duration began at 15 minutes and systematically increased by 5 minutes every 3 weeks to a maximum of 35 minutes.	Quality of life: FACT-G, FACT-B Cardiopulmonary fitness: peak oxygen consumption L/min and peak oxygen consumption Vo_2 ml/kg/min Physical functioning: FACT Physical well-being Fatigue: Piper Fatigue Scale Body composition: body weight and body mass index (BMI), sum of skin folds. Other outcomes: happiness	Significant improvements in cardiopulmonary function, QOL, fatigue, and happiness
Crowley 2003 US	22 women aged 35-60 years with Stages I-II breast cancer undergoing adriamycin and cyclophosphamide chemotherapy	**Home-based exercise vs. control** Exercise subjects participated in a mixed aerobic (walking) and strength training (tubing) program 3-5x per week for 13 weeks. The exercise intensity was based on 60% of target heart rate and was individualized.	Quality of life: MOS SF36 Cardiopulmonary fitness: peak oxygen consumption Vo_2 ml/kg/min Fatigue: Revised Piper Fatigue Scale Other outcomes: 1 repetition maximum: chest press and leg press	Significant improvements in cardiopulmonary fitness in favor of exercise group

Continued

Table 20-1 CHARACTERISTICS OF EXERCISE STUDIES IN WOMEN WITH BREAST CANCER—CONT'D

Study	Participants	Intervention/Comparison	Outcomes	Results
Drouin 2002 US	23 women aged 50 (± 8.2) years with Stages 0-III breast cancer undergoing adjuvant radiation therapy	**Home-based exercise vs. placebo stretching** Exercise subjects participated in an aerobic walking program (self-monitored with HR monitor) 3-5x per week for 7 weeks. The exercise intensity was prescribed at 50%-70% of heart rate (HR) maximum, based on the results of the baseline symptom-limited graded exercise test (SLGXT). Each session was 20-45 minutes per session. Subjects in the placebo group followed a home stretching program 3-5x per week for 7 weeks.	Cardiopulmonary fitness: Peak oxygen consumption Vo2 ml/kg/min Fatigue: Revised Piper Fatigue Scale Body composition: body weight and body mass index (BMI) Other outcomes: sum of skin folds, mood, immune parameters Analysis: without intention-to-treat analysis	Significant improvements in cardiopulmonary fitness in favor of exercise group
MacVicar 1989 US	45 women aged 45 (± 9.9) years with Stage II breast cancer undergoing adjuvant chemotherapy/ hormonal therapy	**Supervised exercise vs. placebo vs. control** Subjects participated in interval training on a stationary cycle ergometer 3x per week for 10 weeks. The exercise intensity was 60%-85% of heart rate reserve, based on the results of the SLGXT. Subjects in the placebo group performed stretching and flexibility exercises for 10 weeks.	Cardiopulmonary fitness: Peak oxygen consumption L/min Other outcomes: heart rate, maximum test time, maximum workload Analysis: without intention-to-treat analysis	Significant improvements in cardiopulmonary fitness in favor of exercise group

McKenzie 2003 (Kalda, 1999)	14 women aged 56 (±9) with Stages I and II breast cancer in the posttreatment phase. All subjects had unilateral arm lymphedema.	**Supervised exercise vs. control** Subjects participated in a resistance exercise program and an upper body aerobic exercise via arm ergometer, 3x per week for 8 weeks (aerobic component weeks 2 to 8) The intensity was based on resistance watts/HR-monitored. The aerobic component progressed from 5x 1-minute bouts to 20 minutes continuous. The resistance exercise started with light weights and progressed as tolerated.	Quality of life: MOS: SF 36 short form Physical functioning: SF 36 Physical functioning scale Weight/height: baseline data only Other outcomes: arm volume, arm circumference	Significant improvements in physical functioning in favor of exercise group
Mock 2004 US	119 sedentary women aged 52 (±9) years with Stages 0-III breast cancer undergoing adjuvant chemotherapy or radiation therapy	**Home-based exercise vs. control** Subjects participated in a walking program 5x-6x per week. The length on the program for subjects undergoing radiation therapy was 6 weeks and 3-6 months for subjects undergoing chemotherapy. The intensity was approximately 50%-70% maximum HR, and sessions were progressed from 15 to 30 minutes.	Fatigue: Piper Fatigue Scale Cardiopulmonary: 12-minute walk test Physical functioning: SF 36 physical functioning scale	No significant differences between groups in any outcomes When data were analyzed by exercise participation level, significant differences were found in favor of exercise in reducing fatigue.

Continued

Table 20-1 Characteristics of Exercise Studies in Women with Breast Cancer—cont'd

Study	Participants	Intervention/Comparison	Outcomes	Results
Mustian 2003 US	27 women aged 52 (±9) years with Stages 0-III breast cancer in the posttreatment phase	**Supervised exercise vs. support group** Exercise subjects participated in tai chi chuan 3x per week for 12 weeks. Each exercise session was 60 minutes in duration. Support group subjects participated in sessions focusing on educational/peer support/coping strategies, 3x per week for 12 weeks. Sessions for both groups were 60 minutes in duration.	Cardiopulmonary: submaximal 6-minute walk test = estimated bioelectrical impedance max Body composition: BMI Other outcomes: muscular fitness: biodex isokinetic dynamometer; self-esteem, self-efficacy, bioelectrical impedance, handgrip.	Significant improvements in global self-esteem Significant within-group differences for 6-minute walk for exercise group
Nieman 1995 US	16 women aged 35-72 years with Stages I-III breast cancer in the posttreatment phase	**Supervised exercise vs. control** Exercise subjects participated in a supervised walking program with resistance weight training (2 sets of 12 repetitions for 7 exercises) 3x per week for 8 weeks. The intensity of the exercise was not stated. Each exercise session was 30 minutes in duration.	Cardiopulmonary: 6-minute walk test Other outcomes: leg extension strength; natural killer cell cytotoxic activity	Significant improvement in 6-minute walk in favor of exercise group
Segal 2001 Canada	123 women aged 50.9 (±9) years with Stages I-II breast cancer undergoing adjuvant treatment (chemotherapy, radiation therapy, or hormonal therapy)	**Supervised exercise (SE) and self-directed exercise (SD) vs. control** Exercise subjects in both the self-directed and supervised groups participated in an aerobic walking program 5x per week for 26 weeks. The SE group was supervised for 3x per wk with 2x per wk self-directed. The intensity of the exercise was based on 50%-60% of predicted Vo_2 max and was progressive. The duration was not reported.	Quality of life: MOS SF 36, FACT-G, FACT-B Physical functioning: SF36 Cardiopulmonary: Aerobic capacity: Modified Canadian Aerobic Fitness Test = estimated Vo_2 max Body composition: body weight	Significant increases in physical functioning in self-directed exercise group when compared to control group Supervised exercise improved aerobic capacity and reduced body weight compared with control but only in participants not receiving chemotherapy.

composition (such as increases in muscle mass and decreases in fat mass) occurred as a result of the exercise intervention. Results for other, less commonly studied, outcomes are presented in Table 20-1.

Overall, the findings on exercise interventions in women cancer survivors are primarily positive. Most studies reported changes in important outcomes in the desired direction even if the changes were not always statistically significant. Moreover, few studies reported any major safety issues or serious adverse events associated with exercise testing or training. Lastly, the adherence rates were quite acceptable in these studies, indicating the feasibility of an exercise intervention in women cancer survivors.

Despite these positive findings, there are important limitations that need to be highlighted. First, the quality of the randomized controlled trials was not optimal, and the reporting of important methodologic issues was sketchy (e.g., randomization, blinding, analytical plan). Second, the sample sizes were relatively small, leaving the studies underpowered. Third, the length of the interventions was fairly short, and there was no long-term follow-up. Fourth, many studies included participants on various treatment protocols, making it unclear if exercise is equally feasible and beneficial during different adjuvant therapies (e.g., chemotherapy, radiation therapy, hormone therapy). Finally, all studies focused on breast cancer survivors, making the generalizability of the findings to women survivors of other cancers tenuous (e.g., lung, pancreatic, ovarian).

Given the restricted focus of exercise studies on breast cancer, the only study to date that exclusively examined women survivors of any other cancer is reviewed (even though it was not a randomized controlled trial). Courneya and others[12] examined the association between exercise and QOL in 386 endometrial cancer survivors using a mailed survey methodology. These researchers found that endometrial cancer survivors meeting public health exercise guidelines (i.e., at least 60 minutes of strenuous exercise or 150 minutes of moderate-to-strenuous exercise per week) reported statistically and clinically better QOL than survivors not meeting guidelines. The authors concluded that a randomized controlled trial designed to test the causal effects of exercise on QOL in endometrial cancer survivors is warranted.

STUDIES THAT INCLUDED WOMEN CANCER SURVIVORS

Exercise trials involving mixed-sex cancers are reviewed to determine (a) how well women were represented in these trials, and (b) if any of these trials presented the data separately for women. Thirteen controlled trials of mixed-sex cancers that focused on either single cancer sites[3,13-17] or mixed cancer sites were reviewed.[18-24] The single cancer sites consisted of colorectal, multiple myeloma, lung, stomach, leukemia, and head and neck cancer. The review showed that women were well represented in these trials, comprising 42% to 84% (mean of 66%) of participants in the mixed-site cancer studies and 18% to 46% (mean of 30%) of participants in the single-site cancer studies. Although the findings for the mixed-sex studies were also primarily positive (see Stevinson and others[25] and Irwin and others[26] for recent reviews), no study analyzed the effects of the exercise intervention separately for men and women (i.e., examined sex as a moderator). To explore this issue here, the authors report an ancillary subanalysis from a previously published trial—the Colorectal Cancer and Home-Based Physical Exercise (CAN-HOPE) trial.[27-29]

Ancillary Analysis from the CAN-HOPE Trial

The CAN-HOPE trial was a randomized controlled trial that examined if a home-based exercise program could improve QOL in colorectal cancer survivors who had recently completed surgery (over half of whom were receiving adjuvant therapy at the time of the exercise intervention). Participants (N = 102) were randomly assigned in a 2:1 ratio to either an exercise (n = 69) or a control (n = 33) group. The exercise group was asked to exercise independently 3 to 5 times per week for 16 weeks at a moderate-to-vigorous intensity (60% to 80% of estimated maximum heart rate) for at least 20 to 30 minutes each time. The primary endpoints were QOL (assessed by self-report scales) and cardiovascular fitness (assessed by a submaximal treadmill test).

The authors reported a 91% completion rate (93/102) and a 76% adherence rate among those who completed the trial (i.e., excluding drop-outs). The authors also reported that 52% of the control group reported regular exercise. Intention to treat analyses on those who had completed the trial showed no statistically significant differences between the two arms. In an "as treated" ancillary analyses, participants who increased their fitness over the course of the intervention had more favorable changes in anxiety, depression, overall QOL, and satisfaction with life compared to those whose fitness decreased over the course of the intervention.

For the present chapter, data were reanalyzed using sex as a moderator. Fifty-four men (58%) and 39 women (42%) participated in the trial. Using the intention to treat analysis, we found one significant group by sex interaction and it was for treadmill time [$F(1,89) = 5.9$; $p = 0.017$]. Independent t-tests on change scores within each sex category indicated that women improved their fitness with our home-based exercise program whereas men did not improve their fitness (Table 20-2; Figure 20-1). Although speculative, it is possible that the lower-intensity exercise program (mainly walking) was sufficient to improve the fitness of women but not men. This speculation is further supported by the fact that the women did not exercise more than the men during the intervention but did have a lower fitness level at baseline. In any case, these data should be interpreted with caution, given the post hoc nature of these analyses, the relatively small sample sizes, and the multiple analyses that could lead to a chance finding.

Using the "as-treated" analysis, borderline significance was found in sex by group interactions for fatigue [$F(1,89) = 3.2$; $p = 0.079$] and physical well-being [$F(1,89) = 3.7$; $p = 0.057$]. Independent t-tests on change scores within each sex category indicated that fitness changes in women were more positively associated with changes in physical well-being (Figure 20-2) and fatigue (Figure 20-3) than fitness changes in men (Table 20-2). The group that did particularly poorly was the women whose fitness levels decreased over the course of the intervention. This difference could be due to the possibility that the women had less physical reserve than men at baseline, and therefore any further losses in fitness may have had more profound effects for the women. Again, these data should be interpreted with caution, given the post hoc nature of these analyses, the relatively small sample sizes, multiple analyses, and the ancillary "as-treated" analysis, which reduces the strength of the causal inference. Nevertheless, these data at least suggest that one should be open to the possibility that women may respond differently to different exercise interventions (and fitness changes) than men with the same cancer.

EFFECTS OF EXERCISE IMPORTANT TO WOMEN CANCER SURVIVORS

There are many outcomes important to women cancer survivors that have not been adequately addressed in current exercise and cancer trials. Here, the authors offer a brief overview of some of the most important outcomes (e.g., lymphedema, menopausal symptoms, body composition, osteoporosis, cognitive function, and body image) and how exercise may affect such outcomes. Research in women cancer survivors was used when available but we also include research with other groups of women, where needed.

Lymphedema

Lymphedema is an important issue for women after cancer treatment (see Chapter 12). Guidelines for the prevention of lymphedema have been developed and often include a proscription of strenuous exercise.[30,31] Women are cautioned against strenuous exercise because it may increase arterial blood flow to the limb and/or region. In theory, exercise may negatively disrupt the

Table 20-2 Effects of a Home-Based Exercise Program on Physical Fitness, Physical Well-Being, and Fatigue in Male and Female Colorectal Cancer Survivors[a]

	Baseline	P Value[a]	Posttest	Mean Change	Difference between Groups in Mean Change [95% CI]	P Value[b]
MALES (N = 54)						
Treadmill time						
Exercise group (n = 34)	441 (274)	0.173	525 (310)	84 (224)	-61 [-194 to 71]	0.356
Control group (n = 20)	334 (279)		479 (300)	145 (251)		
Physical well-being (0-28)						
Increased fitness (n = 33)	23.3 (4.2)	0.890	23.4 (4.8)	0.2 (5.6)	0.3 [-2.6 to 3.2]	0.845
Decreased fitness (n = 21)	23.1 (5.2)		23.0 (5.4)	-0.1 (4.3)		
Fatigue (0-52)						
Increased fitness (n = 33)	10.7 (8.6)	0.159	9.2 (8.8)	-1.4 (9.6)	0.8 [-2.4 to 5.6]	0.723
Decreased fitness (n = 21)	14.8 (12.8)		12.6 (9.7)	-2.3 (7.8)		
FEMALES (N = 39)						
Treadmill time						
Exercise group (n = 28)	320 (311)	0.786	534 (314)	214 (288)	225 [15 to 436]	0.037
Control group (n = 11)	291 (255)		280 (253)	-11 (301)		
Physical well-being (0-28)						
Increased fitness (n = 25)	23.0 (4.7)	0.924	23.8 (3.4)	0.7 (3.6)	4.9 [-0.4 to 10.2]	0.066
Decreased fitness (n = 14)	23.2 (2.6)		19.0 (8.1)	-4.2 (8.9)		
Fatigue (0-52)						
Increased fitness (n = 25)	13.5 (10.4)	0.894	12.6 (9.8)	-0.9 (10.3)	7.8 [-3.4 to 18.9]	0.160
Decreased fitness (n = 14)	13.0 (9.8)		19.9 (15.2)	6.9 (18.2)		

[a]P value for difference between groups at baseline; [b]P value for differences in change scores between groups from baseline to posttest.

CI, Confidence interval.

Data are from the Colorectal Cancer and Home-Based Physical Exercise (CAN-HOPE) trial and reported by Courneya KS and others: A randomized trial of exercise and quality of life in colorectal cancer survivors, *Eur J Cancer Care (Engl)* 12:347, 2003.

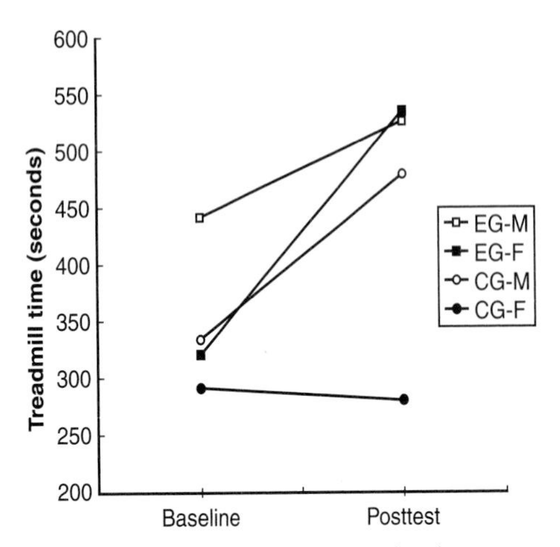

FIGURE 20-1 Significant Interaction between Experimental Group and Sex on Treadmill Time from the CAN-HOPE Trial.
EG-M = exercise group—males; EG-F = exercise group—females; CG-M = control group—males; CG-F = control group—females.
(Data from Courneya KS and others: A randomized trial of exercise and quality of life in colorectal cancer survivors, *Eur J Cancer Care (Engl)* 12:347, 2003.)

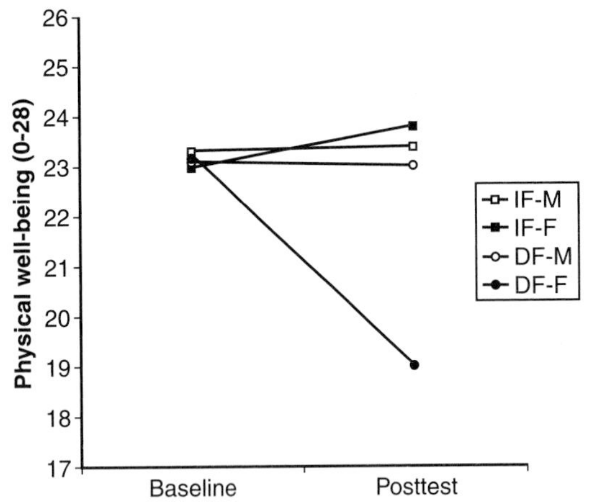

FIGURE 20-2 Borderline Significant Interaction between Fitness Group and Sex on Physical Well-Being from the CAN-HOPE Trial.
IF-M = increased fitness—males; IF-F = increased fitness—females; DF-M = decreased fitness—males; DF-F = decreased fitness—females.
(Data from Courneya KS and others: A randomized trial of exercise and quality of life in colorectal cancer survivors, *Eur J Cancer Care (Engl)* 12:347, 2003.)

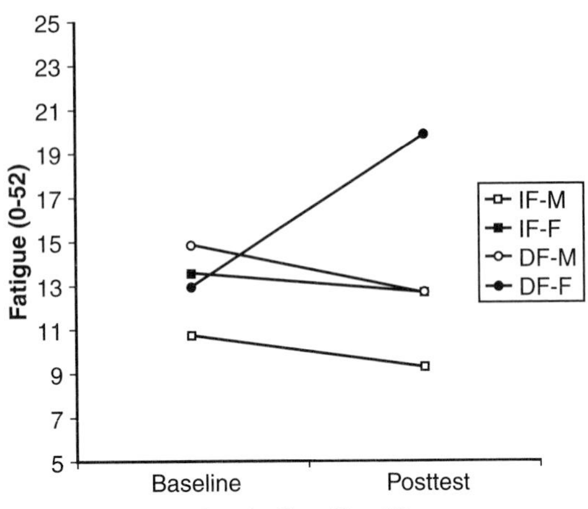

FIGURE 20-3 Borderline Significant Interaction between Fitness Group and Sex on Fatigue from the CAN-HOPE Trial.
IF-M = increased fitness—males; IF-F = increased fitness—females; DF-M = decreased fitness—males; DF-F = decreased fitness—females.
(Data from Courneya KS and others: A randomized trial of exercise and quality of life in colorectal cancer survivors, *Eur J Cancer Care (Engl)* 12:347, 2003.)

balance between capillary filtration and lymphatic drainage and result in increased swelling of the limb.[30] This guideline is supported by anecdotal clinical evidence that patients often report a transient increase in limb tension, heaviness, and/or swelling with functional activities and with exercise.[32]

In contrast, however, it is also known that skeletal muscle contraction is a primary force propelling lymph fluid through the lymphatic system,[33] and that consequently it might be of benefit to lymphatic drainage. Furthermore, changes in intrathoracic pressure that occur during the respiratory cycle, and specifically with abdominal breathing, also increase lymphatic flow.[32] Aerobic exercise, in theory, could potentially facilitate this process. Furthermore, obesity, which can be successfully reduced with physical activity and/or exercise, is a known risk factor in the development of lymphedema.[34] Given this background, two important questions to pose are the following: (a) Will exercise prevent or precipitate the development of lymphedema? and (b) Will exercise ameliorate or exacerbate existing lymphedema?

No randomized controlled trials have examined the effect of exercise specifically on the development of lymphedema. However, early evidence does suggest that most breast cancer survivors can safely participate in activities involving strenuous upper extremity exercise without developing lymphedema.[7,35] Harris and Niesen-Vertommen,[35] in a case series, followed 20 breast cancer survivors participating in dragon boat racing and reported no clinically significant difference in arm circumference from the beginning of training to the end of the season.

Only two randomized controlled trials have monitored and/or reported the occurrence of lymphedema as an adverse event in clinical exercise trials. Courneya and others[3] examined the effects of aerobic exercise training in postmenopausal breast cancer survivors and reported a trend towards a higher incidence of lymphedema occurring in the exercise group. Crowley and others[4] examined the effects of a mixed aerobic/resistance exercise program on breast cancer survivors undergoing adjuvant chemotherapy. The authors reported a single case of lymphedema developing, and it was in the exercise group. At present, there is insufficient evidence on the effect of exercise on limb volume to provide clear guidelines to cancer survivors. Clearly, however, monitoring of limb volume in studies examining exercise interventions is warranted.

Similarly, there has been only one study that has examined the effects of exercise on cancer survivors with existing lymphedema. In a pilot randomized controlled trial, McKenzie and Kalda[7] examined the effects of an 8-week upper body resistance and aerobic exercise program on arm volume in 14 women with breast cancer–related lymphedema. All participants wore compression sleeves throughout the study period. The program consisted of a combined aerobic and resistance exercise program designed to strengthen the larger muscles of the upper extremity. Arm volume was measured by arm circumference measurement and water displacement volumetry every 2 weeks over the 8-week program. Although the exercise intervention did not result in a reduction of lymphedema in the arm, there was no significant increase in arm volume, either. The findings of this pilot study suggest that women with breast cancer–related lymphedema who wear a compression sleeve while exercising can participate in combined aerobic and resistance upper body exercise programs without deleterious effects on their lymphedema. Although these preliminary results are promising, randomized controlled trials with larger samples are needed before definitive conclusions can be drawn.

Menopausal Symptoms

Managing menopausal symptoms in women cancer survivors is an important challenge, and many women are interested in nonpharmacologic options.[36] Physical activity is often recommended as a strategy to reduce menopausal symptoms, but there is limited evidence supporting this advice. Observational research suggests that lower levels of self-reported physical activity are associated with more hot flashes[37] and that physical activity started in perimenopause may decrease the occurrence of hot flashes and night sweats.[38] Nevertheless, Aiello and others[39] conducted the only randomized controlled trial to date to isolate the effects of exercise on menopausal symptoms. The trial randomized 87 women to a 12-month, moderate-intensity exercise intervention and 86 women to a stretching control group. The exercise intervention consisted of an average of 171 minutes of moderate-intensity exercise over 3.7 days per week.

Over the 12-month period, there was actually a significant **increase** in hot flash severity in exercisers compared to controls. Exercisers did have a decrease in memory problems, and there were no reported differences in depressive feelings or sleep problems. The authors suggest that the increase in hot flashes may have been due to the decrease in total body fat, which lowers circulating estrogen levels, or to the increase in core body temperature that results from exercise.

Based on the current literature, there does not appear to be compelling evidence that exercise can reduce menopausal symptoms. Moderate-intensity physical activity may even increase some menopausal symptoms, such as hot flashes, but more research is needed to look at different types of physical activity, a wider scope of menopausal symptoms, and women cancer survivors in particular.

Body Composition

Weight gain is a common side effect in women receiving adjuvant chemotherapy for breast cancer[40] and may be linked to recurrence and survival.[41] Proposed mechanisms for this observation include decreased physical activity or energy expenditure, alterations in resting metabolic rate, increase in dietary intake, and increase in edema or water weight.[40,42,43] There is consistent evidence that physical activity levels drop during cancer treatment.[44-49] This suggests that strategies to maintain or increase levels of physical activity during adjuvant treatment may help to reduce weight gain. However, few studies to date have examined body weight or composition endpoints in women cancer survivors. A review of exercise interventions in cancer survivors,[25] not limited to women, suggests no change in body weight but a possible improvement in body **composition** (i.e., fat loss offset by an increase in lean body mass). Goodwin and others[50] undertook a specific weight management trial for women newly diagnosed with breast cancer, which involved group sessions, nutrition counseling, and an exercise program. Fifty-five women entered the trial and averaged 63.5 minutes of moderate aerobic activity per week over 12 months. Overall, the women lost a mean of only 0.5 kg, whereas those who were initially overweight (BMI ≥25 kg/m^2) lost a mean of 1.6 kg. A combination of physical activity and healthful eating for weight loss/maintenance is advocated by an expert panel from the American Cancer Society.[51] Clearly, trials examining the effects of diet and/or exercise on weight loss/maintenance in women cancer survivors during and after treatments are warranted.

Osteoporosis

Osteoporosis is a significant issue for women after cancer (see Chapter 11). In the general population, physical activity is recommended to slow or prevent bone loss and osteoporosis.[52-54] Specifically, exercise that places a strain on bone, such as resistance training, stimulates bone formation.[55] To date, very little is known about the effects of resistance training, or any physical activity, on preserving bone mass in women cancer survivors. Five studies have examined bone mineral density (BMD) outcomes in relation to exercise in cancer survivors.[56-60] Of these studies, only two involved adult women.[57-59]

One of these studies was cross-sectional and involved 27 postmenopausal breast cancer survivors.[57] No significant associations were found between light, moderate, or hard exercise and BMD. The second study was an uncontrolled trial involving 21 postmenopausal breast cancer survivors.[59] Participants followed a 12-month, home-based strength training program as well as took alendronate, calcium, and vitamin D.[59] Results indicated significant improvements in BMD of the spine and hip after the exercise intervention. The results of these studies are difficult to interpret, given serious limitations such as small sample sizes, uncontrolled designs, and the possibility of other confounding variables.

In nonclinical populations, weight-bearing exercise has been found to have a beneficial effect on BMD in a number of cross-sectional and intervention studies.[61] A review by Bonaiuti and others[62] found 18 randomized controlled trials of exercise and BMD in postmenopausal women. Results showed that aerobic, resistance, and walking interventions of 1 year or longer were all effective in improving spinal BMD in postmenopausal women.[62] In addition, walking interventions were found to improve BMD of the hip, and aerobic interventions improved BMD of the wrist.

A recent randomized controlled trial examined BMD outcomes in 120 premenopausal women.[63] Participants were randomly assigned to either an exercise group or a control group. The exercise group performed high-impact aerobic activity

3 times per week for 60 minutes for a 12-month period. BMD was assessed at the lumbar spine, the proximal femur, and the distal forearm at baseline and postintervention. Significant improvements in BMD were found in the femoral neck, the intertrochanter, and the total femur in the exercise group compared to the control group. Results suggest that high-impact aerobic exercise may have utility in improving BMD in the lumbar spine and upper femur in premenopausal women. Although these data are quite convincing, randomized controlled trials of exercise and BMD in women cancer survivors are warranted because of the unique issues in this population.

Cognitive Function

Several studies have suggested that impairments in neuropsychologic or cognitive functioning may occur following adjuvant cancer treatment. These cognitive side effects may include difficulty concentrating, impaired verbal and visual memory, difficulty organizing information, decreased motor skills, and language problems (e.g., word retrieval difficulty).[64] This dysfunction is often referred to as "chemo brain" or "chemo fog."[65] While these deficits may be subtle, they can have a significant impact on QOL and are of great concern to women cancer survivors.[64]

The majority of studies reporting cognitive deficits following cancer treatment have focused on women who received chemotherapy for breast cancer. The rate of cognitive dysfunction in these controlled studies has ranged from 16% to 50%.[65] Cognitive dysfunction has also been reported following adjuvant treatment for other cancers such as lymphoma, colorectal, renal, ovarian, lung, CNS, melanoma and leukemia.[64] Although there is uncertainty about the exact mechanisms that lead to cognitive dysfunction, proposed mechanisms include changes in sex hormones and inflammatory cytokines, and vascular effects.[65] Moreover, cognitive dysfunction may be related to affective factors such as depression, fatigue, and anxiety.[65]

Treatments for chemotherapy-induced cognitive dysfunction have primarily focused on pharmacologic agents (e.g., erythropoietin, aspirin, and methylphenidate). Suggested rehabilitative interventions have included education (on potential problems in cognitive functioning with treatment), stress management, and compensatory strategies for memory and attention problems.[65] Exercise is another intervention that may potentially attenuate cognitive dysfunction, but no studies have specifically examined the effects of exercise on cognitive dysfunction in cancer survivors.[66,67] Many studies have, however, examined the effect of exercise on cognitive dysfunction in other older adult populations.

A recent metaanalysis by Colcombe and others[68] examined the effects of exercise on cognitive dysfunction in older sedentary adults. Using metaanalytic techniques, the authors reported significant, though selective, benefits for cognition. The greatest benefits occurred for **executive control processes,** namely, coordination, inhibition, scheduling, planning, and working memory (tasks that do not become automatic over time and require constant central mediation). Exercisers also improved on **controlled processing** (automatic processing with consistent practice), **speed** tasks (e.g., finger-tapping speed) and **spatial** tasks (transforming or remembering visual and spatial information). Interestingly, the review suggested that these benefits were greater in women.[68] The authors also noted a larger beneficial effect on cognition from certain exercise program factors. Specifically, the magnitude of effects on cognition was greater with combined aerobic and resistance exercise programs and in studies with longer-duration programs (longer than 6 months) and longer intervention sessions (more than 30 minutes per session). These findings serve to provide some insight into the potential role of exercise on cognitive dysfunction and highlight the need for research on this topic in women cancer survivors.

Body Image

Body image is another important issue for women cancer survivors (see Chapter 16). Some evidence suggests that exercise may have utility in improving body image in cancer survivors, possibly by improving muscle strength and tone, aiding in weight loss, and increasing the perception of healthiness.[69] Mock and others[8] reported, in a randomized controlled trial of 14 breast cancer survivors on chemotherapy, that women in the exercise arm (a structured walking program) maintained their body image scores whereas those in the control group (usual care) showed a deterioration in body image. Similarly, Pinto and others,[70] in a randomized controlled trial of 24 breast cancer survivors, found improvements in body image scores in the exercise group compared to the control group after a 12-week supervised aerobic exercise intervention.

In the general population, exercise has also been found to improve body image.[71,72] For example, Stoll and Alfermann[71] examined body self-concept in a quasi-experimental study of 101 older adults. Participants in the study were divided into three groups: an exercise group, a placebo group, and a control group. The exercise group followed a 14-week intervention of 60 to 75 minutes once per week of aerobic and strength training. The placebo group took part in a foreign language course once per week for 90 minutes. Results indicated that the exercise group showed an improvement in body self-concept after the intervention. Additional trials of exercise and body image in women cancer survivors are warranted.

EXERCISE MOTIVATION AND BEHAVIOR CHANGE IN WOMEN CANCER SURVIVORS

The growing evidence that exercise may be an important self-care behavior for women cancer survivors has spurred some preliminary research into the prevalence and determinants of this behavior in women cancer survivors. In terms of prevalence, a recent survey of 806 breast cancer survivors reported that only 32% of the sample were meeting public health exercise guidelines.[26] Similarly, Blanchard and others[73] reported that 23% of breast cancer survivors were meeting public health exercise guidelines. In the only study of women survivors of a cancer other than breast, Courneya and others[12] surveyed 386 endometrial cancer survivors and reported that only 30% were meeting public health exercise guidelines. These studies suggest that women cancer survivors, like many other segments of the population, are not obtaining adequate exercise for health benefits.

Given this state of affairs, research has also begun to examine the determinants of exercise motivation and behavior in women cancer survivors. These studies have clearly shown that adjuvant therapy has a negative effect on exercise levels. For example, an early study reported that exercise levels declined significantly during breast cancer treatments and did not return to prediagnosis levels even years after treatments had been completed.[74] A more recent survey found that breast cancer survivors who received a combination of surgery, chemotherapy, and radiation had more substantial decreases in physical activity than patients who had surgery only or patients who had surgery plus radiation.[75] Nevertheless, the key determinants of exercise behavior in women cancer survivors appear to be social cognitive factors such as attitudes, social support, perceptions of control, and intentions.[76-78]

Only one study to date has attempted an exercise behavior change intervention in women cancer survivors, and it focused on the potential role of the oncologist.[79,80] In the Oncologist Recommendation to Exercise (ONCORE) trial, 450 newly diagnosed breast cancer survivors were randomly assigned to receive an oncologist's exercise recommendation, an oncologist's recommendation plus referral to an exercise specialist, or to usual care during their first adjuvant treatment consultation. The primary outcome of the trial was self-reported exercise behavior 5 weeks after the consultation. Results from the trial showed that the recommendation-only group reported significantly more exercise than the usual care group, suggesting that oncologists may play a small but important role in encouraging exercise in breast cancer survivors.

FUTURE RESEARCH DIRECTIONS

It is obvious from our review that what we know about exercise in women cancer survivors is derived exclusively from breast cancer survivors.

Although breast cancer is by far the most common cancer diagnosed in American women, it still accounts for only about one third of cancers in women.[81] The obvious converse of this fact is that cancers other than breast account for about two thirds of all cancers diagnosed in American women. After breast cancer, the most common cancers in American women are lung (see Chapter 4), colorectal (see Chapter 9), endometrial (see Chapter 8), ovarian (see Chapter 7), non-Hodgkin's lymphoma (see Chapter 10), and skin melanoma.[81] These six cancers account for about 40% of all the cancers diagnosed in American women (a combined total more than breast) and about 60% of all the non–breast cancers.

The disproportionate focus of exercise researchers on breast cancer may have arisen for several reasons. First, breast cancer is the most common cancer in women, which allows for an adequate sample size to conduct a single center study on a single cancer site. Second, the generally good prognosis of breast cancer makes QOL an important issue and makes exercise interventions more feasible. Third, the greater abundance of funding for breast cancer–specific research may have enticed exercise researchers into this area. Nevertheless, an important future direction for exercise researchers is to extend their research to women survivors of cancers other than breast. This goal may be achieved by examining other cancers that exclusively affect women (e.g., endometrial, ovarian, cervical) or by focusing on women with cancers that include high proportions of women (e.g., colorectal, lung, lymphomas).

For studies that do not target women cancer survivors specifically, it may be possible to conduct subgroup analyses for women. Such analyses may help to determine if women and men who are being treated for, or have survived, the same cancer respond similarly to the same exercise training intervention. The post hoc secondary analyses we conducted in this chapter suggest that men and women colorectal cancer survivors may respond differently to exercise, although our study was not designed or powered to answer such a question. If possible, it would be ideal to power a study a priori to conduct such a subgroup analysis by stratifying on sex ahead of randomization and by attempting to recruit equal numbers of men and women cancer survivors.

In addition to simply starting research programs in various groups of women cancer survivors, it will be important to examine the effects of exercise interventions on all aspects of women's QOL including physical, functional, emotional, spiritual, and social well-being. It will also be important to determine if exercise can help control some of the side effects of cancer treatments that are particularly important to women cancer survivors such as lymphedema, menopausal symptoms, weight gain, osteoporosis, cognitive dysfunction, and body image. Other important clinical endpoints that should be examined include disease recurrence, other diseases (e.g., cardiovascular disease, diabetes), mortality, treatment compliance, and treatment efficacy.[82] Moreover, for all of the above questions, it will be important to determine the optimal type (e.g., walking, aerobic, resistance), volume (i.e., frequency, intensity, and duration), periodization, and context (e.g., center-based versus home-based, individual versus group format) of exercise that is most beneficial and feasible for women cancer survivors. This information will allow practitioners to tailor their exercise interventions to appeal to the widest cross-section of women cancer survivors.

Clinical Implications

Based on the current evidence, the American Cancer Society has recommended regular exercise to all cancer survivors.[51] As indicated in the present review, the evidence is most compelling for breast cancer survivors. However, there are several special precautions for cancer survivors, and the reader is referred to previous published guidelines for these safety issues.[83,84] In general, exercise during adjuvant therapy will be a major struggle for women cancer survivors,[85] but it is still feasible and likely that benefits can be realized.[67] The authors recommend low- to moderate-intensity exercise performed 3 to 5 days per week for 20 to 30 minutes each time, depending on baseline fitness levels and treatment toxicities.[83,84] The exercise should be of moderate intensity in the range of 55% to 75% of maximal heart rate. Unfortunately, many women cancer survivors receiving chemotherapy experience tachycardia, which makes heart rate alone an unreliable indicator of exercise intensity. Consequently, it may be useful to also monitor intensity with a rating of perceived exertion scale using the range of "somewhat hard" to "hard." The preferred exercise choice in women cancer survivors is walking,[86] and this activity will likely be sufficient to meet the recommended intensity for most women cancer survivors on adjuvant therapy. Exercise periodization during adjuvant therapy is unpredictable and does not always follow a linear course, given the accumulating side effects of most cancer therapies. Women cancer survivors should exercise to tolerance during adjuvant therapy, including reducing intensity and performing exercise in shorter durations (e.g., 10 minutes) if needed. Resistance exercise training may be particularly helpful to women cancer survivors during adjuvant therapy, but there are very few data at the present time to support such a recommendation.

After treatments, when most acute toxicities have dissipated, most women cancer survivors can probably be recommended to follow the public health exercise guidelines from the American College of Sports Medicine and the US Centers for Disease Control.[87] These guidelines propose two different exercise prescriptions for general health. The more traditional prescription is to perform at least 20 minutes of continuous, vigorous-intensity exercise (i.e., ≥75% of maximal heart rate) on at least 3 days per week. The alternative prescription is to accumulate at least 30 minutes of moderate-intensity exercise (i.e., 50% to 75% of maximal heart rate) in durations of at least 10 minutes on most (i.e., at least 5), and preferably all, days of the week. Exercise trials in women cancer survivors have generally followed the traditional prescription, and there is some evidence that QOL benefits may be enhanced if cardiovascular adaptations occur.[3] Nevertheless, in the absence of clinical trials comparing the two prescriptions in women cancer survivors, it seems reasonable to expect both exercise prescriptions to yield health benefits. The key issue is providing an exercise program that women cancer survivors are able and willing to follow. Again, resistance training will likely be an important addition to any aerobic-based exercise program.

SUMMARY

There is a growing interest in the potential role of exercise in enhancing QOL in women cancer survivors. Preliminary research suggests that exercise may be an effective intervention to increase fitness and QOL in breast cancer survivors, but the evidence for women with other cancers is sparse (e.g., endometrial, ovarian) or undetermined because of combined analyses in mixed-sex studies (e.g., colorectal). Future research is needed to provide important information on the role of exercise in addressing many of the health issues facing women cancer survivors. Moreover, it will be important to learn how best to motivate, facilitate, and reach this growing population with effective and feasible exercise programs.

REFERENCES

1. Bouchard C, Shephard RJ: Physical activity, fitness, and health: the model and key concepts. In: Quinney HA, Gauvin L, Wall AE, editors: *Physical activity, fitness, and health: international proceedings and consensus statement,* Champaign, 1994, Human Kinetics.
2. Campbell A and others: A pilot study of a supervised group exercise program as a rehabilitation treatment for women with breast cancer receiving adjuvant treatment, *Eur J Oncol Nurs* 9:56-63, 2005.
3. Courneya KS and others: Randomized controlled trial of exercise training in postmenopausal breast cancer survivors: cardiopulmonary and quality of life outcomes, *J Clin Oncol* 21:1660, 2003.
4. Crowley SA: *The effect of a structured exercise program on fatigue, strength, endurance, physical self-efficacy, and functional wellness in women with early stage breast cancer,* Ann Arbor, 2003, University of Michigan.
5. Drouin J: *Aerobic exercise training effects on physical function, fatigue and mood, immune status, and oxidative stress in subjects undergoing radiation treatment for breast cancer,* Detroit, 2002, Wayne State University.
6. MacVicar MG, Winningham ML, Nickel JL: Effects of

aerobic interval training on cancer patients' functional capacity, *Nurs Res* 38:348, 1989.
7. McKenzie DC, Kalda AL: Effect of upper extremity exercise on secondary lymphedema in breast cancer patients: a pilot study, *J Clin Oncol* 21:463, 2003.
8. Mock V and others: A nursing rehabilitation program for women with breast cancer receiving adjuvant chemotherapy, *Oncol Nurs Forum* 21:899, 1994.
9. Mustian K. *Breast cancer, tai chi chuan, and self-esteem*, Greensboro, 2003, University of North Carolina.
10. Nieman DC and others: Moderate exercise training and natural killer cell cytotoxic activity in breast cancer patients, *Int J Sports Med* 16:334, 1995.
11. Segal R and others: Structured exercise improves physical functioning in women with stages I and II breast cancer: results of a randomized controlled trial, *J Clin Oncol* 19:657, 2001.
12. Courneya KS and others: Associations among exercise, body weight, and quality of life in a population-based sample of endometrial cancer survivors, *Gynecol Oncol* in press.
13. Coleman EA and others: Facilitating exercise adherence for patients with multiple myeloma, *Clin J Oncol Nurs* 7:529, 2003.
14. Cunningham BA and others: Effects of resistive exercise on skeletal muscle in marrow transplant recipients receiving total parental nutrition, *JPEN J Parenter Enteral Nutr* 10:558, 1986.
15. McNeely ML and others: A pilot study of a randomized controlled trial to evaluate the effects of progressive resistance exercise training on shoulder dysfunction caused by spinal accessory neurapraxia/neurectomy in head and neck cancer survivors, *Head Neck* 26:518, 2004.
16. Wall LM: Changes in hope and power in lung cancer patients who exercise, *Nurs Sci Q* 13:234, 2000.
17. Na YM and others: Exercise therapy effect on natural killer cell cytotoxic activity in stomach cancer patients after curative surgery, *Arch Phys Med Rehabil* 81:777, 2000.
18. Burnham TR, Wilcox A: Effects of exercise on physiological and psychological variables in cancer survivors, *Med Sci Sports Exerc* 34:1863, 2002.
19. Courneya KS and others: The group psychotherapy and home-based physical exercise (group-hope) trial in cancer survivors: physical fitness and quality of life outcomes, *Psychooncology* 12:357, 2003.
20. Dimeo F and others: Effects of aerobic exercise on the physical performance and incidence of treatment-related complications after high-dose chemotherapy, *Blood* 90: 3390, 1997.
21. Dimeo FC and others: Aerobic exercise in the rehabilitation of cancer patients after high dose chemotherapy and autologous peripheral stem cell transplantation, *Cancer* 79:1717, 1997.
22. Hayes SC and others: Role of a mixed type, moderate intensity exercise programme after peripheral blood stem cell transplantation, *Br J Sports Med* 38:304, 2004.
23. Mello M, Tanaka C, Dulley FL: Effects of an exercise program on muscle performance in patients undergoing allogeneic bone marrow transplantation, *Bone Marrow Transplant* 32:723, 2003.
24. Petersson LM and others: Differential effects of cancer rehabilitation depending on diagnosis and patients' cognitive coping style, *Psychosom Med* 64:971, 2002.
25. Stevinson C, Lawlor DA, Fox KR: Exercise interventions for cancer patients: systematic review of controlled trials, *Cancer Causes Control* 15:1035, 2004.
26. Irwin ML, Ainsworth BE: Physical activity interventions following cancer diagnosis: methodologic challenges to delivery and assessment, *Cancer Invest* 22:30, 2004.
27. Courneya KS and others: A longitudinal study of exercise barriers in colorectal cancer survivors participating in a randomized controlled trial, *Ann Behav Med*, 29:147, 2005.
28. Courneya KS and others: A randomized trial of exercise and quality of life in colorectal cancer survivors, *Eur J Cancer Care (Engl)* 12:347, 2003.
29. Courneya KS and others: Predictors of adherence and contamination in a randomized trial of exercise in colorectal cancer survivors, *Psychooncology* 13:857, 2004.
30. Ridner SH: Breast cancer lymphedema: pathophysiology and risk reduction guidelines, *Oncol Nurs Forum* 29:1285, 2002.
31. Runowicz CD and others: American Cancer Society Lymphedema Workshop. Workgroup II: patient education pre- and posttreatment, *Cancer* 83:2880, 1998.
32. Miller L: Lymphedema: unlocking the doors to successful treatment, *Innov Oncol Nurs* 10:53, 1994.
33. Loscalzo J, Creager MA, Dzau VJ: *Vascular Medicine*, Boston, 1992, Little, Brown.
34. Kopanski Z and others: Influence of some anthropometric parameters on the risk of development of distal complications after mastectomy carried out because of breast carcinoma, *Am J Hum Biol* 15:433, 2003.
35. Harris SR and others: Clinical practice guidelines for the care and treatment of breast cancer: lymphedema, *CMAJ* 164:191, 2001.
36. Hunter MS and others: Menopausal symptoms in women with breast cancer: prevalence and treatment preferences, *Psychooncology* 13:769, 2004.
37. Gold EB and others: Relation of demographic and lifestyle factors to symptoms in a multi-racial/ethnic population of women 40-55 years of age, *Am J Epidemiol* 152:463, 2000.
38. Sternfeld B, Quesenberry CP, Jr., Husson G: Habitual physical activity and menopausal symptoms: a case-control study, *J Womens Health* 8:115, 1999.
39. Aiello EJ and others: Effect of a yearlong, moderate-intensity exercise intervention on the occurrence and severity of menopause symptoms in postmenopausal women, *Menopause* 11:382, 2004.
40. Demark-Wahnefried W, Rimer B, Winer E: Weight gain in women diagnosed with breast cancer, *J Am Diet Assoc* 97:519, 1997.
41. Chlebowski RT, Aiello E, McTiernan A: Weight loss in breast cancer patient management, *J Clin Oncol* 20:1128, 2002.
42. Aslani A and others: Changes in body composition during breast cancer chemotherapy with the CMF-regimen, *Breast Cancer Res Treat* 57:285, 1999.
43. Demark-Wahnefried W and others: Reduced rates of metabolism and decreased physical activity in breast cancer patients receiving adjuvant chemotherapy, *Am J Clin Nutr* 65:1495, 1997.
44. Courneya KS, Friedenreich CM: Relationship between

exercise pattern across the cancer experience and current quality of life in colorectal cancer survivors, *J Altern Complement Med* 3:215-226, 1997.

45. Irwin ML and others: Effect of exercise on total and intra-abdominal body fat in postmenopausal women: a randomized controlled trial, *JAMA* 289:323, 2003.
46. Demark-Wahnefried W and others: Reduced rates of metabolism and decreased physical activity in breast cancer patients receiving adjuvant chemotherapy, *Am J Clin Nutr* 65:1495, 1997.
47. Demark-Wahnefried W and others: Changes in weight, body composition, and factors influencing energy balance among premenopausal breast cancer patients receiving adjuvant chemotherapy, *J Clin Oncol* 19:2381, 2001.
48. Kutynec CL and others: Energy balance in women with breast cancer during adjuvant treatment, *J Am Diet Assoc* 99:1222, 1999.
49. Rock C and others: Factors associated with weight gain in women after diagnosis of breast cancer. Women's Healthy Eating and Living Study Group, *J Am Diet Assoc* 99:1212, 1999.
50. Goodwin P and others: Multidisciplinary weight management in locoregional breast cancer: results of a phase II study, *Breast Cancer Res Treat* 48:53, 1998.
51. Brown JK and others: Nutrition and physical activity during and after cancer treatment: an American Cancer Society guide for informed choices, *CA Cancer J Clin* 53:268, 2003.
52. ACSM: Position stand on osteoporosis and exercise, *Med Sci Sports Exerc* 27:i, 1995.
53. Rapado A: Prevention early after menopause: non-hormonal intervention. In: Geusens P, editor: *Osteoporosis in clinical practice: a practical guide for diagnosis and treatment*, Glasgow, 1998, Springer-Verlag London.
54. Slemenda CW: Adult bone loss. In: Marcus R, editor: *Osteoporosis*, Cambridge, 1994, Blackwell Scientific.
55. Rubin CT, Lanyon LE: Regulation of bone formation by applied dynamic loads, *J Bone Joint Surg* 66:397, 1984.
56. Daniell HW and others: Progressive osteoporosis during androgen deprivation therapy, *J Urol* 163:181, 2000.
57. Gross GJ and others: Postmenopausal breast cancer survivors at risk for osteoporosis: physical activity, vigor, and vitality, *Oncol Nurs Forum* 29:1295, 2002.
58. Tillmann V and others: Male sex and low physical activity are associated with reduced spine bone mineral density in survivors of childhood acute lymphoblastic leukemia, *J Bone Miner Res* 17:1073, 2002.
59. Waltman NL and others: Testing an intervention for preventing osteoporosis in postmenopausal breast cancer survivors, *J Nurs Scholarsh* 35:333, 2003.
60. Warner JT and others: Relative osteopenia after treatment for acute lymphoblastic leukemia, *Pediatr Res* 45:544, 1999.
61. Rutherford OM: Is there a role for exercise in the prevention of osteoporotic fractures?, *Br J Sports Med* 33:378, 1999.
62. Bonaiuti D and others: Exercise for preventing and treating osteoporosis in postmenopausal women, *Cochrane Database of Syst Rev* 3:CD000333, 2002.
63. Vainionpaa A and others: Effects of high-impact exercise on bone mineral density: a randomized controlled trial in premenopausal women, *Osteoporosis Int* 16:191-197, 2005.
64. Anderson-Hanley C and others: Neuropsychological effects of treatments for adults with cancer: a meta-analysis and review of the literature, *J Int Neuropsychol Soc* 9:967, 2003.
65. Tannock IF and others: Cognitive impairment associated with chemotherapy for cancer: report of a workshop, *J Clin Oncol* 22:2233, 2004.
66. Karki A and others: Efficacy of physical therapy methods and exercise after a breast cancer option: a systematic review, *Crit Rev Phys Rehab Med* 13:159, 2001.
67. Courneya KS: Exercise in cancer survivors: an overview of research, *Med Sci Sports Exerc* 35:1846, 2003.
68. Colcombe S, Kramer AF: Fitness effects on the cognitive function of older adults: a meta-analytic study, *Psychol Sci* 14:125, 2003.
69. Pinto BM, Maruyama NC: Exercise in the rehabilitation of breast cancer survivors, *Psychooncology* 8:191, 1999.
70. Pinto BM and others: Psychological and fitness changes associated with exercise participation among women with breast cancer, *Psychooncology* 12:118, 2003.
71. Stoll O, Alfermann D: Effects of physical exercise on resources evaluation, body self-concept and well-being among older adults, *Anxiety, Stress & Coping* 15:311, 2002.
72. Adame DD and others: Physical fitness in relation to amount of physical exercise, body image, and locus of control among college men and women, *Percept Mot Skills* 70:1347, 1990.
73. Blanchard CM and others: A comparison of physical activity of posttreatment breast cancer survivors and noncancer controls, *Behav Med* 28:140, 2003.
74. Courneya KS, Friedenreich CM: Relationship between exercise during treatment and current quality of life among survivors of breast cancer, *J Psychosoc Oncol* 15:35, 1997.
75. Irwin ML and others: Physical activity levels before and after a diagnosis of breast carcinoma: the Health, Eating, Activity, and Lifestyle (HEAL) study, *Cancer* 97:1746, 2003.
76. Blanchard CM and others: Determinants of exercise intention and behavior in survivors of breast and prostate cancer: an application of the theory of planned behavior, *Cancer Nurs* 25:88, 2002.
77. Courneya KS, Blanchard CM, Laing DM: Exercise adherence in breast cancer survivors training for a dragon boat race competition: a preliminary investigation, *Psychooncology* 10:444, 2001.
78. Courneya KS, Friedenreich CM: Utility of the theory of planned behavior for understanding exercise during breast cancer treatment, *Psychooncology* 8:112, 1999.
79. Jones LW and others: Effects of an oncologist's recommendation to exercise on self-reported exercise behavior in newly diagnoses breast cancer survivors: a single-blind, randomized controlled trial, *Ann Behav Med* 28:105, 2004.
80. Jones LW and others: Does the theory of planned behavior mediate the effects of an oncologist's recommendation to exercise in newly diagnosed breast cancer survivors? Results from a randomized controlled trial, *Health Psychol* 24:189, 2005.
81. American Cancer Society: *Cancer facts and figures 2004*, Atlanta, 2004, American Cancer Society.
82. Courneya KS and others: Physical activity in cancer survivors: implications for recurrence and mortality, *Cancer Ther* 2:1, 2004.

83. Courneya KS, Mackey JR, Quinney HA: Neoplasms. In Humphrey R, editor: *ACSM's resources for clinical exercise physiology: musculoskeletal, neuromuscular, neoplastic, immunologic, and hematologic conditions*, Baltimore, 2002, Lippincott Williams & Wilkins.
84. Courneya KS, Mackey JR, McKenzie DC: Exercise for breast cancer survivors: research evidence and clinical guidelines, *Physician Sportsmed* 30:33, 2002.
85. Courneya KS, Friedenreich CM: Relationship between exercise pattern across the cancer experience and current quality of life in colorectal cancer survivors, *J Altern Complement Med* 215, 1997.
86. Jones LW, Courneya KS: Exercise counseling and programming preferences of cancer survivors, *Cancer Pract* 10:208, 2002.
87. Pate RR and others: Physical activity and public health. A recommendation from the Centers for Disease Control and Prevention and the American College of Sports Medicine, *JAMA* 273:402, 1995.

CHAPTER

21 Complementary and Alternative Medicine (CAM)

Georgia M. Decker

INTRODUCTION AND OVERVIEW

There are multiple definitions for complementary and alternative medicine (CAM) therapies. A selection of these definitions is presented in Table 21-1.

It is the interchangeable use of the terms *complementary* and *alternative* that has contributed to miscommunication and misunderstanding between patients and health care professionals. CAM is referred to as *integrative*, *integrated*, or *complementary* when therapies are *combined* with conventional approaches, and it is termed *alternative* or *unconventional* when these therapies are used *instead* of conventional approaches. The Oncology Nursing Society (ONS) Position Paper entitled "The Use of Complementary and Alternative Therapies in Cancer Care" promotes standardizing terminology to enhance communication.[1]

There is a continued and lasting interest in CAM therapies in the US that has been confirmed by national surveys.[2,3] Medical advances, legislative action and public education in the mid 1970s to the 1980s did not dissuade patients from seeking CAM in the US.[4] The Office of Alternative Medicine (OAM) was established in 1992 and later, in 1998, became the National Center for Complementary and Alternative Medicine (NCCAM) to address the ever-increasing number of significant issues associated with CAM. NCCAM is one of 27 institutes and centers that make up the National Institutes of Health (NIH), and the NIH is one of eight agencies under the Public Health Service (PHS) in the Department of Health and Human Services (DHHS). There are four focus areas for NCCAM: research (clinical and basic science research), training and career development and exhibits, the information clearinghouse, and integration (of scientifically proven CAM practices into conventional medicine).[1,5] To enhance quality cancer research and information about CAM use, the National Cancer Institute (NCI) established the Office of Cancer Complementary and Alternative Medicine (OCCAM) in 1998. The OCCAM promotes and supports research within CAM disciplines and therapies as they relate to the prevention, diagnosis, and treatment of cancer, cancer-related symptoms, and side effects of conventional cancer treatment. The OCCAM coordinates the NCI's CAM research and informational activities and collaboration with other governmental and nongovernmental organizations on cancer CAM issues, and provides an interface with health practitioners and researchers regarding cancer CAM issues.[6,7]

In March 2000, the White House Commission on Complementary and Alternative Medicine Policy (WHCCAMP) was established to address those issues related to access and delivery of CAM, research priorities, and the need for public and professional education. WHCCAMP endorsed 10 principles described in Box 21-1.[8]

Table 21-1 Definitions of CAM

Source	Definition
Gevitz[44]	Practices that are not accepted as correct, proper, or appropriate or not in conformity with the beliefs or standards of the dominant group of medical practitioners in a society
Eisenberg and others[2]	Interventions not taught widely in medical schools or generally available in hospitals
Segen[45]	Alternative health care systems constitute an array of treatments and ideologies that are based on no common or consistent philosophy. Three groups of philosophies are (1) formal therapeutic systems such as traditional Chinese medicine, (2) informal therapeutic systems such as mind-body medicine, and (3) quackery involving potentially predatory practices in which the therapist or developed has been found guilty of fraud.
Cassileth and Vickers and Vickers and Cassileth[46,47]	CAM is an umbrella term used to describe diverse techniques. Unproven methods (alternative therapies for cancer treatment) should be distinguished from complementary methods applied to mainstream care for symptom management and to enhance QOL.
Ernst[48]	CAM is any approach to improve a health problem that is not used or taught routinely to conventional Western practitioners. Alternative cancer treatments are CAM therapies that reduce tumor burden or replace mainstream therapy.
Oncology Nursing Society[1]	CAM involves the interchangeable use of the terms "complementary," "alternative," and "integrative" therapies reflecting what may describe a therapy rather than how it is used. "Complementary" describes a therapy that is used with a conventional therapy, whereas "alternative" describes a therapy that is used "instead of" conventional therapy. "Integrative care" is defined as a combination of complementary and conventional approaches to care.
NCCAM[5]	CAM is a group of diverse medical and health care systems, practices, and products that are not currently considered to be a part of conventional medicine. Complementary medicine is used with conventional medicine. Alternative medicine is used in place of conventional medicine. Integrative medicine combines mainstream and CAM therapies for which scientific evidence of safety and efficacy exists.
Institute of Medicine, 2005 (www.iom.edu/report.asp?id=24487)	Complementary and alternative medicine (CAM) is a broad domain of resources that encompass health systems, modalities, and practices and their accompanying theories and beliefs, other than those intrinsic to the dominant health system of a particular society or culture in a given historical period. CAM includes such resources perceived by their users as associated with positive health outcomes. Boundaries within CAM and between the CAM domain and the domain of the dominant system are not always sharp or fixed.

The Institute of Medicine (IOM) of the National Academies (a nongovernmental agency) was established in 1970 and guarantees unbiased, evidence-based information and advice concerning health and science policy to policy-makers, health care professionals, and the public. In 2003 and 2004, the IOM sponsored seven committee meetings to explore scientific, policy, and practice questions that arise from the increasing use of CAM by the American public.[9]

Box 21-1 The White House Commission on CAM Guiding Principles[8,28]

- A wholeness orientation in health care delivery: delivery of high quality health care must include supportive care of the whole person.
- Evidence of safety and efficacy: use science to generate evidence that protects and promotes public health.
- Healing capacity of a person: support capacity for recovery and self-healing.
- Respect for individuality: each person has the right to health care that is responsive, respects preferences, and preserves dignity.
- Right to choose treatment: each person has the right to choose freely among safe and effective approaches and among qualified practitioners.
- Emphasis on health promotion and self-care: good health care emphasizes self-care and early interventions for maintaining and promoting health.
- Partnerships in integrated health care: good health care requires teamwork among patients, HCP, and researchers committed to creating healing environments and respecting diversity of health care traditions.
- Education as a fundamental health care service: education about prevention, healthy lifestyles, and self-healing should be part of the curriculum of all HCP and made available to the public.
- Dissemination of comprehensive, timely information: health care quality is enhanced by examination of the evidence on which CAM systems, practices, and products are based. This information should be widely, rapidly, and easily available.
- Integral public involvement: input from informed consumers must be incorporated in proposing priorities for health care, research, and policy decisions.

HCP, Health care professional.

BACKGROUND EVIDENCE

What we know about these therapies is increasing. Nevertheless, much remains to be determined concerning the safety, efficacy, potential benefits, and adverse effects of specific CAM therapies in connection with specific diseases and treatments in specific populations. Initial surveys were not disease- or population-specific. By the end of the 1990s we knew more about the use of CAM by specific populations with cancer.[10-13] Additional research described CAM use specific to those in urban, suburban, and rural areas and the elderly.[14-19]

A CAM therapy survey in patients with cancer who were participating in clinical trials reported in 2000 that these patients used the following: spirituality (94%), imagery (86%), massage (80%), lifestyle, diet and nutrition interventions (60%), herbal/botanical (20%), and high-dose vitamins (14%).[20] Other researchers have reported use of these therapies at a rate of 50% to 83%.[21] Bridevaux[22] reported that mean out-of-pocket payments per visit for specific CAM therapies include $9.00 for spiritual healing, $23.00 for herbal therapies, $33.00 for massage, $44.00 for acupuncture, and $49.00 for nutritional counseling. This author suggests that the value placed on these therapies is reflected in the amount of money a consumer is willing to pay.[22] Consumers spent $27 billion out-of-pocket dollars on CAM practitioner services from 1990 to 1997. This reflected an increase of 45.2% in dollars spent from 1990 to 1997.[3]

Individuals who use CAM are more likely to be female and better educated, and have higher incomes.[3] Swisher[11] used a cross-sectional design in studying CAM use among women with gynecologic cancer and reported that characteristics associated with CAM use included annual incomes greater than $30,000, cancer site of origin other than cervix, and use of CAM before cancer diagnosis. Respondent reasons for using CAM were (1) hope of improved well-being and (2) possible anticancer effects of the particular CAM modalities used. Reported reasons for seeking CAM therapies remain consistent. These include the sharing of similar philosophical beliefs about what constitutes the active patient role, use of natural and less toxic treatments, similar spiritual beliefs, positive relationship with the therapist (e.g., time for discussion, including of emotional aspects), and increased well-being.[16,23,24] Some authors suggest that the appeal of CAM is related to a perceived association of CAM with nature, focus on energy forces promoting vitalism, intellectual traditions, sophisticated philosophies, and the blending of the physical and spiritual realms.[23,25] Reasons for the reduction in the use of conventional medicine in favor of CAM included dissatisfaction with contemporary health care system (ineffective therapies, adverse effects, poor communication), insufficient time with and insufficient access to health care professionals, desperation, and cost of care.[23,24] Stevinson[23] reports that patients have consistently expressed a desire to manage their health by actively participating in treatment decisions that involve solely conventional, solely CAM, or a combination of both therapies.

The NCCAM[5] classifies CAM therapies into 5 domains: 1) alternative medical systems, 2) biologically based therapies, 3) mind-body interventions, 4) manipulative and body-based methods, and 5) energy therapies. The NCI's OCCAM increased the NCCAM domains to include 3 additional categories: movement therapy and pharmacologic and biologic treatments, with a subcategory of complex natural products and a miscellaneous domain.[6] Table 21-2 describes these domains and identifies those modalities currently in clinical trials.

EVIDENCE-BASED PRACTICE AND CAM

A common criticism of CAM made by conventional biomedical practitioners is the lack of scientifically conducted research. Evidence of effectiveness is critical to widespread support of the use of CAM just as with conventional interventions.[26] Researchers and clinicians rely on levels of evidence to evaluate the extent to which interventions meet preestablished criteria. Clinical practice guidelines are an outcome of level of evidence data and are used as a foundation for recommendations for the care of patients with specific conditions.[27] Although these guidelines involve value judgments as to how patients should be managed, the basis is a systematic review of the research focusing on the strength of the evidence. Previously, guidelines focused on the effectiveness of interventions. Recently, more attention has been given to the magnitude of the effect and the balance between the effect and any harm and costs to the patient.[28] The classification system developed by the NCI PDQ Adult Treatment Editorial Board ranks human cancer treatment studies according to the statistical strength of the study design and specific scientific strength of the treatment outcomes. The NCI PDQ classification has been adopted for human studies involving CAM treatments. The strength of a study is rank-ordered in descending order from 1 to 4.

Randomized controlled clinical trials (double-blinded or nonblinded) are the gold standard of study design, including CAM studies. Nonrandomized controlled clinical trials include any strategy that would make the patient known to the researcher. Case series, ranking numbers 3 and 4, either population-based or non–population based to a best-case series, are the weakest form of study design. For some CAM modalities, case series may be the only available or practical study design. Table 21-2 lists CAM therapies currently in clinical trials.

Table 21-3 provides examples of the types of current clinical trials that involve conventional and CAM modalities for cancer treatment.[28,29] Levels of evidence in CAM are generated in the same way as in conventional medicine. Positive and negative clinical trial results form the foundation for systematic reviews and metaanalysis. These, in turn, contribute to the development of evidence-based practice and practice guidelines. Levels of evidence are used by organizations such as the ONS (PRISM project), NCI (clinical trials), as well as appearing in databases such as Natural Medicine Comprehensive Database,[30] Natural Standard Database,[31] and the Oxford Centre for Evidence-based Medicine.[32]

Table **21-2** OCCAM DOMAINS OF CAM AND MODALITIES IN CLINICAL TRIALS[28,29]

Domain	Definition	Example(s)	Modality in Clinical Trials[5,49]
Alternative medical systems	Systems built upon completed systems of theory and practice	Traditional Chinese medicine (acupuncture), Ayurveda, homeopathy, naturopathy, Tibetan medicine	Acupuncture Acupressure Electroacupuncture *Traumeel S*
Mind-body interventions	Techniques designed to enhance the mind's capacity to affect bodily function and symptoms	Medication, hypnosis, art therapy, biofeedback, mental healing, imagery, relaxation therapy, support groups, music therapy, cognitive-behavioral therapy, prayer, dance therapy, psychoneuroimmunology, aromatherapy, animal-assisted therapy	Massage therapy
Movement therapy	Assortment of nutrients and nonnutrient and bioactive food components that are used as chemopreventive agents, and the use of specific foods or diets as cancer prevention or treatment strategies	Dietary regimens such as macrobiotics, vegetarian, Gerson therapy, Kelley/Gonzalez regimen, vitamins, dietary macronutrients, supplements, antioxidants, melatonin, selenium, coenzyme Q10, ephedrine, orthomolecular medicine	Energy healing Energy therapy Reiki Touch
Manipulative and body-based methods	Methods based on manipulation and/or movement of one or more parts of the body	Chiropractic, therapeutic massage, osteopathy, reflexology	Distance healing Exercise-based counseling Group therapy Healing touch Music therapy Spirituality, Religiosity Standard counseling Stress management training
Energy therapies	Therapies involving the use of energy fields	QiGong, Reiki, therapeutic touch, pulsed fields, magnet therapy	
Nutritional therapies	Modalities used to improve patterns of bodily movement	T'ai Chi, Feldenkrais, hathayoga, Alexander technique, dance therapy, QiGong, rolfing, Trager method, applied kinesiology,	Black cohosh Creatine Curcumin Flax seed Folic acid Fruit and vegetable extracts Garlic Ginger Herbal therapy

Table 21-2 OCCAM Domains of CAM and Modalities in Clinical Trials[28,29]—cont'd

Domain	Definition	Example(s)	Modality in Clinical Trials[5,49]
Nutritional therapies			Hypericum perforatum Juven L-carnitine Low-fat diet Lycopene Macrobiotic diet Noni fruit extract Nutritional supplements Pomegranate juice Selenium Soy protein isolate *Valeriana officinalis* Vitamins C and E Zinc sulfate
Pharmacologic and biologic treatments	Drugs, complex natural products, vaccines, and other biologic interventions not yet accepted in mainstream medicine, off-label use of prescription drugs	Antineoplastons, products from honey bees, mistletoe, 714-X, low-dose naltrexone, met-enkephalin, immunoaugmentative therapy, laetrile, hydrazine sulfate, Newcastle virus, melatonin, ozone therapy, thymus therapy, enzyme therapy, high-dose vitamin C	Antineoplastons Mistletoe Pancreatic Proteolytic enzymes
Complex natural products	Subcategory of pharmacologic and biologic treatments consisting of an assortment of plant samples (botanicals), extracts of crude natural substances, and unfractionated extracts from marine organisms used for healing and treatment of disease	Herbs and herbal extracts, mixtures of tea polyphenols, shark cartilage, essiac tea, cordyceps, Sun soup, MGN-3	Chinese herbal extract Green tea extract (polyphenon E) Kanglaite injection Milk thistle *Pycnogenol* Shark cartilage *Virulizin*
Miscellaneous	Interventions that have conventional therapeutic applications, are not generally used for cancer treatment promoted by cancer CAM practitioners	Hyperbaric oxygen	Hyperbaric oxygen

Table **21-3** SAMPLE CLINICAL TRIALS INVOLVING CONVENTIONAL AND CAM MODALITIES FOR CANCER TREATMENT[28,29]

Type	Description	Example of Conventional Biomedical Trial	Example of Cancer CAM Trial
Prevention Trials	Study ways to reduce risk of developing cancer	Phase IIB/III randomized chemoprevention study of celexicob in patients with superficial transitional cell carcinoma of the bladder at high risk for recurrence	Phase III randomized study of selenium and vitamin E for the prevention of prostate cancer (SELECT Trial)
Screening Trials	Study ways to detect cancer in people who do not have any symptoms of cancer	Phase II pilot study of CA 125 screening in patients at high risk for ovarian cancer	None at this time
Diagnostic	Study tests or procedures that identify cancer earlier	Phase II/III diagnostic study of C11-methionine and FDG PET imaging in patients with progressive prostate cancer	None at this time
Treatment	Study new therapies or new indications of drug, vaccines, approaches to treatment	Phase II/III randomized study of paclitaxel and carboplatin with or without bevacizumab in patients with advanced, metastatic, or recurrent NSCLC	Phase II study of supplemental treatment with mistletoe in patients with stage IV NSCLC receiving palliative chemotherapy
Supportive care (includes quality of life)	Study ways to improve cancer-related symptoms and quality of life	Phase III randomized study of ocreotide vs. standard care for chemotherapy-induced diarrhea in patients with colorectal cancer	Phase II/III randomized study of ginger for chemotherapy-related nausea in patients with cancer
Genetic studies	Study ways in which genetic makeup can affect detection, diagnosis or treatment response	Genetic study of familial factors in patients with colon cancer	None at this time

FDG, 2(^{18}F) fluoro-2-deoxy-D-glucose; *PET,* positron emission tomography scan; *NSCLC,* non small cell lung cancer.

Evidenced-based practice (EBP) is caring for patients by letting clinical decision-making be guided by the best available evidence resulting from research. This includes defining the question, accessing the information, judging the credibility of the results, and applying these results to the care of patients.[27] Defining EBP for certain CAM therapies can be similar to the same process in conventional medicine and a result of the integration of clinical expertise, epidemiologic studies, and anecdotal evidence. Some authors contend that there cannot be two kinds of medicine—conventional and alternative.[33] Rather, there is one type of medicine: one that is adequately tested (versus one that has not been tested); the reasoning being that once a treatment has been tested rigorously, it does not matter if it was considered *alternative* at the outset. If a modality is found to be reasonable, safe, and effective, it can be accepted into clinical practice. Assertions, speculations, and testimonials are not a substitute for evidence.[33]

The concept of an evidence-based approach to CAM is still in its initial stages. There are data validating an increase in the use of CAM therapies in the US and abroad. However, there remain limited data on safety, efficacy, and mechanism of action of many individual CAM therapies, and until recently most available information was based on theoretical opinion or testimonials rather than evidence. Recommending CAM therapies remains a challenge for health care professionals. More and more, health care professionals receive requests from patients for information regarding CAM therapies for prevention or treatment of medical conditions. Eisenberg[34] offered an algorithm for physicians who must advise patients regarding CAM. The algorithm provides consideration for nurses and other health care professionals.[35] The patient's interest in CAM therapies may intensify when traditional therapies are not providing the desired result.[36] A desire for CAM therapies is complicated by the amount of information available from a variety of nonprofessional sources including the Internet and well-meaning friends and family. Unfortunately, much of this information is inaccurate. Opinions differ, and methods for rating therapies vary even among experts.

Ernst and colleagues strove to establish a base of evidence for CAM and offered a direction-of-evidence model.[37] Ernst uses "direction of evidence" (clearly positive; tentatively positive; uncertain; tentatively negative; clearly negative) and "weight of evidence" (Low; Moderate; High). Eisenberg uses "recommend," "tolerate," and "avoid."[38]

Natural Standard uses an evidence-based validated grading rationale: level of evidence grade reflects the level of available scientific evidence in support of efficacy. Expert opinion and folklore and evidence of harm are shown in a separate section of individual monographs. Table 21-4 describes the Natural Standards level of evidence grades. Selected sources of reliable cancer CAM information are listed in Box 21-2.

Many patients with cancer want to participate in medical decision making. A collaborative approach to decision making will be affected by a variety of factors including age, educational level, social structure of the family, and influence of friends.[39] Obtaining relevant and reliable information can be a challenge for anyone, but for the person who is recently diagnosed and feeling overwhelmed and perhaps fearful, it can be too complicated to manage.[40] The following describes some of the variables that influence a patient's response to the subject of CAM modalities including culture, religion, and age. For example, an older adult may be concerned with modalities that involve touch. This is exemplified by the patient we will call Edith in Box 21-3.

Oncology nurses are participating with greater frequency in conversations with patients regarding the role of nutrition, herbal medicine, and complementary approaches in cancer care. Conversations such as these are leading many oncology health care professionals to consider their moral, ethical, and legal obligation to remain aware of the best available evidence in CAM, present the evidence in patient-friendly terms, and address choices from a comprehensive perspective.[1,41]

Patients with cancer use CAM therapies for cancer treatment and/or symptom management. Oncology nurses are experts in cancer symptom management. And, many believe that an herb or supplement taken for a comorbidity does not endanger the efficacy of their cancer therapy. Montbriand describes categories of herbs and natural products that have the following effects: decrease cancer growth; have the potential to increase cancer growth or recurrence; interfere with cancer therapy; protect against cancer growth;[42] and, possibly, cause cancer and do harm.[43]

Table 21-5 provides examples of herbs and supplements that may influence cancers in women.

COMMONLY USED CAM MODALITIES

Alternative Systems: Acupuncture

In the US, physicians, dentists, and acupuncturists perform acupuncture for a number of health

Table 21-4 NATURAL STANDARD EVIDENCE-BASED VALIDATED GRADING RATIONALE[31]

Level of Evidence Grade	Criteria
A (strong scientific evidence)	Statistically significant evidence of benefit from >2 properly randomized trials (RCTs), OR evidence from one properly conducted RCT AND one properly conducted metaanalysis, OR evidence from multiple RCTs with a clear majority of the properly conducted trials showing statistically significant evidence of benefit AND with supporting evidence in basic science, animal studies, or theory
B (good scientific evidence)	Statistically significant evidence of benefit from 1-2 properly randomized trials, OR evidence of benefit from ≥1 properly conducted metaanalysis OR evidence of benefit from >1 cohort/case-control/nonrandomized trials AND with supporting evidence in basic science, animal studies, or theory
C (unclear or conflicting scientific evidence)	Evidence of benefit from ≥1 small RCT(s) without adequate size, power, statistical significance, or quality of design by objective criteria,* OR conflicting evidence from multiple RCTs without a clear majority of the properly conducted trials showing evidence of benefit or ineffectiveness, OR evidence of benefit from ≥1 cohort/case-control/nonrandomized trials AND without supporting evidence in basic science, animal studies, or theory, OR evidence of efficacy only from basic science, animal studies, or theory
D (fair negative scientific evidence)	Statistically significant negative evidence (i.e., lack of evidence of benefit) from cohort/case-control/nonrandomized trials, AND evidence in basic science, animal studies, or theory suggesting a lack of benefit
F (strong negative scientific evidence)	Statistically significant negative evidence (i.e., lack of evidence of benefit) from ≥1 properly randomized adequately powered trial(s) of high-quality design by objective criteria*
Lack of evidence	Unable to evaluate efficacy due to lack of adequate available human data

*Objective criteria are derived from validated instruments for evaluating study quality, including the 5-point scale developed by Jadad and others.[31]

conditions. The foundation of the therapy is that *qi* (pronounced "chee," meaning *energy*) is present at birth and is maintained throughout one's life. *Qi* flows throughout the body via 12 major pathways known as *meridians*. There are approximately 350 acupoints along 12 meridians, with additional acupoints that occur outside the meridian pathways. Typically, it involves insertion of a needle into the skin in a number of specific sites (acupoints) along a *meridian*. Acupoint stimulation may also be accomplished through the use of electrical current, laser, moxibustion, pressure, ultrasound, and vibration. There are Japanese, Korean, and Chinese types of acupuncture. Health is believed to be a balance of yin and yang (opposite forces present in everyone), and *disease* is a result of imbalance caused by a blockage or deficiency of energy. Acupuncture theory is based on the belief that stimulating the appropriate acupoints helps the body to correct any imbalance in the flow of energy and restores balance. It is important that changes in the balance of energy and flow of *qi* be identified before disease has developed. Therefore, acupuncture has a role in the prevention of illness and maintenance of health. It is routinely used in Eastern countries and has also been integrated with allopathic and osteopathic medicine in the US.[14,37]

Strength of Evidence

The diagnostic value of acupuncture has not been established.[36,37] Although there is no evidence of the physical existence of *qi* or meridians, there is

Box 21-2 Selected Sources of Reliable Cancer CAM Information

SPONSORED WEBSITES

American Cancer Society
www.cancer.org

American Society for Clinical Oncology
www.asco.org

National Institutes of Health
www.nih.gov

Cancer Information Service
http://cis.nci.nih.gov

Office of Cancer Complementary and Alternative Medicine
www.cancer.gov/occam

National Center for Complementary and Alternative Medicine
www.nccam.nih.gov

Office of Dietary Supplements
www.ods.od.nih.gov

Medline Plus
www.medlineplus.gov

Cancer Patient Education Network
www.cancerpatienteducation.org

People Living with Cancer
www.plwc.org

The Rosenthal Center for Complementary and Alternative Medicine
www.rosenthal.hs.columbia.edu

SELECTED SPONSORED DATABASES

ClinicalTrials.gov
www.clinicaltrials.gov/ct

Complementary and Alternative Medicine and Pain Database (University of Maryland School of Medicine)
www.campain.umm.edu/News.html

Food & Drug Administration
www.fda.gov

American Botanical Council's Herbalgram.org
www.herbalgram.org

Office of Dietary Supplements: International Bibliographic Information on Dietary Supplements
http://dietary-supplements.info.nih.gov/databases/ibids.html

Micromedex Healthcare Series
www.micromedex.com/products/hcs

Natural Medicine
www.naturaldatabase.com

Natural Standard
www.naturalstandard.com

PDQ: NCI's Comprehensive Cancer Database
www.cancer.gov/cancerinfo/pdq

The Cochrane Collaboration
www.cochrane.org/index0.htm

Box 21-3 CAM Exemplar

At the time of our meeting, Edith was 80 years young and had chronic myalgias and arthralgias related to her diagnoses of osteoporosis and fibromyalgia. Edith is a long-time breast cancer (more than 20 years) and colon cancer (15 years) survivor who had been persuaded by her youngest child, Patricia, to try Reiki therapy. Edith was saying Reiki but was thinking, massage. At the time of her appointment, Edith was very shocked and relieved to learn that she could keep her clothing on during the session. As the Reiki Master positioned herself, it became apparent to Edith that there had been some sort of misunderstanding, and she was fairly certain that this misunderstanding was ours. The Reiki Master again explained the components of the session, and Edith was stunned. She had envisioned a massage session and she had not heard the differences when they were explained. She politely said that she would "pass" on her gift certificate. We offered her the opportunity to observe a Reiki session and she agreed—reluctantly. She appeared to be awed when watching the Reiki Master and would repeatedly put her hands between the "patient" and the hands of the practitioner. She said she was trying to feel the universal energy (see Table 21-6). She ultimately decided to experience Reiki and subsequently became increasing enamored with it. Edith is now 84 years young and a Reiki practitioner working toward a Reiki Master.[50]

Table 21-5 Examples of Commonly Used Herbs or Natural Products[42,43,91]

Herb/ Supplement	Has Been Used for/as	Implications for Oncology	Other Potential Adverse Reactions
Alfalfa	Diuretic, diabetes, thyroid dysfunction, kidney and bladder conditions	Can interfere with hormone-sensitive cancers; high doses associated with pancytopenia	Photosensitivity
Beer and alcoholic beverages	Prevention of heart disease, Alzheimer's disease, cancer, gallstones, kidney stones	More than 1 drink per day increases mortality among women with breast cancer, increases risk for cancer of the larynx, mouth, esophagus, and larynx	3 or more per day can lead to physical dependence, malnutrition, amnesia, dementia, somnolence, cardiomyopathy, cirrhosis
Beta carotene	To decrease exercise-induced asthma, for age-related macular degeneration, prevent cardiovascular disease, and cancer	Smokers who take more than 20 mg per day increase their risk for lung cancer	Oranging of skin
Black cohosh/ blue cohosh	"Natural" hormone replacement, menopausal symptoms	Laboratory tests show no proliferation of estrogen-positive breast cancer cells; human studies needed; may interfere with tamoxifen	
Chasteberry	Menopause and menopausal symptoms, acne, infertility (female) fibrocystic breasts, and prevention of miscarriage	Influences estrogen levels	Minor changes in menstrual flow
Coffee	Fatigue, mental clarity	May increase the risk for breast cancer in obese women and ovarian and pancreatic cancers in all women	Increases total cholesterol when consumption exceed 1 liter/day; also increases LDL and triglycerides
DHEA	Prevention of heart disease, breast cancer, and diabetes	Involved in metabolism of precursor of estrogens and androgens and should be avoided by women with hormone sensitive cancers	Acne, hair loss, hirsutism, voice deepening, insulin resistance, hepatic dysfunction, abdominal pain, hypertension

Table 21-5 Examples of Commonly Used Herbs or Natural Products[42,43,91]—cont'd

Herb/ Supplement	Has Been Used for/as	Implications for Oncology	Other Potential Adverse Reactions
Flax seed oil	Constipation; bladder inflammations; antiestrogen effects may inhibit the growth of hormone-dependent cancer; may protect postmenopausal women against breast cancer by causing increase in excretion of estrogen metabolites	Hormone-sensitive breast cancer	Impairs the absorption of all oral drugs, without adequate fluids seeds can cause intestinal blockage
Folic acid (folate)	Wellness	Prevention of colon and cervical cancers	High doses can worsen neuropathy associated with B12 deficiency
Ginseng (American, Siberian, Panax)	Atherosclerosis, blood disorders, cancer, colitis, memory loss, fatigue	All types are estrogenic and should be avoided by women with hormone-sensitive cancer	Interferes with antidiabetic agents; has anticoagulant properties, therefore avoid with herbs and drugs with anticoagulant action/ properties; insomnia; mastalgia, vaginal bleeding
Glucosamine (hydrochloride, sulfate)	Osteoarthritis, weight loss	Can induce resistance to etoposide and doxorubicin (by inhibiting topoisomerase II (needed for DNA replication in tumor cells); demonstrated in colon, ovarian and breast cancers	None reported
Green tea	Prevention of cancer and immune enhancement	May be preventive for colon, breast and gastric cancers in small quantities; large quantities associated with esophageal cancer	Headache, diuresis, anxiety, insomnia, tremor, arrythmias, nausea, vomiting, tinnitus, elevated blood sugar, convulsions, delirium

Continued

Table 21-5 Examples of Commonly Used Herbs or Natural Products[42,43,91]—cont'd

Herb/ Supplement	Has Been Used for/as	Implications for Oncology	Other Potential Adverse Reactions
Melatonin	Treatment of the breast, lung, brain, head, gastrointestinal tract	Can decrease cytokine-induced hypotension in patients with cancer, beneficial in stabilizing solid tumor disease when not responsive to treatment, improves survival in advanced solid tumors of the breast, gastrointestinal tract, kidney, liver, lung, melanoma Has been used with chemotherapy, radiation therapy for cancer treatment	Can cause headaches, transient depression, daytime fatigue, drowsiness, abdominal pain, irritability
Milk thistle	Gastrointestinal and hepatic conditions, prostate cancer	Parts of plant enhance estradiol binding to estrogen receptors, thereby enhancing estradiol-induced transcription activity in estrogen-responsive cells; therefore should be avoided by women with hormone-sensitive tumors	Allergic reactions including pruritis, rash, urticaria, eczema, anaphylaxis
Omega-6 fatty acids (vegetable oils)	Prevention of heart disease, lower cholesterol, and reduce risk for cancer	Some studies suggest they may play a role in the development of breast cancer, whereas others suggest a prevention of breast and prostate cancers	
Pau d'arco	Treatment of breast cancer, Candida albicans, vital and parasitic infections	May be helpful in the treatment of sarcomas	High doses associated with diarrhea, dizziness, anemia, and/or hemorrhage
Shark liver oil	Treatment of leukemia and other cancers	Has antiangiogenetic properties in certain cancers: cutaneous lesions, kidney and urinary bladder cancers	

Table **21-5** EXAMPLES OF COMMONLY USED HERBS OR NATURAL PRODUCTS[42,43,91]—CONT'D

Herb/ Supplement	Has Been Used for/as	Implications for Oncology	Other Potential Adverse Reactions
St. John's wort	Mood disturbances, anxiety, mild to moderate depression	A component (hyperforin) appears to inhibit certain cancer cells	Contraindicated in severe depression; interferes with drugs including etoposide, paclitaxel, vinblatine, vincristine, vindesine, calcium channel blockers, glucocorticoids, fentanyl, ondansetron, and many others

LDL, Low-density lipoproteins; *DHEA*, dehydroepiandrosterone.

evidence that the effects of acupuncture are more than placebo.[37] Opioid peptides, serotonin, and other neurotransmitters are released by acupuncture.[52-54] Acupuncture is used for pain and other musculoskeletal system disorders, headaches, stress, ENT conditions including sinusitis, tinnitus and vertigo, allergies, dental pain, addictions, and immune system support. It is commonly used for chronic pain. Conclusive evidence exists that acupuncture is effective in the treatment of dental pain and postoperative nausea.[55] Evidence is considered by some authors inconclusive for acupuncture use in the treatment of asthma, neck pain, drug dependency, fibromyalgia, migraine and tension headaches, neck pain, osteoarthritis, menopausal symptoms, and stroke.[36] Others suggest that the evidence is equivocal and/or promising for some indications, including addiction, stroke rehabilitation, postoperative and chemotherapy related nausea and vomiting, tennis elbow, carpal tunnel syndrome, and asthma[53-56]

Contraindications

The "needling" technique is contraindicated in patients with severe bleeding disorders or those at increased risk for infection as in neutropenia. Treatment for nausea may be an exception.[57] Some authors suggest that patients with cardiac pacemakers should not be treated with electrical stimulation.[58] Caution is advised and some authors recommend that the first treatment be administered with the patient supine. Some patients become drowsy and therefore should be cautioned to take care in operating machinery after a treatment. Needles should not be reused and strict asepsis must be maintained. Side effects may include bleeding, bruising, pain with needling, and worsening of symptoms. Reported adverse events are rare but include pneumothorax and death.[58]

Opportunities

There is evidence that, with accurate diagnosis, acupuncture is safe under certain conditions. It may be more effective than placebo when administered by an appropriately trained practitioner.[37]

Practitioners

In the US, acupuncturists can be certified in two ways: through completion of a formal, full-time educational program that includes both classroom and clinical hours; or participation in an apprenticeship program. The acupuncturist must also complete a "clean needle technique" approved course. Medical doctors with training in acupuncture can also obtain board certification. The National Certification Commission of Acupuncture and Oriental Medicine (NCCAOM) established standards for certification that are accepted by some states for licensure. Some states require medical referral, while others allow nonmedical practitioners to see patients without a referral (www.nccaom.org). A comparison of licensed vs. certified acupuncturists is available at www.asny.org. Medical doctors must possess a valid medical license and be certified through the American Academy of Medical Acupuncture (www.medicalacupuncture.org).

Energy Therapies: QiGong

QiGong (pronounced "Chi Kung") means "Energy Cultivation" and refers to movements believed to improve health, longevity, and harmony within oneself and the world.[59] There are thousands of such movements, and QiGong may include any done with the intention of enhancing energy. It is based on four common principles, sometimes referred to as the "secrets" of QiGong: mind (the presence of intention), eyes (the focus of intention), movement (the action of intention), and breath (the flow of intention).There are numerous styles that may include meditation, exercise, and self massage.[37] Mastery is achieved through harmonious existence and action in all situations. Mastery exhibits as a willingness to continue learning despite the level of expertise. There are numerous books and teachers professing to teach the secrets of QiGong. Authors agree that it is actually defined by a person's willing to practice and experience.[37,59] There are 24 rules for QiGong practice.[60]

Strength of Evidence

There are approximately 100 randomized clinical trials reported in Medline from 1997 to 2004 using QiGong for various conditions. Two trials involved patients with cancer (inspiratory muscle training and relief of breathlessness). Four meta-analyses from 1997 to 2004 examine the use of QiGong for respiratory-related conditions.[61,62]

Contraindications

Psychosis has been reported. It is not known if this was a latent condition.[37,63]

Opportunities

Yang has predicted the use of QiGong in the treatment of arthritis.[60] Ernst and colleagues suggest that QiGong can be used for health promotion, as well as for functional disorders and symptom control.[37]

Practitioners

Because it is considered a form of Chinese medicine, those credentialed in acupuncture and/or Asian medicine are appropriate practitioners.

Energy Therapies: Reiki

Reiki means *universal life energy*. It is an ancient form of healing. The practitioner is a conduit for the movement of energy. It is energy—not the healer—that influences healing. In this respect, Reiki differs from other healing systems; energy travels through and not from the healer. It is said to alleviate physical, emotional, and spiritual blockages.[64] Energy is considered pure because it is not influenced by the practitioner's faith or religion.[64] The practitioner gently places his/her hands on the client in a particular series of positions. Typically, up to 5 minutes are spent on each of the 12 positions, although this may vary based on a client's needs. The client remains fully clothed at all times and there is no pressure, massage, or manipulation applied. The environment is kept quiet and soothing, and the client should emerge feeling relaxed. Reiki is considered to be capable of healing because it works at the very fundamental levels of reality. Even though the capability is there, it is not always successful. Limits seem to be in the recipient's willingness to cast off old habits and patterns, to accept change, and to accept healing.[37] Ernst and colleagues[36] consider Reiki to be a form of spiritual healing.

Strength of Evidence

Reiki is believed to be helpful in the treatment of chronic pain and emotional problems,[37] decreasing stress, and increasing vitality.[64] It can be used when massage is not possible or is contraindicated.[64] A significant body of anecdotal literature and two randomized controlled trials suggest that Reiki may be an effective treatment for fibromyalgia by relieving pain and improving psychologic well-being.[64]

Contraindications

None are known.[37] Caution must be used in choosing a practitioner.

Opportunities

Reiki appears to have no adverse effects and can eventually be self-administered, making it a low-risk, low-cost, potentially patient-empowering intervention.[5] There are clinical trials sponsored by the National Center for Complementary and Alternative Medicine.

Practitioners

Reiki is taught in three parts. Reiki I may be the most intense due to the volume of content: history of Reiki, Reiki hand positions, Reiki symbols including their names and how to draw and use them for specific conditions, and meditation manifestation. Reiki II is intense training using advanced techniques. Reiki II usually includes a review of Reiki I. Reiki III (Master) includes a review of previous training and information for long-distance healing, scanning techniques, more meditation techniques, and an additional Reiki symbol. Typically, there is a Reiki attunement at the end of the course in addition to others during the course. Information on Reiki and Reiki practitioners is at Awareness I at the Reiki Institute.

Energy Therapies: Magnetic Field Therapy

In magnetic field therapy, magnetic fields are applied to parts of the body that may be permanent or pulsed. It is sometimes used in conjunction with acupuncture.[37] Permanent magnetic fields are sometimes referred to as electromagnets.[65] Some enthusiasts for this therapy feel that it has enormous therapeutic potential.[66]

Strength of Evidence

Animal studies have suggested that there is a possible application of magnetic field therapy in the treatment of stroke. Most controlled studies used magnetic field therapy for diagnosis, not treatment.[36] Currently, magnets are accepted and incorporated into medical practice in Germany, Japan, Israel, Russia, and about 45 other countries for treatment of arthritis, back pain, bursitis, carpal tunnel syndrome, headaches, and other inflammatory conditions.[65] There is growing evidence that magnetic field therapy is an effective approach to pain treatment.[66]

Contraindications

Magnetic field therapy is contraindicated during pregnancy and in those with pacemakers, myasthenia gravis, and bleeding disorders.[37]

Opportunities

The FDA has approved magnetic field therapy for use with nonunion of fractures.[37,66]

Practitioners

Magnetic field therapy is used primarily in conjunction with acupuncture or by licensed acupuncturists.

Mind-body Interventions: Aromatherapy

Aromatherapy is the controlled use of plant essences for therapeutic purposes.[52] *Essential oil* is the aromatic essence of a plant in oil or resin form derived from plant leaf, stalk, bark, root, flower, fruit, or seeds. *Carrier* is the diluent used to dilute concentrated essential oil for application. The *neat* is the direct application of essential oil compound (essential oil plus carrier) to the skin. The *note* is the unique aromatic variable of essential oil used when blending combinations of essential oil compounds: *top note* is bright, *middle note* is lingering, and *base note* is grounding.[67] Essential oils can be applied directly to the skin through compress or massage, inhaled via a diffuser or steaming water, or added directly to bath water. There are about 150 essential oils.[68] The mechanism of the action begins with the olfactory sense. After sensing smell, the limbic system is activated into retrieving learned memories. Essential oils are also absorbed via the dermal route and subcutaneous fat into the bloodstream. Entry via the oral route into the digestive system is not recommended. Aromatherapy is often practiced with massage and used in palliative-care settings to improve quality of life for patients with cancer.[37]

Strength of Evidence

Published data on dosing, comparative methods of administration, and therapeutic outcomes for aromatherapy is limited. In a systematic review of 12 clinical trials, 6 suggested it had a relaxing effect.[69,70] There were measured responses of 17 patients with cancer to humidified essential lavender oil, with a positive change noted in blood pressure, pulse, pain, anxiety, depression, and sense of well-being after both humidified water treatment and lavender treatment.[71] Studies have compared drop size between 6 different essential oils and reported bottles differed in delivery method and have recommended universal measure standardization to ensure equity and safety in administration. Massage and aromatherapy massage offer short-term benefits for psychologic well-being, with the effect on anxiety supported by limited evidence.[72] There is conflicting evidence as to whether aromatherapy enhances the effects of massage.[72] In 2003, a Cochrane Database was performed involving aromatherapy for dementia.[73]

Contraindications

Contraindications for aromatherapy include pregnancy, contagious disease, epilepsy, venous thrombosis, varicose veins, allergies, open wounds or skin sites, and any type of recent surgeries. It should not be administered orally or applied undiluted on the skin. Possible adverse events include photosensitivity, allergic reactions, nausea, and headache. Many essential oils have the potential to either enhance or reduce the effects of prescribed medications including antibiotics, tranquilizers, antihistamines, anticonvulsants, barbiturates, morphine, and quinidine.[37] Cases of potentially serious reactions are reported in two individuals without known allergies or sensitivities before exposure.[74]

Opportunities

Campbell and others[75] offer guidelines for safe integration of aromatherapy in clinical practice:

- Identify certified staff to serve as resources and educators.
- Conduct patient assessment.
- Select essential oils with low known risk potential.
- Choose one supplier with stringent product testing.
- Develop range of oils and methods of application that can be used consistently.
- When blending oils, consider symptoms, patient allergies, preference of aroma.
- Obtain a verbal consent.
- Place oil on tissue for patients in semiprivate rooms.
- Document outcome of intervention.
- Avoid vaporizers in clinical settings.[74,75,76]

Practitioners

Aromatherapy can be practiced in combination with massage therapy and holistic nursing care programs. Certification is available through the National Association for Holistic Aromatherapy Standards of Aromatherapy Training (NAHA, www.naha.org) Schools must provide 200 hours of training in aromatherapy, essential oil studies, anatomy, and physiology. In addition, students must submit a research paper, 10 case histories, and pass a written examination. Holistic nursing certification is available through the American Holistic Nurses' Certification Corporation (AHNCC, http://ahna.org/edu/certification.html). Requirements include a Baccalaureate of Science in Nursing, continuing education, 1 year of practice, and passing a written exam. Certification in aromatherapy or holistic nursing does not qualify a nurse to work independently, nor does it necessarily meet institutional requirements for practice.[77]

Mind-body Interventions: Meditation

Meditation is the systematic mental focus on particular aspects of an inner or outer experience, originally developed within a spiritual context aiming for spiritual growth, personal transformation, or transcendental experience. Transcendental meditation (repeating a mantra with the goal of quieting) and mindfulness meditation (giving spontaneous rise to thoughts, emotions, sensations, and perceptions) are the most extensively researched forms of meditation.[78] Mindfulness meditation is a self-regulatory approach to stress and emotion management.[37,78]

Strength of Evidence

There are no published meta-analyses on mindfulness meditation. There were 11 randomized clinical trials from 1973 to 2004. In 2 randomized clinical trials involving patients with cancer, mindfulness meditation was effective in reducing mood disturbance and stress symptoms in male and female patients.[37]

Contraindications

Meditation and guided imagery is contraindicated in those with a history of depression, bipolar disorder, and/or schizophrenia.[37]

Opportunities

For patients with cancer, mindfulness (and other types of meditation) may offer an opportunity to reduce mood disturbance and symptoms of stress.[37,78]

Practitioners

Trained practitioners may administer this modality in groups or individually.

Antioxidants

Commonly used antioxidant vitamins E, C, and beta carotene are believed to have health-promoting properties. Coenzyme Q 10 (ubiquinone) is an antioxidant found in all living cells and is believed to have potent effects. Cancer patients typically take antioxidants at doses higher than recommended daily allowances (RDAs).[79,80] Antioxidants scavenge free radicals. The most commonly used antioxidant is Vitamin C. Debate surrounding antioxidants and chemotherapy focuses on cancer therapy purposefully creating free radicals through cytotoxic mechanism, such as alkylating agents, antimetabolites, and radiation therapy. Limited research supports the belief that chemotherapy diminishes total antioxidant status,[81] but inconsistencies based on cancer site, cancer therapy, research methodologies, patient populations, variability in doses, duration of supplementation, and timing of interventions prevent formulation of conclusions.[82]

Strength of Evidence

Antioxidants and cancer therapy debate is not new. The association between beta carotene and increased risk of lung cancer in smokers is well known.[83,84] Some researchers believe selective inhibition of tumor cell growth is the action of antioxidants, and that they may also promote cellular differentiation with enhanced cytotoxic effects.[85] Ray and colleagues[86] suggest that typically recommended doses may be insufficient to cover the higher production of reactive oxygen metabolites. It has also been maintained that inadequate coverage may actually contribute to malignant cell proliferation.[85] Researchers have been concerned that, while antioxidants may decrease some kinds of toxicity associated with cancer chemotherapy, the therapeutic benefit of cancer therapy may be compromised.

Ladas and colleagues[82] reviewed over 100 citations on antioxidant status and cancer outcomes and antioxidant use among patients receiving chemotherapy with or without radiation therapy. Of the 52 studies that met research criteria, 31 were observational studies and 21 were intervention trials. Findings showed a decline in total antioxidant status of patients receiving cancer therapy, but conflicting and inconsistent results regarding the effect of chemotherapy on antioxidant status in patients receiving cancer therapy.[82]

Supplementation with vitamin E altered metabolism of doxorubicin. Some researchers question whether this means decreased treatment efficacy, arguing that adjunctive agents such as mesna and amifostine are used to reduce free radicals and do not appear to interfere in therapeutic benefit.[82] Among patients receiving chemotherapy for bone marrow transplant and total-body irradiation, serum vitamin E levels decreased even among those receiving through total parenteral nutrition.[87] Two randomized studies treating patients that had gynecologic cancers with doxorubicin, cyclophosphamide, cisplatin with ftorafure or mehalan and selenium, vitamin E, selenium and vitamin E, or placebo demonstrated increased serum selenium levels, but not vitamin E levels after supplementation.[88]

Studies among patients with breast cancer reveal the possible direct effect of selenium supplementation on serum and whole blood selenium.[82] RDAs appear inadequate for maintaining plasma antioxidant levels in patients receiving high-dose chemotherapy before stem cell transplant.[82] Antioxidants may have role in cancer prevention. Holm and colleagues[89] and Ingram and colleagues[80,90] suggest that high vitamin C intake before diagnosis of breast cancer has positive effect on mortality. Brawley and Parnes[90] report selenium and vitamin E supplementation may reduce risk of prostate cancer. Formal conclusions and recommendations could not be reached owing to variability in doses, duration of supplementation, and timing of doses.[82]

Contraindications

Contraindications for specific antioxidants are related to those known, e.g., beta carotene and lung cancer risk among smokers.

Vitamin C. Potential interactions: Aluminum antacids, cyclosporine, statins, calcium channel blockers and protease inhibitors, iron and vitamin E.[91]

Vitamin E. Potential interactions: Cholestramine, colestipol, mineral oil, anticonvulsants, anticoagulants, verapamil.[91]

Beta carotene. Potential interactions: Cholestyramine, colestipol, mineral oil, orlistat[91]

Opportunities

There are only opportunities within the context of clinical trials. Conclusive recommendations as well as contraindications for cancer patient are not established for the category of antioxidants.

Practitioners

Registered dieticians (RDs) have minimum bachelors degree in dietetics. Certified Clinical Nutritionists (CNCs) have education and training in clinical nutrition and may be a nurse or other health care professional. Caution should be used when choosing a nutrition practitioner. Be certain that he or she has expertise in cancer care as well as supplements and nutrition.

Shark Cartilage

Shark cartilage is also known as arthrelam or carticin. It is a derivative of the fin of a hammerhead or spiny dogfish shark. The use of bovine and shark cartilage for the treatment of cancer has been studied for >30 years.[29] As a result, numerous commercial products are available.

Strength of Evidence

There have been 3 angiogenic inhibitors identified from 1995 to 2004. Seven randomized clinical trials reported using shark cartilage for a variety of conditions. Human studies are limited, and the results are reported as inconclusive.[29] In animal studies, shark cartilage has been administered orally, by injection, by surgically implanted devices, and topically. Miller and colleagues[92] challenge oral administration because the molecules of shark cartilage are too large to allow absorption from intestines. There are further studies being conducted at this time.[29]

Contraindications

There is a lack of standardization of products available, and this raises concern for purity of the products on the market. Cases of hepatitis have been reported that are believed to be caused by shark cartilage.[93]

Opportunities

There are clinical trials being conducted at this time for those patients who wish to include this in their treatment regimen.

Practitioners

Recommendations for using shark or bovine cartilage should not be made until more conclusive evidence has been established.

REFERENCES

1. Oncology Nursing Society: *The use of complementary and alternative therapies in cancer care*, Pittsburgh, 2002, The Society.

2. Eisenberg DM and others: Unconventional medicine in the United States. Prevalence, costs, and patterns of use, *N Engl J Med* 328(4):246-252, 1993.
3. Eisenberg DM and others: Trends in alternative medicine use in the United States, 1990-1997: results of a follow-up national survey, *JAMA* 280(18):1569-1575, 1998.
4. Antman K and others: Complementary and alternative medicine: the role of the cancer center, *J Clin Oncol* 19(18 Suppl):55S-60S, 2001.
5. NCCAM, National Center for Complementary and Alternative Medicine; available online at http://nccam.nih.gov/. Accessed May 8, 2004.
6. OCCAM, Office of Cancer Complementary and Alternative Medicine. National Cancer Institute; available online at http://www3.cancer.gov/occam/. Accessed May 8, 2004.
7. White JD: Complementary and alternative medicine research: a National Cancer Institute perspective, *Semin Oncol* 29(6):546-551, 2002.
8. WHCCAMP, White House Commission on Complementary and Alternative Medicine Policy, United States Department of Health and Human Services, NIH Publication No. 03-5411, Washington, D.C., 2003.
9. IOM: Use of Complementary and Alternative Medicine (CAM) by the American Public. Institute of Medicine of the National Academies. Retrieved 5/16/04 from www.iom.edu/project.asp?id=4829.
10. Ashikaga T and others: Use of complimentary and alternative medicine by breast cancer patients: prevalence, patterns and communication with physicians, *Support Care Cancer* 10(7):542-548, 2002.
11. Swisher EM and others: Use of complementary and alternative medicine among women with gynecologic cancers, *Gynecol Oncol* 84(3):363-367, 2002.
12. Maskarinec G and others: Ethnic differences in complementary and alternative medicine use among cancer patients, *J Altern Complement Med* 6(6):531-538, 2000.
13. Lengacher CA and others: Frequency of use of complementary and alternative medicine in women with breast cancer, *Oncol Nurs Forum* 29(10):1445-1452, 2002.
14. Ernst E, Cassileth BR: The prevalence of complementary/alternative medicine in cancer: a systematic review, *Cancer* 83(4):777-782, 1998.
15 Bennett M, Lengacher C: Use of complementary therapies in a rural cancer population, *Oncol Nurs Forum* 26(8):1287-1294, 1999.
16. Bernstein BJ, Grasso T: Prevalence of complementary and alternative medicine use in cancer patients, *Oncology (Huntingt)* 15(10):1267-1272; discussion 1272-1268, 1283, 2001.
17. Vallerand AH, Fouladbakhsh JM, Templin T: The use of complementary/alternative medicine therapies for the self-treatment of pain among residents of urban, suburban, and rural communities, *Am J Public Health* 93(6):923-925, 2003.
18. Najm W and others: Use of complementary and alternative medicine among the ethnic elderly, *Altern Ther Health Med* 9(3):50-57, 2003.
19. Herron M, Glasser M: Use of and attitudes toward complementary and alternative medicine among family practice patients in small rural Illinois communities, *J Rural Health* 19(3):279-284, 2003.
20. Sparber A and others: Use of complementary medicine by adult patients participating in cancer clinical trials, *Oncol Nurs Forum* 27(4):623-630, 2000.
21. Basch U: Prevalence of CAM use among US cancer patients: an update, *J Cancer Integr Med* 2(1):13-14, 2004.
22. Bridevaux IP: A survey of patients' out-of-pocket payments for complementary and alternative medicine therapies, *Compl Ther Med* 12(1):48-50, 2004.
23. Stevinson C: Why patients use complementary and alternative medicine. In Ernst E, editor: *The desktop guide to complementary and alternative medicine: an evidence-based approach,* Edinburgh, 2001, Harcourt.
24. Furnham A: Why do people choose and use complementary therapies? In Ernst E, editor: *Complementary medicine: an objective appraisal,* Oxford, 1996, Butterworth Heinemann.
25. Kaptchuk TJ, Eisenberg DM: The persuasive appeal of alternative medicine, *Ann Intern Med* 129(12):1061-1065, 1998.
26. Hilsden RJ, Verhoef MJ: Complementary therapies: evaluating their effectiveness in cancer, *Patient Educ Couns* 38(2):101-108, 1999.
27. Fletcher RH: Clinical practice guidelines. Retrieved 3/17/04 from www.uptodateonline.com/application/topic/topicText.asp?file=genr_med/.
28. Decker G, Lee C: Complementary and alternative medicine (CAM) therapies. In Yarbro CH, Goodman M, Frogge M, editors: *Cancer nursing: principles and practice,* ed 6, pp. 590-620, Sudbury, Mass., 2005, Jones and Bartlett.
29. PDQ, PDQ® Cancer information summaries: complementary and alternative medicine; available at http://www.cancer.gov/cancerinfo/pdq/cam. Accessed April 13, 2004.
30. NMCD, Natural medicines comprehensive database [electronic database]. Retrieved 5/12/04 from www.naturaldatabase.com/.
31. Jadad AR and others: Assessing the quality of reports of randomized clinical trials: is blinding necessary? *Controlled Clinical Trials* 17(1): 1-12. NaturalStandard, Natural Standard Database, University of Texas M.D. Anderson Cancer Center. Retrieved 5/8/04 from www.naturalstandard.com/. Accessed May 8, 2004.
32. CEBM, Oxford Centre for Evidence-Based Medicine, University Department of Psychiatry, Warneford Hospital, Headington, Oxford; available online at http://www. cebm.net.
33. Angell M, Kassirer JP: Alternative medicine—the risks of untested and unregulated remedies, *N Engl J Med* 339(12):839-841, 1998.
34. Eisenberg DM: Advising patients who seek alternative medical therapies, *Ann Intern Med* 127(1):61-69, 1997.
35. Decker G: Integrating complementary and alternative medicine therapies into an ambulatory practice. In Buchsel P, Yarbro, CH, editors: *Oncology nursing in the ambulatory setting,* Sudbury, Mass., 2004, Jones and Bartlett.
36. Ernst E: Research into complementary/alternative medicine: an attempt to dispel the myths, *Int J Clin Pract* 55(6): 376-379, 2001.
37. Ernst E, editor: *The desktop guide to complementary and alternative medicine: an evidence-based approach,* Edinburgh, 2001, Mosby.
38. Eisenberg DM and others: Complementary and alternative medicine—an Annals series, *Ann Intern Med* 135(3):208, 2001.

39. Degner LF and others: Information needs and decision-making preferences in women with breast cancer, *JAMA* 277:1485-1492, 1997.
40. Brett H: Aromatherapy in the care of older people, *Nurs Times* 95(33):56-57, 1999.
41. Cohen MH: Legal and ethical issues in complementary and alternative medicine. In Ernst E, editor: *The desktop guide to complementary and alternative medicine: an evidenced-based approach,* Edinburgh, 2001, Harcourt.
42. Montbriand MJ: Herbs or natural products that protect against cancer growth, *Oncol Nurs Forum* 31(6):127-146, 2004.
43. Montbriand MJ: Herbs or natural products that may cause cancer and harm, *Oncol Nurs Forum* 32(1):20-29, 2005.
44. Gevitz N: *Other healers: unorthodox medicine in America,* Baltimore, Md., 1988, John's Hopkins University Press.
45. Segen JC: *Dictionary of alternative medicine,* Stamford, Conn., 1998, Appleton & Lange; 1998.
46. Vickers AJ, Cassileth BR: Unconventional therapies for cancer and cancer-related symptoms, *Lancet Oncol* 2(4):226-232, 2001.
47. Cassileth BR, Vickers AJ: Complementary and alternative therapies, *Urol Clin North Am* 30(2):369-376, 2003.
48. Ernst E: Complementary therapies for cancer. Retrieved 4/12/04 from www.uptodateonline.com/application/topic/print.asp?file=genl_onc/8402.
49. PDQ; retrieved 4/13/04 from www.cancer.gov/cancerinfo/pdq/.
50. Decker G: Complementary and alternative medicine therapy use in the older adult with cancer. In Cope D, Reb A, editors: *An evidence-based approach to the treatment and care of the older adult with cancer,* Pittsburgh, 2005, Oncology Nursing Press.
51. Blumenthal M and others, editors: *The complete German commission E monographs: therapeutic guide to herbal medicines,* Boston, 1998, American Botanical Council.
52. Ernst E: The current position of complementary/alternative medicine in cancer, *Eur J Cancer* 39(16):2273-2277, 2003.
53. Andersson S, Lundeberg T: Acupuncture—from empiricism to science: functional background to acupuncture effects in pain and disease, *Med Hypotheses* 45(3):271-281, 1995.
54. Han JS, Terenius L: Neurochemical basis of acupuncture analgesia, *Annu Rev Pharmacol Toxicol* 22:193-220, 1982.
55. Ernst E, Pittler MH: The effectiveness of acupuncture in treating acute dental pain: a systematic review, *Br Dent J* 184(9):443-447, 1998.
56. Mayer DJ: Acupuncture: an evidence-based review of the clinical literature, *Annu Rev Med* 51:49-63, 2000.
57. Aikins Murphy P: Alternative therapies for nausea and vomiting of pregnancy, *Obstet Gynecol* 91(1):149-155, 1998.
58. Ernst E, White A: Life-threatening adverse reactions after acupuncture? A systematic review, *Pain* 71(2):123-126, 1997.
59. Eichelberger B: A Qi Gong primer. Acupuncture.com; available online at http://www.acupuncture.com. Accessed May 19, 2004.
60. Yang JM: A brief history of QiGong. Acupuncture.com. Retrieved 5/10/04 from www.acupuncture.com.
61. Weiner P and others: The effect of incentive spirometry and inspiratory muscle training on pulmonary function after lung resection, *J Thorac Cardiovasc Surg* 113(3):552-557, 1997.
62. Corner J and others: Non-pharmacological intervention for breathlessness in lung cancer, *Palliat Med* 10(4):299-305, 1996.
63. Wu CY: [Spontaneous dynamic qigong and mental disorders], *Zhong Xi Yi Jie He Za Zhi* 10(8):497-498, 1990.
64. Finley S: Secrets of Reiki, *Health Healing* (March/April): 1992.
65. Whitaker JM, Adderly BD: *The pain relief breakthrough: the power of magnets to relieve backaches, arthritis pain, menstrual cramps, carpal tunnel syndrome, sports injuries and more.* Boston, 1998, Little, Brown.
66. Rosenfeld I: *Dr. Rosenfeld's guide to alternative medicine,* New York, 1996, Knopf.
67. Perez C: Clinical aromatherapy. Part I: an introduction into nursing practice, *Clin J Oncol Nurs* 7(5):595-596, 2003.
68. Thomas DV: Aromatherapy: mythical, magical, or medicinal? *Holist Nurs Pract* 16(5):8-16, 2002.
69. Cooke B, Ernst E: Aromatherapy: a systematic review, *Br J Gen Pract* 50(455):493-496, 2000.
70. Louis M, Kowalski SD: Use of aromatherapy with hospice patients to decrease pain, anxiety, and depression and to promote an increased sense of well-being, *Am J Hosp Palliat Care* 19(6):381-386, 2002.
71. Olleveant NA, Humphris G, Roe B: How big is a drop? A volumetric assay of essential oils, *J Clin Nurs* 8(3):299-304, 1999.
72. Fellowes D, Barnes K, Wilkinson S: Aromatherapy and massage for symptom relief in patients with cancer, *Cochrane Database Syst Rev* (2):CD002287, 2004.
73. Cochrane, The Cochrane Collaboration [electronic database. Retrieved 5/8/04 from www.cochrane.org/index0.htm.
74. Maddocks-Jennings W: Critical incident: idiosyncratic allergic reactions to essential oils, *Complement Ther Nurs Midwifery* 10(1):58-60, 2004.
75. Campbell L, Pollard A, Roeton C: The development of clinical practice guidelines for the use of aromatherapy in a cancer setting, *Aust J Holist* Nurs 8(1):14-22, 2001.
76. Avis A: Aromatherapy in practice, *Nurs Stand* 13(24):14-15, 1999.
77. Lee CO: Clinical aromatherapy. Part II: safe guidelines for integration into clinical practice, *Clin J Oncol Nurs* 7(5):597-598, 2003.
78. Astin JA And others: Mind-body medicine: state of the science, implications for practice, *J Am Board Fam Pract* 16(2):131-147, 2003.
79. VandeCreek L, Rogers E, Lester J: Use of alternative therapies among breast cancer outpatients compared with the general population, *Altern Ther Health Med* 5(1):71-76, 1999.
80. Ingram D: Diet and subsequent survival in women with breast cancer, *Br J Cancer* 69(3):592-595, 1994.
81. Durken M and others: Impaired plasma antioxidative defense and increased nontransferrin-bound iron during high-dose chemotherapy and radiochemotherapy preceding bone marrow transplantation, *Free Radic Biol Med* 28(6):887-894, 2000.
82. Ladas EJ and others: Antioxidants and cancer therapy: a

systematic review, *J Clin Oncol* 22(3):517-528, 2004.

83. Omenn GS and others: Effects of a combination of beta carotene and vitamin A on lung cancer and cardiovascular disease, *N Engl J Med* 334(18):1150-1155, 1996.
84. Albanes D and others: Effects of alpha-tocopherol and beta-carotene supplements on cancer incidence in the Alpha-Tocopherol Beta-Carotene Cancer Prevention Study, *Am J Clin Nutr* 62(6 Suppl):1427S-1430S, 1995.
85. Conklin KA: Dietary antioxidants during cancer chemotherapy: impact on chemotherapeutic effectiveness and development of side effects, *Nutr Cancer* 37(1):1-18, 2000.
86. Ray SD and others: In vivo protection of DNA damage associated apoptotic and necrotic cell deaths during acetaminophen-induced nephrotoxicity, amiodarone-induced lung toxicity and doxorubicin-induced cardiotoxicity by a novel IH636 grape seed proanthocyanidin extract, *Res Commun Mol Pathol Pharmacol* 107(1-2):137-166, 2000.
87. Jonas CR and others: Plasma antioxidant status after high-dose chemotherapy: a randomized trial of parenteral nutrition in bone marrow transplantation patients, *Am J Clin Nutr* 72(1):181-189, 2000.
88. Sundstrom H and others: Supplementation with selenium, vitamin E and their combination in gynaecological cancer during cytotoxic chemotherapy, *Carcinogenesis* 10(2):273-278, 1989.
89. Holm LE and others: Treatment failure and dietary habits in women with breast cancer, *J Natl Cancer Inst* 85(1):32-36, 1993.
90. Brawley OW, Parnes H: Prostate cancer prevention trials in the USA, *Eur J Cancer* 36(10):1312-1315, 2000.
91. PDR, *PDR for nutritional supplements,* Montvale, N.J., 2001, Medical Economics Company.
92. Miller FG and others: Ethical issues concerning research in complementary and alternative medicine, *JAMA* 291(5):599-604, 2004.
93. Gotay CC, Dumitriu D: Health food store recommendations for breast cancer patients, *Arch Fam Med* 9(8):692-699, 2000.

UNIT V

Impact of Cancer on Social and Family Life

CHAPTER

22 Spouse and Family Considerations

Margaret I. Fitch

INTRODUCTION

When a woman is diagnosed with cancer, there is more than a physical impact. A cancer diagnosis and its subsequent treatment also has emotional, psychologic, social, spiritual, and practical consequences.[1] It is an ongoing challenge for women to experience these consequences and cope with the subsequent impact on their lives.

In addition, when cancer strikes, her family and friends also feel the impact and challenges. They too experience emotional and psychosocial reactions, worrying about the woman who is diagnosed with the disease as well as worrying about themselves.[2] A cancer diagnosis means life is irrevocably changed for the individual woman and the significant others in her life. They too will have to cope with a myriad of changes. How they manage to deal with these challenges and adjust will have an influence on how the woman deals with her illness.

This chapter will highlight perspectives regarding spousal and family experiences with a woman's diagnosis and treatment of cancer. Armed with an increased understanding of the range of perspectives that may emerge, a health care provider is in a better position to appreciate what may be influencing a specific person's response or behavior and determine what intervention may be most useful in a particular situation. The material for this chapter is drawn from the literature as well as research conducted in the Psychosocial and Behavioral Research Unit in Toronto, Canada.

BACKGROUND: THE CONTEXT OF CANCER

From the moment an individual thinks something might be wrong in her body, and throughout the course of diagnostic investigation, treatment, and follow-up care, the experience of living with cancer is a continuous one for that person and her family members. The spectrum of cancer-related events is embedded in their daily lives. The illness becomes part of everyday living and decision making. It is an ever-present specter, not a separate entity that can easily be set aside and ignored. As illness-related events occur, there is a connectedness, from one event to another, for the woman and her family. What happens within the context of one event may influence the next event and the individual's responses to it. Each event unfolds within the full context of that person's life and within her family.

This reality has significant implications for health care providers. Firstly, most aspects of a woman's life and family living have the potential to be touched and altered throughout the course of the cancer experience. Health care assessments must be comprehensive, if providers are to fully understand the impact illness-related events are having within that cancer journey. Secondly, when a woman or family member interacts with any of the numerous cancer care providers they may encounter in the health care system, the individual is carrying along all past experiences and perspectives. For the woman or family member, the interaction is one more in a chain of interconnected events, whereas the health care provider may only focus on the interaction during that specific patient episode. The patient is responding and reacting within the context of a lifetime of events, while the health care provider may be working within the context of a single event. To fully understand, or comprehend, a patient or family member's reactions, the health care provider needs to appreciate how the event that is occurring at a point in time (i.e., learning one has cancer) is embedded in and linked to the unique life journey of the individual.

According to Lazarus and Folkman, no two individuals will respond to a difficult situation in exactly the same way.[3] The explanation for the individual variation in responses has emerged from the work concerning cognitive appraisal. Cognitive appraisal is the process whereby an individual thinks about and categorizes an event and its various aspects, and judges its effects on his or her well-being. It is largely an evaluative process, focused on meaning, and occurs constantly during waking hours. When confronted with an event, the individual engages in primary appraisal and judges the event as irrelevant, benign, positive, or stressful by answering the question, "Am I in trouble or will I benefit, now or in the future?" Secondary appraisal involves answering the question, "What can be done about this situation?" and assessing the options available to cope with the demands imposed by the event or situation. These appraisals can be conscious or unconscious and are influenced by an individual's existing knowledge, past experiences, self-concept, needs, attitudes, culture, and life goals. The individual judges the situation using his or her own unique frame of reference (cognitive map) and personal ideas about what is important.

Illness-related events evoke subjective pressures or demands.[4] It is the perception of an individual, not the objective characteristics of some aspect of an event, that affects how that person responds and is affected by the event.[5]

When a woman and her family members are faced with a diagnosis of cancer, each will respond in his or her own manner to the situation. Each will have concerns, issues, and needs related to himself or herself as an individual and will hold his or her own perspective about what ought to happen. In turn, each may behave differently from the others and choose to cope with that same event in different ways. Over time, some will mobilize their own resources and manage successfully, whereas others will experience ongoing distress and difficulty, requiring additional assistance or intervention. Clearly, different family members can use divergent processes to manage the situation.

At the same time, the individuals within a family form a social unit or system. Family structures vary, and each family has its own cultural attitudes, values, and beliefs. Each has its own set of rules, ways of working together, and expectations about roles and responsibilities. Just as with individuals, there is a life cycle with stages of growth and development for families. At each stage of development, certain critical tasks must be accomplished for the family to function effectively as a unit and for its members to support one another. When illness strikes, the family's usual way of functioning is often disturbed. Usual roles and responsibilities of family members can be thrown into disarray, and the family unit may not be able to meet the needs of its members. This may be the case particularly when situations arise unexpectedly or from a source external to the family. A diagnosis of life-threatening illness can be such an event.[2] Families need to find a way to balance their coping with illness-related events and their coping with their everyday functioning. In turn, this may require learning new skills and new ways of working together.[6]

IMPACT OF CANCER ON FAMILIES

During the past 15 years, there has been a substantial increase in the body of knowledge about the quantitative impact of cancer on the family. Although a cancer diagnosis is an intensely personal experience for the individual with the disease, it is clearly a family experience as well.[7] Lewis described how this work has evolved through discernible stages.[8] The first and early phase included clinical papers describing the potential psychosocial morbidity in cancer patients and ramifications for family members. Husbands reported various emotional problems in response to their wives' mastectomies as well as sleeping disturbances, eating disorders, and problems at work.[9] These issues served to raise the level of awareness about the value of involving spouses in communication exchanges and decision-making.[9-12]

The second phase of research about families and cancer emerged in the 1970s and 1980s. The focus of this work was on describing and measuring, using standardized instruments, psychosocial distress in both the patient and the spouse.[13-15] Much of this work was conducted with women living with breast cancer and their partners, and reported moderate to high levels of emotional distress in the partners following the diagnosis. By using longitudinal designs, the patterns of distress over time were identified. Baider and De-Nour documented that husbands had higher levels of distress over time (up to 3 years after surgery) and lower levels of adjustment than did the diagnosed women.[16] Maguire found husbands of women with malignancy had higher distress than those of women with benign disease.[12]

The third phase of studies used statistical modeling techniques to test hypotheses about the impact of breast cancer on the family.[6,17-19] This type of work began to attend to the complexity of family life as they took multiple variables and outcomes into account. Based on these empirical studies, *The Relational Model of Family Functioning with Cancer* has been described and offered as a framework for oncology nursing practice.[6]

The Relationship Model of Family Functioning with Cancer describes cancer as a psychosocial transition in which family members work to find a balance in their ongoing life as a family and their life with cancer. Seven concepts provide the basis for the model: the family members' perceived illness-related demands, the child's frame of reference for understanding the cancer, the parent's mood and affect, parenting quality, social support available to the family, marital adjustment, and family member coping and management strategies.

A family has the potential to be an active manager of its own resources, ways of working, interactions with each other, and negotiations with the community. When illness strikes a parent, the family is required to maintain stability in its routine internal arrangements and activities as well as restructure its interactions and activities to manage the ongoing demands of the illness.[2,20] Their desire is to maintain some sense of control and predictability over what is happening to them.[21] In some instances, this can involve delusions of control.[22]

However, the very nature of cancer and its course of treatment engender uncertainty and put pressure on the family. The negative mood, symptom state, and diminished capacity of the person with cancer affects other family members, and the illness-related demands can have a deleterious consequence on the marital relationship.[23,24] In turn, this heightened tension in the marital relationship can have deleterious consequences on the household.[17,25] Clearly, attention to the illness-related demands of cancer is of vital importance if tension and problems are to be resolved or avoided.

Health care providers caring for women with cancer must embrace the family as the unit of care and a system of intimate, interacting, and interdependent members.[7] Responding to the family as a family system and to the members as individuals with their own needs will promote healing for the patient as well as for the family. An important initial step in achieving this goal is to understand the nature of the impact cancer has on the family members from their own perspectives. Much of the research to date has focused on understanding that impact from patients' perspectives. However, a growing body of qualitative work is shedding light on the perspectives and experiences of the family members. It can inform the practice of health care professionals caring for women with cancer.

PERSPECTIVES FROM PARTNERS/FAMILY MEMBERS

Cancer patients and their family members often talk about their experiences with cancer in terms of being on a journey. Significant events and perspectives of transitions mark this journey.

In the author's work at the Psychosocial and Behavioral Research Unit (Toronto Sunnybrook Regional Cancer Centre, Canada) patients identified specific points of transition (see Box 22-1).

Our research makes use of in-depth interviews with patients, survivors, and family members and aims to document the respective experiences and perspectives about living with cancer.[26-31] The narratives or stories that patients and families shared within the research studies provided a poignant and salient picture of the viewpoints they held about their cancer-related events, often in marked contrast to those held by health care providers.

For the purposes of this chapter, material from a variety of the studies will be used to illustrate partner and family responses to the unfolding series of events that constitute the cancer journey. It is anticipated that these illustrations will assist care providers to broaden their assessment and focus on the family as the unit of concern. Perspectives on major challenges at each transition point will be presented.

Finding an Abnormality (Initial Event)

One of the key challenges concerning this initial event on the cancer journey is the understanding of what constitutes a change or difference in the way the body functions that would herald cancer. Overall, many patients and partners reflect after the diagnosis on changes that may have occurred, but reveal they often had not assigned their interpretation that cancer was the reason why the changes occurred. For example, in the words of a partner of a woman with ovarian cancer:

> Looking back, I had no idea that what was happening could have been cancer. I did not even think about it. I mean, we were both under a lot of stress, with jobs and family, and all the things that happen when you get older. I mean, women's bodies just change. We just thought was all just menopause.

In some instances, partners actually discover the abnormality. This is particularly the situation with breast cancer. The awareness of what ought to be done and how quickly action ought to be taken is a function of what couples know about signs and symptoms of the various cancers and their respective readiness to take action. A tension that may arise is that associated with one partner encouraging action and the other not following through. For example, in the words of one partner of a breast cancer patient:

> You know, when I look back on that time before we had the diagnosis, when we knew there was a hard spot but she had not seen the doctor, I was so angry with her. Why didn't she go, get it checked out? I just knew something was wrong, but she didn't make the appointment for ages. I kept asking her about it.

Discovery of an abnormality may also take place during a routine doctor's office visit or while undergoing a routine screening procedure. In these situations, the partner is often not present and only learns about the situation later. This can lead to some feelings of remorse or guilt for not being present when their partner found out something was wrong, or a sense of being left out or left behind.

In general, once an abnormality is acknowledged as serious and requiring attention, both partners share a level of concern about the situation.[32] However, the fundamental issue seems to be deciding that something is serious enough for investigation. For example, as one partner described:

> I knew something was different. She had symptoms I guess over the couple of years. She was tired all the time and intercourse was

Box 22-1 Times of Transition

- finding an abnormality
- seeking an opinion/diagnostic testing
- hearing a diagnosis
- starting treatment
- getting back to normal
- experiencing a recurrence
- requiring palliative care
- approaching death
- dying... death
- grieving the loss

painful. She had no energy. But we are getting older. I guess we didn't know much about ovarian cancer then or how serious this could be.

Finally, the response of health care professionals to patients' concerns plays a role at this time in patients' and partners' subsequent reactions. When symptoms are somewhat vague and physicians do not suggest further investigation, women often do not pursue additional testing once they have seen their physician. For some, it was only the persistence of symptoms over time that took them back for another appointment. On the other hand, if the family doctor directed them initially to further testing, and emphasized the potential for cancer as a diagnosis, diagnostic investigation was undertaken. When patients and partners reflect back on the early days, many cite the initial responses of the family doctor as very important to their understanding of what could be happening and to their sense of being heard and supported.[28]

Seeking an Opinion/Undergoing Diagnostic Tests

The second event in the cancer journey is the interval of diagnostic testing. This interval has been identified as one of the most distressing times for women and their partners. For many, this is a time of hearing new words and being exposed to new people and places. Referral often occurs from the family physician to various laboratories or other specialists. There are waits for test appointments and subsequent waits for test results. For many patients and partners, there are numerous questions that begin to arise, as they anticipate the possible outcomes of the tests, and a lack of clarity about where to find the answers. As one example, one partner described his feelings at that time:

> I can remember waking up at night and thinking about all the possibilities. What if it was cancer? What would that mean? Would she die right away? Who would take care of the children? What would I do? But then, not wanting to think about any of that and not wanting to upset her any more, so I didn't say anything. I didn't tell anyone at work. And we didn't say anything at all to the kids.

When partners reflect back upon this time, many will say that there is not much that health care professionals can do for them. They sense that more can be done for them after the results are known. However, some want to be more involved in the diagnostic process. As one husband commented, "It would have been more helpful to be called into the examining room instead of being left in the waiting room." These men, like their wives, talked about wanting information that was factual, complete, and easy to understand. They wanted to know about the biopsy procedure and its potential results. Not having relevant information can contribute to feelings of being left out or pushed aside.

Although some partners do acknowledge their own emotional distress, many focus on the well-being of their wives. In the words of one man:

> The biggest thing that the spouse has to deal with is the mental well-being of his wife. The mental strain that it puts on her, gets put on me... What do I say? What do I do for her? What is the best thing? How do I support her? It's hard enough for me, but it's worse for her.

Partners have described wanting to know what they can expect in terms of emotional responses both during this diagnostic interval and later. Phrases like "She was a basket case because of the wait" and "The waiting and not knowing was agony" are not unusual. When asked what would be helpful, many partners suggest shortening the wait times to get into test appointments and get the results back.

The responses of health care providers are seen as important during this interval. Patients and partners will describe how this experience is new for them and filled with anxiety. They realize that for health care providers it may be a daily event and one that is routine. The potential for providers to be dismissive of the patient's or partner's anxiety is heightened in this type of situation and must be guarded against.

Hearing the Diagnosis

Partners describe the event of hearing a definitive diagnosis with words like "shocking," "devastating," "unreal," "scary," and "overwhelming." Even if there had been a clear indication that cancer was a possible diagnosis, the definitive result was upsetting. In the words of partners:

> It was devastating. I felt so helpless in that there was nothing I could do. I knew a lot about breast cancer from what I saw in the media, and at first I thought she was going to die. That is what you often see in the media. And for a while I was quite depressed... It took a while, but I started feeling better.
>
> It was unreal. I was just in shock... I was pretty naive then, too. I mean, the only thing I could think about was that she will survive. If I knew then what I know now, my emotional state would have been a lot worse.
>
> I was really unprepared for it all. I really felt caught off guard. I didn't know about the disease, or the treatment options, or anything. If it was happening again today, we'd seek another opinion and check out treatment options a lot more.
>
> Cancer is a scary word. I really did not know much about it then. I did not understand about prognosis or what that meant. I'd say this is the worst thing I've ever gone through, all the unknowns... it is like a bad dream.

The other major challenge at this time was making a decision about treatment. Partners often expressed concerns about having all the information needed to make an informed decision and experiencing difficulty knowing where to find it. Many partners felt they were dependent on their wives for information. Much of the information that did exist was directed at their wives and not at them as partners. Many felt there was little they could do for their wives. As one example, one partner talked about the experience of feeling helpless:

> There is a feeling of helplessness about it all. It's sort of like childbirth. Similar to it. You sit on the sidelines and really there is nothing much you can do... There is nothing you can give up that will make a difference.

Other partners described actively pursuing information on the Internet, at libraries, and from organizations such as the American Cancer Society and the Canadian Cancer Society. This activity was perceived as doing something, but there was also some frustration at the difficulties in finding relevant information and sorting through all the opinions. Frequently the language was hard to comprehend and the implications were unclear. In the words of one partner:

> Oh, I found lots of information, but none of it agreed. It is so discouraging. What do you pay attention to? How can you sort through it all? She was so young and nothing was available about cancer in that age. Why was this happening to us?

Partners who had good communication with health care providers and who were able to talk about their questions and concerns, overall, found this to be useful. In organized cancer programs the access to information was easier; however, for many this becomes available only after referrals to cancer treatment.

Starting Treatment

Once the decision has been made to begin a specific course of treatment, much of the energy on the part of patients and partners is devoted to coping with the treatment impact. The specific nature of that impact will depend, to a large extent, on the need for surgery, radiation, chemotherapy, or combined approaches. Understanding what is anticipated and the likely course of events during treatment is important if people are going to be able to plan ahead. For example, a partner described how he and his wife managed with her chemotherapy cycles:

> The nurse told us up front that my wife would have bad days and good days. Right after her chemo she'd have a few bad days. Then she'd start to feel a little better. And that would continue until her next dose... So we organized around that. I took a day off work, or her Mom came over on the bad days and got the kids looked after. When she could do it herself, then she did.

For many patients and partners, treatment is a matter of dealing with multiple symptoms and trying to cope with their impact. The treatment course can be arduous. At the very least, it is disruptive of family life. Roles and responsibilities often have to be reorganized, and this can lead to tensions within a family. This impact will be felt to a greater or lesser degree based on how much change any one individual has to undergo. For example, one partner illustrated the lack of impact on him:

> I'd say it hardly changed my life on a day-to-day basis. I think that is basically because of how she handled it. The children are in their teens and quite independent, and she was not working. So I'd say I really did not have to change much.

Another partner depicts a contrasting situation:

> I had to pick up all the slack quite literally. I had to do more and more chores as she did not have the energy. It really cut into my sleep time and I got more and more tired... I really got tired answering all the questions about how she was doing. Only one person asked about me and how I was doing.

Working through these changes in roles and responsibilities can be challenging. If there is little clarity about how long the changes will be necessary or if there are few extended family members or friends to help, additional strain can easily develop. Depending on the ages of any children, challenges can arise in caring for the children, sharing the diagnosis with them, or expecting older siblings to support younger ones. Communication between partners and negotiating responsibility change is an important arena. One woman's narrative illustrates this challenge:

> My husband and I go through stages... It's sort of like a roller-coaster where at times little stuff doesn't matter, you know, all those trivial, little fights. We didn't fight for a long time after my diagnosis, because who cares if you picked up your clothes off the floor... because we are in love and we have each other, and we don't know how long that will last, and that kind of stuff. And we go from that to under so much stress because of it and feeling so much fear that we're at each other's throats. You know, just feeling really stressed out about stuff. And sometimes not wanting to tell each other how fearful we are. He does not want to pull me down and upset me about his fears and what's going on in his head. Yet being really stressed and you get into arguments all the time. So it's put a lot of stress on our relationship. But it's also brought us closer together at the same time.

Stopping Treatment/Getting Back to Normal

When the course of treatment is finished, another transition begins to unfold for patients and their family members. A new time of waiting begins, since there may not yet be dependable evidence the treatment has been effective. Suddenly, patients are confronted with "no longer doing anything active about the cancer" and feeling a growing sense of unease. Many only now begin to reflect upon their experiences with cancer, what it has meant, and what it means for their future. Meanwhile, many family members are feeling a sense of relief that the treatment is over and "things can get back to normal." The tensions arise when these two perspectives unfold without communication between partners and family members.

Of interest are the unfolding perspectives about self that patients experience. Whereas some will describe themselves and their bodies as "new," "forever altered," and "changed," others perceive the changes as temporary. They describe a "waiting until things go back to the way they were before." In the latter case, if changes do not revert, subsequent disappointment and frustration can emerge. Long-term side effects such as lymphedema, treatment-induced menopause, and cognitive dysfunction can be particularly challenging.

Issues of sexuality can emerge during this interval. Changes in body image (e.g., scars) and self-esteem (e.g., no longer feeling like a woman) can have an impact on a woman's sense of desirability. In turn, the partner's response to these changes has the potential to influence the woman's adjustment and, subsequently, the couple's continued intimacy. There are mixed reports on the value of open communication, and in large measure the degree depends on the couple's previous communication patterns before the diagnosis. Communication and disclosure must be handled in light of the needs for information by each partner and not forced inappropriately.

In the story of one partner, the change is poignantly illustrated:

> Really, right now, I am not dealing well with it all. Her moods and reactions are really wearing me down. I can deal with the disease, but I am

> having extreme difficulty dealing with her. I can understand her frustrations, but I wish she wouldn't take them out on me. I really wonder how long I can continue. Her attitude has pushed me to the limit. Sex is at zero, too. I don't think it will ever return.

In contrast, relationships can grow stronger between couples:

> We are really a lot closer now than ever before. We talk a lot more. Really, you don't realize how important someone is to you until you wind up potentially losing her. It makes you reassess your priorities, what you are doing with your life and what's important to you... I was shocked at the scar in the beginning and sex is a little different now... but you adjust. You get used to it... it is better than the alternative.

Facing Recurrence/Facing It All Again

The fear of recurrence is an ever present fear for those living after the diagnosis of cancer. When recurrence occurs it begins a cycle that patients and families describe as "facing it all again." They now have the past experiences of decision making and treatment, as well as dealing with side effects and changes in their home life. They also have a sense of their options being narrowed. However, they also have more experience gathering information, sorting through that information, and taking charge of their care. In many cases, this can result in more active engagement in decision making about treatment and assertive communication styles with health care professionals. The challenges partners talk about include learning to live with unknowns and uncertainties, staying positive and optimistic, carrying on with life, and keeping the stress down. In the words of one man:

> You've just got to learn to live with it. What other option do you have? I wish it hadn't happened, but it did. You have to play the hand you were dealt. You have to deal with the realities.

During this time, roles and responsibilities often have to be altered again. If limited alteration occurred previously, more pronounced change emerges as the woman deals with progressive disease and limitations. Often changes are needed with regard to work schedules, household schedules, child care arrangements, and social activities. Often these responsibilities fall to the spouse to organize, especially if there are frequent hospitalizations and younger children. Generally, greater success will occur through more open communication and greater flexibility in role allocation.

Dealing with Advancing Disease/Death

As death becomes imminent, issues arise regarding pain and symptom management, location of care and death, and the burden of care on family members. One of the prominent concerns for family members is the care and comfort of their loved one who is dying. They look for reassurance that their loved one is not in undue discomfort and for guidance regarding what they can do to aid in alleviating discomfort. Regardless of whether the person who is dying is in the hospital or at home, family members will benefit from learning about what they can do to reduce their loved one's suffering.

Preparing for death through talking can be of benefit, although difficult. As one partner offered:

> Death is more difficult to talk about now because of the way the treatments and everything has gone; things have not gone well. Death is a real possibility now. It is closer than before.

Couples vary in their willingness and capacity for open communication about this difficult topic. Some never talk about it directly. Others will use humor. Others will actively plan the funeral. Some are able to talk about the anticipated loss and its implications. In the words of one partner:

> We talked about her leaving, that the best friendship is over and will be breaking up. We talked about our child and how he will not have a mother any more. It's so hard, I hardly want to talk about it.

Grieving the Loss

Even when death has occurred, the journey is not yet over for the family. In a sense, a new journey is beginning. Initially the feelings of loss and grief are intense and all-consuming. Physical and psychosocial changes are frequently observed (e.g., sleep, eating, concentration, emotions). Gradually those will ease but only as the work of grieving is accomplished. As one partner describes:

> I look back and I missed her desperately at first. I could barely stay alone at night in the house. There were just so many memories... I really never thought she'd die... but now it's a little better. I still think I'll sell the house. There is just too much of her here to be around every day.

Yet at the same time family members can experience a sense of relief that the suffering is over for their loved one. This perspective is often used to begin the healing process for themselves. As one partner shared:

> You know, cancer is such a terrible disease, really. You are watching the disease take over, watching the body being destroyed, watching the person you love being destroyed. It is almost unbearable. So when it's over, it is a relief in some ways for everyone.

SUMMARY

Confronting and coping with life-threatening illness is a challenge for the person who is diagnosed with the disease and for the family members. Balancing everyday living as a family and meeting the demands imposed by the disease requires considerable energy and capacity on the part of all the individuals concerned.

Health care providers can assist individuals with the realities of cancer and cancer treatment through their capacity to understand that reality from the perspective of the patient and the family member. Sensitive communication, provision of relevant easy-to-understand information, and meaningful inclusion in decision making about care are key interventions that health care providers can offer throughout the cancer journey. A focus on the family as the unit of care and as a system of interconnected relationships is vitally important for healing of both the patient and the other family members.

REFERENCES

1. Canadian Cancer Society: *Final report on the needs of persons living with cancer across Canada,* Toronto, 1992, The Society.
2. Davis-Ali SH, Chesler MA, Chesney BK: Recognizing cancer as a family disease: worries and support reported by patients and spouses, *Soc Work Health Care* 19(2):45-65, 1993.
3. Lazarus R, Folkman S: *Stress, appraisal and coping,* New York, 1984, Springer.
4. Haberman MR, Woods NF Packard NJ: Demands of chronic illness: reliability and validity assessment of a demands of illness inventory, *Holist Nurs Pract* 5(1):25-35, 1990.
5. Compas BE and others: When Mom or Dad has cancer: markers of psychological distress in cancer patients, spouses, and children, *Health Psychol* 13(6):507-515, 1994.
6. Lewis FM, Hammond MA, Woods NF: The family's functioning with newly diagnosed breast cancer in the mother: the development of an exploratory model, *J Behav Med* 16:351-370, 1993.
7. Yates P: Family coping: Issues and challenges for cancer nursing, *Cancer Nurs* 22(1):63-71, 1999.
8. Lewis FM, Hammond MA: Psychosocial adjustment of the family to breast cancer: a longitudinal analysis, *J Am Med Women's Assoc* 47:194-200, 1992.
9. Wellisch DK, Jamison KR, Pasnau RO: Psychosocial aspects of mastectomy II: the man's perspective, *Am J Psychiatr* 135:543-546, 1978.
10. Kent S: Coping with sexual identity crises after mastectomy, *Geriatrics* 30:145-146, 1975.
11. Ervin Jr C: Psychologic adjustment to mastectomy, *Med Aspects Hum Sex* 7:42-65, 1973.
12. Maguire P: The repercussions of mastectomy on the family, *Int J of Fam Psychiatry* 1:485-503, 1981.
13. Northhouse L: Social support in patients' and husbands' adjustment to breast cancer, *Nurs Res* 37:91-95, 1988.
14. Northouse L, Swain MA: Adjustment of patients and husbands to the initial impact of breast cancer, *Nurs Res* 36:221-225, 1987.
15. Oberst MT, James RH: Going home: patient and spouse adjustment following cancer surgery, *Topics in Clin Nurs* 7:46-57, 1985.
16. Baider L, De-Nour AK: Couples' reactions and adjustment to mastectomy: a preliminary report, *J Psychiatr Med* 14:265-276, 1984.
17. Lewis FM, Hammond MA: The father's, mother's and adolescent's adjustment to a mother's breast cancer, *Fam Relats* 45:456-465, 1996.
18. Lewis FM and others: The family's functioning with chronic illness in the mother: the spouse's perspective, *Soc Sci Med* 29:1261-1269, 1989.
19. Woods NF, Lewis FM: Living with chronic illness: women's perspectives on their families' adaptation, *Health Care Women Int* 16:135-148, 1995.
20. Hough EE, Lewis FM, Woods NF: Family response to mother's chronic illness: case studies of well- and poorly-adjusted families, *West J Nurs Res* 13(5):568-596, 1991.
21. Lewis FM, Daltroy L: How causal explanations influence health behaviour: attribution theory. In Glanz K, Lewis FM, Rimer B (editors): *Health behaviour and health*

education: theory, research and practice, San Francisco, 1990, Jossey-Bass.
22. Lewis FM, Deal LW: Balancing our lives: a study of the married couple's experience with breast cancer recurrence, *Oncol Nurs Forum* 22(6):943-953, 1995.
23. Morse SR, Fife B: Coping with a partner's cancer: adjustment at four stages of the illness trajectory, *Oncol Nurs Forum* 25(4):751-760, 1998.
24. Fuller S, Swensen CH: Marital quality and quality of life among cancer patients and their spouses, *J Psychosoc Oncol* 10(3):41-56, 1992.
25. Zahlis EH, Shands ME: Breast cancer: demands of illness on the patient's partner, *J Psychosoc Oncol* 9:75-93, 1991.
26. Fitch MI: Psychosocial management of patients with recurrent ovarian cancer: treating the whole patient to improve quality of life, *Sem Oncol Nurs* 19(3):40-53, 2003.
27. Fitch M, Deane K, Howell D: Living with ovarian cancer: women's perspectives on treatment and treatment decision-making, *Can Oncol Nurs J* 13(1):8-13, 2003.
28. Fitch M, Deane K, Howell D, Gray RE: Women's experiences with ovarian cancer: reflections on being diagnosed, *Can Oncol Nurs J* 12(3):152-159, 2002.
29. Gray RE and others: Managing the impact of illness: the experiences of men with prostate cancer and their spouses, *J Health Psychol* 5:525-542, 2000.
30. Gould J and others: Nothing fit me: cross-support needs of young women with breast cancer, *Psychooncology* 12(4)(Suppl):S146-147, 2003.
31. Mitchell T and others: Living life to the limits: dragon boaters and breast cancer, *Psychooncology* 12(4)(Suppl): S172-173, 2003.
32. Northouse LL, Tocco KM, West P: Coping with a breast biopsy: how health cancer professionals can help women and their husbands, *Oncol Nurs Forum* 24(3):473-480, 1997.

CHAPTER

23 Work Considerations

Cheryl Brohard-Holbert

More people in the US are surviving cancer. The person with cancer faces many challenges during the immediate days and weeks after their diagnosis that are very different from the challenges of survivorship. The survivors' focus shifts from fear of death and dying, fighting for a cure, or adjusting life's activities around cancer treatment, to long-term issues of survival. This chapter explores the issues of work—employment, finance, and insurance.

SURVIVORSHIP AND BREAST CANCER

According to 2005 statistics from the American Cancer Society (ACS), an estimated 9.8 million Americans alive in 2001 had a history of cancer.[1] This statistic has progressively increased over the past 30 years. Combined 5-year relative survival rates for all cancers diagnosed between 1995 and 2000 is 64%. Survival has steadily increased because of knowledge gained through clinical research, the development of new technologies designed to target cancer (e.g., tomotherapy, pharmaceutical agents), and refined diagnostic testing.

About 5% to 10% of cancers are clearly inherited. As the Human Genome Project sponsored by the National Institutes of Health (NIH) came to completion in April 2003, the next focus was on mapping genes identified with common diseases such as cancer.[2] The goal is to develop diagnostic tests and eventually develop vaccines and treatments. In the meantime, more Americans are identifying their family's risk of developing a hereditary disease and seeking genetic counseling. Genetic counselors are advising patients to seek regular screenings and perform risk-reducing behaviors. With the help of the emerging science of molecular epidemiology, the relationships between genetics, environment, and cancer will be uncovered and lead to improvements in early detection, treatment, and ultimately a decrease in mortality.

The ACS Guidelines for Screening Breast Cancer (for women) include the following: yearly mammograms starting at age 40, clinical breast exam starting between 20 and 30 years of age, and self–breast exams starting in a woman's 20s. Women with an increased risk for breast cancer are identified by their family history of breast cancer, past history of breast cancer, or a genetic tendency. The ACS recommends that women talk with their health care providers about their risk factors and make a plan for early detection such as a screening mammogram at an earlier age and/or more frequent examinations.[1]

If the cancer is diagnosed when it is in a localized state, the relative survival rate climbs to 95% for the 5-year period. The 5-year relative survival rate has reached an all-time high of 98% for localized breast cancer; for regional disease the survival rate is 80%; for distant metastasis the survival rate is 26%. The 5-year survival rate for all stages of cancers is 88%, and at 10 years the survival rate is 77%. Early detection and screenings for cancer are helping to increase the 5-year survival rate, now nearing 85%. When patients seek advice on what they can do to lower their risk of cancer, this is a prime opportunity for the nurse to educate the patient and family members.[1]

Nurses are educated to support patients while coping with the day-to-day challenges of the diagnosis and treatment. Once the focus of care shifts from curing their cancer to living with it, the survivors begin to reintegrate themselves back into society and into their established lifestyles. They will face a different set of challenges in areas such as work, personal finances, employment decisions, and health care insurance. As the volume of cancer survivors grow, these issues will magnified in complexity and require nursing interventions regarding specific survivorship education.

WORKPLACE DISCRIMINATION LAWS

Two federal laws were enacted in the 1990s to protect people with cancer from workplace discrimination. The Americans with Disability Act (ADA) of 1990 and the Family and Medical Leave Act (FMLA) of 1993 were approved by the US Congress as a means to reduce employment-related issues.[3,4] A disability is defined as a limitation or inability to perform functions or tasks as a result of a medical condition, injury, or impairment.[3] Cancer is cited as one of the medical conditions identified by the ADA.[3] Under the ADA, an individual with a disability is one who has: a physical or mental impairment that limits one or more major life activities, has a record of the impairment, or is regarded as having such impairment.[3]

The ADA guarantees the civil rights of people with disabilities. The ADA mandates that employers cannot discriminate against an employee on the basis of an employee's disability for the purposes or hiring or employment, and the employer must provide "reasonable accommodation" to employees with disabilities without causing "undue hardship on the employer." Not all employers are mandated to provide such accommodations. There are specific parameters to be taken into account such as the size of the workforce, employment status, worked hours, and others that govern the employers' participation (Box 23-1).

The FMLA mandates employers to allow employees up to 12 weeks of unpaid leave in a 12-month period when a serious health condition exists. It also mandates that the employee's health care benefits must be continued. There are two issues addressed in this act, family leave and medical leave. As with the ADA, certain employee stipulations must be met before the law is enforced; they are summarized in Box 23-2.

EMPLOYMENT EXPERIENCES

Studies conducted before the workplace laws were enacted found discrimination.[5-8] As reported by patients with cancer, the discrimination manifested itself in the form of promotion denials, unfavorable transfers, demotions, and unfair hiring practices. Employer concerns ranged from lower job performances and lower productivity to higher absenteeism, increased financial burden for the employer, higher worker's

Box **23-1** 1993 American Disability Act (ADA) Stipulations

1. Applies to employers with 15 or more employees for each working day for at least 20 weeks in the current or preceding calendar year.
2. Excludes employees of the federal government or its subdivisions, private membership clubs, or Native Americans.
3. Employers cannot ask job applicants questions that are medical-related, relate to private medical records, relate to a need to leave the workplace for medical treatment, or any matters related to a disability.
4. Employers may have an extremely limited leave of absence policy or no policy
5. Employers are required to provide "reasonable accommodation" of the disability unless the accommodation would impose an "undue hardship" on the employer.

Box 23-2 Family and Medical Leave Act (FMLA) Stipulations

1. The employee must have completed 12 months of service before the FMLA coverage begins.
2. The employee must have worked for the employer for 1250 hours with the 12 months immediately preceding the FMLA leave.
3. The worksite must be within a 75-mile radius of 50 or more of the same employer's employees.
4. State and federal government employees are covered.
5. The following are FMLA types of leave:
   a. Employee has serious health condition.
   b. The leave is associated with birth, adoption, or foster placement of a child.
   c. The leave is required so the employee can care for a spouse, child, or parent with a serious health condition.

compensation expenses, and higher disability insurance premiums.

Research conducted before the enactment of the ADA and the FMLA shows the extent of the problem in the workplace. However, there were limited numbers of research studies conducted with patients with cancer and the issues addressed by ADA and FMLA before the legislation was enacted. A few examples of research conducted after the laws were enacted will demonstrate the employers' compliance with the laws. Again, there are limited numbers of research studies conducted on patients with cancer and these laws.

A 1992 National Health Interview Survey asked questions regarding survivorship issues and cancer prevalence.[5] Survey results showed that 3.9% of the US population had a history of cancer (excluding skin cancer). Approximately 11% had been denied health or life insurance coverage because of cancer. Over 18% of the individuals reported being employed before and after their diagnosis, and they reported at least one of these problems: couldn't take a new job because of a change in insurance related to cancer, felt they couldn't change jobs because of the cancer, faced on-the-job problem from their employer directly because of the cancer, refrained from applying for the next job because they did not want their medical records made public, and were fired or laid off from their jobs because of the cancer. Patients with health insurance were more likely to seek a second opinion than those without health insurance.

Four hundred patients with cancer were surveyed regarding employment discrimination.[6] Rothstein and others found over 225 respondents reported that cancer treatment did not interfere with their ability to perform their job functions. Over 300 patients responded that they could work a flexible schedule. Police, health care services, and personal service occupations were cited as more likely to offer a flexible schedule. Respondents who were employed as laborers were found less likely to be offered flexible work time. The findings showed that employers, regardless of the size, offered their employees flexible schedules during their cancer treatments. Employers were not required to provide flexible scheduling to employees under the 1993 ADA law. In the same study, the researchers reported that 27% of the responders had been fired from their job. The researchers did not explore the reasons for the terminations.

In a more recent study with long-term survivors of cancer, Hounshell and others surveyed 31 persons diagnosed with hairy cell leukemia.[7] At the time of the survey, the median survival time was 7.8 years and 50% of the group was employed. Approximately 23% of the patients had taken a leave of absence from work because of their disease and treatment but returned to work after treatment. When the researchers asked if there had been any health insurance issues, 76% of the respondents said that their health care insurance premiums did not change. The majority of the patients has private insurance or employer insurance plans. Only four patients had their benefits stopped or coverage refused because of their leukemia diagnosis. The significance of this study is the insight it gives nurses into two significant survivorship issues, employment and health insurance. Because of the limited number of study patients, the findings can not be generalized.

In 2004, researchers investigated discrimination and employment issues in a cohort of women in Quebec, Canada.[8] Maunsell and others sent questionnaires to two groups of cancer survivors identified from the Quebec Tumor Registry and a comparison group of women never diagnosed with cancer identified in the provincial health care files. They found that at the start of follow-up, survivors with a new breast cancer event (n = 79) worked more hours than disease-free survivors (n = 567), and both groups worked more hours than women in the comparison group (n = 890). Three years after diagnosis, survivors decreased the mean work hours per week by 1.8 hours, whereas women in the comparison group increased their mean work hours per week by 0.8 hours. Both groups decreased their number of work hours at their second jobs. Survivors earned more before and 3 years after their diagnosis than the comparison group. Women who decided not to return to work did so out of personal choice, not the choice of employers or as a result of discrimination.

Patients with cancer were denied health insurance before the enactment of the ADA and the FMLA. Patients have continued to work while undergoing cancer treatments. A flexible schedule is an excellent strategy to maintain employment for the patient and the employer. Nurses can encourage patients to discuss this option with their employers. The productivity of patients with cancer or survivors can be the same or better than people without cancer.

PHYSICAL LIMITATIONS AND DISABILITY ASSOCIATED WITH CANCER

Taylor and colleagues showed that patients with breast cancer are not the only group affected with disabilities secondary to cancer treatment.[9] In a study of patients with head and neck cancer, the variables of chemotherapy, neck dissections, stage of the disease, and high pain scores increased the odds of being disabled. Patients experienced disabilities with neuropathies, dysphagia, and loss of taste. Patients undergoing chemotherapy were 3 times more likely to have disability than those not undergoing chemotherapy. The disabilities developed as a result of a prolonged period of cancer treatment. Neck dissections without other cancer treatments disabled more than 50% of the patients in this sample at a rate of 2 times greater than those not undergoing a neck dissection. Patients with increased pain showed a 20% increase in disability. Overall, 52% of the patients in this study were disabled because of cancer therapy. Patients can become disabled at any time during their cancer treatment. Nurses should assess for physically debilitation and limitations before the initiation of therapy and throughout the course of therapy.

A 2002 pilot study investigated the feasibility of gathering employment, disability, and cancer treatment data.[10] The researchers concluded that it was feasible to conduct this type of trial. They measured four types of cancer, but we will discuss the 73 women diagnosed with breast cancer. The mean age for the group was 58.5 years, 70% had at least a high school education or higher, 71% were staged as local cancer, and approximately 29% were staged as regional cancer. Cancer treatment included surgery only (34%); surgery and radiation (31%); surgery and chemotherapy (19%); and surgery, radiation, and chemotherapy (15%). Over 88% of participants reported that they were insured through their health plan or their spouses' health plan. Respondents reported at least one physical limitation such as heavy lifting, stooping, kneeling, crouching, concentrating, analyzing data, learning new things, or keeping pace with co-workers.[10] Even though these problems are not considered disabilities as defined by ADA, they can be physically limiting. Women in this study pointed out several side effects of therapy that could affect their work and employment. To understand the level of complexity between physical limitations and employment, further research studies are warranted.

Predictor of Disability and Cancer

A survey conducted in 1989 described key factors in predicting work disabilities.[11] Patients with four different cancers were assessed using multiple tools to evaluate illness, job, skills, education, income, age, sex, and more. Results showed that three key factors predicted whether a person with cancer will become disabled. The key factors are physical dimensions of illness, physical demands of the job, and time discretion. Physical dimension of illness included stage of disease, physical demands of the job, intensity of cancer treatment(s), and pain. Time discretion was described as the time it took to complete the work, the pace, and the time period available in which to complete the work. Time discretion, skill discretion, education, and income appeared to be positive predictors for staying in the work force. Aspects of social background such as sex, age, income, and education had little effect on work disability. Time discretion was the consistent predictor of continued employment. Time discretion was measured by questions on flexible work schedule, flexible hours, and setting the pace of the work. The employee who has a flexible work schedule, is autonomous in determining his or her pace of work, and can work a few hours at a time is the worker who will continue to be employed during cancer therapy.

In a study conducted with a relatively small sampling of women diagnosed with breast cancer and undergoing radiation therapy, fatigue was the most common symptom reported and was cited in all age groups as a problem.[12] Of the 10 women who were working full-time at the time of diagnosis, 40% took paid leave, 30% took disability, and 30% took unpaid leave or decided to stay at home. One way of combating fatigue is to empower women with the autonomy to set their own schedule and pace; then fatigue can become a manageable symptom.

RETURN TO WORK

Approximately 80% of patients with cancer who are employed at the time of diagnosis will attempt to return to work.[10,13,14] Some patients elect to delay their return to work until after cancer treatment. Nurses are encouraged to learn about FMLA laws to assist patients and families.[15]

As early as 1992, Berry and Catanzaro wrote that nursing interventions were key factors in patients returning to work.[15] They identified three crucial areas: personal factors, environmental factors, and human responses. By understanding the key factor to the patient's in returning to work, the nurse could intervene and positively influence the patient's continued employment. Nursing interventions could include (a) patient education about the disease, treatment, and side effects; (b) discussion of work and its meaning to the patient and family; (c) exploration of health insurance and employment benefits; (d) communication with workplace officials regarding the disease, its course, treatment schedules, and accommodations; (e) discussions of work options or alternatives during treatment; and (f) preschedule updates with employers about when the patient will be returning to work.

When survivors of cancer elect other employment options, do they keep their medical history private?[16] Do they focus on their current ability to perform the job functions? It is reasoned that if they have an impairment such as lymphedema that will affect their job, these conditions are disclosed to the potential employer. It is recommended that benefits questions should not be approached until after the employer has extended an offer for the position. In many circumstances, the human resource department is responsible for reviewing and negotiating benefits with employees, and one strategy that may be beneficial for persons with cancer is to keep these issues separate from actual job issues and discuss them privately with human resources as opposed to disclosing to their immediate supervisor.

In several studies published in the last few years, there have been consistent measurements, definitions, and methodologies that make for easier cross-comparisons. In one study, 80% of the survivors (n = 200) were employed at diagnosis.[17] Of those survivors, 89% (n = 177) returned to work and 81% (n = 142) were still employed after 5 years. Twenty-three people did not return to work; the majority of these cited reasons of physical and medical illness (n = 17) that prevented them from working. Another set of employees (34%) completed their treatment before returning to work. Approximately 60% of survivors remained with the same employer for over 5 years. In another larger cohort study conducted in 2004, approximately 61% of 4,100 breast cancer survivors identified from the Finnish Cancer Registry were employed 2 to 3 years after diagnosis.[18]

Over 4,350 long-term cancer survivors were surveyed regarding their ability to work, job discrimination, and quality of life.[19] Approximately 35% of the cancer survivors were working at the time of the patient survey, with more men than women working. More Hispanic (47.3%) and Asian (52.2%) survivors were working than white (31.2%) and black (34.6%) survivors. The younger the survivor was at the time of diagnosis, the more likely he or she was to be working. Over 8.5% reported they were not able to work because of diagnosis or treatment; of those, there were more blacks (23.2%) than Hispanics (9.7%), whites (8.0%), and Asians (4.3%). Of special interest were the 300 breast cancer survivors who responded to the survey: of these, 68 women (18.4%) reported they were unable to work. Some 110 patients (less than 2%) responded they experienced job discrimination. There were 10 individuals who reported being fired or forced to quit, 4 who were denied promotions, 7 who were denied employment, and 5 who were denied health insurance.

A 2005 study found that 73% of patients with cancer returned to work 1 year after their diagnosis, and 84% of patients returned to work after 4 years.[20] Researchers interviewed approximately 1,400 patients with a diagnosis of cancer identified in Pennsylvania and Maryland. Those patients not returning to work cited disability as the reason. The recommendation is to focus on symptom management, rehabilitation, and disability accommodation to provide assistance for patients wanting to return to work.

Employment Productivity

Two myths of productivity are being dispelled through research.[8,21] The first myth is that persons with cancer are less productive, and the second myth is that persons with cancer have a negative impact on the labor force. The findings tend to support that women with breast cancer contribute to their employment during and after diagnosis. The women's employment choices were not hindered by the fear of losing the job, not being able to find another job, or job discrimination. They made personal choices regarding their employment independent of having a diagnosis of cancer or being a survivor of cancer.

Bradley and others linked the 1992 Health and Retirement Study (HRS) and employment elements together.[22] They focused on a cohort of 51- to 61-year-olds with one member of the family surviving at least 3 years with female breast cancer. The sample of 5,974 women included 156 women with breast cancer. Women with a history of breast cancer had a mean age of 55 and averaged 7 years from their diagnosis, with 75% having survived at least 3 or more years. These women worked a mean of 41.42 hours/week, and they earned an average of $11.49/hour. In comparing the breast cancer survivors and the women without breast cancer, the survivors worked 3.39 more hours/week, had 13% higher wages, and earned on average $2,350 more per year. The study did not explore the reasons for the survivors of breast cancer to work more hours.

In 2005, researchers reported the results of a survey of 837 women diagnosed with breast cancer and 613 women without breast cancer.[23] Women in the Detroit area were surveyed between the summer of 2001 and 2002; the researchers controlled for age, marital status, education, number of children, and household income. A subset of employed women in both study and control groups were employed at the time of the first survey; 69% and 84% of the working women with breast cancer and control group were employed at the second interview. Women with breast cancer worked on average of 39 hours/week at the time of the first interview (6 months after diagnosis) and an average of 33 hours/week at the second interview. Results showed that patients with stages III and IV disease reduced their hours by an average of 10 hours/week. The control group were working an average of 37 hours/week at the first interview and an average of 38 hours/week at the second interview. For women not returning to work after a diagnosis of breast cancer, 74% reported the cause to be illness and 19% as "other," 6% were laid off, and 1% attributed not working to a personal reason. The researchers contend that 50% of the working women with breast cancer will have some type of labor market consequences, and that the late-stage cancers are account for the majority of negative effects on the labor market.

FINANCIAL IMPACT OF CANCER

The NIH estimated the financial impact and overall cost for cancer in 2003 to be $189.9 billion.[1] This is a staggering number by any standard. Direct medical costs accounts for $69.4 billion; $16.9 billion for indirect morbidity costs (lost productivity because of illness); and $103.5 billion for indirect mortality costs (lost productivity owing to premature death). Researchers investigated a targeted population of persons over the age of 70 years from a cohort of the HRS.[24] The team noted there was a greater expenditure of health care dollars for patients undergoing cancer treatment than persons previously diagnosed or who had never had cancer.

A surprise finding was the difference in expenditures among the three study groups. Patients with a history of cancer had a median total expenditure for health care of $640, whereas patients currently in treatment for cancer had a median total expenditure of $920 and patients without cancer had a median total expenditure of $570. The greatest difference in health care expenditure among the three groups was in outpatient services; there was a median of $270 spent on patients with cancer receiving current treatment, whereas a median of $160 was spent on patients without cancer. These outpatient services included physician office appointments, dental visits, and outpatient surgery. From the patient's perspective the cost of cancer care can be staggering. The need for insurance coverage and continued employment is vitally important to the welfare of the patient and family.

A patient's health care expenditures can reach well into the hundreds of thousands of dollars depending on the treatment plan. For example, bone marrow transplants exceed $100,000.[25] When this amount is combined with the charges for surgery, antineoplastic agents, growth factors, outpatient services, and physician's fees, the patient is faced with reaching or exceeding maximum benefit limits. Employers can establish a maximum annual benefit and a maximum lifetime benefit as a condition of a health insurance policy. These are typically between $250,000 and $1 million. The year-to-date and lifetime amounts are usually provided on the explanation of benefits form.

The Internal Revenue Service (IRS) provides information that can help determine the individual's responsibility for health care expense.[26] The IRS defines medical expenses as the costs associated with diagnosis, cure, symptom management (mitigation), and treatment; this includes equipment and diagnostic medical devices, supplies, and dental expenses. For 2004, the IRS calculated this responsibility as 7.5% of the adjusted gross income. An itemized deduction form must be submitted to the IRS to take advantage of the deduction. For example: if one's adjusted gross income is $50,000, then the patient's responsibility is for 7.5% of that, or $3,750. One can deduct that portion of paid medical expenses that exceed $3,750.

Health Insurance and Insurance Reform

The percentage of Americans under the age of 65 with no health insurance coverage is estimated to be 17%, according to the 2003 National Health Interview Survey.[27] Another 33% of Americans 65 years or older have Medicare coverage only. In the 18- to 64-year-old age group, 18% of

Americans do not have a regular source of health insurance; and of that group, 6% cite cost as the barrier to obtaining health care.

Poverty is an important factor influencing survival.[1] The delay in obtaining medical care, the lack of early detection, and the lack of or limited health insurance coverage add to the higher percentage of late-stage diagnosis. The National Cancer Institute's Surveillance, Epidemiology, and End Results (SEER) program cites that women in high-poverty areas were 1.7 times more likely to be diagnosed with metastatic breast cancer than their counterparts in low-poverty areas.[1] Poverty level was derived from the 1990 decennial census. Rate is defined as the percentage of the population below the poverty level: low-poverty areas are census tracts with less than 10% of the population below poverty level and high-poverty areas have 20% below poverty level or more.[1] From 1988 to 1994, the 5-year survival for all cancers in the lower-poverty areas was 63% and 53% in high-poverty areas.

In 1974, Congress passed the Employee Retirement Income Security Act (ERISA), which regulates self-insured health insurance plans and employee benefit plans.[28] The act requires employers to provide a health plan to employees and a summary health plan document including details of the plan's rules, financial information, operations, and management. The act prohibits the employer from discriminating against an employee for the purpose of preventing him or her from collecting benefits from the employee benefit plan.

In 1986, the US Congress passed the Consolidated Omnibus Reconciliation Act (COBRA), requiring employers to offer medical coverage at group rates to an employee who loses coverage by voluntary resignation, retirement, termination, or reduced work hours.[29] Employer stipulations include having at least 20 employees and cover both public and private employers, and coverage must be extended to surviving, divorced, or separated spouses and dependent children. Group insurance through COBRA is commonly more expensive than for an active employee enrolled in the health plan; however, self-insured plans are less expensive than individual health plans obtained through a health insurance company. Medical coverage typically covers surgery, hospitalization, outpatient medical services, dental care, and vision care, and prescription plans are an added expense if offered at all; services and benefits are defined by the plan. Patients with cancer may need to purchase COBRA insurance to ensure continuous medical coverage and no gaps in insurance.

It is important for people with a cancer history to avoid any gaps or lapses of insurance coverage. Future employers may have a preexisting condition clause in their health insurance plan. A preexisting condition is defined as a health-related condition that was diagnosed before the employment with the company. If there are gaps in insurance, the health plan can decide whether or not to cover the preexisting conditions. There are specific pieces of insurance legislation and regulations governing health maintenance organizations and other types of health insurance carriers. Each individual's case is reviewed by the health plan's benefits administrator. The waiting period for preexisting conditions can range from months up to 1 year.

In 1996, Congress passed the Health Insurance Portability and Accountability Act (HIPAA), protecting the employee's rights to health insurance coverage when the employee changes jobs or loses his or her job.[30] This portability portion of the act has four main components. The type of previous health care coverage, the impact of preexisting conditions, the length of time of exclusions for preexisting conditions, and the type of coverage protection are determined by the individual circumstances of the patient. The insurance reform act is complex; a referral to the health plan's benefits administrator or insurance specialist may be beneficial for the patient.

If the patient with cancer is eligible for HIPAA and applies for health coverage within 63 days of losing the previous employer's insurance, then under the act the patient is guaranteed eligible to purchase health care insurance, receives at least two health coverage choices, and is not subject to any exclusionary period for preexisting conditions. Patients with cancer who are faced with a change in employment status need to seek assistance. In 2005, Centers for Medicare and Medicaid Services (CMS) suggests that to be eligible for a HIPAA guarantee, a person must meet the following requirements: the person has at least 18 months of creditable continuous health care insurance coverage; the coverage is through a group plan; the person is not eligible for government insurance programs or group insurance plan; the person did not lose insurance coverage as a result of fraud or not paying premiums; the person accepted and used up all COBRA continuation of coverage.[30] Information can be obtained on the HIPAA web site at www.cms.hhs.gov/hipaa.

The CMS and the federal government developed an interactive Internet tool called HIPAA OnLine, accessible online at www.cms.hhs.gov/hipaa/online.[31] This website is focused on the insurance portability. Another government Internet site is provided by the Office of Civil Rights, www.hhs.gov/ocr/hipaa, focused on the medical privacy of personal health information.

Another piece of legislation has helped patients with cancer. In 1998, Congress passed the Women's Health and Cancer Rights Act (WHCRA), which protects the rights of women who have elected to have a mastectomy.[32] The act provides medical and surgical benefits for the mastectomy operation and all stages of reconstruction, procedures to the contralateral breast for symmetry, prosthesis, and treatment of physical complications (e.g., lymphedema). The act stipulates that group health plans and their insurers or health maintenance organizations must provide such coverage.

Employment and Health Insurance

In a study published in 1996 by Ganz and colleagues, 139 patients were recruited during their first year after primary treatment for breast cancer.[33] A mailed survey was sent 2 years after the initial surgery. The survey was conducted between 1990 and 1992, before the enactment of ADA and FMLA, with women with breast cancer who remained employed. At the time of diagnosis, approximately 90% of the women reported adequate health insurance. Coverage for health insurance fell from 80% to 60% between the second and third years after diagnosis; this decrease was attributed to increases in premiums, loss of COBRA, or decreases in benefits. Two years after their diagnosis, over 46% of the women were employed in professional or white collar jobs and cited the benefits of a flexible schedule and time off from work. This group referenced the ability to communicate with their employers and did not experience discrimination.

In a patient-oriented VHS videotape entitled Back to Work after Breast Cancer, six women who are survivors of breast cancer tell of their experience with employment, co-workers and insurance.[34] There is one vignette that illustrates the ethical dilemma of disclosing a history of cancer. The research literature shows that the effects of disclosing cancer to employers has been minimal since ADA regulations were passed. In short, it is illegal to discriminate against a person with cancer. In one vignette a theology student in her late 30s found herself at the time of diagnosis with inadequate health care coverage. After treatment was completed, she obtained employment with excellent health care benefits. She settled for a job that held little interest for her but gave her the health care benefits she desired. Months later, she found an opportunity within the same university and changed jobs. The video depicted her weighing the advantages of disclosing her cancer to a future employer. This woman did not disclose her past history of cancer. Her story explored the practical aspects of employment and demonstrates the need for health insurance coverage and the lengths to which some women go to ensure that coverage for themselves and their families.

Professional Responsibility

In multiple studies, it is evident that people with health insurance often know little of their benefits until illness is upon them. The stories of friends and neighbors, myths, misconceptions, and the lack of experience with insurance and catastrophic illness fuel the fears of a newly diagnosed patient with cancer. This is evident in patient comments about insurance and employment. It is in the best interest of the patient for health care professionals to learn as much about these issues as possible and to refer patients to financial counselors and/or social service professionals for assistance. However, the oncology team should possess a basic knowledge about these issues.

A primer was published in 1999 entitled Cancer Survivors' Employment and Insurance Rights.[35-37] The article provided oncologists and their team with a summary of patient employment issues, the impact of cancer on health insurance, and survivor rights including ADA, FMLA, and health insurance. Particularly enlightening is the review of HIPAA and its impact on the insured patient's ability to change jobs without losing coverage, even if the patient has previously been diagnosed with cancer. Common insurance terminology is clearly defined in terms that the oncologist and team can understand. The article provided vital information to the cancer specialist, addressed the positive impact of the ADA in the workplace and employment and insurability problems, and explored unique problems faced by pediatric cancer survivors.

In the Oncology Nursing Society Nursing (ONS) Sensitive Outcome paper published in 2003, symptom experience, functional status, safety (prevention), psychologic distress, and economics were identified as the sensitive outcomes.[38] The paper asserts that economics is to be incorporated into all the other categories. This is a clear signal of the importance that economics has on the patient outcomes and the potential impact of oncology nurses. With this ONS endorsement, oncology nurses are mandated to explore economic issues through nursing research. Measurements of economic outcomes included length of stay, numbers of unexpected readmissions and emergency visits, out-of-pocket costs (family), costs per patient day or per episode of care, time lost from work by patients and caregivers, and others.

Patient Education Resources on Employment and Finances

Patients are more active than ever in educating themselves on services and information that will help them deal with the cancer experience. Information comes from the Internet and organizations such as the National Cancer Institute and the American Cancer Society, oncologists and oncology nurses, mass media, and written educational materials.

There are numerous patient education resources regarding cancer. Many are listed in Box 23-3. Before recommending a web site, an educational pamphlet, or a book to a patient or support group, a nurse should investigate it. Questions should be asked such as these: what is the goal of the web site, who is the target audience, what message is the site projecting, is there a content expert who monitors the site and answers questions or clarifies misconceptions, is the site updated on a regular basis, does it have timely updates, who is the administrator, and what groups support the site. What do other professional nursing organizations think about the resource? Is the resource produced by the a government agency, a pharmaceutical company, or a person surviving with cancer? These are some key factors to question when recommending this type of resource.

An example of a web site is "Living with It," an Internet site produced by Aventis Pharmaceuticals. It focuses on survivors of cancer and is accessible in English or Spanish. Topics include diet and exercise, financial matters, lifestyle, medical options, and survivor stories. Additional website access options include support groups, resources, journaling, cancer organizations, and coping with cancer. Financial issues such as health insurance, laws governing health insurance, financial issues, and employment rights are also presented. The web address for this site is www.livingwithit.com.

The American Cancer Society internet site can be accessed at www.cancer.org and has more than 10 sets of patient-oriented educational materials ranging from ADA, health insurance, COBRA, working during treatment, employment discrimination, and other work-related topics.

Comical, whimsical, and understandable: the Cancer S.O.S. book is a survival guidebook for women diagnosed with cancer. It has a particularly hopeful outlook as it navigates the reader from diagnosis and treatment to image control and mind and body issues through finance and life resources.

Women's Cancers is a self-help book for women written by two seasoned oncology nurses.[39] The book explores a variety of women's cancers: breast, gynecologic, lung, and others. Making informed choices and empowerment are key concepts in every chapter. The text and writing style are easy to read and friendly as the chapters unfold from diagnostic tests to cancer treatments. The "Systemic Treatment for Cancer" chapter touches on costs associated with clinical trials and paying for cancer treatment. Readers are encouraged to seek counselors during their hospitalization for any type of social or financial worry or consult with the physician's office staff in the outpatient setting. Some financial information is given within the book.

One of many patient newsletters supported by nonprofit organizations is Lymphoma Today.[40] An educational newsletter, it published an article in the summer of 2002 on ADA and FMLA. The article provides simple explanations and examples for patients and professionals. In addition, it recommended that patients discuss issues with the human resources department or the employer because of the intricacies of the discrimination laws.[41]

Media productions sponsored by pharmaceutical companies are available on their Internet sites or by writing the companies. Many pharmaceutical companies offer a medication assistance program, or indigent program. These programs can be very beneficial to people with limited means of support or lower incomes. Patients are required to follow a process and apply for medical assistance. Each case is reviewed based on criteria such as insurance coverage, income, and medical necessity. Often, cancer centers will have dedicated staff in the pharmacy to assist patients in completing applications. This expedites the process not only for the patient but for the facility.

Box 23-3 Internet Sites with a Focus on Employment and Financial Issues

American Cancer Society
www.cancer.org

The Association of Cancer Online Resources
www.acor.org

Cancercare
www.cancercare.org

CancerLinks
www.cancerlinks.com

Family and Medical Leave Act
www.dol.gov/dol/topic/benefits-leave/fmla.htm

Living Beyond Breast Cancer
www.lbbc.org

Living With It
www.livingwithit.org

National Asian Women's Health Organization
www.komen.org

National Breast Care Coalition
www.stopbreastcancer.org

National Coalition for Cancer Survivorship
www.canceradvocacy.org

National Partnership for Women & Families
www.nationalpartnership.org

Patient Advocate Foundation
www.patientadvocate.org

Pharmaceutical Research and Manufacturers of America
www.phrma.org

The Susan G. Komen Breast Cancer Foundation
www.komen.org

Sisters Network
www.sistersnetworkinc.org

Young Survival Coalition
www.youngsurvival.org

Y-Me National Breast Cancer Organization
www.y-me.org

Compassionate medication programs are also advertised on many pharmaceutical company's web sites. The larger pharmaceutical companies offer rebates or discounted drug cards to patients regardless of income. Some companies provide free medications on an international level to developing countries. The range of services provided by the pharmaceutical industry is broad. The nurse should be familiar with the medication assistance programs of the pharmaceutical agents commonly used in their work setting and be knowledgeable about the referral process. Pharmaceutical companies provide literature explaining their medication programs.

FUTURE IMPLICATIONS

Great strides have been made to protect survivors' rights in the area of work, health insurance, and finances, but more is needed. Further research studies focusing on patients with cancer are needed to establish the predictors of disability and to develop interventions geared toward factors that lead to disability. In 2005, the first major changes in the FMLA were proposed since its origination. The proposal is coming from business groups, which cite the administrative time consumed by the requirements of the 76 FMLA regulations. The proposal would restrict the current definition of serious health condition, change the consequence days from 3 to 10 for an illness, and limit the employee to not less than a half a day of intermittent leave. The debate in Congress should be closely monitored, since the approval of any of the proposals will affect patients with cancer. An area that we know little about is the interaction between co-workers and patients with cancer who continue to work during treatment. It is an interesting area of research given reported survivorship concerns about fatigue, short-term memory and cognitive impairments, and other symptoms.

SUMMARY

In summary, this chapter has explored issues of work, in particular, employment, finance, and insurance concerns facing persons with cancer. While the majority of research concerns persons with cancer in general, specific information about women with cancer and work-related issues is derived from experience with the breast cancer population. Return to work, employment productivity, and laws protecting cancer survivors from discrimination will continue to be an area of increased concern in cancer survivorship.

REFERENCES

1. American Cancer Society: *Cancer Facts and Figures 2005,* Atlanta, 2005, American Cancer Society.
2. Jemal A and others: Cancer Statistics, 2005, *CA Cancer J Clin* 55:1, 2005.
3. United States Department of Justice, Americans with Disabilities Act; on the Web at www.usdoj.gov/crt/ada.
4. United States Department of Labor, Family and Medical Leave Act; on the Web at www.dol.gov/esa/whd/fmla.
5. Hewitt M, Breen N, Devesa, S: Cancer prevalence and survivorship issues: analysis of the 1992 national health interview survey, *J Natl Cancer Inst* 91:17, 1999.
6. Rothstein MA, Kennedy K, Ritchie KJ: Are cancer patients subject to employment discrimination? *Oncology* 9(12): 1303-1315, 1995.
7. Hounshell J and others: Changes in finances, insurance, employment and lifestyle among persons diagnosed with hairy cell leukemia, *Oncologist* 6:435-440, 2001.
8. Maunsell E and others: Work situation after breast cancer: results from a population-based story, *J Natl Cancer Inst* 96(24):1813-1822, 2004.
9. Taylor JC and others: Disability in patients with head and neck cancer, *Arch Otolaryngol Head Neck Surg* 130: 764-769, 2004.
10. Bradley CJ, Bednarek HL: Employment patterns of long-term cancer survivors, *Psycho-Oncology* 11:188-198, 2002.
11. Greenwald HP: Work disability among cancer patients, *Soc Sci Med* 29(11):1253-1259, 1989.
12. Burnie C: Breast cancer: a study of the psychosocial issues faced by women undergoing radiation therapy, *Can J Med Radiat Tech* 2000, 31(3):119-128, 2000.
13. Berry DL: Return to work experience of people with cancer, *ONF* 20(6):905-911, 1993.
14. Bloom JR and others: Then and now: quality of life of young breast cancer survivors, *Psycho-Oncology* (13): 147-160, 2004.
15. Berry DL, Catanzaro M: Persons with cancer and their return to the workplace, *Cancer Nurs* 15(1):40-46, 1992.
16. Welsh R, Grandahl S: Keep financial, insurance and legal concerns in check, *Cancer S.O.S. strategies in survival,* ed 1, Lake Mary, Fla., 1998, Alva.
17. Sanchez KM, Richardson JL, Mason HRC: The return to work experiences of colorectal cancer survivors, *AAOHN J* 52(12):500-510, 2004.
18. Taskila-Abrandt T and others: The impact of education and occupation on the employment status of cancer survivors, *Eur J Cancer* 40:2488-2493, 2004.
19. Schultz PN and others: Cancer survivors. Work related issues, *AAOHN J* 50(5):220-226, 2002.
20. Short PF, Vasey JJ, Tuncelli K: Employment pathways in a large cohort of adult cancer survivors, *Cancer* 103(6):1292-1301, 2005.

21. Bradley CJ, Bednarek HL, Neumark D: Breast cancer and women's labor supply, *Health Services Res* 37(5): 1309-1328, 2002.
22. Bradley CJ, Bednarek HL, Neumark D: Breast cancer survival, work and earnings, *J Health Econ* 21:757-779, 2002.
23. Bradley CJ and others: Short-term effects of breast cancer on labor market attachment: results from a longitudinal study, *J Health Econ* 24:137-160, 2005.
24. Singh GK and others: Area socioeconomic variations in U.S. cancer incidence, mortality, stage, treatment, and survival 1975-1999, Number 4, Bethesda MD, 2003, NCI Cancer Surveillance Monograph Series.
25. Stewart SK: *Bone marrow transplants*, Highland Park, Ill., 1992, BMT Newsletter.
26. United States Department of the Treasury, Internal Revenue Service; available online at www.irs.gov.
27. Langa KM and others: Out-of-pocket health-care expenditures among older Americans with cancer, *Value in Health* 7(2):186-194, 2004.
28. United States Department of Labor, Employee Retirement Income Security Act; on the Web at www.dol.gov/dol/topic/health-plans/erisa.
29. United States Department of Labor, Consolidated Omnibus Reconciliation Act; on the Web www.dol.gov/dol/topic/health-plans/cobra.
30. United States Department of Health and Human Services, Office of Civil Rights; on the Web at www.hhs.gov/ocr/hippa.
31. United States Department of Health and Human Services, The Centers for Medicare and Medicaid Services; available online at www.cms.hhs.gov.
32. United States Department of Health and Human Services, The Centers for Medicare and Medicaid Services: Women's Health and Cancer Rights Act, on the Web at www.cms.hhs.gov/hipaa/hipaa1/content/whcra.
33. Ganz PA, Coscarelli A, Fred C: Breast cancer survivors: psychosocial concerns and quality of life, *Breast Cancer Res Treatment* 38:183-199, 1996.
34. Nessim-Keeney, S (producer): Back to work after breast cancer, *Aventis Oncology* 2003, videotape, TxT-Bx-11483-1.
35. Hoffman, B: Cancer survivors' employment and insurance rights: a primer for oncologists, *Oncology* 13(6):841-846, 1999.
36. Moore D: The Hoffman article reviewed, *Oncology* 13(6):846, 1999.
37. Hobbie WL: Hoffman article reviewed, *Oncology* 13(6): 849,852, 1999.
38. Given B and others: ONS Nursing Sensitive Outcomes, *Oncology Nursing Society* 2003, white paper, on the Web at www.ons.org/research/outcomes.
39. McGinn, K: The systemic treatment for cancer. In McGinn KA and Haylock PJ: *Women's cancers*, ed 2, Alameda, Calif, 1998, Hunter House.
40. Schwerin BU: Taking time off for treatment: your rights, *Lymphoma Today* 1(2):7, 2002.
41. Boyer GC: Legal barriers against employment discrimination for the breast cancer patient, *Innov Breast Cancer Care* 2(1):13-16, 1996.

UNIT VI

Reaching Culturally and Ethnically Diverse Women

CHAPTER

24 Hidden Populations of Women

Victoria Wochna Loerzel

INTRODUCTION

This chapter focuses on the uniqueness of women in relation to cancer. Health professionals are very aware of women as a diverse population. Differences include age, race, ethnicity, socioeconomic status, educational level, sexual orientation, and employment status. Because of these differences, women will respond to cancer-related prevention, diagnosis, treatment, and survivorship in different ways. Not only do women respond differently, they are responded to in diverse ways by health care professionals. Health care professionals do not always recognize these differences in women, or their own preconceptions and biases. This lack of awareness may prevent women from receiving appropriate recommendations for early detection of disease, treatment decisions, and referrals to support services.

The purpose of this chapter is to introduce cancer-related issues involving different populations of women who have specific concerns and needs. The author acknowledges that much of the research that focuses on women and cancer involves women with breast cancer and gynecologic cancers. This is an obvious and plentiful population with which to conduct research because of the number of women diagnosed with these specific diseases. However, excluding women with other cancers is not intentional. In addition, the women discussed in this chapter are not the only groups of diverse women that health professionals will encounter. Still, they do represent a substantial portion of the population.

LESBIANS AND CANCER

Lesbians have been defined as a minority group with specific needs and concerns. They also make up a population that is vulnerable and at risk for discrimination.[1] *Healthy People 2010* identifies gay and lesbian persons to be at risk for disparities in health and health care, which can directly affect their risk for developing cancer.[2]

The US Census Bureau counted 601,209 same-sex unmarried, but partnered, households in the US in the year 2000. It is estimated that this statistic could be undercounted by as much as 62%.[3] Gay and lesbian families live all over the US, and it is likely that health care professionals encounter this population in medical practice whether they are aware of it or not. Lesbians may be a hidden population whose needs are underaddressed, which leads to increased health disparities.

Because of the many misperceptions involving lesbians, health, and health care, it is important to highlight this population. Many health care professionals may not realize that lesbians are at risk for certain cancers based on their lifestyle, when in fact lesbians may be at increased risk for certain cancers resulting from past and present lifestyle and health behaviors. Lesbians have higher rates of smoking, alcohol

Acknowledgement
The author would like to thank Christopher Blackwell, RN, PhD, ARNP, for his thoughtful review of this manuscript.

abuse, obesity, and stress than their heterosexual counterparts. In addition, lesbians can be solely partnered with women throughout their lives or may have had sexual relationships with men at some point in their lives.[4] The combination of lifestyle behaviors and previous sexual relationships place lesbian women in higher risk categories for some cancers. These experiences, coupled with fears of homophobia from physicians and medical staff, may affect health-seeking behaviors in lesbians and lead to late diagnosis and treatment of cancer in this population.

Risk Factors for Specific Cancers

Lesbian women may be at increased risk for developing certain types of cancers. Factors that influence risk include reproductive history, history of cancer-related screening, lack of education concerning personal risk for developing cancer, and misperceptions of the medical community regarding health risk in lesbian patients. The majority of research concerning lesbians and cancer has been conducted in relation to breast and gynecologic cancers.

Breast Cancer

The risk factors for developing breast cancer are well known. These include increasing age, personal or family history, early menses and late menopause, history of or biopsy-confirmed atypical hyperplasia, dense breast tissue, postmenopausal obesity, use of chemical hormones (birth control pills or hormone replacement), having a first child after the age of 30 or having no children, and consuming one or more alcoholic beverages a day. Protective factors include breastfeeding, moderate exercise, and maintaining an ideal body weight.[5]

Although the overall risk for lesbians developing breast cancer compared to heterosexual women is unclear,[6] several studies in the literature suggest that lesbians are at increased risk for developing breast cancer because of reproductive choices that include nulliparity or being of an older age when having their first child, and behavioral choices that include increased incidence of obesity and increased alcohol consumption.[7,8] One study that compared breast cancer risk between lesbians and their heterosexual sisters indicated that lesbians had a significantly higher five year ($p < 0.0001$) and lifetime ($p = 0.001$) risk of developing breast cancer compared to their sisters.[9] Number of pregnancies, higher body mass indices, and higher incidence of a past history of smoking were attributed to the increased risk. In addition, lesbians are less likely than heterosexual women to participate in cancer-related screening activities such as breast self-exam and mammography, which may translate into late detection of breast cancer and higher mortality rates.[7,8]

Gynecologic Cancer

Risk factors for *cervical cancer* are also well known. These include having sex at an early age, having multiple sex partners, sexually transmitted human papilloma virus (HPV) infection, and smoking. Women who are overweight are more likely to die from cervical cancer than women within their ideal weight range. Risk factors for developing *ovarian cancer* include family history, nulliparity, and using estrogen alone as hormone replacement after menopause. Protective effects include pregnancy, tubal ligation, and use of birth control pills.[5]

Clearly, lesbians may be affected by both of these cancers. Current and past social behaviors may increase their risk for cervical cancer. Further, lesbians are less likely to have used birth control pills and have fewer pregnancies and children than their heterosexual counterparts, so they do not enjoy a protective benefit against endometrial or ovarian cancer.[7,10] In addition, lesbians are less likely than heterosexual women to have received recent or annual screening for gynecologic (GYN) cancers.[4,8] Lack of recent screening may translate into later diagnosis and higher mortality rates for GYN-related cancers.

Health Care Behaviors in Lesbians

The American Cancer Society has well-established recommendations for early detection and screening for breast and gynecologic cancer. Women who detect breast, ovarian, and cervical cancer early have increased rates of cure and decreased mortality rates associated with cancer compared to women diagnosed in later stages of disease.[5] Unfortunately, lesbians are less likely than heterosexual women to participate in preventive and screening services.[4,6-8,11] Reasons for low rates of participation in screening activities are multifactorial.

Many barriers to accessing appropriate screening tests are similar in lesbian and heterosexual populations. Regardless of sexual orientation, reasons for not participating in screening tests include being uncomfortable with the test procedure, perceived low-risk status, and access issues such as lack of health insurance.[4] Additional factors may include misperceptions by health care providers regarding risk for cancers such as cervical cancer, which may translate into fewer referrals to gynecologists for gynecologic cancer screening tests.[4,12,13]

Fish and Wilkinson[6] examined lesbians' practice of breast self-examination in the United Kingdom and found perception of risk and lack of education as barriers to this practice. In a sample of 1,066 lesbian women, 218 (20%) reported that they have never practiced breast self-examination. Reasons for not practicing breast self-examination included not knowing what they were looking for (34%); never getting into the habit or not wanting to be bothered (21%); fear (12%); and belief that they were not at risk (11%). This belief was mostly seen in younger lesbians who felt they were too young to have breast cancer. Older lesbians did perceive that they were at risk because of their age. Admittedly, many of these reasons are also shared by heterosexual women; however, this study stresses the need for education to lesbians regarding screening and early detection tests in light of their risk factors for developing breast cancer.

Other studies have examined the screening behaviors of lesbians for cervical cancer. Lesbians were less likely (49%) to have had a routine Pap tests in the last 3 years when compared to heterosexual women (66%), even when they reported behaviors known to increase risk for developing cervical cancer.[4] Lesbians (n = 550) in this study reported earlier age at first intercourse, higher number of sexual partners, and never practicing safe sex, as compared to heterosexual women (n = 279). Older lesbians were more likely to participate in cervical screening than younger lesbians. Overall, the reasons for differences in Pap screening between lesbian and heterosexual women are unclear. The researchers propose that the lower reproductive needs and need for medications such as birth control pills reduces visits to a gynecologist, who usually performs screening tests. Further, lesbians who are in relationships with women may not realize their risk of developing cervical cancer and the need to see a gynecologist based on past sexual experiences.

Homophobia, Heterosexism and Discrimination in Health Care

Unique factors specific to lesbians not seeking appropriate screening tests for cancer include fears related to homophobia and discrimination in the general and medical populations.[14] Many lesbians have had previous negative encounters with medical and health care professionals[1,7,9] and have perceived bias regarding their sexual orientation, and other lesbians have perceived hostility from medical personnel.[15]

Disclosure of sexual orientation is of great concern to lesbians;[16] however, it is unclear what impact it may have on health care in this population.[12] Diamant, Schuster, and Lever[12] did not find that disclosing sexual orientation had a negative effect on receiving preventive health services. However, in their study that examined preventive health care services received by lesbians (n = 6935), women who were comfortable disclosing their sexual orientation with physicians were more likely to have received a Pap test in the last 2 years than those women who were not comfortable with sharing this information (82% versus 64%). The researchers discussed that being comfortable with disclosing sexual orientation may lead to women being more comfortable discussing their sexual histories, including experiences with men. Disclosure may prompt the physician to make the appropriate cancer screening referrals based on risk factors. The receipt of mammograms was not affected by disclosure of sexual orientation.

In other studies, lesbians did not feel that it was necessary to disclose their sexual orientation to all of their health care providers. Instead they preferred to disclose their orientation to those physicians they saw on a regular basis, unless there was a reason to do otherwise.[16] When lesbians did disclose their sexual orientation during treatment to their oncologists and staff, they did not report any change in care or quality of their treatment or attitudes towards them by the medical professionals. Many lesbians did introduce their partners to their oncology team to ensure that their partner received the same consideration a heterosexual spouse would receive.[16]

Satisfaction with Health Care and Support

Several studies examined lesbians' perceptions of their interactions with their oncologists, medical staff, and other resources available to them. Matthews and colleagues[16] compared lesbians' experience with breast cancer with the experience of heterosexual women. Overall, lesbians tended to be less satisfied with their care than heterosexual women (75% versus 96%, $p < 0.05$). They also reported being slightly less satisfied (although the difference was not statistically significant) with the care given by nurses; about emotional support given by their providers and significant others; and about the inclusion of themselves and their partners in medical decisions.

Both lesbian and heterosexual women reported experiences with social support and support groups; however, heterosexual women were more likely to be currently involved in formal support groups (57% versus 18%). In focus groups, lesbians reported that they did not feel comfortable disclosing their sexual orientation with other support group participants and that the support groups dealt with issues that did not apply to them; for example, discussions that concerned men's attraction to female breasts.[16] Interestingly, lesbians reported a higher incidence of participation in individual counseling because of cancer-related issues than heterosexual women (69% versus 39%). Lesbians in this study were also concerned with the lack of resources tailored to their needs and the needs of their partner during their experience with cancer.

UNMARRIED AND UNPARTNERED WOMEN AND CANCER

Single women with cancer are a population with unique needs during diagnosis, treatment, and survivorship. These women may be older or younger, never married, separated, divorced, or widowed from their husband or partner. Unfortunately, unmarried women and the concerns they have related to cancer have not been well studied. Many issues encountered by single women are related to social relationships and support, concerns about fertility, and care of current children.

Research examined the impact of social support on both married and unmarried women. Perception regarding lack of support among single women is inconclusive.[17] In general, being married has been equated with having greater support. Studies have associated marital status with incidence of depression,[18] with unmarried individuals reporting higher rates of depression. Being unmarried is also associated with more reports of worse physical symptoms from treatment and more psychologic distress when compared to married people.[19,20] Other studies have reported that unmarried women perceive high levels of social support and low incidence of psychosocial adjustment problems.[21]

Gluhoski and colleagues[17] address the challenges for young single women with breast cancer (average age was 33.5 years). In this qualitative study, 16 unmarried women identified stressors that were associated with being an unmarried breast cancer survivor. These stressors were organized into the following themes:

- Being pessimistic about future relationships. Dating was an important concern. The women believed that the number of partners available

to them was limited because of their breast cancer and its possible ramifications for the future. Some women thought they were more selective than before their cancer. Other women believed men would now find them less appealing.
- Concern and fears related to disclosing their illness to future partners. Women were concerned with when and how to disclose the fact that they had had breast cancer to a new partner. Some women expressed that being uncomfortable talking about their cancer and the fear of rejection from a new partner caused them to avoid new relationships.
- Impaired sexuality and negative body image. Disfigurement caused by surgery for breast cancer led to a negative view of their sexuality and desirability. Fear of rejection led to a reluctance to begin new sexual relationships. Women discussed the emphasis some men place on women's breasts and their own discomfort at revealing an altered body to a new partner.
- Pain of being rejected by partners. Several women in this study were rejected by their partners as a result of their diagnosis. The illness and its possible long-term impact were overwhelming for some of the men they were in relationships with.
- Lack of support and a sense of isolation after illness. Several women in this study felt alone and desired a close companion or confidant during their illness. Lack of a partner left these women without day-to-day assistance and emotional support during their illness.

Holmberg and colleagues[22] support many of these concerns. In a small study (n = 15) that examined relationship issues of women of various ages with breast cancer, unpartnered women had significant concerns with body image, sexuality, self-esteem, and future relationships. Unpartnered women were very concerned about how and when to introduce their cancer diagnosis and the physical changes from surgery in a new relationship. Additional concerns such as fear of rejection, being viewed as undesirable, and believing they will never be involved in a relationship again were also supported by the participants.

Fertility Concerns

Fertility and family planning has been reported as a concern among young cancer survivors,[17,23] especially unmarried women of child-bearing age. Many of the treatments available to treat cancer can have a significant impact of a woman's reproductive capabilities. Women treated for breast cancer with the standard treatment regimes that include cyclophosphamide and doxorubicin are at risk for amenorrhea and damage to the ovaries. Both of these factors increase the risk of infertility in women after treatment. Hormonal therapy with agents such as tamoxifen also has an impact on starting or continuing a family, since women are often advised to wait at least 2 years after treatment before attempting to become pregnant.[23] As the age increases, fertility may decrease; women undergoing breast cancer therapy who are unmarried may be at increased risk for infertility by the time they find a partner with whom they would like to have a family.

Custody Planning

Many women are raising children independently. In some instances, women may be the sole caretaker of their children as a result of a spouse's death. In other instances women may be partnered with their children's nonbiologic or legal father. A diagnosis of cancer, especially in later stages, may force women to think about how their children will be cared for in the event of their death. Child custody is a topic that many people may put off discussing for fear of not being hopeful about their recovery from cancer, and of causing distress to their children and other family members. Realistically, it is a topic that some women should think about from the very beginning of their treatment. Oftentimes, health care professionals are in a position to initiate this conversation, which may be met with resistance from women under treatment.[24]

In a retrospective study concerning custody planning for oncology patients conducted by Willis and colleagues,[24] half of the families studied did not have an established custody plan for their children, and in 40% of the cases, custody of the children went to individuals to whom the parent had been adamantly opposed while he or she was alive. In addition, children reported increased stress when they did not know who would be caring for them in the future. Discussing custody planning with children can also ensure that they will be taken care of by guardians with whom they find it acceptable to spend the rest of their dependent years.

OLDER WOMEN AND CANCER

Although many of the issues women face during and after treatment for cancer are similar, each woman may experience unique concerns and issues. Older women are no exception. There are many differences between older women and younger women in relation to cancer diagnosis, treatment, survivorship, and psychosocial needs.

In a review of literature, Sammarco[25] indicated that women will experience breast cancer differently based on their psychosocial life stage. Older women may need extra time with the physician or nurse and may need to be encouraged to participate in their treatment decisions. On the other hand, several qualitative studies have shown that older women do want to be included in treatment decisions.[26,27] Although older women may not be as distressed about their diagnosis as younger women, they may require other interventions to meet their needs, both physical and social.[25] Many older women live alone and may need help identifying resources.

Overall, it appears that older women have more variable treatment than younger women and are often undertreated for their disease.[28-34] Most of the research concerning the differences in treatment among elderly and younger patients have taken place in women with breast cancer because of the readily available population; however these differences in treatment have also been seen in populations with lung cancer, colorectal cancer, and lymphoma.[34]

Many of the differences can be attributed to misperceptions and erroneous beliefs of health care professionals and of patients themselves: that breast cancer in the elderly is less aggressive; that the elderly have limited life expectancy because of other chronic comorbid conditions; and that breast cancer is not as big of a problem compared to other causes of mortality.[28] Further, many health care professionals may be under the impression that elderly women are frail and cannot handle standard treatments. Age alone should not be used as a determining factor for optimal treatment regimens.[35]

Differences between the cancer experiences of elderly women and of younger women can be noted from the moment of diagnosis. Busch and colleagues[29] compared women aged 75 years and older to women younger than 75 (n = 41,033). Approximately 22% of those in this sample were older than 75. Older women have fewer cancers detected by mammogram and fewer needle localizations, and had more advanced disease stage at diagnosis. Bouchardy and colleagues[28] studied 407 women in Switzerland over the age of 85 and noted many inconsistencies with both diagnosis and treatment. Diagnosis was made by clinical examination in 14% of the population, and the majority of the women had no histologic assessment of their disease. Estrogen receptor status was unknown in 74% of the population. The majority of these women were diagnosed with stage II disease or higher (78%).

Treatment differences were notable. Busch and colleagues[29] noted that if older women received breast-conserving surgery, they were less likely to receive radiation therapy. Woodard and colleagues[33] observed that the older women were less likely than younger women to receive chemotherapy as part of their treatment. Women of ages 50 to 65 were 6 times as likely to not receive chemotherapy, and women over the age of 65 were 62 times as likely not to receive chemotherapy, when compared to women under age 50. The researchers concluded that age bias contributed to the undertreatment of this patient population.

Bouchardy and colleagues[28] noted no standardization of treatment in older women. Women opted for no treatment (12%); tamoxifen only (32%); breast-conserving surgery and radiation (7%); and mastectomy (14%). Tamoxifen was given to women regardless of their estrogen receptor status. The researchers determined that 50% of these women had suboptimal treatment that contributed to increased mortality related to breast cancer. In this sample, 47% of older women received standard treatment, as compared to 91% of women aged 50 to 79 years.

WOMEN WITH A FAMILY HISTORY OF CANCER

Nurses and other health care professionals must be aware of the needs of women with a family history of cancer and integrate information into teaching strategies. A more thorough discussion of genetics and cancer in women is found in Chapter 3. Women with a family history of breast, ovarian, and colon cancers are at increased risk for developing a similar or related cancer as compared to the average woman.[36] Subsequently, these women and their families have additional educational and psychosocial needs as compared to women without a family history of cancer.[37] Many women do not realize their risk for developing a family-related cancer and inconsistently participate in screening programs.[38,39] This puts women at risk for late diagnosis.

Every woman who has a family history of cancer does not necessarily have a genetic predisposition to developing cancer. Approximately 5% of all breast cancer diagnoses are related to *BRCA1* and *BRCA2* mutations, and these mutations have also been seem in some women with ovarian cancer.[36] Although the likelihood of carrying this mutation is small, many women choose to undergo genetic counseling and testing to determine if they carry the *BRCA1* or *BRCA2* genetic mutation. Deciding to undergo genetic testing is an individual decision and has implications for the entire family.

Knowing *BRCA* status allows women to make choices regarding their participation in screening programs for breast and ovarian cancer and prophylactic treatment options, and possibly may cause them to alter their life plan and make reproductive choices to reduce the risk of passing on the genetic mutation to their children.[39] Knowing *BRCA* status is very empowering for many women but in others can create very high levels of anxiety, negatively affecting quality of life.[39,40]

Regardless of known genetic status, informational needs of women with a family history of cancer are high. In a study that examined informational and support needs of daughters and sisters of women with breast cancer, Chalmers and collegues[41] asked participants to rate their informational needs. The highest rated item was the need for information regarding their own personal risk for developing breast cancer. Other highly ranked items included the need for information concerning early detection, risk factors, and strategies to decrease their risk for developing breast cancer.

Worry about developing cancer among women with a family history varies from one study to another, ranging from low worry to a great deal of worry. Loescher[42] evaluated worry in women with hereditary risk factors for breast cancer and found that the women in her study experienced low worry overall, but that worry was increased when they had cancer-specific symptoms such as an abnormal mammography finding or pending biopsy. Chalmers and colleagues[41] reported that over half of the women in their study worried either somewhat or a great deal about getting breast cancer.

One method of coping with the worry and anxiety associated with a having a family history of cancer or genetic mutations is prophylactic surgery. It has been established that bilateral prophylactic mastectomy can reduce a women's risk of developing breast cancer by 95% if she has a *BRCA1* or *BRCA2* mutation.[43] Women who have received this procedure have reported reduced distress and positive satisfaction with their decision.[44,45]

Although women with a family history of cancer are encouraged to participate in cancer-screening activities, participating in screening programs may increase anxiety and distress among women. Andrykowski and collegues[46] demonstrated the psychologic impact of abnormal screening results for ovarian cancer. Women with either a personal or family history of breast

Box 24-1 Resources

The Susan G. Komen Breast Cancer Foundation (www.komen.org) is an excellent resource for all women and health care professionals. Several informational pamphlets have been developed by the Komen Foundation for lesbian education, and a workbook has been designed to assist providers in developing patient educational materials for women who partner with women.

The Mautner Project (www.mautnerproject.org)
This is the only national organization specifically dedicated to lesbians with cancer, their caregivers, and their partners. This organization provides education, services, and support to lesbians with cancer. It also promotes research concerning lesbian health and acts as an advocate for the lesbian community.

The Gay and Lesbian Medical Association (www.glma.org)
Dedicated to promoting equality in health care for gay, lesbian, bisexual, and transgendered individuals, this organization is actively involved in professional and public education, public policy, and promoting research that focuses on issues specific to gay and lesbian populations.

Young Survival Coalition (www.youngsurvival.org)
This is an organization dedicated to the concerns of young women with breast cancer

Cancercare.org (www.cancercare.org)
Cancercare offers free, professional support services to anyone affected by cancer and provides information for women concerned with sexuality and relationship issues after cancer.

National Cancer Institute (www.cancer.gov)
In addition to providing a wealth of information on general cancer issues, the NCI has numerous publications and informational brochures on sexuality and fertility and coping with cancer.

The American Cancer Society (www.cancer.org)
The ACS offers many different support programs for women with cancer.

The National Ovarian Cancer Coalition (www.ovarian.org)
The coalition provides a variety of information on ovarian cancer, treatment, and survivorship. The web site also offers a wide range of links to resources of interest to women with ovarian cancer or those who are interested in learning more.

Women's Cancer Network (www.wcn.org)
The network is dedicated to informing women and empowering them to be their own health advocates. The web site provides information on cancer risk, clinical trials, and survivorship.

National Cervical Cancer Coalition (www.nccc-online.org)
The web site provides educational information for women interested in learning more about their risk for cervical cancer, diagnosis and treatment, and survivorship. This organization also maintains an ongoing support system for women diagnosed with cervical cancer.

cancer or a family history of ovarian cancer, and asymptomatic women over the age of 50, were offered transvaginal ultrasound screening for ovarian cancer. Abnormal results were clearly distressing to all women and lasted for several months. However, women without a family history of ovarian cancer were more distressed than women with a family history. The authors reasoned that women without a family history were not aware of their risk for developing this cancer, and this caused them to brood over the thought. Women with a family history experienced less distress, possibly as a result of thinking about the possibility throughout their lives, which enabled them to avoid thinking about a possible diagnosis with abnormal ultrasound results.

Health care professionals are in a position to assist women who have a family history of cancers such as breast or ovarian with education, screening, and treatment decisions. Promoting healthy behaviors and being supportive of treatment decisions is imperative when discussing risk and treatment options with women who have a family history of cancer.

RESOURCES

Resources for women with specific needs such as lesbians, single and unmarried women, older women, and women with a family history of cancer are often scarce. Health care professionals often have to seek out specific resources for their patients, or their needs go unmet. Box 24-1 lists organizations that assist health care professionals in providing appropriate and sensitive information to patients.

SUMMARY

Health care providers encounter women with different needs and concerns every day; however, recognizing the unique needs of women may be challenging. Not recognizing the differences in the patient populations they see may lead to inappropriate referral for cancer screening programs or support services, or lack of it altogether. This in turn may lead to later diagnosis of cancer and increased emotional distress in women. Health care professionals must familiarize themselves with their patient population and the needs they have.

REFERENCES

1. O'Hanlan KA and others: Advocacy for women's health should include lesbian health, *J Womens Health* 13(2): 227-234, 2004.
2. U.S. Department of Health and Human Services: *Healthy People 2010: A systematic approach to health improvement,* Washington, D.C., 2001, U.S. Department of Health and Human Services, Government Printing Office. Retrieved 3/3/05 from www.healthypeople.gov/Document/html/uih/uih_2.htm#goals.
3. Smith DM, Gates G: Same-sex unmarried partner households. Retrieved 3/5/05 from www.urban.org/Template.cfm?NavMenuID=24&template=/TaggedContent/ViewPublication.cfm&PublicationID=8425.
4. Matthews AK and others: Correlates of underutilization of gynecological cancer screening among lesbian and heterosexual women, *Prev Med* 38(1):105-113, 2004.
5. American Cancer Society: *Cancer Facts and Figures 2004,* Atlanta, 2004, The Author. Retrieved 3/21/05 from www.cancer.org.
6. Fish J, Wilkinson S: Understanding lesbians' healthcare behaviour the case of breast self-examination. *Soc Sci Med* 56(2):235-245, 2003.
7. Cochran SD and others: Cancer-related risk indicators and preventive screening behaviors among lesbians and bisexual women, *Am J Public Health* 91(4):591-597, 2001.
8. Dibble SL, Roberts SA: Improving cancer screening among lesbians over 50: results of a pilot study, *Oncol Nurs Forum* 30(4):E71-79, 2003.
9. Dibble SL, Roberts SA, Nussey B: Comparing breast cancer risk between lesbians and their heterosexual sisters, *Womens Health Issues* 14(2):60-68, 2004.
10. Dibble SL and others: Risk factors for ovarian cancer: lesbian and heterosexual women, *Oncol Nurs Forum* 29(1):E1-7. 2002.
11. McGregor BA and others: Distress and internalized homophobia among lesbian women treated for early stage breast cancer, *Psychol Women Q* 25(1):1-9. 2001.
12. Diamant AL, Schuster MA, Lever J: Receipt of preventive health care services by lesbians, *Am J Prev Med* 19(3): 141-148, 2000.
13. Stine K: Discrimination's impact of public health practices, *J Gay Lesbian Med Assoc* 6(2):79-83, 2002.
14. Clark MA and others: The cancer screening project for women: experiences of women who partner with women and women who partner with men, *Womens Health* 28(2):19-33, 2003.
15. Matthews AK: Lesbians and cancer support: clinical issues for cancer patients, *Health Care for Women Internatl* 19:193-203, 1998.
16. Matthews AK and others: A qualitative exploration of the experiences of lesbian and heterosexual patients with breast cancer, *Oncol Nurs Forum* 29(10):1455-1462, 2002.
17. Gluhoski VL, Siegel K, Gorey E: Unique stressors experienced by unmarried women with breast cancer, *J Psychosoc Oncol* 15(3-4):173-183, 1997.
18. Kugaya A and others: Correlates of depressed mood in ambulatory head and neck cancer patients, *Psychooncology* 8(6):494-499, 1999.
19. Lewis FM And others: The functioning of single women with breast cancer and their school-aged children, *Cancer Pract* 4(1):15-24, 1996.
20. Rodrigue JR, Park TL: General and illness-specific adjustment to cancer: relationship to marital status and marital quality, *J Psychosom Res* 40(1):29-36, 1996.
21. Budin WC: Psychosocial adjustment to breast cancer in unmarried women, *Res Nurs Health* 21(2):155-166, 1998.
22. Holmberg SK And others: Relationship issues of women with breast cancer, *Cancer Nurs* 24(1):53-60, 2001.
23. Dow KH, Kuhn D: Fertility options in young breast cancer survivors: a review of the literature, *Oncol Nurs Forum* 31(3):E46-E53, 2004.
24. Willis L and others: Custody planning. a retrospective review of oncology patients who were single parents, *J Pain Symptom Manage* 21(5):380-384, 2001.
25. Sammarco A: Psychosocial stages and quality of life of women with breast cancer, *Cancer Nurs* 24(4):272-277, 2001.
26. Crooks DL: Older women with breast cancer: new understandings through grounded theory research, *Health Care Women Int* 22(1-2):99-114, 2001.
27. Overcash JA: Using narrative research to understand the quality of life of older women with breast cancer, *Oncol Nurs Forum* 31(6):1153-1159, 2004.
28. Bouchardy C and others: Undertreatment strongly decreases prognosis of breast cancer in elderly women, *J Clin Oncol* 21(19):3580-3587, 2003.
29. Busch E and others: Patterns of breast cancer care in the elderly, *Cancer* 78(1):101-111, 1996.

30. Gajdos C And others: The consequence of undertreating breast cancer in the elderly, *J Am Coll Surg* 192(6): 698-707, 2001.
31. Giordano SH and others: Breast cancer treatment guidelines in older women, *J Clin Oncol* 23(4):783-791, 2005.
32. Silliman RA: What constitutes optimal care for older women with breast cancer? *J Clin Oncol* 21(19): 3554-3556, 2003.
33. Woodard S and others: Older women with breast carcinoma are less likely to receive adjuvant chemotherapy: evidence of possible age bias? *Cancer* 98(6):1141-1149, 2003.
34. Dale DC: Poor prognosis in elderly patients with cancer: the role of bias and undertreatment, *J Support Oncol* 1(4 suppl 2):11-17, 2003.
35. Muss HB and others: Adjuvant chemotherapy in older and younger women with lymph node-positive breast cancer, *JAMA* 293(9):1073-1081, 2005.
36. American Cancer Society: *Cancer Facts and Figures 2005,* Atlanta, 2005, The Author. Retrieved 3/21/05 from www.cancer.org.
37. Conto SI, Myers JS: Risk factors and health promotion in families of patients with breast cancer, *Clin J Oncol Nurs* 6(2):83-87, 2002.
38. Andersen MR and others: Awareness and concern about ovarian cancer among women at risk because of a family history of breast or ovarian cancer, *Am J Obstetr Gynecol* 189(4):S42-47, 2003.
39. Hutson SP: Attitudes and psychological impact of genetic testing, genetic counseling, and breast cancer risk assessment among women at increased risk, *Oncol Nurs Forum* 30(2):241-246, 2003.
40. Kenen R, Arden-Jones A, Eeles R: Healthy women from suspected hereditary breast and ovarian cancer families: the significant others in their lives, *Eur J Cancer Care* 13(2):169-179, 2004.
41. Chalmers K and others: Reports of information and support needs of daughters and sisters of women with breast cancer, *Eur J Cancer Care (Engl)* 12(1):81-90, 2003.
42. Loescher LJ: Cancer worry in women with hereditary risk factors for breast cancer, *Oncol Nurs Forum* 30(5): 767-772, 2003.
43. Rebbeck TR and others: Bilateral prophylactic mastectomy reduces breast cancer risk in BRCA1 and BRCA2 mutation carriers: the PROSE Study Group, *J Clin Oncol* 22(6):1055-1062, 2004.
44. Metcalfe KA: Prophylactic bilateral mastectomy for breast cancer prevention, *J Womens Health (Larchmt)* 13(7): 822-829, 2004.
45. Metcalfe KA and others: Psychosocial functioning in women who have undergone bilateral prophylactic mastectomy, *Psychooncology* 13(1):14-25, 2004.
46. Andrykowski MA and others: Psychological response to test results in an ovarian cancer screening program: a prospective, longitudinal study, *Health Psychol* 23(6): 622-630, 2004.

CHAPTER

25 African American Women and Cancer

Margaret Chamberlain Wilmoth and Lutchmie Narine

INTRODUCTION

The American Cancer Society estimates that 211, 240 American women will be diagnosed with breast cancer in 2005 and 40, 410 will die from the disease.[1] African American women have a lower incidence of breast cancer than Caucasian American women (119.9% vs. 141.7%), but a higher mortality rate (35.4% vs. 26.4%).[1] African American women have both higher incidence and mortality rates of other cancers than Caucasian American women, including cancers of the stomach, colorectal, stomach, and cervix. A variety of reasons is postulated to explain how the incidence of breast cancer in African American women can be lower and the mortality rate higher, including less access to health care, lack of health insurance, lower socioeconomic status (SES), communication barriers, and fatalistic views of cancer.[2-4]

Healthy People 2010 identified the elimination of health care disparities as the number two goal to improve the health of Americans. This goal includes reducing disparities based on sex, race and ethnicity, income, and education, among others.[5] Eliminating the disparities in cancer prevention, early detection, and treatment is a key focus area for public health efforts for this decade. Furthermore, this document calls for culturally competent, community-based health care systems to ensure comprehensive care for all Americans.

This chapter will briefly explore some of the important factors involved in making contact with African American women and seeking to increase their participation in early detection programs for a variety of cancers. Programs and strategies that have been successful in this population will be highlighted. Implications for nurses working in the area of cancer detection and prevention will be presented as well as resources that may be of assistance in providing high quality, holistic care while overcoming barriers.

CONTEXTUAL FACTORS

Contextual factors that contribute to the difficulties in getting African American women to participate in cancer prevention/early detection activities are complex, but can be generally divided into the following areas: health care environment, patient, and clinician factors.[4] Selected health care environment factors that have had a negative effect on quality of health care include the lack of health insurance, racial discrimination, and negative racial attitudes that continue to persist long after passage of the Civil Rights Act of 1965. The disproportionately small numbers of minority health care providers has also had a negative effect on gaining access to these populations for clinical trials research.[4]

Patient context factors include the pervasive impact that the abuse of ethnic minorities in research (most notably the Tuskegee syphilis study) has had on the African American community as well as the mistrust that has developed toward medical institutions based on claims that minorities are genetically inferior to Caucasians.[6] Knowledge that they receive lower rates of the more effective, higher-technology diagnostic tests and treatments, and higher rates of less effective procedures than Caucasians contributes to minorities' distrust in the recommendations made by majority population health care providers.[4]

Finally, clinician factors that add to the contextual background include the clinician's ethnicity, and type and site of his or her clinical practice. Minority physicians are more likely to have hospital-based practices or to engage in family practice in a staff-model HMO than nonminority physicians,[4] thus reducing their ability to engage in primary cancer detection activities. African American nurses make up less than 5% of all registered nurses in the US, despite concerted efforts by schools of nursing to attract and retain minority students. The small number of minority health care providers contributes a great deal to the lack of cultural appreciation for the cultural, social, and economic factors that provide the context in provision of care. Linguistic or communications barriers also play a role in the context of health care for African Americans. Phrases or even single words can be interpreted differently by White health care providers, leading them to misinterpret the significance of symptoms or the meaning of the symptom to the individual.[7] These contextual factors are important to consider when planning outreach to African American women.

CULTURAL AND HEALTH FACTORS

Religion and Spirituality

Concepts of spirituality and religious affiliation are fundamental to African American women's worldview of health and the disease process. Spirituality is an important element in understanding behaviors of African Americans in relation to health and disease. Many African Americans believe that their degree of health or the presence of illness is God's will.[8] Spirituality provides a foundation for both coping with disease and overcoming distrust of the dominant health care system.[9] Many breast cancer outreach programs are based on the role spirituality and personal faith play in lives of African Americans, particularly in the southeastern portion of the US.[10] These spiritually-based programs teach women health-promoting behaviors within the context of their faith, assuming that their confidence and grounding in their spiritual beliefs will have a positive effect on self-efficacy in wellness and health promotion.[10]

Traditionally African American women have had strong religious orientations. The church was a major institution in the lives of slaves and continues to be one of the few indigenous institutions in African American communities. Thus sources of authority (e.g., ministers) in the church can be quite influential in the lives of African American women and the decisions they make about their cancer care. In investigating how African American women cope, Lena Wright Myers[11] interviewed 200 black women from across the country and found that most of her subjects felt the church and religion helped prepare them for getting ahead in life. Responses showing how the church and religion were of help included "The Lord would always show me the way to go"; "Got to have something to believe in, in order to get ahead, and I believe in spiritual things." Similarly, Wilson-Ford,[12] in her study of 407 African American women in rural North Carolina, identified prayer and belief in God as the second most important health-protective behavior.

As a result of their cultural heritage, furthermore, African American women have retained a holistic philosophy of health, mind, and body perceived as inseparable with the total person in interaction with the environment. Illness is thought to result from disharmony or conflicts in some area of a person's life. Ill health can be seen as a sign of being out of favor with God or a "spirit," and African American women may seek for a traditional minister or unconventional spiritualists and healers to intercede with prayer. Indeed, folk medicine and similar practices based on African American women's belief of the etiology of their cancer are often used in conjunction with conventional healers like nurses and physicians.[13] Consequently, in order to better meet the needs of African American women, nurse providers must assess the importance of religion and spirituality in the lives of these women and how this can affect the design of outreach activities.

Distrust of the Medical System

One of the major barriers to cancer outreach programs among African American women is their almost innate distrust of the medical system. Dulla,[14] in an article titled "African American Suspicion of the Health System Is Justified: What Do We Do about It?" has documented some of the very real factors that have contributed to African Americans distrust of the medical system. These include the following:

i) Past abuses of slaves as experimental and teaching material
ii) Tuskegee syphilis experiment
iii) Involuntary sterilization
iv) Attitudes about the cause of AIDS
v) Research about violence among males

Suspicion and distrust of the US medical system among African Americans has its origins in the time of slavery. Slaves were often used for medical experiments and research, and put on display as instructional material for medical students.[14] In 1932, the Tuskegee experiment was launched to understand the effects of untreated syphilis. However, researchers failed to educate the participants about their risks or treat them adequately. There is also the perception that state-supported family planning clinics in the past have performed involuntary sterilizations on African American women.[14,15] Also, in response to the high rate of AIDS among African Americans there has been speculation among members of the African American community that the AIDS epidemic may be part of a genocidal plot by the white power structure to deliberately infect them with the AIDS virus.[14,15] Through oral and written history, many African American women have come to know of past abuse of their community by researchers and medical profession—which continues to this day.[16] Indeed, in a survey of African American and European American women, Mouton and colleagues[17] found that 32.1% of African American women agreed or strongly agreed that scientists cannot be trusted, as compared to only 4.1% of European American women. In addition, 28.6% of African American women agreed or strongly agreed that researchers did not care about them, whereas only 13.7% of European American women shared this view. This and other studies confirm that there is a strong cultural norm in the African American community not to trust the medical community and not to participate in medical research.

This distrust makes African American women hesitant to get screened for cancer or initiate early treatment. However, of even more concern are the low participation rates of African American women in clinical cancer trials. Clinical trials are perhaps the most important way to develop more effective cancer treatments, yet it has been estimated that only 0.005% of African American women have ever participated in one.[18] This has serious consequences because many cutting-edge treatments are only available through clinical trials. Thus African American women who do not participate in clinical trials will lose out on opportunities to benefit from new cancer treatments. Apart from missing out on treatments, the lack of participation of African American women in clinical trials also results in poor understanding among the medical community about the unique effects of new cancer treatments in this population. Many cancers manifest themselves differently in women in general and African American women specifically. Thus to know whether a treatment (e.g., a drug) is effective or to what degree it is effective among African American female cancer patients requires their participation in medical research.[18]

Alternative Medical Practices

Partly as a result of the mistrust of the medical system discussed in the previous section, and partly because of other factors, African American women tend to seek alternative sources of health care, either as the only choice or in combination with more traditional options. In some instances the use of alternative medical practitioners is a result of previous discrimination where African American women were denied services or felt they received substandard care from the established medical system. In other cases they may lack economic resources or insurance to pay for cancer care. Thus folk remedies may be the only alternative some African American women have to costly cancer treatments provided by the mainstream medical system.[15]

In addition, there are important historical underpinnings to the use of alternative healers and therapies in the African American population. Most African Americans are primarily the descendents of West African people who have their own native beliefs about health and medical treatment. There is documented evidence that these West African health practices have been handed down and maintained among contemporary African American women. Thus in many cases folk remedies used by African American caregivers have received a stamp of approval and legitimacy by having been passed down through the generations.[15] Another reason for the use of alternative sources of care is the sense that it provides to cancer sufferers that they are coping with their problem in the context of their own resources, and within their own social and cultural environment. Most ethnic groups, including African American women, like to use a health network they perceive as more "in tune" with their culture rather than that of the formalized and less culturally friendly health care system.

The alternative health practices used by African American women include herbs and home remedies such as sugar and turpentine for stomach problems, poultices applied to body parts to treat infection and pain, herb teas for gastrointestinal problems, soda for chest pain, vinegar and garlic for blood afflictions, and hot tea with lemon and honey or a dash of brandy for respiratory problems. There are basically two types of alternative indigenous health practitioners who serve the African American community—independent and cultic practitioners. Independent practitioners usually operate as individuals and are affiliated with an alternative or occult supply store. The cultic practitioner is usually affiliated with some religious group and can practice his or her healing arts in either public or private settings. One variation of the independent practitioner is the neighborhood prophet, or Old Lady.[15] She does not often dispense therapies but serves as an advisor about what herbal and home therapies are appropriate for a condition and how to concoct these remedies. Most of the time the Old Lady or neighborhood prophet does not require money but will be paid for her services with gifts of food or expressions of gratitude.

The implications of the alternative health practices of African American women for cancer outreach are manifold. The simple fact that they use alternative healers may make them reluctant to consider help from representatives of the formal health care system. The use of herbal and home remedies used in combination with more traditional medications may hamper the effectiveness of treatments, if there are drug interactions, or may actually cause harm to the patient. To the extent that African American women see alternative care as having a higher potential for success or offering more immediate attention, they can develop attitudes that inhibit traditional cancer outreach activities. For example, African American women who use alternative care sources can develop an attitude and behavior of presenting their cancer difficulties to mainstream practitioners only as a last resort, or they may view preventive cancer services as not being worth their time and effort.[19]

Place in Social and Family Structure

Despite their presence at all socioeconomic levels in American society African American females tend to be disproportionately represented in the lower classes. The Census 2000 indicated that 22.7% of all African Americans were below the poverty level, as compared with 7.8% for non-Hispanic Whites.[20] Thus on the basis of socioeconomics, African American women tend to be found on the lower rungs of the social order. This is further exacerbated by the place women hold in African American society. While they are often essential breadwinners in the family and more educated than their male counterparts, African American women are still subject to the same stereotypes and sexism that afflict women in the larger American society.[21] The diminished social position experienced by many African American women can present special challenges to those trying to direct outreach activities to them. Often these diminished roles mean they come to the health care setting with a low sense of agency about their ability to affect their health and health care. Also, occupying low income levels means African American women are primarily concerned with immediate economic and social needs. Cancer or other illness becomes a priority only when African American women become very ill and find it difficult to carry out their usual social and economic roles.[22]

Most African Americans seem to have a nuclear family model, but underlying this is the concept of the extended family. Kennedy,[23] in a study of southern African American families, found they were an extended kinship network with complex patterns of relationships among a wide range of people who were not necessarily related by blood or marriage. The extended family is based on a sense of obligation and can be called upon for support and advice when an individual is faced with health problems. Martin and Martin,[24] in interviews with 30 extended African American families, found the typical household consisted of at least four generations that were looked upon for emotional, social, and material support. They also that found that a dominant figure kept the family together. However African American families are typically egalitarian in their roles, and the dominant figure and decision maker could be a female or male. Thus African American women do not make cancer care decisions in a vacuum. Their decisions are often based on the role of family in their lives and on the needs of the family. This consideration of the role and needs of family is factored in as they consider the level of risk posed by various factors in their lives including the possibility of having cancer.[22] Thus cancer outreach programs to African American women need to take into consideration a woman's family situation and in particular the key decision makers in her life that can affect her judgment about whether to participate in cancer screening or to seek treatment for cancer.

Health Beliefs

African American beliefs about health and health practices include ideas about the origins of disease, hot and cold, blood, and surgery.[13] Some African American women believe in a dichotomous classification of the cause of illness into natural and unnatural, which determines where an individual will seek health care. Unnatural causes are said to be due to forces like "worriation" (worry), stress, evil influences, and sorcery, and care is likely to be sought from alternative folk healers. Cold surroundings are thought to be the source of illness, especially those associated with the respiratory system. Some women are suspicious of having too many blood tests taken because blood is a substance that can be used in witchcraft. This of course can present difficulties in cancer screening efforts. With respect to cancer treatment, many African American women may be reluctant to have surgery, since they believe exposing cancer cells to air causes the cancer's spread. Another important belief that can affect cancer outreach efforts is the thinking that if a condition does not interfere with activities it is not important enough to seek care. Further, there is a strong preference for care that can be administered over a short rather than a longer period of time.[13,19]

A sense of fatalism and the inevitability of death upon diagnosis with cancer is another culturally specific facet of health beliefs that must be addressed when working with African Americans.[25] Powe, Ntekop, and Barron[26] posit that fatalism about cancer develops over time as an individual witnesses cancer being diagnosed in its late stages in family and friends, with concomitantly limited treatment options and, ultimately, death. The researchers also suggest that fatalism regarding the ultimate outcome after receiving a diagnosis of cancer represents a situational manifestation of a perceptual paradigm of hopelessness, meaninglessness, and despair. Although there appears to be agreement in the literature that cancer fatalism plays a role in the barriers to cancer screening, it is not clear how much of a factor it is.[27] Furthermore, there does not appear to be solid science on the ways to effectively overcome this barrier to screening or to participating in cancer clinical trials.

Social Support

Social support is generally defined in the literature as provision of information that makes the patient feel as though she is valued and a member of a network of communication and mutual obligation.[28] Results of focus groups with older African American women living with breast cancer suggest that they benefit from social support from other women with the disease, but that their opportunities are limited.[29] Data supporting this finding indicates that higher levels of perceived emotional support have a significant association with increased survival in both African American and Caucasian women who were diagnosed with breast cancer.[27] In addition, recent research suggests that African American women with breast cancer may not benefit from social support as typically defined, for example by means of disease-oriented support groups, and recommends that social support measures must be refined for appropriateness in African Americans.[30]

Empowerment

A significant barrier to cancer outreach to African American women can be the lack of empowerment and helplessness they feel about the health care system, cancer treatment, and their ability to prevent or control cancer.[15,17] This sense of a lack of empowerment has its origins in a variety of sources involving large societal issues as well as experiences with the health care system. On the larger societal stage, mention has already been made of the subordinate economic and social position in which African American women often find themselves both in general society and within their own community. This general subordination is further reinforced by the negativity they may be subjected to when their images are compared to those of their white counterparts.[19] The dominant culture in which they live broadly values the features of white women. Thus when compared with this standard, African American women are often judged and in turn tend to judge themselves as unattractive and hence inferior. Indeed, there is a close connection between feelings of attractiveness and feelings of self-worth among African American women. Greene[21] has observed that among the African American women in her practice "...there are few who do not report experiencing some degree of emotion regarding physical self-image, from mild dissatisfaction to shame."

The lack of empowerment felt by African American women due to large societal forces is further compounded by their experience with the health care system. In many cases, African American women's interaction with the health care system is not positive. Many of them approach the system with a healthy distrust, which, in many cases, is confirmed by the lack of sensitivity shown by their cancer care providers. Examples of the type of insensitivity include perceptions of a usually white genetic counselors taking a judgmental attitude or a physician not taking time to explain more about a diagnosis at the first visit.[18] Eley and collegues[31] reported that approximately 25% of differences in breast cancer mortality between African American women and Caucasian women remained unexplained even after adjusting for socioeconomic and other potentially explanatory variables. Similarly, Breen and collegues[32] found that health care providers did not consistently offer optimal care alternatives to African American breast cancer patients as compared to the treatments offered to their white counterparts. The combination of insensitivity and inequality in the standard of care provided further contributes to feelings of a lack of empowerment and helplessness among African American women.

It is important for those conducting cancer outreach among African American women to address feelings of lack of empowerment and helplessness, because the issue can underlie an absent sense of agency (i.e., that one has the ability to manage one's life including one's illness).[17] This lack of agency can make it difficult to get African American women to participate in cancer outreach, to make decisions about seeking cancer prevention care, or to play an active part in their treatment. Indeed, Lythcott, Green, and Brown[18] suggest that African American women who lack agency may be likely to "avoid screening activities or to drop of out of detection activities prior to diagnosis."

HEALTH PROMOTION AND EDUCATION STRATEGIES

Cultural tailoring and cultural targeting have been described as two broad methodologies that can be employed in providing health education to a variety of ethnic and cultural groups.[33] Cultural tailoring has been defined as "any combination of information or change strategies intended to reach one specific person, based on characteristics that are unique to that person, related to the outcome of interest and have been derived from an individual assessment."[34] Thus, tailoring of educational materials occurs on the individual level based on the health care provider's assessment of that individual.

Conversely, cultural targeting occurs on a macro level and may be defined as "the use of a single intervention approach for a defined population subgroup that takes into account characteristics shared by the subgroup's members."[33] Targeting assumes that everyone in the cultural subgroup holds the same values and that all will respond to the same approach to providing information, and that this will lead to the desired behavior change. Strategies commonly used in this approach involve the use of one or more of the following: use of peripheral strategies, evidential strategies, linguistic strategies, constituent-involving strategies, and sociocultural strategies.[33]

Peripheral strategies include packaging print materials using colors and design that appeal to a specific cultural group whereas evidential strategies provide evidence for the relevance of a specific health problem in a specified culture. In cancer care, there is much publication of the lower incidence and nonetheless higher mortality rate of breast cancer in African American women. Peripheral strategies are employed when print information uses colors associated with the African American culture (yellow, red, green) and photos of African American women who are breast cancer survivors. For example, two different groups of researchers used focus groups to assist in the development of booklets emphasizing the need to engage in breast cancer screening.[35,36] Another researcher used similar strategies in the development of a video to encourage screening for colorectal cancer.[37] Linguistic strategies would take this print material one step further and use terms more closely aligned with the culture being targeted. For Hispanics, this would involve providing the material in Spanish.

Constituent-involving strategies were used in the Save Our Sisters Project in North Carolina. This breast cancer outreach program used "natural helpers" in getting the word out to other African American women about breast cancer.[38] Natural helpers are part of the same culture being targeted for outreach; they are recognized within their community as leaders and thus are viewed as powerful women who can get others to adapt the healthy behaviors being targeted. However, there are problems with using lay or natural helpers, particularly the fact that there may be a waxing and waning of their outreach efforts that may be affected by other health and situational demands.[39]

Finally, socio-cultural strategies have been employed by the Witness Project, which is a program grounded in African American cultural values, spiritual beliefs, and health care beliefs and which are reinforced in all aspects of the outreach and support program. The Witness Project combats the fatalistic view many African American women hold about breast cancer and recruits survivors to share how they overcame and lived through the cancer diagnosis.[10,40,41] Culturally relevant programs such as the Witness Project uses women recognized as spiritual leaders, natural healers, or survivors of breast cancer to encourage cancer screening in the African American community.[10,39] These peer educators (PE) "witness" in a manner similar to the witnessing done in many fundamentalist Christian churches in an attempt to meet the women's beliefs rather than to change their beliefs.

There are many ideas about how to implement successful cancer outreach programs to African American women. However, the authors' review of the literature on this topic suggests that there are a few factors that need to be considered in the design of effective, culturally sensitive outreach programs. The first is the understanding that outreach approaches have to go beyond symbolic attempts to identify with African American women. Resnicow and colleagues[42] have pointed out that cultural sensitivity can be thought of in terms of two primary dimensions—surface structure and deep structure. Outreach strategies that address surface structure seek to match materials and messages to observable behavioral and social characteristics of African American women. Deep structure strategies seek to reflect how cultural, environmental, historical, psychologic, and social factors influence the cancer health behaviors of African American women. Thus simply having an outreach approach that uses educational materials that highlight other African American women or include their specific jargon is not sufficient to constitute a culturally tailored intervention. An effective intervention would also have to incorporate deep structure features that contextualize outreach efforts within the socio-cultural framework of the lived experience of African American women. It is said that outreach programs that address surface structure can increase the receptivity and acceptance of messages, but that real salience is achieved when deep structure features are incorporated.[43] Thus surface structure may establish the feasibility and acceptance of outreach, but it is deep structure that ensures program impact.

A related issue is the need to appreciate the importance of collectivism in the lives of African American women and how that can affect the impact of outreach programs.[43] The culture of African American women includes high levels of interdependence with others in their community, conformity to group norms, and sacrifice for the good of others. Therefore it is important to note that African American women often do not make cancer health decisions as individuals in a vacuum, but rather decision making is done with reference to larger social and cultural contexts.[22] However, many outreach efforts, especially those that are guided by psychologic theories of behavior change, focus on individual factors and can be limited in impact by the their neglecting to address such factors as familial influences, religious referents, and other factors that have been discussed earlier in this chapter. Thus it is important that when directing outreach efforts to African American women, emphasis is placed on appeals to collective goals and outcomes such as "Get screened for you, your family, and your people," or "We need more healthy sisters for the struggle,"[29,43] rather than focus placed exclusively on individual efficacy or self-centered motivation to change behavior.

Given the importance of relationships and the influence of social networks on African American women's behaviors, another factor that is important to effective outreach is the involvement of peers. Many successful outreach programs are peer-led and involve the recruitment and training of African American women, who are similar to the group that one wants to reach, to serve as leaders, educators, and counselors about cancer issues.[15,44] Peers are often more effective at delivering messages to other African American women who are like them, they can be influential and credible role models since they are members of the same social milieu, and they are better positioned to offer social support to other women who may be at risk for cancer.

Jennings[44] formulated many of these considerations into a set of six practical strategies for nursing professionals who are developing culturally sensitive outreach programs for African American women. These strategies are appreciate, negotiate, integrate, educate, advocate, and evaluate. *Appreciate* refers to seeking to relate, sister to sister, to the African American women one wishes to reach out to. *Negotiate* is about gaining the trust of the community and creating a sense of kinship with those who are influential with the groups that one wants to reach. *Integrate* focuses on combing multiple approaches such as using individual and collective strategies in outreach programs. *Educate* refers to empowering African American women by providing them with knowledge about cancer risks and treatments. *Advocate* means taking an approach that conveys a caring attitude and being willing to act as a support to women with cancer; it can be simply summarized as "I've got your back." Finally, *evaluate* refers to assessing the application of the nursing process in advancing outreach to African American women and making changes when needed to improve outreach strategies.

Resources for Nurse Providers

Many majority culture (i.e., white) nurses are engaging in cancer prevention and early detection programs in the effort to improve morbidity and mortality from cancer. In addition to addressing the barriers to participation discussed above, nurses also must consider how they will try to gain access to and be considered "trustworthy" by those they are trying to reach. This is commonly called the "insider/outsider" dilemma,[45] and although most often seen and discussed in the research literature, it does have an impact on nurses in clinical settings. Kaufman[46] suggests that no matter whether the nurse is an insider or outsider (e.g., of the same ethnicity or culture as one's patient's or not), the fundamental processes of building and maintaining trust are critical to the success of the nursing care being delivered, the educational program, or research. The importance to attaining the goals of care of the participants' trust in the nurse cannot be underestimated.

Researchers or those developing cancer outreach programs must take the time to learn cultural values and mores to facilitate program success; for example, knowing the rules of etiquette particular to the group of insiders to which one desires access, being nonjudgmental, and taking time to listen to what is important to the group. An additional strategy is to identify "key informers" who are liked and respected by the insider group and seek their advice are critical activities.[46] For example, when trying to establish a breast cancer screening program in a church comprised primarily of African Americans, the preacher indicated that there were several women who had to be consulted; the implication was that once they gave their consent, then others would come on board and support the project (this material comes from the author's personal files).

There are a number of resources and tools available to nurses that can help nurses improve their ability to provide culturally sensitive care. These resources have been developed by a variety of nursing organizations, agencies of the federal government, and nongovernmental organizations (Table 25-1). There are also specific tools that can

Table **25-1** RESOURCES TO ASSIST NURSES IN REDUCING CARE DISPARITIES

Organization	Purpose of Resource	Web Access
Oncology Nursing Society	To assist cancer nurses in providing culturally competent care	www.ons.org
Intercultural Cancer Council	To promote polices, programs, research, and partnerships to eliminate the unequal burden of cancer among minority and underserved populations	http://iccnetwork.org
Office of Minority Health	Provides resources for nurses to use to increase their ability to provide culturally competent care	www.hrsa.gov/omh
National Coalition of Cancer Survivorship	Has developed a Minority Guide that addresses issues of concern to minority cancer patients	www.canceradvocacy.org
Health Research and Educational Trust	Resource to aid hospitals in collecting critical information about minority patients with the aim of improving the care available to them	www.hretdisparities.org

be very helpful to nurses in developing culturally sensitive cancer outreach programs. One technique is the use of focus groups for developing culturally sensitive outreach messages. During the formative stage of planning a cancer outreach program, it is necessary to get information about the population being targeted. Some of this information can come from the previous literature. However, to obtain current and detailed information about the target audience, it has become common to convene subgroups and use focus group techniques to uncover experiences, assumptions, preferences, and enabling and constraining factors that can affect the implementation of outreach strategies.[43]

Basch[47] and Krueger[48] provide more information and some specific guidelines for conducting focus groups that can be useful in planning cancer outreach programs. Another tool that can provide useful information on the potential of culturally based messages in cancer outreach programs is "ethnic mapping." Ethnic mapping involves having members of the target audience rate aspects of behavior that are relevant to outreach strategies along a visual continuum ranging, for example, from "mostly black thing" to "equally a black or white thing" and so on.[42] This kind of mapping allows planners to delineate the cultural attributes that are most relevant to cancer outreach activities.

For information that goes beyond preferences expressed in focus groups or ethnic mapping, nurses can use tools such as the Cultural Status Exam[49] or Purnell and Paulanka's[50] organizing framework. These methods help nurses to better understand the full socio-cultural context within which African American women with cancer are embedded. The Cultural Status Exam is a brief tool consisting of six questions that elicit information about the impact and significance of the family, the degree of adaptation or assimilation into mainstream culture, health and medical practices, and cultural beliefs and attitudes.

Purnell and Paulanka's[50] organizing framework is more involved than the Cultural Status Exam in that it provides a comprehensive approach to conducting cultural assessments among African American women or other cultural groups. The framework or model examines the culture of an individual or group through the collection of data from 12 domains of socio-cultural context including communication, family roles and organization, work force concerns, biocultural ecology, high-risk behaviors, nutrition, pregnancy and childbearing practices, health care practitioners, and health care practices. The information gathered from this type of assessment can then be used to develop cancer-related outreach programs that target African American women and other ethnically diverse groups.

Finally, nurses can learn more about African American women by reading African American authors such as bell hooks, Toni Morrison, Maya Angelou, and others. The African American Literature Book Club found online at http://authors.aalbc.com/author1.htm provides a thorough listing of African American authors.

Nurses can and should play a pivotal role in reducing health care disparities in this country. They have a professional obligation, based on Provision 1 and Provision 8 of the *Nurses Code of Ethics*,[51] to ensure that quality health care is provided to all Americans.

REFERENCES

1. American Cancer Society: *Cancer Facts and Figures 2005,* Atlanta, 2005, The Author. On the Web at www.cancer.org/downloads/STT/CAFF2005f4PWSecured.pdf
2. Paskett ED and others: Racial differences in knowledge, attitudes, and cancer screening practices among a triracial rural population, *Cancer* 101:2650-2659, 2004.
3. Schwartz KL and others: Race, socioeconomic status and stage at diagnosis for five common malignancies, *Cancer Causes Control* 14:761-766, 2003.
4. Smedley BD, Stith AY, Nelson AR, editors: *Unequal treatment: confronting racial and ethnic disparities in health care,* Washington, D.C., 2003, The National Academies Press.
5. U.S. Department of Health and Human Services: *Healthy People 2010: Understanding and Improving Health.* Washington, D.C., 2000, U.S. Department of Health and Human Services, Government Printing Office.
6. Haynes MA, Smedley BD: *The unequal burden of cancer: an assessment of NIH research and programs for ethnic minorities and the medically underserved,* Washington, D.C., 1999, National Academy Press.
7. Davis B: personal communication, June 16, 2004.
8. Gregg J, Curry RH: Explanatory models for cancer among African-American women at two Atlanta neighborhood health centers: the implications for a cancer screening program, *Soc Sci Med* 39:519-526, 1994.

9. Abrums M: "Jesus will fix it after awhile": meanings and health, *Soc Sc Med* 50:89-105, 2000.
10. Erwin DO, Spatz TS, Turturro CL: Development of an African-American role model intervention to increase breast self-examination and mammography, *J Cancer Ed* 7:311-319, 1992.
11. Fryar ILB: The roots of coping behavior for African American Women: a literary perspective. In Fisher Collins C, editor: *African American women's health and social issues*, Westport, 1996, Auburn House.
12. Wilson-Ford V: Health protective behaviors of rural black elderly women, *Health Soc Work* 17(1):28, 1992.
13. Lassiter SM: *Multicultural clients—a professional handbook for health care providers and social workers*, Westport, Conn., 1995, Greenwood Press.
14. Dulla A: African American suspicion of the healthcare system is justified: what do we do about it?, *Camb Q Healthc Ethics* 3:347, 1994.
15. Bailey EJ: *Medical anthropology and African American health*, Westport, Conn., 2000, Bergin & Garvey.
16. Gilchrist L: personal communication, March 3, 2005.
17. Mouton C and others: Barriers to black women's participation in cancer clinical trials, *J Natl Med Assoc* 89:721, 1997.
18. Lythcott G, Green BL, Brown ZK: The perspectives of African-American breast cancer survivor-advocates, *Cancer* 97(1 Suppl):324, 2003.
19. Telfair J, Nash KB: African American culture. In Fisher NL, editor: *Cultural and ethnic diversity—a guide for genetics professionals*, Baltimore, 1996, The Johns Hopkins University Press.
20. Bureau of the Census: U.S. Census Bureau News CB04-144, Washington, D.C., 2004, U.S. Department of Commerce.
21. Greene B: African American Women. In Comas-Diaz L, Greene B, editors: *Women of color: integrating ethnic and gender identities in psychotherapy*, New York, 1994, The Guilford Press.
22. Guldry JJ, Matthews-Juarez P, Copeland VA: Barriers to breast cancer control for African-American women, *Cancer* 97(1 Suppl):318, 2003.
23. Kennedy T: *You gotta deal with it: black family relations in a southern community*, New York, 1980, Oxford University Press.
24. Martin EP, Martin JM: *The black extended family*, Chicago, 1978, University of Chicago Press.
25. Powe BD: Fatalism among elderly African Americans. Effects on colorectal cancer screening, *Cancer Nurs* 18(5):385-392, 1995.
26. Powe BD, Ntekop E, Barron M: An intervention study to increase colorectal cancer knowledge and screening among community elders, *Public Health Nurs 21*(5):435-442, 2004.
27. Soler-Vila H, Kasl SV, Jones BA: Prognostic significance of psychosocial factors in African-American and white breast cancer patients: a population-based study, *Cancer* 98(6): 1299-1308, 2003.
28. Cobb S: Social support as a moderator of life stress, *Psychosom Med* 38(5):300-314, 1976.
29. Wilmoth MC, Sanders LD: Accept me for myself: African American women's issues after breast cancer, *Oncol Nurs Forum* 28(5):875-879, 2001.
30. Hamilton JB, Sandelowski M: Types of social support in African Americans with cancer, *Oncol Nurs Forum* 31: 792-800, 2004.
31. Eley JW and others: Racial differences in survival from breast cancer: results of the National Cancer Institute Black-White Cancer Survival Study, *JAMA* 272:947-954, 1994.
32. Breen N and others: The relationship of socioeconomic status and access to minimum expected therapy among female breast cancer patients in the National Cancer Institute Black-White Cancer Survival Study, *Ethn Dis* 9:111-125, 1999.
33. Kreuter MW and others: Achieving cultural appropriateness in health promotion programs: targeted and tailored approaches, *Health Ed Behav* 30(2):133-146, 2002.
34. Kreuter M, Strecher V, Glassman B: One size does not fit all: the case for tailoring print materials, *Ann Behav Med* 21:1-9, 1999.
35. Coleman EA and others: Developing and testing lay literature about breast cancer screening for African American women, *Clin J Oncol Nurs* 7:66-71, 2003.
36. Holt CL and others: Development of a spiritually based breast cancer educational booklet for African American women, *Cancer Control Cancer Cult Lit Suppl* 10:37-44, 2003.
37. Powe BD, Weinrich S: An intervention to decrease cancer fatalism among rural elders, *Oncol Nurs Forum* 26(3): 583-588, 1999.
38. Earp JAL and others: Lay health advisors: A strategy for getting the word out about breast cancer, *Health Ed Behav* 24:432-451, 1997.
39. Altpeter M and others: Lay health advisor activity levels: Definitions from the field, *Health Ed Behav* 26:495-512, 1999.
40. Phillips JM: Breast cancer and African American women: moving beyond fear, fatalism, and silence, *Oncol Nurs Forum* 26:1001-1007, 1999.
41. Phillips JM, Cohen MZ, Moses G: Breast cancer screening and African American women: fear, fatalism, and silence, *Oncol Nurs Forum* 26:561-571, 1999.
42. Resnicow K and others: Cultural sensitivity in public health: defined and demystified, *Ethn Dis* 9:10, 1999.
43. Resnicow K and others: Applying theory to culturally diverse and unique populations. In Glanz K, Rimer BK, Lewis MF, editors: *Health behavior and health education: theory, research, and practice*, ed 3, San Francisco, 2002, Josey-Bass.
44. Jennings K: Getting black women to screen for cancer: incorporating health beliefs into practice, *J Am Acad Nurse Pract* 8(2):53-59, 1996.
45. Merton RK. Insiders and outsiders: a chapter in the sociology of knowledge, *Am J Sociol* 7:9-45, 1970.
46. Kauffman KS: The insider/outsider dilemma: field experience of a white researcher "getting in" a poor black community, *Nurs Res* 43(3):179-183, 1994.
47. Basch C: Focus group interview: an underutilized research technique for improving theory and practice in health education, *Health Ed Q* 14:411-448, 1988.
48. Krueger RA: *Focus groups: a practical guide for applied research*, Thousand Oaks, 1988, Sage.
49. Pfefferling JH: A cultural prescription for medicocentrism. In Eisenberg L, Kleinman A, editors: *The relevance of social science to medicine*, Boston, 1981, D. Rendel.
50. Purnell LD, Paulanka BJ: *Transcultural health care: a culturally competent approach*, Philadelphia, 1998, F.A. Davis.
51. American Nurses Association: Code of ethics for nurses; on the Web at http://www.nursingworld.org/ethics/ecode.htm. Accessed March 15, 2005.

CHAPTER

26 Asian Women and Cancer

Dianne N. Ishida

INTRODUCTION

Although cancer in Asian (and Pacific Islander) women is considered low for all body sites when collectively compared to Caucasians and African Americans,[1] there is increasing evidence to cause concern. As Asian groups are separated out from the general population, incidence and mortality rates have begun to provide startling evidence of rising rates and health disparities with specific cancers in different Asian American groups. The chapter explores the recent literature (primarily from 2000) on Asian women and cancer after an overview of the Asian population in the US.

OVERVIEW OF THE ASIAN AMERICAN POPULATION

Asians, according to the US Census, comprise 11.8 million, or 4.2%, of the US population.[2] This represents a 72% increase since 1990. The term "Asian" refers to people whose origins are from the Far East, Southeast Asia, or the Indian subcontinent. While there are more than 25 Asian groups in the US, the US census provides detailed information on only the 11 largest groups, with the rest listed as "other"[3] (Table 26-1). In descending order in the "Asian alone" listing, the groups are Chinese (23.8%), Filipino (18.3%), Asian Indian (16.2%), Vietnamese (10.9%), Korean (10.5%), Japanese (7.8%), other Asian (4.7%), Cambodian (1.8%), Hmong (1.7%), Laotian (1.6%), Pakistani (1.5%), and Thai (1.1%). The five largest Asian groups account for 80% of the Asian population. Over half of the Asians live in the western US (49%), with declining percentages in the Northeast (20%), the South (19%) and in the Midwest (12%). Over 51% of Asians live in three states: California, New York, and Hawaii.[2]

Asians have been coming to the US for several hundreds of years off of trade ships, as contract workers, and as people seeking economic and educational opportunities unavailable in their homelands. Since the mid-1960s and until recently, others have also come as political refugees (e.g., from the Philippines after Marcos declared martial law in 1972, after the Vietnam war, and after the Tiananmen Square incident in 1989 in China). Also, as immigration laws eased after 1965, more highly educated professionals and specialists began immigrating into the US. About 75% of Asian Americans are recent immigrants or refugees.[4]

As a group, the Asian population is younger than the national average by 2 years, with a median age of 33 years. The majority are in their young to middle adulthood. There is great variation on median age in different Asian groups. Japanese have the oldest median age at 43 years and Hmong the youngest at 16 years. The older age group is pertinent to cancer, since age increases the risk of specific cancers. There may be a shift as this population ages in the coming decades. Only 8% of Asians in the detailed census groups were aged 65 years or older, as compared to 12% of the US population. The exceptions are Chinese, Filipino,

Table **26-1** ASIAN POPULATION BY ASIAN GROUP ALONE OR IN COMBINATION: 2000

Asian Group	Number	Percentage of Asian Population	Percent of US Population
Total	**11,859,446**	**100.0**	**4.21**
Asian Indian	1,855,590	16.2	0.66
Cambodian	212,633	1.8	0.08
Chinese	2,858,291	23.8	1.02
Filipino	2,385,216	18.3	0.85
Hmong	184,842	1.7	0.07
Japanese	1,152,324	7.8	0.41
Korean	1,226,825	10.5	0.44
Laotian	196,893	1.6	0.07
Pakistani	209,273	1.5	0.07
Thai	150,093	1.1	0.05
Vietnamese	1,212,465	10.9	0.43
Other Asian	561,485	4.7	0.20

From Reeves TJ, Bennett CE: *We the people: Asians in the United States*. Washington, D.C., 2004, U.S. Census Bureau; available online at www.census.gov/prod/2004pubs/censr-17.pdf. Retrieved on January 11, 2005.

and Japanese. The Japanese have the highest proportion of persons aged over 65 years, 20%, which is 1.6 times greater than the national percentage.[3]

Asian households are more likely to be comprised of married couple families (60%) than the total population (54%). However, Cambodian households have the highest proportion of no-husband households at 21%. In terms of place of birth, only 31% of Asians are native born, as compared to 90% of the total US population. There are an equal proportion of Asians who are naturalized and noncitizens. Thus an overwhelming number of Asians (69%) are foreign born. This varies by group, with the Japanese at a low 40% that is foreign born to Asian Indians, Vietnamese, Koreans, Pakistani, and Thai, in which 75% are foreign born. The period during which each Asian group migrated to the US varies, but over 75% foreign-born Asians came in the past 2 decades. Over half of the foreign-born Asian Indians, Japanese, and Pakistanis entered the US relatively recently, between 1990 and 2000. The number of Asians who speak a language other than English at home ranged from 47% for the Japanese to 96% for the Hmong. This accounts for almost 80% of Asians speaking languages other than English at home, which has implications for linguistic needs when they interact with society at large in their daily lives. On the positive side, about 60% of Asians have noted in the census data that they speak English "very well."[3]

Educational attainment of high school, while varying between Asian groups, is approximately 80% for Asians 25 years and older, with a higher proportion (44%) attaining a bachelor's degree as compared to the total population (24%). Asian Indians have the highest percentage (64%) with a bachelor's degree. The Hmong, Cambodians, and Laotians have 60% or less with a high school education.[3] This bimodal pattern seen in education is also reflected in income.

Asians are more likely to be in management, professional, and related occupations (45%) as compared to the total population (34%). Asians who work full time and year-round have higher median earnings than all full-time year-round workers. This figure does not take into account multiple wage earners in a family or multiple jobs held by a worker. Thus it is not surprising that the median annual income of Asian families is higher than all US families. However, there are some Asian groups (Hmong, Cambodian, Korean, Laotian, Pakistani, Thai, and Vietnamese) with substantially lower median incomes. In fact, poverty rates for Asians and the total US population are similar. The participation of women in the labor force also varies by group. Filipino women have the highest employment rate at 65% and Pakistani women the lowest (40%). Home ownership may reflect the ability to accrue income. Asians have lower owner-occupied housing (53%) than the total US population. Japanese, Chinese, and Filipinos have the highest proportion of owner-occupied housing, whereas Hmong, Koreans, Pakistanis, and Cambodians had the highest renter-occupied housing.[3] The effect of socioeconomic status has been positively associated with female breast cancer, ovarian cancer, and cancer of the corpus uteri.[5] In fact, the influence of socioeconomic status was stronger for breast cancer for Hispanics and Asians than for Caucasians and Africans Americans.[6] Many of the statistics, when averaged out for Asian groups, cloud the differences between Asian groups. The picture becomes even more fuzzy when Asians are categorized together with Pacific Islanders, which is frequently the case in multiethnic cancer studies.

National data on cancer incidence and mortality rates of Asians has historically been limited. Asians are diverse groups that are frequently categorized with Pacific Islanders, another diverse group. Though a fast-growing group, Asians still hold a small percentage of the US population. The National Institute of Cancer's Surveillance, Epidemiology, and End Results (SEER) made some inroads in providing cancer data at specific regional areas of the country on five major Asian groups from 1988 to 1992.[7] The most recent SEER publication lumps Asians and Pacific Islanders (API) together again.[8] The overall cancer death rates for all ethnic/racial populations decreased from 1993-2001, but in men (1.5%) they were almost twice that in women (0.8%). However, of note is that cancer is the leading cause of death among Asian American women. Cancer is followed by heart disease, cerebrovascular disease, injuries and accidents, diabetes mellitus, and chronic liver disease and cirrhosis.[9] Major cancer sites in women were generally breast, colon/rectum, and lung. Breast cancer incidence rates were increasing in Caucasian and API women. Other major cancer sites varied according to Asian group; significant sites were ovary for the Chinese and South Asians, uterus for Filipinos, Chinese, and Japanese, and stomach for the Japanese and Vietnamese. Among Vietnamese, Laotian, and Cambodian women, cervical cancer was the first or second most common cancer. Thyroid cancer was common among Vietnamese, Cambodian, and Filipino women.[9]

APIs had a higher incidence for stomach, liver, thyroid (women),[8] and cervix cancers[9] than other racial/ethnic populations. However, when all cancers were combined to look at survival rates 5 years after diagnosis, non-Hispanic Caucasians and API women had the highest survival rates at 67% to 68.7%, with significant subgroup variations. However, APIs had the lowest survival rates for leukemia of all groups.[8]

Cancer data for Asian Americans have come from tumor registries where there are large concentrations of Asians. Since the last SEER monograph was published in 1996,[7] there have been no comparative SEER data published. Thus some of the data presented is from specific geographical regions or states, and not all Asian groups are noted.

Cancer Incidence Rates

The most current data on the leading cancers for Asian groups come from California and Hawaii cancer surveillance programs. Table 26-2 lists cancer distribution by site for Asian females from 1988 to 2001 from California.[10] According to this data, Japanese Americans have surpassed non-Latino Caucasians in breast cancer incidence. This percent increase in the Japanese is even higher in the Hawaii data (Table 26-3). In fact, cancer incidence has been steadily rising in Hawaii for all races/ethnicities since 1994, which may reflect better screening rates. Of the ethnic groups cited (Caucasian, Native Hawaiian, Japanese, Filipino, and others), Japanese in Hawaii had the highest percentage of those having ever had a mammogram (95.2%) and having had that mammography within the past year (81%). In six groups, over 70% reported having had a mammography within the past year.[11]

Table 26-2 Five Leading Cancers by Sites for Asian Females in California, 1988-2001[10]

Asian Group	1	2	3	4	5
Chinese	Breast (28%)	Colorectal (14.8%)	Lung (11.2%)	Corpus Uteri (4.7%)	Stomach (4.3%)
Japanese	Breast (32.7%)	Colorectal (16.8%)	Lung (8.8%)	Stomach (6%)	Corpus Uteri (5.4%)
Filipino	Breast (32.2%)	Colorectal (9.1%)	Lung (7.3%)	Corpus Uteri (6.1%)	Cervix Uteri (4.6%)
Korean	Breast (21.2%)	Colorectal (12.4%)	Stomach (11%)	Lung (8.1%)	Cervix Uteri (7.3%)
Vietnamese	Breast (22.9%)	Cervix Uteri (9.9%)	Colorectal (9.8%)	Lung (9.4%)	Stomach (5.0%)
South Asian	Breast (35.5%)	Colorectal (6.9%)	Ovary (5.8%)	Corpus Uteri (4.1%)	Non-Hodgkin's Lymphoma (4.5%)
Non-Latino White (Comparison)	**Breast (32.5%)**	**Lung (13.9%)**	**Colorectal (11.4%)**	**Corpus Uteri (6.0%)**	**Ovary (3.6%)**

Table 26-3 Five Leading Cancers by Sites for Asian Women in Hawai'i, 1995-2000

Asian Group	1	2	3	4	5
Chinese	Breast (32.4%)	Colorectal (14.3%)	Lung (9.9%)	Corpus Uteri (5.0%)	Thyroid (4.1%)
Japanese	Breast (36%)	Colorectal (16.1%)	Lung (7.8%)	Corpus Uteri (6.4%)	Stomach (5.1%)
Filipino	Breast (30.5%)	Colorectal (10.1%)	Lung (10.0%)	Thyroid (8.1%)	Corpus Uteri (7.7%)

From American Cancer Society, Cancer Research Center of Hawai'i and Hawai'i Department of Health. Hawai'i Cancer Facts & Figures 2003-2004. Honolulu (HI): Hawai'i Pacific, Inc. of the American Cancer Society; Hawai'i Tumor Registry, Cancer Research Center of Hawai'i, University of Hawai'i; and Hawai'i Department of Health, 2003.
Source: Hawai'i Tumor Registry, Cancer Research Center of Hawai'i, University of Hawai'i. Reprinted with permission, Hawai'i Cancer Facts & Figures 2003-2004.

As noted, the Hawaii cancer incidence data are slightly different than the California data for the five most common cancers. There is a higher percentage of Chinese and Japanese in Hawaii with breast cancer and a lower percentage with lung cancer. The colorectal cancer incidence remains relatively the same between the states. However, thyroid cancer appears in the top five cancer sites for the Chinese and Filipino women in Hawaii. A thyroid cancer study noted the thyroid cancer rates in Filipino migrants in the Bay area to be twice as high as in women in the Philippines or in Caucasian women.[12] High rates were also noted in South Asian women. The higher prevalence of thyroid nodules or goiter and dietary factors were implicated.

In a study of a multiethnic cohort in Hawaii and Los Angeles that looked at relative risk-factor–adjusted incidence of breast cancer among over a thousand postmenopausal women,[13] Caucasians had a relative risk (RR) of 1.0, African Americans of 0.98, Native Hawaiians of 1.65, and Japanese of 1.11. The authors noted that the slightly greater risk of Japanese was balanced by the very low rates in "traditional" Japanese women and Japanese migrants. The Los Angeles Cancer Surveillance Program has noted rapidly increasing rates of breast cancer for Japanese Americans.[14] The researchers noted that the breast cancer risk for Japanese and Filipino women is twice that of Chinese and Korean women in the US. In another study in the San Francisco Bay area, Vietnamese women were younger at diagnosis than other racial/ethnic groups, with 49.6% being diagnosed at younger than 50 years of age.[15]

The North American Association of Central Cancer Registries data from 1992-1997 on ovarian cancer in the US has noted that although this type of cancer is less prevalent among Asians than Caucasians, the incidence rates in 15- to 24-year-old API women were higher than in Caucasian and African American women.[16]

Cancer Survival Rates

API women have shown significantly better 5-year survival rates from 1988 to 1997 than Caucasian women when all cancer sites are combined. However, there were low survival rates for API women with liver and intrahepatic bile duct cancers, melanomas of the skin, and leukemias. Relative survival rates have improved from 1973 to 1990 for most cancers, except cervical and lung cancer (for Chinese and Japanese).[4]

When looking at immigrant populations, Singh and Miller[17] found that male and female immigrants have 3.4 and 2.5 years longer life expectancy respectively than the US-born. However, Chinese, Japanese, and Filipino immigrants had lower life expectancy. Although these Asian immigrants experienced much higher stomach, liver, and cervical cancer mortality than their US counterparts, they had significantly lower mortality from lung, colorectal, breast, prostate, and esophageal cancers, as well as from cardiovascular disease, cirrhosis, diabetes, respiratory diseases, HIV and AIDS, and suicide.

Not all Asian American groups have similar survival rates. Looking at breast cancer survival among Chinese, Japanese, Filipino, and Caucasian American women, Pineda and colleagues[18] found Japanese women had significantly better survival rates than the other groups. Even when adjusted for age, year of diagnosis, stage of disease, SEER region, or type of treatment, the survival advantage of Japanese women persisted. The authors suggested a vigorous host response to breast cancer as a possible reason. Filipino women had a younger median age at diagnosis and a significantly poorer survival in premenopausal (younger than 50 years old) women than premenopausal Japanese women.[18] Survival differences were also seen with colorectal and cervical as well as breast cancer. Colorectal cancer was more likely to be diagnosed at a later stage in Chinese women than in Japanese and Filipino women, with resulting worse survival rates. Chinese women also had worse survival after early-stage cervical cancer. Japanese women were likely to be diagnosed at early stages and experienced better survival for colorectal and breast cancers regardless of stage.[19] Japanese and Chinese bladder cancer patients have higher survival rates than Caucasian, Filipino, and Hawaiian patients.[20]

Survival data comparing Asians with Caucasians and African Americans have shown some advantages with specific cancers. Asians with pancreatic cancer have longer survival, which can be partly explained by the higher proportion of a less aggressive form of pancreatic carcinomas (papillary or mucinous cystadenocarcinomas rather than ductal adenocarcinomas).[21] Similarly, Asians with gastric adenocarcinomas have significantly higher survival than non-Asians.[22] This overall better survival was attributed to Asians being less likely to have distant metastases and having more resectable cancers. Non-Asians (Caucasians, Latinos, and African Americans) were younger and more likely to have cancers of the gastroesophageal junction, a difficult area for resection.

Migration and Cancer

The effects of migration can be seen vividly in some cancers in some Asian groups as rates either increase or decrease. As noted, earlier immigrants generally have a longer life expectancy than the US-born.[17] American-born Japanese women had a 40% higher incidence of colorectal cancer than Japanese women born in Japan or US-born

Caucasian women. In contrast, Chinese women had a rate that was 30% to 40% lower than US-born Caucasian women, regardless of their place of birth. Filipino women, whether U.S.-born or foreign-born, had a 20% to 50% the incidence rates of U.S.-born Caucasians.[23] When looking at endometrial cancer in the same Asian groups, a lower incidence was found among Chinese American and Japanese American women born in Asia than in those born in the US. However, no difference was found between Filipino women born in the US and those born in Asia.[24]

In analyzing incidence trends among Japanese in Japan and Japanese in Hawaii between 1960 and 1997, the migrant effect was strongest for colon and stomach cancers, but less so with prostate and breast cancers. Migration led to lower risk of stomach, esophageal, pancreatic, liver, and cervical cancers, but increased rates of all other cancers. The authors concluded that the persistent incidence over several generations after migration supports that living in a host country alone is insufficient to modify cancer risk to the level of the host population for all cancer sites.[25]

When comparing Vietnamese in the US with Vietnamese in Hanoi, Vietnam, marked differences can be seen in the cervical cancer burden in the US. An exceptional rise in incidence was noted in US. Vietnamese between the ages of 50 and 64 years, nearly sevenfold that of US Caucasian women. Cancers with the greatest differences between geographic regions were reproductive cancers (breast, cervix, uterus, and ovary) and gastrointestional cancers (pancreas, colorectal). Cancer rates were lower in US Vietnamese than in US Caucasians except for stomach, liver, nasopharyngeal, and cervical cancers. However, even these lower rates for Vietnamese in the US were higher than for those in Hanoi.[26]

Cancer incidence patterns for Korean Americans and for Koreans in South Korea were compared. Breast and colon cancer were considerable higher in US Koreans than in South Koreans, though still not as high as for Caucasians. Cervical and stomach cancers were highest in South Koreans, and rectal cancer in women was twice as common as in US Korean women.[27]

Looking at leukemia incidence and Asian migrants, no appreciable difference was seen between US-born and foreign-born Asian Americans of Chinese, Japanese, and Filipino descent.[28] In another study looking at Hodgkin's disease (HD), which is generally rare in Asians, the incidence of HD was compared between Japanese, Chinese, Filipinos, and Asian Indians in the US and their Asian counterparts. Rates were low for both groups, although Japanese and Chinese had lower rates than Filipinos and Asian Indians. The authors suggest that the consistently low rates of HD point to a genetic resistance to development of the disease.[29]

CANCER SCREENING AND BARRIERS TO REACHING ASIAN WOMEN

General

The bulk of the literature on Asian women and cancer is in the area of cancer screening. Several studies have noted that Asian American Pacific Islanders (AAPI) have lower screening rates than Caucasians. APPI women were less likely to have cervical cancer screening,[30] mammography, and colorectal screening if they were foreign-born.[31] Reasons cited for the underutilization of early cancer screening by Asian American women as include cultural, psychosocial, linguistic, and economic barriers.[32] Given the demographic data previously presented, these reasons seem reasonable. However, barriers vary according to Asian subgroups and for how many generations they have lived in the US. Generalizations cannot be made with impunity. A study in San Diego of six Asian groups (Asian Indians, Chinese, Filipino, Japanese, Korean, and Vietnamese) found statistically significant variations in breast cancer knowledge, attitudes, and screening behaviors in the groups studied.[33] For instance, of the six Asian groups, Koreans and Vietnamese had the lowest percentage (22% to 39%) of annual mammography compared to Japanese and Asian Indians (64% to 81%). But regarding perceptions of whether they had sufficient information on breast cancer, Vietnamese women were the most likely to report sufficient information (45%) and the Koreans least likely (17%). There was also significant variation between groups on how they wished to receive health information. Adherence to screening follow-up after the initial contact in women aged 50 years and older revealed significant group variation, with 60% of Chinese and 52% of Vietnamese following screening guidelines, but no change seen in Asian Indians and Japanese, who had the highest screening rates. The authors surmised that the latter groups had a subset of women resistant to adopting the Western screening methods.

The concepts of "health" and "prevention" may have different meaning for different populations. Western medicine's cancer screening tests may be unfamiliar to foreign-born migrants especially if they are not fluent in English. The practice of hot and cold conceptualized by some Asian cultures can be observed in their views on cause of disease (an imbalance), or how they approach preventive measures or treatment.[34,35] Other cultural and religious beliefs about disease causation and preventive actions can also be at odds with Western screening.[35] Chinese and Korean American women noted a sense of fatalism when discussing cancer prevention that may affect their willingness to engage in cancer screening.[34,36,37] They also cited other barriers such as transportation difficulties, lack of English capability,[34] and lack of knowledge of cancer screening tests.[38] Lack of knowledge of common signs, symptoms, and risk factors for breast and cervical cancer as well as misconceptions on causes was also noted with Vietnamese women.[39] Korean women were also unclear on causative factors and preventive strategies for cervical cancer.[36]

Community stigmatization of cancer can affect women's willingness to have cancer screening and thus the chances of early diagnosis. Beliefs that cancer is contagious (25.7%), is caused by immoral behavior, or is a punishment for ancestor conduct (15%) were found in Chinese immigrants in San Francisco.[40] South Asian women also felt that breast cancer could be caught, that women could bring it upon themselves by having negative lifestyles, or that it could be caused by by means of the careless words or curses of others, or by divine power.[41]

When Chinese women were ask about barriers to seeking additional educational sessions, they cited lack of time (49%), limitations of language (14%) and money (6%), not important (5%), did not want to think about breast cancer (4%), topic embarrassing to discuss (3%), and transportation difficulties (2%).[42] Korean women also mentioned lack of time (53%), language barriers (34.1%), not believing education was important (5.7%), and not wanting to think about breast cancer (4.9%).[43]

Physician Influence

The influence of physicians on cancer screening was noted in several studies. Chinese Americans women identified physician recommendation as the most important factor for cancer screening.[34] This was supported for mammography screening by Tu and associates,[35] who noted a strong association between screening with physician and nurse recommendation. Chinese women who had a female physician who spoke their Chinese dialect had the greatest likelihood of prior and recent mammogram screening. However, language concordance with a Chinese male physician did not increase screening.[35] For colorectal screening, urban Japanese Americans were more likely to do screening with a physician recommendation.[44] Although having a physician of the same ethnicity is generally preferred, Korean American women in California demonstrated that having a non-Korean doctor was associated with greater likelihood of having a Pap smear, mammogram, and clinical breast exam than having a Korean doctor.[45] The sex of the physicians is not specified in this study. Another study of Korean women indicated that having a physician recommendation was a facilitator in cervical cancer screening.[46] A study of Asian Indian physicians also revealed that this group of physicians was less likely to make use of preventive screenings than those in the general US population, except for mammography.[47] A study of Cambodian women showed significant association between screening stage of women and physician characteristics, with Asian American female physicians increasing the likelihood of Cambodian women being in the maintenance stage of screening for breast cancer.[48]

Colorectal Cancer Screening

In a large national study on colorectal screening in the US that included API, the lowest rates of screening were reported by Hispanics and API; those with less than ninth-grade education, with no health care insurance, or on Medicaid; those who smoked every day; and those with no routine physician visit in the last year.[49] Predictors for screening were health care coverage and a routine doctor's visit. For Japanese Americans, screening was associated with physician recommendation, acculturation, and health insurance (for sigmoidoscopy or colonoscopy).[44] While having lower screening rates, fewer Vietnamese (22%) would find endoscopic test uncomfortable compared to 79% of Caucasians, they were less likely to find fecal occult blood testing (FOBT) embarrassing, and they were more likely than Caucasians to plan to have a sigmoidoscopy in the next 5 years.[50] For Chinese Americans, factors associated with having FOBT were fewer years in the US, fewer worries or fears of the results, and a higher perceived susceptibility to colorectal cancer (CRC).[51] Having a flexible sigmoidoscopy was associated with more education, in addition to fewer worries or fears of the results and higher perceived susceptibility to CRC.

Cervical Cancer Screening

Data in California showed that 9.09% of API women had invasive cervical cancer at final diagnosis. This is twice the rate of African American (3.97%) and 3 times that of Latinas (2.74%). The API women were also significantly less likely to have had a prior Pap smear, were older, and were less likely to be self-referred.[52]

South Asian women in the US in a cross-sectional study had a Pap smear rate lower than the national recommendation, with 73% having a Pap smear within the last 3 years despite their high socioeconomic strata (income and education). South Asian women were more likely to have had a Pap smear if they were married and educated, had a regular source of health care, and were more acculturated.[53]

In a randomized controlled intervention trial to promote cervical cancer screening among Chinese women in Seattle and Vancouver, British Columbia, there was a significant reported increase in Pap testing with the outreach worker and the direct mail arms than the control group.[54] The authors concluded that having culturally and linguistically appropriate interventions (e.g., bilingual workers, Chinese language videos and materials) can increase Pap testing in this population. Another Seattle study of Chinese women noted factors associated with having at least one Pap test as being married, belief that the test is necessary for the sexually inactive, less embarrassment or concern about a cancer diagnosis, physician or family recommendation, receipt of family planning services, and having a regular health care provider.[55]

For Korean women, factors associated with having a Pap smear were female sex with age less than 50 years, having lived longer in the US, and being married and employed.[56] Also facilitating Korean women's having Pap tests were knowledge of screening guidelines, physician recommendation, health insurance, and having friends or family who had received Pap smears.[45]

Southeast Asian women also have low levels of cervical cancer screening. With Cambodian American women, barriers to cervical cancer screening were found to be a traditional orientation to prevention, causation, and treatment of disease; lack of knowledge about cervical cancer and early detection; concerns about the Pap procedure; and issues of health care access.[57] The use of outreach workers in Cambodian neighborhoods resulted in statistically significant increases in cervical cancer screening.[58] After reclassifying Hmong cases using population-based California Cancer Registry data on cervical cancer diagnosis, Hmong women experienced higher average annual age-adjusted incidence (38.7 per 100,000) as compared to API women (13.1 per 100,000) and non-Hispanic Caucasian women (8.6 per 100,000).[59] Similarly, the annual average mortality rates were also much higher at

10.5 per 100,000 for Hmong women, 3.7 per 100,000 for API and 2.5 per 100,000 for non-Hispanic Caucasians.

Breast Cancer Screening

Breast cancer is the number one cancer for Asian women. More studies have been done on breast cancer screening than other types of screening for Asian women. Similar to other cancer screenings, non-Caucasian women including Asians were significantly less likely to meet breast cancer screening recommendations.[60] The women who tended not to adhere were of younger age, less educated, underinsured/uninsured, and women with no family history of breast cancer. Breast cancer screening will be presented by Asian group in the following sections.

For Chinese women recruited from senior centers in two large east coast cities, significant predictors of having had one mammogram were insurance coverage and acculturation, whereas predictors for having a mammogram in the past year were how recent physical examination had been performed and having low perceived need or lack of physician recommendation.[61] Longer acculturation and decreased sense of modesty were predictors for having a clinical breast examination at least once. A Seattle study of Chinese women showed a strong association between mammogram screening and recommendation by physicians and nurses.[35] These researchers noted that about a third of the women reported that the best way to detect breast cancer was other than mammogram. In assessing knowledge of breast cancer risk factors, Chinese women in New York with better knowledge were twice as likely to have higher income and more education, although no significant relationship was found to acculturation.[62] With Taiwanese immigrant women, those who were more knowledgeable, confident, and health cautious, and who perceived fewer barriers were likely to initiate and/or continue regular breast cancer screening.[63] The results from Yu and associates[64] reiterate that knowledge of mammography, ability to speak English, and health insurance were significantly associated with Chinese (and Korean) women's use of mammography.

Korean women have low rates of clinical breast exams (48.4%) and mammograms within the past 12 months (21.9%).[43] Although they were willing to receive educational information, over half (55.3%) reported lack of time. This is reflected in their choice of how they preferred receiving the educational information: 76.4% by mail, 35.1% by telephone, and 35.8% by educational program. As noted previously, Korean women were more likely to be screened for breast cancer with a non-Korean physician than a Korean physician.[45] Another study showed that having a mammogram was associated with Korean women being under 50 years of age and with English-language proficiency.[56]

In a small Japanese sample, Japanese American women had high adherence to mammography screening guidelines, but less than optimal adherence to clinical breast examination (CBE) and monthly breast self-exam (BSE).[65] All the Asian women in this study were willing to share what health education knowledge they gained with their loved ones.

Regardless of their language proficiency, Filipino women's reliance on their health care provider determined whether they would take part in screening.[66] A significant lack of knowledge on screening guidelines and information on breast cancer was reported, although only by one woman. Of the women aged 40 years and above, 37% reported having a mammogram within the past year, and 65% reported ever having had one. The Filipino women's source of cancer information was generally the health care provider (61%), printed media (43%), television (20%), friends (12.5%), and health education programs, community centers, or school (9%). Like in other Asian groups the major barrier was lack of time for participating in educational programs.

With the Vietnamese women, Nguyen and associates[67] showed that a media- and neighborhood-based intervention had little effect on Vietnamese American women's recognizing symptoms or planning for clinical breast exam or mammography as compared to the control group.[67] Comparing this to their previous success using media-based interventions and lay health care workers, the researchers noted that the current study had a project coordinator and 31 unpaid volunteers who worked with a dispersed Vietnamese population, whereas the previous successful media-based intervention study had 84 paid, intensively trained lay health care workers in a concentrated urban area.

With the Hmong women in California, only 52% ever had a CBE, and only 30% ever had a mammography.[68] In a study of Vietnamese, Cambodian, and Hispanic women, all three groups were more likely to perceive barriers to receiving a mammogram than Caucasians.[69] Cambodian and Hispanic women shared similar health beliefs and behaviors when compared to Vietnamese women, thus reawakening the need to caution against collapsing all Asian groups together.

With Asian Indian women, the rate of BSE adherence was low, at 40.7%, but that of having a mammogram within the past 12 months was relatively high—between 61.3% and 70%, as compared to other ethnic minorities.[70]

Summary on Cancer Screening

Although gaps in early detection have narrowed, minority women including Asian Americans still fall behind expected levels.[71] Increased use of cancer screening by Asian women appears to be associated with English fluency, education, the source of medical care,[38] and having health insurance[49,72] and bilingual health outreach workers.[73] Likewise, barriers were lack of time, lack of knowledge of guidelines and cancer screening methods, lack of English proficiency, transportation difficulties, and lack of health insurance. Physician characteristics may influence screening rates. Generally higher screening rates were noted in specific Asian groups when physicians followed the screening guidelines with Asian women.

TREATMENT

A disproportionate number of cancer deaths occur among all racial/ethnic minorities. Many studies have shown that treatment differences were associated with adverse health outcomes of racial/ethnic minorities.[74] These outcomes included more frequent recurrence, shorter disease-free survival, and higher mortality. Fatalistic beliefs, misconceptions about cancer, and lack of health insurance and a health care provider may delay screening, diagnosis, and treatment of Asian women. Studies on the treatment of Asian American women are overwhelmingly on breast cancer, and thus the primary focus here is on this disease.

Various factors may influence an Asian woman's receptivity to seeking therapy. These may differ with each ethnic group or with individual characteristics, for example first-generation or sixth-generation status. For instance, first-generation Chinese Americans were reported to have a "sense of invulnerability to breast cancer." They tend to link breast cancer with "tragic luck" and thus are more likely to delay Western therapies, preferring Chinese medicine.[37] The need or expectation to be self-sacrificing and nurturing to their family[75] may affect treatment decision making and the type of family support they receive during treatment.

Factors that influence treatment patterns may not be clear. While there has been a steady increase in the incidence of ductal carcinoma in situ (DCIS) in the US, Asian Pacific Islander women have experienced the steepest increase, particularly in the 50- to 60-years-of-age group. Certain patterns of treatment have been noted in Asian women. Younger women and API women were more likely to undergo mastectomies.[76,77] Vietnamese women were younger at diagnosis (49.6% under 50 years), but were significantly more likely to receive a mastectomy for in situ and localized tumors (61.1%) than other racial or ethnic subgroups.[15] Similarly, Chinese women with in situ or localized tumors (under 4 cm) were also more likely than Caucasians to have a mastectomy rather than breast-conserving surgery (BCS) or no surgery. However, those Chinese women who did receive BCS or no surgery were older than the Caucasians who received similar treatment.[78] A lower rate of BCS was also noted in Filipino women.[79] In fact, twice as many Chinese and Filipino women had mastectomies as Caucasian women.[80] It is not clear whether choices were made based on cultural differences in body image, insufficient information or understanding of choices, amount of time needed for treatment options, the influence played by family role obligations, access and transportation issues, cost, or fear. The authors of the later study surmised that socioeconomic factors or immigration and acculturation issues may be associated with the choices made. Another study found that factors associated with lower use of BCS were older age, Asian or Hispanic race/ethnicity, late-stage diagnosis, and residence in a neighborhood with an undereducated population.[81]

In looking at breast reconstruction after mastectomy, Asian women were significantly less likely to have reconstruction as compared to Caucasian women.[82,83] The reason for this has not been examined.

In Chinese women who had BSC and were estrogen receptor–positive, there was a significantly lower rate of having radiation, hormonal, or adjuvant therapy as compared with Caucasian women. This treatment pattern can affect recurrence and overall survival in the women.[79,80] When compared to a Western cohort, Chinese women with early breast cancer in Hong Kong had a higher myelotoxicity while on doxorubicin and cyclophosphamide. It was felt that the toxicity may be related to ethnic variation in susceptibility to chemotherapy toxicity, lower body mass index with higher percentage of body fat composition, and concurrent use of traditional medicine during chemotherapy.[84]

As far as alternative and complementary medicine is concerned, different ethnic/racial groups tend to take different alternative therapies.[85] Chinese women with breast cancer most often used herbal therapies (22%), whereas Caucasians used dietary methods and physical methods such as massage and acupuncture. In another study of different ethnic groups, the rates of use of complementary and alternative medicine were highest among Filipino and Caucasian women, intermediate among Native Hawaiians and Chinese women, and significantly lower among Japanese women.[86] Chinese used herbal medicines, whereas Filipinos used religious healing or prayer.

IMPLICATIONS FOR CARE

Different studies have tried to determine the best strategies to disseminate health information to Asian women. Various Asian groups have preferred means of acquiring health information.[33] Asian Indian women were interested (81%) in receiving information by mail, whereas Vietnamese women were most interested (38%) in receiving information by phone. Chinese women were least likely to prefer phone,[33] but were willing to receive information through the mail.[42] Interest in attending a class was generally low in all the groups (Asian Indian, Chinese, Filipino, Japanese, Korean, and Vietnamese).[33] However, willingness to share knowledge within their cultural group averaged 92%, with a range of 84% among Korean women to 97% among Filipino women.[33] Thus this strategy, which is similar to the American Cancer Society's Tell a Friend Program, can be used to disseminate information within Asian groups.

The use of media campaigns can have an effect on increasing awareness. Japanese patients relied on media such as television, newspapers, books, and magazines.[87] Vietnamese women also used the media for cervical screening information; however, lay outreach health workers were more effective in getting the women to obtain the test.[88] The use of outreach workers also helped increase Cambodian women's rates of Pap testing[58] and those of Vietnamese women for breast and cervical screening.[73]

The use of Asian grocery store–based health education has been reported, with varying degrees of success.[33,42,43,65,66,89] Since saving time was important to many of the Asian women, using sites where Asian women would normally visit in the course of their daily lives, such as the Asian grocery store, seems a good strategy as long as topics and dissemination methods and materials are appropriate to that setting.

The importance of including Asian and other minority groups in clinical trials cannot be overemphasized, since ethnic minorities may have very difference responses to chemotherapy drugs tested on Caucasians. Toxicity levels may be different for different ethnic groups, who may have different ability to metabolize certain drugs, different body mass indexes, or increased susceptibility to chemo-induced toxicities, or who may be taking traditional medicine during their treatments.[84] The health care practitioner must do an assessment of traditional or alternative medicines an Asian woman may be taking or plan to take and assess whether these may interfere with the efficacy or potentiate the toxicities of prescribed Western treatment.

Although it is crucial for Asian women to be recruited for studies on cancer care, they are likely to refuse to participate.[90] Younger Asian American are significantly more likely to participate in clinical trials than older Asians American, resulting in an underrepresentation of those 65 years and older.[91] Thus concerted recruitment strategies must be devised and trusting relationships established with minority communities and families, well ahead of introducing the subject of participation in a clinical trial or study.

SUMMARY

Although Asian Americans represent a small (but growing) proportion of the US population, it is of concern that cancer is **the** leading cause of death for Asian women. Asian groups differ in the incidence and survival rates of different cancers, so desegregating data is important. Data from Los Angeles[14] suggest that Japanese American women have a higher incidence of breast cancer than Caucasians. What can be learned about why some ethnic groups survive certain cancers better than other ethnic groups? What can be learned from why some ethnic groups are more prone to certain cancers or have lower incidence of certain cancers? Migration's impact on cancer incidents can shed light on factors contributing to cancer causation and genetic and environmental interactions. Inroads have been made in the screening of various Asian groups, and these efforts must be continued. The importance of health care providers' following established cancer screening guidelines with Asian clients cannot be underestimated. The differences in treatment, its timing, and its outcome, when minorities are compared to Caucasians, is a national concern. The health care disparities seen with Asian Americans, as well as other minority groups noted in The Institute of Medicine's report,[92] still have to be addressed. Also, poverty and the lack of insurance common among some Asian American groups is associated with poor health outcomes, which necessitate efforts to guarantee all Americans access to quality cancer care.[93] Socioeconomic and cultural variables that affect adaptation and survival from cancer also have to be addressed.[94] Those associated with the health care industry, as well as local and federal governments, must be committed to addressing these concerns to reduce the burden and the cost, both human and financial, that is occurring in the US, particularly among minority populations.

REFERENCES

1. National Cancer Institute. *Surveillance, epidemiology, and end results, 1992-2001,* Washington, D.C. 2001, National Institutes of Health. Retrieved 1/16/05 from seer.cancer.gov/csr/1975_2001/results_single/sect_01_table.17_2pgs.pdf.
2. Barnes JS, Bennett CE: The Asian population: 2000, Washington, D.C., 2002, U.S. Census Bureau. Retrieved 1/11/05 from www.census.gov/prod/2002pubs/scbr01-16-pdf. Retrieved on January 11, 2005.
3. Reeves TJ, Bennett CE: *We the people: Asians in the United States.* Washington, D.C., 2004, U.S. Census Bureau. Retrieved 1/11/05 from www.census.gov/prod/2004pubs/censr-17.pdf. Retrieved on January 11, 2005.
4. National Cancer Institute: *Cancer in Asian American women: Key points.* Retrieved 1/18/05 from www.cancercontrol.cancer.gov/womenofcolor/asian.html.
5. Liu L, Deapen D, Berstein L: Socioeconomic status and cancers of the female breast and reproductive organs: a comparison across racial/ethnic populations in Los Angeles County, California, *Cancer Causes Control* 9:369-380, 1998.
6. Yost K and others: Socioeconomic status and breast cancer incidence in California for different race/ethnic groups, *Cancer Causes Control* 12:703-711, 2001.
7. Miller BA and others: *Racial/ethnic patterns of cancer in the United States 1988-1992, National Cancer Institute.* Bethesda, MD, 1996, NCI. NIH Pub. No. 96-4104.
8. Jemal A and others: Annual report to the nation on the status of cancer, 1975-2001, with a special feature regarding survival, *Cancer* 101:3-27, 2004.
9. National Center for Health Statistics. Surveillance, Epidemiology and End Results (SEER) for leading causes of death for Asian and Pacific islander women in the US. Retrieved 1/18/05 from www.cancercontrol.cancer.gov/womenofcolor/pdfs/asian-tables.pdf.
10. Cockburn M, Deapen D, editors: *Cancer incidence and mortality in California: trends by race/ethnicity 1988-2001,*

Los Angeles, 2004, Los Angeles Cancer Surveillance Program, University of Southern California.
11. Cancer Research Center of Hawai'i: *Hawai'i cancer facts and figures 2003-2004*, Honolulu, 2004, American Cancer Society.
12. Haselkorn T, Stewart SL, Horn-Ross PL: Why are thyroid cancer rates so high in Southeastern Asian women living in the United States? The Bay Area Thyroid Cancer Study, *Cancer Epidemiol Biomarkers Prev* 12:144-150, 2003.
13. Pike MC and others: Breast cancer in a multiethnic cohort in Hawai'i and Los Angeles: risk factor-adjusted incidence in Japanese equals and in Hawaiians exceeds that in whites, *Cancer Epidemiol Biomarkers Prev* ll:795-800, 2002.
14. Deapen D and others: Rapidly rising breast cancer incidence rates among Asian-American women, *Int J Cancer* 99: 747-750, 2002.
15. Lin SS, Phan JC, Lin AY: Breast cancer characteristics of Vietnamese women in the Great San Francisco Bay Area, *Wes J Med* 176:87-91, 2002.
16. Goodman MT and others: Incidence of ovarian cancer by race and ethnicity in the United States, 1992-1997, *Cancer* 97(10 Suppl):2676-2685, 2003.
17. Singh GK, Miller BA: Health, life expectancy, and mortality patterns among immigrant populations in the United States, *Can J Public Health* 95:114-121, 2004.
18. Pineda MD and others: Asian breast cancer survival in the US: a comparison between Asian immigrants, US-born Asian Americans and Caucasians, *Int J Epidemiol* 30: 976-982, 2001.
19. Lin SS and others: Survival differences among Asian subpopulations in the United States after prostate, colorectal, breast, and cervical carcinomas, *Cancer* 94:1175-1182, 2002.
20. Hashibe M and others: Comparison of bladder cancer survival among Japanese, Chinese, Filipino, Hawaiian and Caucasian populations in the United States, *Asian Pac J Cancer Prev* 4:267-273, 2003.
21. Longnecker DS and others: Racial differences in pancreatic cancer: Comparison of survival and histologic types of pancreatic carcinoma in Asians, blacks and whites in the United States, *Pancreas* 21:338-343, 2000.
22. Theuer CP: Asian gastric cancer patients at a southern California comprehensive cancer center are diagnosed with less advanced disease and have superior stage-stratified survival, *Am Surg* 66:821-826, 2000.
23. Flood DM and others: Colorectal cancer incidence in Asian migrants to the United States and their descendants, *Cancer Causes Control* 11:403-411, 2000.
24. Liao CK and others: Endometrial cancer in Asian migrants to the United States and their descendants, *Cancer Causes Control* 14:357-360, 2003.
25. Maskarinec G, Noh JJ: The effect of migration on cancer incidence among Japanese in Hawai'i, *Ethn Dis* 14:431-439, 2004.
26. Le GM and others: Cancer incidence patterns among Vietnamese in the United States and Ha Noi, Vietnam, *Int J Cancer* 102:412-417, 2002.
27. Gomez SL and others: Cancer incidence patterns in Koreans in the U.S. and in Kangwha, South Korea, *Cancer Causes Control* 14:167-174, 2003.
28. Pan JW and others: Incidence of leukemia in Asian migrants to the United States and their descendants, *Cancer Causes Control* 13:791-795, 2002.
29. Glaser SL, Hsu JL: Hodgkin's disease in Asians: Incidence patterns and risk factors population-based data, *Leuk Res* 26:261-269, 2002.
30. Chen JY and others: Disaggregating data on Asian and Pacific Islander women to assess cancer screening, *Am J Prev Med* 27:139-145, 2004.
31. Goel MS and others: Racial and ethnic disparities in cancer screening: the importance of foreign birth as a barrier to care, *J Gen Intern Med* 18:1028-1035, 2003.
32. Yu MY and others: Cancer screening promotion among medically underserved Asian American women: integration of research and practice, *Res Theory Nurs Pract* 16:237-248, 2002.
33. Sadler GR and others: Heterogeneity within the Asian American community, *Int J Equity Health* 2:1-9, 2003.
34. Liang W and others: How do older Chinese women view health and cancer screening? Results from focus groups and implications for interventions, *Ethn Health* 9:283-304, 2004.
35. Tu SP and others: Mammography screening among Chinese-American women, *Cancer* 97:1293-1302, 2003.
36. Lee MC: Knowledge, barriers, and motivators related to cervical cancer screening among Korean-American women. A focus group approach, *Cancer Nurs* 23:168-175, 2000.
37. Facione NC, Giancarlo C, Chan L: Perceived risk and help-seeking behavior for breast cancer: a Chinese-American perspective, *Cancer Nurs* 23:258-267, 2000.
38. Yu ES and others: Breast and cervical cancer screening among Chinese American women, *Cancer Pract* 9:81-91, 2001.
39. Pham CT, McPhee SJ: Knowledge, attitudes, and practices of breast and cervical cancer screening among Vietnamese women, *J Cancer Educ* 7:305-310, 1992.
40. Wong-Kim E, Sun A, DeMattos MC: Assessing cancer beliefs in a Chinese immigrant community, *Cancer Control* 10:22-28, 2003.
41. Johnson JL and others: South Asian women's views on the causes of breast cancer: image and explanations, *Patient Educ Couns* 37:243-254, 1999.
42. Sadler GR and others: Chinese women: Behaviors and attitudes toward breast cancer education and screening, *Women's Health Issues* 10:20-26, 2000.
43. Sadler GR and others: Korean women: Breast cancer knowledge, attitudes and behaviors, *BMC Public Health* 1:1-7, 2001.
44. Honda K: Factors associated with colorectal cancer screening among the urban Japanese population, *Am J Public Health* 94:815-822, 2004.
45. Lew AA and others: Effect of provider status on preventive screening among Korean-American women in Almeda County, California, *Prev Med* 36:141-149, 2003.
46. Juon HS, Seung-Lee C, Klassen AC: Predictors of regular Pap smears among Korean-American women, *Prev Med* 37:585-592, 2003.
47. Misra R, Vadaparampil ST: Personal cancer prevention and screening practices among Asian Indian physicians in the United States, *Cancer Detect Prev* 38:269-276, 2004.
48. Tu SP and others: Breast cancer screening: stages of adoption among Cambodian American women, *Cancer Detect Prev* 26:33-41, 2002.
49. Ioannou GN, Chapko MK, Dominitz JA: Predictors of colorectal cancer screening participation in the United States, *Am J Gastroenterol* 98:2082-2091, 2003.

50. Walsh JM and others: Barriers to colorectal cancer screening in Latino and Vietnamese Americans compared with non-Latino white Americans, *J Gen Intern Med* 19:156-166, 2004.
51. Sun WY and others: Factors associated with colorectal cancer screening among Chinese-Americans, *Prev Med* 39:323-329, 2004.
52. Arnsberger P and others: Cervical intraepithelial lesions and cervical cancer among Asian Pacific Islander women in a cervical cancer screening program, *Health Care Women Int* 23:450-459, 2002.
53. Chaudhry S and others: Utilization of Papanicolaou smears by South Asian women living in the United States, *J Gen Intern Med* 18:377-384, 2003.
54. Taylor VM and others: A randomized controlled trial of interventions to promote cervical cancer screening among Chinese women in North America, *J Natl Cancer Inst* 94:670-677, 2002.
55. Taylor VM and others: Cervical cancer screening among Chinese Americans, *Cancer Detect Prev* 26:139-145, 2002.
56. Juon HS, Choi Y, Kim MT: Cancer screening behaviors among Korean-American women, *Cancer Detect Prev* 24:589-601, 2000.
57. Jackson JC and others: Development of a cervical cancer intervention program for Cambodian American women, *Community Health* 25:359-375, 2000.
58. Taylor VM and others: Evaluation of an outreach intervention to promote cervical cancer screening in Cambodian American women, *Cancer Detect Prev* 26: 320-327, 2002.
59. Yang RC, Mills PK, Riordan DG: Cervical cancer among Hmong women in California, 1988 to 2000, *Am J Prev Med* 27:132-138, 2004.
60. Strzelczyk JJ, Dignan MB: Disparities in adherence to recommended followup on screening mammography: interaction of sociodemographic factors, *Ethn Dis* 12: 77-86, 2002.
61. Tang TS, Solomon LJ, McCracken LM: Cultural barriers to mammography, clinical breast exam, and breast self-exam among Chinese-American women 60 and older, *Prev Med* 31:575-585, 2000.
62. Chen WT, Bakken S: Breast cancer knowledge assessment in female Chinese immigrants in New York, *Cancer Nurs* 27:407-412, 2004.
63. Hsu C: *Breast cancer screening behaviors among Taiwanese immigrant women*, Chicago, 2002, University of Illinois at Chicago. (Dissertation).
64. Yu MY, Hong OS, Seetoo AD: Uncovering factors contributing to under-utilization of breast cancer screening by Chinese and Korean women living in the United States, *Ethn Dis* 13:213-219, 2003.
65. Sadler GR and others: Japanese American women: behaviors and attitudes toward breast cancer education and screening, *Health Care Women Int* 24:18-26, 2003.
66. Ko CM and others: Filipina American women's breast cancer knowledge, attitudes, and screening behaviors, *BMC Public Health* 3:27, 2003.
67. Nguyen T and others: Promoting early detection of breast cancer among Vietnamese-American women, *Cancer* 91:267-273, 2001.
68. Tanjasiri SP and others: Breast cancer screening among Hmong women in California, *J Cancer Educ* 16:50-54, 2001.
69. McGravey EL and others: Cancer screening practices and attitudes: comparison of low-income women in three ethnic groups, *Ethn Health* 8:71-82, 2003.
70. Sadler GR and others: Asian Indian women: Knowledge, attitudes and behaviors toward breast cancer early detection, *Public Health Nurs* 18:357-363, 2001.
71. Glanz K and others: Cancer-related health disparities in women, *Am J Public Health* 93:292-298, 2003.
72. Coughlin SS, Uhler RJ: Breast and cervical cancer screening practices among Asian and Pacific Islander women in the United States, 1994-1997, *Cancer Epidemiol Biomarkers Prev* 9:597-603, 2000.
73. Bird JA and others: Opening pathways to cancer screening for Vietnamese-American women: among Vietnamese American women, *Cancer Detect Prev* 27:821-829, 1998.
74. Shavers VL, Brown ML: Racial and ethnic disparities in the receipt of cancer treatment, *J Natl Cancer Inst* 94: 334-357, 2002.
75. Kagawa-Singer M, Wellisch DK: Breast cancer patients' perceptions of their husbands' support in a cross-cultural context, *Psychooncology* 12:24-37, 2003.
76. Innos K, Horn-Ross PL: Recent trends and racial/ethnic differences in the incidence and treatment of ductal carcinoma in situ of the breast in California women, *Cancer* 97:1099-1106, 2003.
77. Ashing-Giwa KT and others: Understanding the breast cancer experience of women: a qualitative study of African American, Asian American, Latina and Caucasian cancer survivors, *Psychooncology* 13:408-428, 2004.
78. Gomez SL, France AM, Lee MM: Socioeconomic status, immigration/acculturation, and ethnic variations in breast conserving surgery, San Francisco Bay area, *Ethn Dis* 14:134-140, 2004.
79. Chui SY, Lyerly HK: Disparities in breast carcinoma treatment in Asian/Pacific Islander women: a challenge to the provider, *Cancer* 95:2257-2259, 2002.
80. Prehn AW and others: Differences in treatment patterns for localized breast carcinomas among Asian/Pacific Islander women, *Cancer* 95:2268-2275, 2002.
81. Morris CR and others: Increasing trends in the use of breast-conserving surgery in California, *Am J Public Health* 90:281-284, 2000.
82. Alderman AK, McMahon L, Wilkins, EG: The national utilization of immediate and early delayed breast reconstruction and the effect of sociodemographic factors, *Plast Reconstr Surg* 111:695-703, 2003.
83. Tseng JF and others: The effect of ethnicity on immediate reconstruction rates after mastectomy for breast cancer, *Cancer* 101:1514-1523, 2004.
84. Ma B and others: Acute toxicity of adjuvant doxorubicin and cyclophosphamide for early breast cancer—a retrospective review of Chinese patients and comparison with an historic Western series, *Radiother Oncol* 62:185-189, 2002.
85. Lee MM and others: Alternative therapies used by women with breast cancer in four ethnic populations, *J Natl Cancer Inst* 92:42-47, 2000.
86. Maskarinec G and others: Ethnic differences in complementary and alternative medicine use among cancer patients, *J Altern Complement Med* 6:531-538, 2000.
87. Kakai H and others: Ethnic differences in choices of health information by cancer patients using complementary and alternative medicine: an exploratory study with correspondence analysis, *Soc Sci Medicine* 56:851-862, 2003.

88. Lam TK and others: Encouraging Vietnamese-American women to obtain Pap tests through lay health workers outreach and media education, *J Gen Intern Med* 18: 516-524, 2003.
89. Sadler GR and others: Breast cancer education program based in Asian grocery stores, *J Cancer Educ* 15:173-177, 2000.
90. Ashing-Giwa KT and others: Breast cancer survivorship in a multiethnic sample—challenges in recruitment and measurement, *Cancer* 101:450-465, 2004.
91. Alexander GA, Chu KC, Ho RC: Representation of Asian Americans in clinical cancer trials, *Ann Epidemiol* 10:S61-67, 2000.
92. Smedley BD, Stith AY, Nelson AR: *Unequal treatment: confronting racial and ethnic disparities in health care,* Washington, D.C., 2003, The National Academies Press.
93. Muss HB: Factors used to select adjuvant therapy of breast cancer in the United States: an overview of age, race, and socioeconomic status, *J Natl Cancer Inst Monogr* 30:52-55, 2001.
94. Aziz NM, Rowland JH: Cancer survivorship research among ethnic minority and medically underserved groups, *Oncol Nurs Forum* 29:789-801, 2002.

CHAPTER

27 American Indian and Alaska Native Women and Cancer

Linda Burhansstipanov

INTRODUCTION AND OVERVIEW

Census Overview of Native Women

The American Indian and Alaska Native (AIAN) population is increasing by about 1.8% a year. According to the 2000 US Census, 4.1 million US residents reported being AIAN or AIAN in combination with one or more races, with 2.2 million reporting themselves AIAN alone. This is an increase of 110% from the 1990 US Census for more than one race; and for those reporting AIAN alone, this is an increase of 26%.

The median age for AIAN population is 28.7 years. In comparison, the median age for the total US population was 35.3 years. The AIAN population is younger in comparison with other racial groups (33% of AIAN population is under 15 years old)[1] and has a shorter life expectancy (the average life span for American Indian women is about 5 years less than for "US All Races" females). Only 11% of AIANs have a bachelor's degree or higher. The AIAN median household income is $32,116, which means that about 24.5% of AIANs live at or below the federal poverty level. Approximately 43% of AIANs live west of the Mississippi, 31% live in the South, 17% live in the Midwest, and 9% live in the east. More than 60% of all AIANs live in urban areas rather than on reservations or in rural areas.

The largest (with 50,000 or more individuals) Tribal Nations are (in rank order) Cherokee, Navajo, Choctaw, Blackfeet, Chippewa, Muscogee, Apache, and Lumbee. The states with more than 100,000 AIANs (in rank order) are California (n = 628,000), Oklahoma (n = 392,000), Arizona, Texas, New Mexico, New York, Washington, North Carolina, Michigan, Alaska, and Florida. Collectively, these states have 62% of the total AIAN population.

Cancer Continues to Increase Among Native Americans

Although cancer incidence is decreasing in the general population, cancer continues to increase among American Indians and Alaska Natives.[2] Incidence rates among Alaska Natives have exceeded "US All Races" rates for most cancer sites and are similarly increasing for Canadian bands.[3,4] Moreover, a persistent gap in self-reported health status remains between AIANs and non-Hispanic Caucasians.[5] According to data summarized in the "Annual Report to the Nation on the Status of Cancer, 1973-1999, Featuring Implications of Age and Aging on the US Cancer Burden," American Indians are not benefiting from the reduced cancer incidence rate as documented for Caucasians.[6] Since World War II, nearly every AIAN community has experienced suffering and death from this disease.[4,7,8] In the last half of the twentieth century, cancer became the leading cause of death for Alaska Native women, and is the second leading cause of death among Alaska Native men.[9-11] Cancer is currently the third leading cause of death for American Indians and Alaska Natives of all ages,[12] and the second leading cause of death among American Indians (both sexes) over age 45. Cancer rates, which were previously reported to be lower in American Indian and Alaska Natives, have been shown to be increasing in the past 20 years.[13] The 5-year relative survival from cancer continues to be among the poorest in comparison to all other ethnic and racial groups in the US.[14-18] When compared to non-Indian peoples in the Southwest, even cancers diagnosed at early stages result in poorer survival in American Indians.[18] The most common sites and kinds of cancer are similar to non-Native populations (e.g., lung, colorectal, breast, cervix).

Many researchers have determined that underreporting of cancer among AIAN is often due to racial misclassification.[19-27] Misclassification occurs for many reasons including factors listed in Box 27-1.[28] Racial misclassification has been one of the most difficult obstacles in the path of getting accurate and informative data for the AIAN population.[28]

Rarely are state data accurate for American Indians or Alaska Natives (exceptions are New Mexico and Alaska). The National Institute of Cancer's Surveillance, Epidemiology, and End Results (SEER) data are primarily based on southwestern tribes, which are not representative of Natives living in other regions of the US. Centers for Disease Control (CDC) data are based on state databases, which are plagued with racial misclassification and coding errors. Thus, also not representative of the urban Indian population, Indian Health Service (IHS) data are considered the most accurate cancer database for Native Americans.

Box 27-1 Factors in Racial Misclassification

- Spanish surnames, often a historical remnant of ancestors who were slaves of missions
- American Indian/Alaska Native (AIAN) not recorded on medical records (e.g., hospital, health clinic) as "American Indian" or "Alaska Native"
- Imprecise and inconsistent definitions of American Indians
- Lack of AIAN option on state/hospital intake forms
- Changing self-identification:
  - Tribe formerly "unrecognized" becoming federally recognized by Congress
  - Tribal enrollment ordinances changing (e.g., minimum blood quantum of 25% versus proof of American Indian ancestry)
- Tribal enrollment ordinances regarding paternal versus maternal lineage
- Errors on birth certificates
- Errors on death certificates
- Personal reasons (e.g., individuals don't want others to know that they are Native)

The nature of cancer varies widely across the country, according to IHS cancer mortality data.[29] Compared to national averages, in IHS regions, AIANs who live in Alaska or the Northern Plains (South and North Dakota, Nebraska) have elevated death rates from cancer. Cancer rates are

Table 27-1 IHS Age-Adjusted Cancer Mortality Data—Females Only[62]

	Breast	Cervix	Colon	Lung
US All Races (includes women from all racial groups in the US)	24	2.6	14.4	33.9
All IHS regions	*14.2	**3.7	*12.0	*22.3
Alaska	20.8	1.5	**35.8	40.2
East (e.g., N.C., N.Y., Ga., Fla.)	*13.4	**4.3	*10.3	*18.0
Northern Plains (e.g., N.D., S.D., Neb., Wyo., Mich., Minn.)	21.6	**4.7	**22.6	**57.6
Pacific coast (Calif., Ore., Wash.)	*16.2	2.4	*7.7	*23.6
Southwest (Ariz., N.M.)	*9.2	**3.9	*8.6	*6.9

*Statistically lower death rates in comparison to US All Races.
**Statistically higher death rates in comparison to US All Races.
IHS, Indian Health Service.

lower among AIANs living on the Pacific coast and in the Southwest. However, even in these regions, cancer continues to increase rather than decrease, as is being seen among the US all races population category.

Compared to national averages, in IHS regions AIANs who live in Alaska and the Northern Plains (South and North Dakota, Nebraska) have elevated age-adjusted mortality rates for the ten most common cancer sites. Most of these rates are statistically significant in comparison with Natives living in other regions of the US as well as in comparison with the US All Races population category. Colon cancer mortality rates vary widely, but are much higher among Alaska Natives and American Indians (AIs) living in the Northern Plains. Cervix cancer mortality is more common (except Alaska and the Pacific coast) in comparison with "US All Races." Both breast and lung cancer are less common except among Alaska Natives and the Northern Plains AIs where the rates are comparable or higher than among Caucasians.

NATIONAL NATIVE AMERICAN CANCER SURVIVORS' SUPPORT NETWORK

Native American Cancer Research (NACR) developed the National Native American Cancer Survivors' Support Network in 1996 through support from the National Susan G. Komen Breast Cancer Foundation [9814 and POP 99-3091] and the Department of Defense [DoD 98-225]. Preliminary data from the network and from literature review relevant to quality of care issues indicate that Native American cancer patients continue to receive poorer quality of care than those in the general population.[30-33] Findings from the Native Survivors Network found that for those without health insurance (two thirds of the study population), most used Tribal or IHS–Contracted Health Services (CHS). None of the latter group had access to a second opinion for diagnosis. Only one of the women who used IHS CHS was offered breast-conserving surgery (lumpectomy with radiation), and none were offered treatment with tamoxifen. Only one woman had benefit of sentinel node surgery. In addition, Native breast cancer patients from one geographic region have not received quality cancer care; no established treatment protocols were followed, no follow-up recommendations were sent back to the patients' home village, no annual check-ups were documented with medical health care records. The average interval from the time of diagnosis (i.e., biopsy) to initiation of treatment was 3 to 6 months.[31]

Network data on Native women living in urban areas were compared with those on women living on reservations. Basically, there was no difference in quality of care received or in the interval between biopsy (diagnosis) and initiation of care.

ACCESS BARRIERS TO QUALITY CANCER CARE

IHS CHS "System of Care"

Indian Health Services (IHS) is severely underfunded and, contrary to common understanding, it is *not* health insurance. All of the more than 565 federally recognized Tribal Nations have individual treaties and agreements through the US Congress for some health services. Although Natives live in all 50 states, IHS/Tribal/urban clinics are only based in 33 of the 50 states, and only the Alaska Native Medical Services includes cancer treatment services. All others use a system of health referrals, called "Contracted Health Services." CHS requires that each Tribal Nation document all of the health conditions that it addresses during each fiscal year and that these conditions be prioritized by Tribal leadership.

The US Congress reviews the Tribal applications for health support each year and underfunds each Tribal Nation by anywhere from 40% to 60% of the documented health care need. This means that each tribe must either find an alternative form of support for the unfunded health issues or decide who within the community will not be referred out for treatment. Such referrals include CHS treatments; and it must be noted that almost all (if not all) cancer treatment services in the lower 48 contiguous states are limited to CHS. Every fiscal year (October 1), Tribal leaders meet to decide which health conditions are of highest priority. Individuals who are diagnosed with those conditions ranked as priorities 1 through 5 are typically referred for care. If the tribe is greatly underfunded (i.e., only funded for 40% of its health problems), the priorities tend to be limited to life and death situations (car accidents, heart attacks), treatments for children to contribute to a healthy next generation, and chronic conditions like alcoholism and diabetes.

Cancer care is usually prioritized within the top five health conditions for less than 20% of all of the federally recognized tribes, but this estimate varies each year. Since most Tribal community members typically believe that cancer is a death sentence rather than a chronic disease (as it is currently becoming), the Tribal leaders may not recommend a cancer patient be referred for care because it is "wasted money, since they are going to die anyway." Most Tribal Nations disburse their CHS monies by late spring. Signs appear on clinic entrances similar to, "CHS referrals available for urgent care only" from May through September.[34]

Insurance Issues

In 2002, 43.3 million Americans were uninsured.[35] Thirty-six percent of AIANs under 200% of Federal Poverty Level were uninsured in 2002, and 35% of AIANs were without health insurance in 1999.[36] Satter and others found only 4.5% of all AIAN adults in California (the state that has the highest numbers of American Indians and Alaska Natives) report being covered by IHS.[37] Having a usual source of care is a key aspect of access to care, providing a place for receipt of preventive services as well as somewhere to go when ill. More than one third of uninsured AIANs report that they do not have a usual source of care, more than 3 times the proportion of those who have some form of health insurance coverage or access to IHS.[38,39]

Of the Native population enrolled in the Native Survivors' Network who have some type of personal health insurance, only a minority have catastrophic health insurance, which requires very high deductibles (e.g., $500). Catastrophic health insurance typically does not include early detection services (e.g., cancer screening). Thus those with catastrophic insurance are less likely to participate in screening. The majority of health insurance plans have copayments of $10 to $20 per visit, which makes it necessary for the individual to have some cash on hand and may contribute to low cancer care participation.

CULTURAL ISSUES AFFECTING AIANS AND CANCER CARE

Cultural Issues Related to Cancer Care

The more than 565 federally recognized Tribal Nations differ greatly from one another.

Many tribes regard cancer as a "white man's disease" because it was a very rare condition before the European presence was established on the North American continent. For many Native cancer patients, the disease is not discussed and is considered a form of punishment, or may be a source of shame and guilt. A few tribes consider cancer to be a condition by which the patient experiences physical challenges to enable the rest of the Tribal members to have fewer health problems (i.e., they wear the pain so that their community will be spared the pain). Some Tribal beliefs indicate that the person with cancer is contagious with the "cancer spirit," and therefore they are ostracized by others in their communities. Other Tribal beliefs prohibit surgery to treat cancer out of the fear that one's body and spirit are missing a "part" after the surgery and that therefore persons undergoing surgery can never find their ancestors when they move to "the other side" (i.e., die). Box 27-2 summarizes examples of cultural beliefs related to cancer diagnosis.[40]

Through culturally acceptable Native American cancer education programs, these perceptions can be addressed in a respectful manner. For example, for the patient who is concerned about her ancestors "from the other side of the river" (or comparable concepts of heaven and afterlife) not being able to find her after she dies, traditional

Box 27-2 Examples of Cultural Perceptions of Cancer Diagnosis

- Cancer is a "white man's disease."
- "I tried to act white when I was young, and that is why the Creator gave me a 'white man's disease.'"
- "Cancer didn't exist until white men brought the disease with them from Europe."
- Cancer is a punishment (from one's actions or a family member's actions)
- "I didn't think I had acted badly, but I must have because now I have cancer."
- "I got cancer because my son drinks and beats his wife; that is why I have cancer—as a punishment for his bad behavior."
- "Wear the pain" to protect other members of one's communities
- "If I carry my cancer with dignity and do not show the pain, I can protect my community and neighbors from something bad."
- "My cancer helps to protect my village, so that is why I do not get Western medicine to treat it. If I was treated, someone else would have to protect my home from danger."
- Cancer is a natural part of one's path and the lessons to learn.
- "Before I was born, my spirit selected cancer for me to learn some lessons ... things that are important for me or my family to learn. "Cancer" is not a bad thing ... it is just part of my path and my lessons. It is not upsetting. It has helped me greatly."
- "My cancer diagnosis was a blessing ... not an easy or pleasant blessing—but now, looking back, it was the best thing that happened to me."

Indian healers perform ceremonies with the patient and her family to help the ancestors recognize her whenever she dies.

Communication Issues Related to Cancer Care

Numerous issues have been raised related to communication issues. Several of these are available on the NACR web page (www.natamcancer.org). An example of these issues is the lack of terminology for cancer within the 217 currently spoken Native languages. Cancer is sometimes translated as "the disease for which there is no cure," "the disease that eats the body," and so on. The difficulty in the terminology is significant because health care providers may be talking with the patient about curing the disease for which there is no cure, which makes no sense to the patient. Most Native languages add the English word *cancer* within translations to patients who do not speak English fluently.

The health care provider frequently uses words and phrases like "oncology," "histologic grade," and "stage of the tumor" that the patient does not understand. Health care providers also are likely to talk fast, in addition to using scientific terminology. Likewise, the Native patient may use words or phrases with different connotations than those generally understood by the provider. Patients who say they will use IHS for cancer care may not understand that such care is only available through CHS. The providers usually assume that IHS is a comprehensive health maintenance organization (HMO) and that the patient will receive timely care (which rarely is true).

Natives also use words like "sovereignty," "93-638 clinics," "intertribal," "blood quantum," and so on, that are unfamiliar for the health care provider. Others are common English, but have a different connotation for Natives. For example, the patient may say she needs to do "ceremony" before she starts her treatment. The health care provider thinks she is talking about having a Novena said in church, whereas the patient may be referring to a very traditional protocol requiring 3 to 6 months of preparation. Another problematic word is "survivor," which NACR staff use regularly. During one training workshop with Native American women cancer patients, a few hours, one of the participants asked, "Am I a survivor?" This question immediately raised a lot of similar questions, such as, "I take care of my sister who has ovarian cancer. Does that make me a survivor?" The NACR staff were surprised and disappointed that even members of the Native

American community were unclear about what the phrase "survivor" refers to in this context. Thus a rule of thumb when working with patients from cultures other than one's own is, assume nothing; and when in doubt, ask for clarification, or explain a concept.

Another common issue is not knowing which type of health care provider the patient is supposed to go to for care. The medical language and terminology are usually uncommon within the lay community, and almost none of these specialties are available at local IHS, Tribal, or urban Indian clinics.

Connotations vary greatly from the Western medical context to that of a Native patient. An example is the different understanding of "positive," as when the health care provider informs the patient that her test is positive. The word positive usually means something good for the Native; however, in this instance the provider means that the tissue had cancer cells present. This type of miscommunication contributes to distrust between the provider and patient.

There are also issues with the number and complexity of health care forms. For a large segment of the elder Native cancer community, the reading level of these forms is too high to be understandable, and the patient needs help filling out the forms.

Outreach Strategies to Improve AIAN Participation in Cancer Programs

Community-Based Participatory (Action) Research (CBPR)

Native communities are very supportive of outreach, recruitment, and retention strategies that evolve as a result of community-based participatory [action] research (CBPR). CBPR, sometimes called "Community-Based Participatory Action Research," is a partnership approach to research that equitably involves community members, organizational representatives, and researchers in all aspects of the research process.[41] It has also been described as "a collaborative process that equitably involves all partners in the research process and recognizes the unique strengths that each brings. CBPR begins with a research topic of importance to the community with the aim of combining knowledge and action for social change to improve community health and eliminate health disparities."[42] CBPR is a current buzz phrase in federal government.[35] However, many researchers mistakenly believe that if their study is conducted in the community or community members are participants, then the study meets the criteria necessary to be considered a CBPR. Mere participation in a study is not the same as being a "partner," and such research does not necessarily meet CBPR criteria.[43,44]

In the mid-1990s in Canada, Aboriginal communities of the Akwasasne Mohawk took a leadership role in helping to clarify principles of CBPR.[45] Partnership roles include the Tribal community having a decision making and leadership role throughout every phase of the research; for example, identifying the priority research questions, hiring and training salaried Native staff for multiple roles in the study, designing, implementing, and evaluating the research project, and disseminating the research findings to the local community and within peer reviewed publications. Native communities are becoming more involved in CBPR projects and are less likely to be involved in a study that only wants to include them as "study participants." Thus health care providers who are interested in increasing the participation of Natives within clinical trials or any other cancer initiative need to develop a trusting working relationship with the community. The process of developing and implementing successful CBPR projects takes 3 to 4 years in most communities.

Community-Driven Interventions

Community-driven interventions are very similar and many times overlapping strategies that emerge directly from the community with few or only minor roles for health care organizations. These will sometimes evolve from local Tribal leadership's promoting more active involvement in addressing a local health issues. For example, Wind River Reservation in Wyoming created the Wind River Cancer Resource Center in Ethete in response to community members who demanded that something be done about the accelerating cancer problem. The resource center is based in a historic building that is easily accessible to a large segment of the reservation residents. The community has identified additional cancer priorities and is gradually seeking funding to attain its goals.

Navigators/Lay Health Outreach Workers/Native Sisters

The navigators model, which evolved from an innovative patient support program implemented by Dr. Harold Freeman in Harlem Hospital,[46] is a good example of an original idea that has been adapted to fit varying conditions.[47-59] In the original Freeman model, the navigator is trained to accompany the patient to follow-up appointments to provide emotional support and patient advocacy. Freeman's navigator support is initiated at the time the patient receives an abnormal cancer test. The navigator supports and assists the patient to access services and obtain appropriate follow-up. Freeman's navigator concept has expanded to include multiple roles such as the following: transporting the patient to and from appointments, meeting the patient at the clinic, escorting or accompanying the patient to all offices where appointments and treatments are scheduled, helping the patient make and keep the appointments, being a friend and confidant to the patient, helping the patient prepare questions to ask the provider during the appointment, helping the patient complete paperwork, helping with language or literacy translation during the appointment, helping the patient get medications prescribed by the health care provider, helping the patient understand how to take prescription and over-the-counter medications, and talking with the family so that they understand the disease and what the patient is experiencing, as well as the patient's changing needs. These roles are typically assumed by a member of the lay community who is trained to provide accurate and efficient support for the patient.

Most programs refer to these individuals as "navigators," "lay health outreach workers," "Native sisters," "patient advocates," "promotores," and "commadries." NACR has been implementing Native sister/patient advocate programs since 1996. Among the factors that help to make these interventions successful is the ability to provide organized training to the staff and to pay these trained individuals a competitive salary. Contrary to other programs, NACR has determined that when one invests the time and effort to train a navigator, this person will quickly be hired by some other program unless one provides a good salary to demonstrate respect for and the placing of value on the navigators' diverse roles.

Additional Strategies

When feasible, it is best to hire female Native cancer survivors as the outreach staff workers. These too are salaried positions. Many cancer survivors volunteer their time to help in programs, but when health care programs are being administered within communities of abject poverty, it is important to pay the workers. So many programs have assumed that just because someone has experienced cancer, they somehow now have some constant, reliable income for daily living expenses. This assumption is certainly not true for most cancer patients, who accumulate massive amounts of economic debt throughout their cancer care.

One-on-one recruitment, outreach, retention, and support is the most effective strategy; and again serving in that function is optimally a female Native cancer survivor. When a survivor is not available for this position, another Native woman from the community is the second best choice. Several health care organizations have learned about the "community health representatives" (CHR) or "community health aides/practitioners" (CHA/Ps) that function within IHS, Tribal, and some urban Indian clinics. The health care organizations have assumed that the CHR or the CHA/P will provide the outreach. However, in most Native settings the CHRs and CHA/Ps are stretched very thin and cannot take on additional roles, particularly if the health care organization assumes that these roles will be integrated into their workload without providing additional financial support. This support is needed to hire and train more CHRs and CHA/Ps so that they can take on these additional roles necessary for successful cancer programs.

For those communities that have access to telephones in the home (about 75% of Tribal communities), it is very effective to have telephone reminder calls to the patients about their upcoming appointments. During this call, it is beneficial to determine if the patient requires help with transportation, child or elder care, or similar needs.

Within Native communities, a large proportion of successful cancer screening programs provide "gifts" after the appointment has been completed. This "gifting" is integrated within the diverse cultures of most of the 565-plus federally recognized Tribal Nations. It is not considered bribery, but rather is perceived as showing respect for the Native woman who models the behaviors required to be a well woman for her children and other members of the community.

The announcement of cancer services by means of Tribal newsletters and newspapers has been effective. Even more effective are announcements of such services on Native radio stations, such as Native American Calling and Raven Radio. Public service announcements that are on either radio or television are significantly more effective when they use local Native women as the "stars" and "speakers" of these promotions.

Unsuccessful Strategies

Less effective strategies include recruiting using voter registration lists, marketing lists, and surveillance databases. Also ineffective are including announcements in general newspapers (e.g., the *Los Angeles Times, USA Today*), unless such announcements are placed on the day and in the section of the paper that provides market discount coupons (e.g., in the "Food" section of the *L.A. Times* on Thursdays). General radio and TV public service announcements that are designed for the general public have little to no effectiveness in Native communities. Likewise, programs such as Sister-to-Sister, which have worked very effectively within African-American churches, have largely been unsuccessful in Indian country. This does not mean that church-based interventions cannot work well, just that there are more failures than successes of such interventions to date. There have been successful church-based breast health programs implemented in two different Oklahoma Tribal communities. Fourteen other church-based efforts have failed in Indian country.

Examples of "Messages" That are Successful

"Messages" refers to the words that are used in the cancer program. Messages that are ineffective tend to use a high literacy level (over grade 8), have a lot of scientific or statistical jargon (e.g., "mortality rate" rather than "deaths"), and emphasize an individual's self. For example, a common message that was developed and promoted by a federal agency is, "Be a well woman, get a mammogram." This message has little to no effect on Native women. It is regarded as being too selfish. To improve the impact of a health message, it must relate back to the family and community. Thus, when NACR staff changed the previous message to "Have a mammogram to show your daughters how a well woman behaves," the community was receptive to receiving more information. Showing the woman who is delivering the message also improves the effectiveness of the message (Figure 27-1).

Messages must be culturally relevant, appropriate, respectful, sensitive, and competent. They

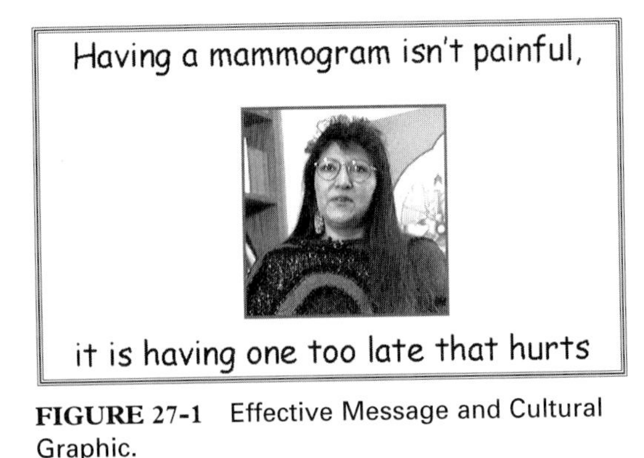

FIGURE 27-1 Effective Message and Cultural Graphic.

also must emphasize behaviors that benefit overall health rather than limiting the benefits to cancer only, such as, "Daily physical activity and healthy diets help prevent cancer, heart disease, and diabetes."

The message is also more effective if the emphasis is on "health" rather than disease; thus "breast health screening" rather than "breast cancer screening."

Examples of Materials That are Successful

Materials include print and video products. There are many effective, easy-to-understand breast and cervix education materials, most of which have been developed by the CDC Tribal breast and cervical cancer programs (e.g., in Hopi Nation, Navajo Nation, Cherokee Nation).[60,61] Both the messages and the artwork reflect the local communities to be most successful in that setting. Successful Native materials also frequently include the use of circles, cultural artwork, and respect for Tribal sacred colors, which are very specific to each Tribal Nation (i.e., in some communities the color red is reserved for sacred artifacts only). A few examples are provided in Figure 27-2 and Figure 27-3.

Storytelling is a very integral component within all of the Native cultures. NACR support materials are dependent on the stories of other survivors to help those newly diagnosed to address or cope with their ongoing experiences. Figure 27-3 shows an excerpt of survivors' support materials from the National Native American Cancer Survivors' Support Network. These materials are available in both print and video formats and are among the most frequently requested from the NACR.

Those materials designed for the general public are frequently laid out in a linear format (e.g., bar graphs). There are times when in using a bar graph, the NACR staff modified the bar graph to include graphics of people, which was more acceptable to the community (Figure 27-4). To make this figure more acceptable, it was also necessary to change "malignant neoplasms" to "cancer."

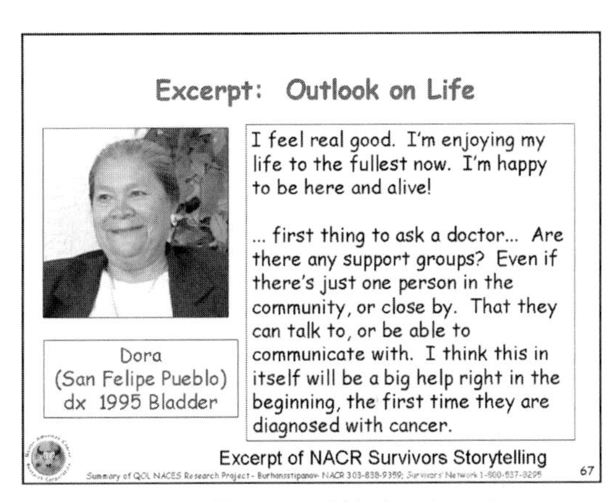

FIGURE 27-3 Excerpt of Native American Cancer Research Survivors Storytelling.

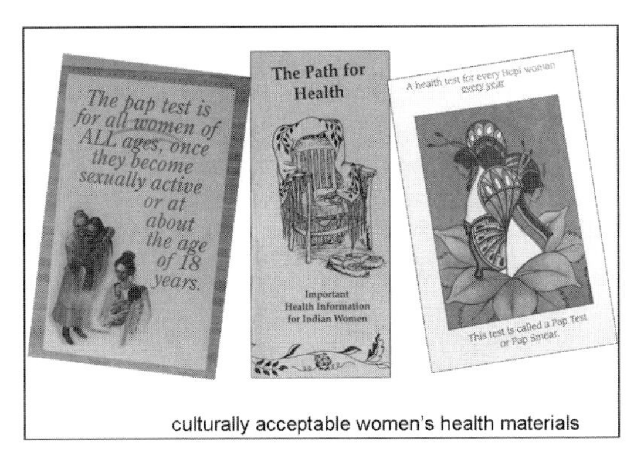

FIGURE 27-2 Culturally Acceptable Women's Health Materials.

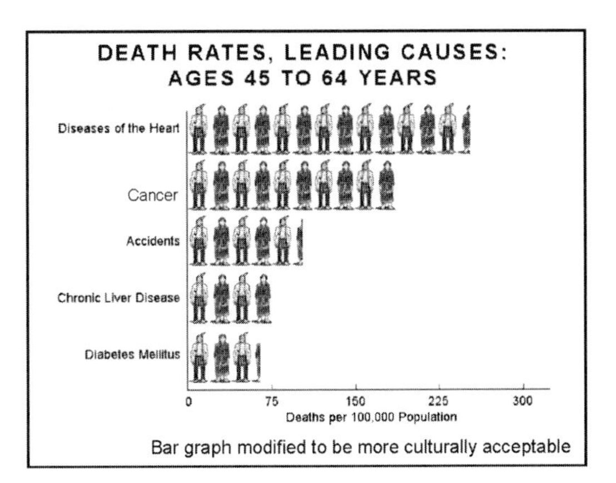

FIGURE 27-4 Bar Graph Modified To Be More Culturally Acceptable.

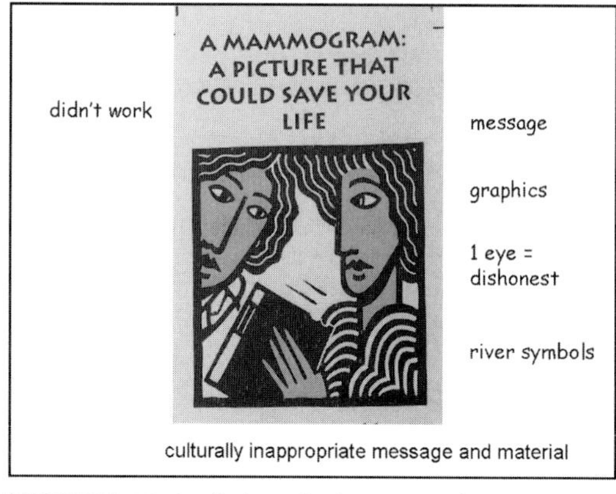

FIGURE 27-5 Culturally Inappropriate Message and Material.

Figure 27-5 is a federal product that has been unsuccessful in *most* Tribal communities. The message is too selfish, and the graphics were not well received: the hair is the same as a river symbol for several tribes that have specific connotations within that Tribal Nation. Showing half of the face indicates dishonesty in other Tribal Nations. This illustrates the need to have the local Tribal community collaborate or take a leadership role in designing cancer materials for its own members. There are subtleties (e.g., the one eye and dishonesty) that people brought up outside of the community are unlikely to know about or to appreciate the significance of.

RESOURCES

Table 27-2 identifies some of the more effective resources that provide accurate and culturally acceptable information about cancer in Indian country. It is not all-inclusive.

Table **27-2** Resources for Native Women

Resource	Description
Mayo Clinic's, "Native CIRCLE" Charlton 6; Room 282 200 First Street S.W. Rochester, MN 55905 Toll-free: 877-372-1617 http://mayoresearch.mayo.edu/mayo/research/cancercenter/native/cfm	The Native Cancer Information Resource Center and Learning Exchange (**C.I.R.C.L.E**), a resource center providing cancer-related materials to health care professionals and lay people involved in the education, care and treatment of American Indians and Alaska Natives.
Native American Cancer Research 3022 South Nova Road Pine, CO 80470-7830 Toll-free: 1-800-537-8295 Headquarters: 303-838-9359 www.NatAmCancer.org	Provides free downloadable print products from its web page after they have been pretested with multiple intertribal groups. These materials are from the following projects or curricula: • NAWWA (energy balance, outreach and referral to screening) • "Genetic Education for Native Americans" • "Get on the Path to Health" (separate slide shows on breast, cervix, colon, lung, and prostate education) • "Clinical Trials Education for Native Americans" (training and resources) • "National Native American Cancer Survivors Support Network" • "Native American Cancer Survivor Support Circles" (training and resources) • "Quality of Life: Native American Cancer Education for Survivors" • "Native American Palliative Care" education

Continued

Table 27-2 Resources for Native Women—cont'd

Resource	Description
Spirit of EAGLES 200 First Street S.W. Rochester, MN 55905 Phone: 507-284-4574 http://mayoresearch.mayo.edu/mayo/research/cancercare/native.cfm	Mayo Clinic's "The American Indian / Alaska Native Initiative on Cancer" ("Spirit of E.A.G.L.E.S." [Survivors, Education, Advocacy, Grants, Leadership, Elders and Scholarships]) [NCI U01 CA86098] provides multiple community-based research opportunities in partnership with Native organizations
Mayo Clinic's "Native WEB" (Women Enjoying the Benefit) 200 First Street S.W. Rochester, MN 55905 Phone: 507-284-4574 http://mayoresearch.mayo.edu/mayo/research/cancercare/native.cfm	Provides culturally and scientifically appropriate women's health screening training for nurses
Mary P. Lovato's "A Gathering of Cancer Support" P.O. Box 83 Santo Domingo Pueblo, NM 84052 Phone: 505-465-0325 Email: NatAmMaryL@aol.com	Provides intensive week-long training program for Tribal communities on cancer survivor support
CeCe Whitewolf's Native People's Circle of Hope 9770 S.W. Ventura Ct. Tigard, OR 97223 Phone: 503-970-8004 Email: c2w2@teleport.com	Provides individualized assistance to Native American cancer survivorship issues, annual conferences and trainings on multiple culturally pertinent topics
The Intercultural Cancer Council 6655 Travis, Suite 322 Houston, TX 77030 Phone: 713-798-4617 www.iccnetwork.org	Provides Fact Sheets on AIAN and opportunities to be more actively involved in regional ICC Network Activities. ICC implements a "Biennial Symposium of Cancer, Minorities and the Medically Underserved" that includes active participation of poor communities and most ethnicities in the US.
Other resources include Tribal programs funded for early detection of breast and cervix cancers from the Centers for Disease Prevention and Promotion; those programs are funded jointly by the National Institutes of Health and IHS for Native American Research Centers for Health (NARCH); as well as other native programs funded by federal agencies (e.g., NCI, DoD) and national foundations (Susan G. Komen, Avon).	

AIAN, American Indian Alaska Native; *HIS*, Indian Health Service; *NCI*, National Cancer Institute; *DoD*, Department of Defense.

REFERENCES

1. Indian Health Service: IHS Trends 1998-1999, Rockville, MD, Pub. No. ISSN 1095-2896.
2. Institute of Medicine: *The unequal burden of cancer: an assessment of NIH research and programs for ethnic minorities and the medically underserved*, Washington, D.C., 1999, National Academy Press.
3. Lanier AP, Bulkow LR, Ireland B: Cancer in Alaska Indians, Eskimos, and Aleuts, 1969-83: implications of etiology and control, *Public Health Report* 104:658-664, 1989.

4. Burhansstipanov L, Olsen S: Cancer prevention and early detection in American Indian and Alaska Native populations. In Marilyn Frank-Stromborg and Sharon J. Olsen, editors: *Cancer prevention in diverse populations: cultural implications for the multi-disciplinary team,* Pittsburgh, 2001, Oncology Nursing Society.
5. U.S. Department of Health and Human Services, Indian Health Service: *Trends in Indian health* 2000-2001 edition, Washington, D.C., 2004, U.S. Government Printing Office.
6. Edwards BK, and others: Annual report to the nation on the status of cancer, 1973-1999, featuring implications of age and aging on the U.S. cancer burden, *Cancer* 94(10):2766-2792, 2002.
7. Lanier AP and others: *Cancer in the Alaska Native population: Eskimo, Aleut, and Indian incidence and trends 1969-1988,* Anchorage, AK, 1993 Alaska Area Native Health Service.
8. Burhansstipanov L, Hampton JW, Tenney MT: American Indian and Alaska Native cancer data issues, *Am Indian Culture Res J* 23(3a):217-241, 1999.
9. Cobb N, Paisano RE: *Cancer mortality among American Indians and Alaska Natives in the United States: regional differences in Indian Health, 1989-1993,* Rockville, MD, 1997, Indian Health Service. IHS Pub. No. 97-615-23.
10. Department of Health and Human Services: *Healthy people 2010: objectives for the nation—draft for public comment,* Washington, D.C., 1998, Government Printing Office.
11. Burhansstipanov L: Cancer: a growing problem among American Indians and Alaska Natives. In Dixon M, Roubideaux Y, editors: *Promises to Keep,* Washington, D.C., 2001, American Public Health Association.
12. Department of Health and Human Services, Office of Planning, Evaluation and Legislation, Indian Health Services: *Regional differences in Indian health:1997,* Rockville, Md., 1997, Indian Health Service.
13. Cobb N, Paisano RE: Patterns of cancer mortality among Native Americans, *Cancer* 83(11):2377-2383, 1988.
14. Department of Health and Human Services, PHS, NIH, NCI: *Report of the Special Action Committee, 1992: program initiatives related to minorities, the underserved and persons aged 65 and over,* (Appendices A, B, C), Washington, D.C., 19912, Government Printing Office.
15. Wilson RT and others: Racial/ethnic differences in breast cancer treatment patterns among American Indian, Hispanic and non-Hispanic White women using SEER-Medicare linked data: New Mexico and Arizona, 1987-1996. Submitted for publication.
16. Burhansstipanov L, Lovato MP, Krebs LV: Native American cancer survivors, *Health Care Women Int* 20:505-515, 1999.
17. Samet JM and others: Survival of American Indian and Hispanic cancer patients in New Mexico and Arizona, 1969-82, *J Natl Cancer Inst* 79(3):457-563, 1987.
18. Bleed DM and others: Cancer incidence and survival among American Indians registered for Indian Health Service care in Montana, 1982-1987, J Natl Cancer Inst 84(19):1500-1505, 1992.
19. Frost F, Shy KK: Racial differences between linked birth and infant death records in Washington State, *Am J Public Health* 70:974-976, 1980.
20. Frost F, Taylor V, Fires E: Racial misclassification of Native Americans in a surveillance, epidemiology and end results cancer registry, J Natl Cancer Instit 84(12):957-962, 1992.
21. Hahn RA, Truman BI, Barker ND: Identify ancestry: the reliability of ancestral identification in the United States by self, proxy, interviewers, and funeral director, *Epidemiology* 7:75-80, 1996.
22. Hahn RA, Mulinare J, Teutsch SM: Inconsistencies in coding of race and ethnicity between birth and death in US infants. A new look at infant mortality, 1983 through 1985, *JAMA* 267(2)259-263, 1992.
23. Hahn RA: The state of federal health statistics on racial and ethnic groups, *JAMA* 267(2):268-271, 1992.
24. Hahn RA: *Differential classification of American Indian race on birth and death certificates, U.S. reservation states, 1983-1985, The Provider,* ,1993, Indian Health Service, Phoenix, Arizona. p. 10.
25. Sugarman JR And others: Racial misclassification of American Indians: its effect on injury rates in Oregon, 1989 through 1990, *AJPH* 83(5):681-684, 1993.
26. Sugarman JR and others: Coding of race on death certificates of patients of an Urban Indian Health Clinic, Washington, 1973-1988, *IHSProvider* July:113-115, 1992.
27. Burhansstipanov L, Hampton JW, Wiggins C: Issues in cancer data and surveillance for American Indian and Alaska Native populations, *J Registry Manage* 29(4):153-157, 1999.
28. Burhansstipanov L, Satter DE: Office of management and budget racial categories and implications for American Indians and Alaska Natives. *AJPH* 90(11):1720-1723, 2000.
29. Espey DK, Paisano RE, Cobb N: Cancer mortality among American Indians and Alaska Natives: regional differences, 1994-1998, Rockville, Md., revised 2003, Indian Health Service. IHS Pub. No. 97-615-21.
30. Burhansstipanov L and others: An innovative path to improving cancer care in Indian country, *Public Health Rep* 116:5, 2002.
31. Burhansstipanov L, Hollow W: Native American cultural aspects of nursing oncology care. *Semin Oncol Nurs* 17(3):206-219, 2001.
32. Gilliland FD, Hunt WC, Key CR: Trends in the survival of American Indian, Hispanic, and non-Hispanic white cancer patients in New Mexico and Arizona, 1969-1994, *Cancer* 82(9):1769-1783, 1998.
33. Hampton JW: The disproportionately lower cancer survival rate with increased incidence and mortality in minorities and underserved Americans, *Cancer* 83(8):1687-1689, 1998.
34. Burhansstipanov L: Personal documentation, 2002.
35. DHHS Progress Review Group. Making cancer health disparities history: report of the Trans-HHS Cancer Health Disparities Progress Review Group, submitted to the Secretary, U.S. Department of Health and Human Services, Washington, D.C., 2004; available online at http://www.chdprg.omhrc.gov. Accessed August 3, 2004.
36. Zuckerman S and others: Health service access, use, and insurance coverage among American Indians/Alaska Natives and Whites: what role does the Indian Health Service play? *Am J Public Health* 94(1):53-59, 2004.
37. Satter DE and others: *Diabetes among American Indians and Alaska Natives in California: prevention is the key,* Los Angeles, 2003, UCLA Center for Health Policy Research.

38. Brown ER, and others: Racial and ethnic disparities in access to health insurance and health care. Los Angeles, Calif. University of California, Los Angeles, Center for Health Policy Research, 2000.
39. Satter DE and others: American Indian and Alaska Natives in California: women's cancer screening and results, *J Cancer Educ* 20(Suppl):58-64, 2005.
40. Burhansstipanov LA: Cancer: a growing problem among American Indians and Alaska Natives. In Dixon M, Roubideaux Y, editors: *Promises to Keep*, Washington, D.C., 2001, American Public Health Association.
41. Israel BA and others, editors: *Multiple methods for conducting community-based participatory research for health*, 2005, San Francisco, Calif, Jossey-Bass.
42. Minkler M and others: Community-based participatory research: implications for public health funding, *AJPH* 93(8):1210-1213, 2003.
43. Israel BA and others: Community-campus partnerships for health. Community-based participatory research: policy recommendations for promoting a partnership approach in health research, *Educ Health (Abingdon)* 14(2):182-197, 2001.
44. Cornwall A, Jewkes R: What is participatory research? *Soc Sci Med* 41:1667-1676, 1995.
45. Macaulay AC and others: Participatory research with Native community of Kahnawake creates innovative code of research ethics, *Can J Public Health* 89(2):105-108, 1998.
46. Freeman HP, Muth BJ, Kerner JF: Expanding access to cancer screening and clinical follow-up among the medically underserved, *Cancer Pract* 3(1):19-30, 1995.
47. Bailey JE, Coombs DW: Effectiveness of an Indonesian model for rapid training of Guatemalan health workers in diarrhea case management, *J Community Health* 21(4):269-276, 1996.
48. Holmes AP, Hatch J, Robinson GA: A lay health educator approach to sickle cell disease education, *J Natl Black Nurses Assoc* 5(2):26-36, 1992.
49. Simmons D and others: Ethnic differences in diabetes knowledge and education: the South Auckland /Diabetes Study, *New Z Med J* 107(978):197-200, 1994.
50. Green B and Werner E. It Works! Breast Cancer Programs for African-American Women. In Weiner , editor: *Cancer in minority and underserved populations*, Westport, CT: Greenwood Publishing Group. 1999 pp. 107-120.
51. McPhee SJ and others: Pathways to early cancer detection for Vietnamese: Suc Khoe La Vang! (Health is gold!), *Health Ed Q* 23(suppl):S60-S75, 1996.
52. Bird JA and others: Tailoring lay health worker interventions for diverse cultures: lessons learned from Vietnamese and Latina communities, *Health Ed Q* 23(suppl):S104-S121, 1996.
53. Eng E, Young R: Lay health advisors as community change agents, *Fam Community Health* 15:24-40, 1992.
54. Navarro AM and others: Por la vida intervention model for cancer prevention in Latinas, *J Natl Cancer Inst Monogr* 18:137-145, 1995.
55. Burhansstipanov L: Developing culturally competent community-based interventions. In Weiner D, editor: *Cancer research interventions among the medically underserved*, Westport, CT, 1999, Greenwood.
56. Burhansstipanov L: Native American cancer programs: recommendations for increased support, *Cancer Suppl* 83(8):1849-1955, 1998.
57. Segal-Matsunaga D and others: Participatory research in a Native Hawaiian community: the Waianae Cancer Research Project, *Cancer* 78(7 Oct. Suppl):1582-1586, 1996.
58. Burhansstipanov L and others: Culturally relevant "navigator" patient support: the Native Sisters, *Cancer Pract* 6:(3):191-194, 1998.
59. Burhansstipanov L and others: Native American recruitment into breast cancer screening: The NAWWA Project, *J Cancer Educ* 15:29-33, 2000.
60. Orians CE and others: Public education strategies for delivering breast and cervical cancer screening in American Indian and Alaska Native populations, *J Public Health Manage Pract* 10(1):46-53, 2004.
61. Lantz PM and others: Implementing women's cancer screening programs in American Indian and Alaska Native populations, *Health Care Women Int* 24(8):674-696, 2003.
62. Burhansstipanov L: Urban Native American health issues, *Cancer* 88:987-993, 2000.

CHAPTER

28 Latino Women and Cancer

Gloria Velez-Barone

GROWTH AND DIVERSITY

Latinos represent over 22 different countries, with a mixture of various racial, ethic, and historic perspectives. How this population self-identifies varies from one group to another; Hispanic is a bureaucratic term that was developed during the Nixon administration to encapsulate this growing population and implies a connection to historic Spain. Latino is a self-defined term that refers more to nationality. The term Latino(a) was used for the first time in Census 2000. The terms have been used interchangeably.

Latinos comprise 12.5% of the US population; this is a 50% increase since 1990.[1] Demographically, of the 12.5% there are 20.5 million Mexican Americans, 3.3 million Puerto Ricans, and 1.1 million Cubans, and 10 million people representing the Dominican Republic, Central America, and South America (Box 28-1).

The majority of Latinos living in the US are concentrated in the West and the South. Almost half live in the West, and approximately one third live in the South, with California and Texas having half of the total Latino population. Other states with a high Latino population are Arizona, Nevada, Colorado, Florida, New York, and New Jersey. Mexican Americans predominantly reside in the Southwest and West, Cuban Americans in the Southeast, and Puerto Ricans in the Northeast. An interesting trend seen in the Census 2000 was the increase in Latino populations in states that traditionally did not have many resident Latinos. Most notable in this regard are Georgia, Illinois, Kansas, Nebraska, North Carolina, Oklahoma, Rhode Island, South Carolina, Tennessee, Utah, and Virginia (Table 28-1). Not only has there been an increase in the numbers of Latinos living in these states, but also an increase and shift in the total percent of the population.

CULTURALLY COMPETENT CARE

The Spaniards brought the Spanish language and Catholicism to the nations they conquered. In many Latino subcultures, there is a blend of Spanish culture and indigenous ones, as well as an African influence in slavery trading posts such as Cuba. Cultural groupings include Afro-Latino (Cuba, Puerto Rico, Hispaniola, influenced by slave trading), Euro-Latino (Argentina and Uruguay, influenced by Germans, English, Welsh, eastern Europeans), Indo-Latino (Central America, influenced by indigenous populations), and Asian-Latinos (influenced by slavery). The diversity of these groups has influenced religion, rituals, and traditions among the subpopulations.[2]

The demographics from Census 2000 and diversity of the Latino subcultures demonstrate the need to provide culturally competent care, particularly in oncology, throughout the continuum of care. Cultural competency involves being sensitive and able to plan care that fits with culture, race, ethnicity, gender, age, socioeconomic status, and sexual preferences.[3] Latinos are a vulnerable population with their own unique issues that can have an adverse impact on health if

Box 28-1 Central and South American Subpopulations

CENTRAL AMERICA (EXCLUDING MEXICANS)
Costa Rican
Guatemalan
Honduran
Nicaraguan
Panamanian
Salvadoran

SOUTH AMERICA
Argentinean
Bolivian
Chilean
Columbian
Ecuadorian
Paraguayan
Peruvian
Uruguayan
Venezuelan

not addressed by health care professionals. Furthermore, the health care model in the US is based on Northern European values that may lead to cultural misunderstandings in the course of providing care. By incorporating and addressing cultural values when developing prevention and screening programs, planning medical care, and discussing end-of-life issues, partnerships are created that lead to enhanced patient outcomes.

LATINOS: A VULNERABLE POPULATION

There are several factors that contribute to Latinos' vulnerability to health disparities. According to Aday,[4] relative risk can be compared by assessing social status, social capital, and human capital. Social status issues place Latinos, along with African Americans, Native Americans, and Asian Americans, at a higher risk compared with Caucasians.

Social networks tend to be strong in the Latino family, and this can be a mediating factor in some cases. For instance, family and friends are involved in treatment and accompany the patient to physician visits. However, if immigrants are in the US illegally or are involved in migratory work, those connections may not be as evident in their day-to-day interactions.

Language, related to social capital, may be another issue. English proficiency, for example, correlates with an individual's degree of acculturation into the society in which he or she lives. Moreover, there is a relationship between acculturation and participation in health screening modalities, such as mammography.[5]

Another concern with language and communication is that there are various dialects among Latinos who speak Spanish, so a translation from English to Spanish may be well interpreted by one

Table 28-1 Latino Population Growth Seen in Nontraditional States[1]

	Population 1990	% Total Population 1990	Population 2000	% Total Population 2000
Georgia	108,922	1.7%	435,227	5.3%
Illinois	904,466	7.9%	1,530,262	12.3%
Kansas	93,670	3.8%	188,252	7.0%
Nebraska	36,969	2.3%	94,425	5.5%
North Carolina	76,726	1.2%	378,963	4.7%
Oklahoma	86,160	2.7%	179,304	5.2%
Rhode Island	45,752	4.6%	90,820	8.7%
South Carolina	30,551	0.9%	95,076	2.4%
Tennessee	32,741	0.7%	123,838	2.2%
Utah	84,597	4.9%	201,559	9.0%
Virginia	160,288	2.6%	329,540	4.7%

subgroup but not another. There also may be no direct translation for a word; for example, "cancer" has no direct equivalent in the Spanish language. When it comes to proficiency in the English language, oral skills may exceed an individual's reading and writing skills. Latinos may be linguistically isolated, which can lead to an increase in health care disparities.

The greatest risk for Latinos lies within the human capital domain. Cubans as a subgroup are the most educated, followed by Mexican Americans, with Puerto Ricans being the least educated of the major Latino groups represented in the US. Half of Latinos 25 years of age and older have not completed high school, one third have less than a ninth-grade education, and less than one tenth have a college education.[6] This lack of education leads to poorly paying jobs or unemployment, low socioeconomic status, poverty, substandard housing, and a lack of adequate health insurance. Thirty-five percent of Latinos have no health insurance,[7] and as a group they are disproportionately uninsured.[8] Traditionally, Latinos have been underrepresented in the health care field. Combined with the stated risk factors and issues with communication, there may be delays in their receiving adequate health care.

An Unequal Cancer Burden

The increased risk and vulnerability of the Latino population is reflected in data collection. The Surveillance, Epidemiology, and End Results (SEER), a National Cancer Institute Program,[9] was developed to estimate the burden of cancer within geographic regions. Misclassification of Latinos has occurred, since Latinos can also be considered as white, black, Asian, Pacific Islander, or Native American. Inadequate cancer surveillance makes it difficult to determine the incidence, mortality, and risk among the Latino subgroups, and the data may not accurately reflect the experience of minority groups throughout the US; data sets that do address specific ethnic groups are limited to recent years.[10]

Cancer is the second leading cause of death among Latinos. In several cancer sites the incidence and mortality rates among Latinos are lower when compared to Caucasians. The disparities are easily noted when specific cancer sites are evaluated (see Tables 28-2 and 28-3). The general incidence of cancer rates for Latinos is 290.5 per 100,000, as compared to 424.4 per 100,000 for white females; mortality rates for Latinos are 105.7 per 100,000 as opposed to 171.2 per 100,000 for white females. Between 1992 and 1999, cancer incidence rates have declined by 1.6% a year for Latinos and 0.9% among whites. The major cancer sites and types for Latinos are breast, colon and rectum, lung and bronchus, uterine cervix, thyroid, ovary, non-Hodgkin's lymphoma, stomach, and pancreas.

Although the breast cancer incidence rate is lower in Latinos than in non-Latinos, it is frequently diagnosed at a more advanced stage[10,11]

Table **28-2** Cancer Incidence Sites for Latinos Compared to White Females[10,11]

Latinos		Whites	
Site	**Percent**	**Site**	**Percent**
Breast	30	Breast	32
Colon and rectum	9	Lung and bronchus	12
Lung and bronchus	6	Colon and rectum	11
Uterine cervix	6	Uterine corpus	6
Uterine corpus	5	Ovary	4
Thyroid	4	Non-Hodgkin's lymphoma	4
Ovary	4	Melanoma	3
Non-Hodgkin's lymphoma	4	Thyroid	3
Stomach	2	Pancreas	2
Pancreas	2	Urinary bladder	2

Table 28-3 LEADING SITES OF CANCER DEATHS FOR LATINOS COMPARED TO WHITE FEMALES[10,11]

Latinos		White Females	
Site	**Percent**	**Site**	**Percent**
Breast	16	Lung and bronchus	25
Lung and bronchus	13	Breast	15
Colon and rectum	11	Colon and rectum	11
Pancreas	6	Pancreas	6
Liver and intrahepatic bile duct	5	Ovary	5
Stomach	5	Non-Hodgkin's lymphoma	4
Non-Hodgkin's lymphoma	5	Uterine corpus	3
Ovary	5	Brian	2
Uterine corpus	5	Multiple myeloma	2
Brain and other	3		
Nervous system	3		

which may lead to poorer outcomes. Hedeen and White[12] examined breast cancer size and stage among Latinos stratified by birthplace. The study found that Latinos had a higher percentage of tumors larger than 1 cm (77.7%) than non-Latino Caucasians (70.3%) and a higher percentage of tumors larger than 2 cm (45.9% as opposed to 33.0%). The results of the study also compared Latinos born in Latin America and Latinos born in the US and found that Latinos from Latin America had a higher percentage of tumors larger than 1 cm (82.2% as opposed to 75.2%) and larger than 2 cm (54.1% as opposed to 41.7%).

Another disparity in Latino women is seen in the incidence and mortality rates of cervical cancer. According to the SEER[9] and Centers for Disease Control (CDC)[13] databases, Latinos living in the US have twice the incidence of cervical cancer as that of non-Latinos. Latinos from Mexico, Central, and South America have triple the rate of cervical cancer as women in the US.[14] Although cervical cancer rates have declined approximately 4% per year from 1992 to 1999, the mortality rate has climbed 4.4% per year.[15]

Risk Factors and Screening

There is a paucity of literature about risk factors for developing cancers in Latinos. Research has now focused on cultural aspects of sexuality, cultural beliefs regarding smoking, alcohol consumption, or nutrition. Current literature tends to overgeneralize risk factors within a highly diverse population.

To date, research activities and scholarly articles have focused on cancer incidence and barriers to screening activities,[16-18] with a preponderance of the literature concentrating on breast cancer.

Research studies have shown that the fear of finding cancer,[19] lacking health insurance and a primary care physician,[20,21] unemployment,[22] knowledge deficits, cultural beliefs,[23,24] degree of acculturation,[5] cost of care, and frustration with complexity of the health care system[25] can lead to underutilization of services, or they can act as barriers to screening.

Outreach Programs

Interventions to help decrease cancer care disparities in Latinos ideally begin with prevention and detection outreach programs that are adapted linguistically and culturally for each Latino subgroup,[17] with respect for cultural values and decision making processes by the individual and family. The values of the individual and cultures should supersede the values and norms of health care. An example is time orientation. The American health care model is time-oriented and time-focused. If an appointment is scheduled for 2:00 and the individual arrives at 2:15, there may be disapproval by the health care professional, and the appointment may even have to be rescheduled. In various subgroups, a 2:00 appointment may represent an approximate timeframe. The health care provider must consider the difficulty the individual may have getting to the appointment. Miscommunication may lead to mistrust and can have an impact on future relationships.

Other avenues to explore are community-based strategies for promoting health. Community-based strategies can assist in building trust between the health care and scientific community and the Latino population. They will also serve to increase the community's knowledge about services offered. Community-based strategies should be culturally appropriate, integrate basic values into the program, and include options for language[26] and literacy skills.[22] The goal is to develop partnerships and systems to assist in future health care needs. According to Cohen,[27] outreach programs for Latinos should be taken out of the hospital setting and placed in the community. Ideally, constituents in the community will identify leaders, whether formal or informal. These leaders should be invited to participate and take the initiative to reach out to members of the community and inform them about the details and value of the program.

Guidelines for and research on community-based strategies for Latinos[27-30] are limited; however, they are beginning to emerge. The Oncology Nursing Society Multicultural Outcomes: Guidelines for Cultural Competence[3] and the Oncology Nursing Society Multicultural Tool Kit can be used when developing outreach programs. Subgroup-specific information on responses to care and general health beliefs can also be found in Culture and Nursing Care: a Pocket Guide.[31-33]

Por La Vida (For Life) is an intervention model that trained community health advisors to conduct educational sessions for their social network.[29] The project was funded by the National Cancer Institute and was well received by the community. The next phase is to evaluate if the program has enhanced nutrition and cancer prevention. Another study found that a group approach to outreach initiatives was more effective then a one-on-one approach.[30]

Cultural Response to Cancer Care

Receiving the diagnosis of cancer and undergoing cancer therapy is universally accepted as a stressor. Coping with cancer is a complex, constantly changing process influenced by the situation, individual differences, and previous experience.[34] There is an abundance of research articles that focus on quality of life issues after the diagnosis of cancer. Few studies have examined the psychosocial impact or the quality of life outcomes among women from diverse backgrounds.[35]

Juarez, Ferrell, and Borneman[36] found that clinicians should devote greater attention to cultural assessment and include cultural beliefs in cancer care to improve quality of life for Latino patients. Furthermore, family and religious beliefs should be included when developing the patient's plan of care. More recently Dirksen and Reed-Erickson[37] compared well-being between Hispanic and non-Hispanic white survivors of breast cancer. Several scales were used to evaluate health care orientation, uncertainty, social support, resourcefulness, self-esteem, and well-being. The study found both groups reported high well-being; however, tools used were not translated into Spanish, and several Latinos were not able to participate because of negative feelings from their spouse regarding the study. Another potential bias in the results of similar studies comes from the fact that the research tools used may not have been able to capture the ethnocultural differences in cancer survivorship.[35]

In providing culturally competent care, the health care professional must view care from the client's perspective. An ethnocentric approach to care may lead to miscommunication and may have a negative impact on outcomes. The US health care system is based on northern European values and is an individualistic in nature.[38] Individualistic cultures value individualism, privacy, and personal care over environment. They are time-oriented, and time-focused, and value women's rights. The self is defined as independent and autonomous, and relationships are secondary.[39] Latinos, in general, value collectivism,[40] where the self is defined as an aspect of a whole. Personal goals are secondary to the needs of the family and group welfare.[40] With Latinos, health care decisions may be addressed, discussed, and decided by the whole family. Potentially, such areas as screening, treatment, and involvement in clinical trials may be hampered if key family members are not involved in the discussions and decision making process. This may be difficult to achieve or may cause ethical dilemmas in a health care environment, which first and foremost has a duty to ensure patient privacy.

Another area, which requires further study and evaluation, is the use of complementary and alternative therapy among Latinos. Integrative therapy focuses on the whole person. It enables self-care, it is an attempt at symptom control, and it can be used to enhance well-being by decreasing anxiety and increasing relaxation.[41]

In a study that evaluated complementary therapies in ethnic groups, the most commonly reported alternative therapies were dietary therapies (27%), spiritual healing (24%), herbal remedies (13%), physical methods (14%), and psychologic methods (9%).[42]

Religion, spirituality, and the use of folk healers are strong elements in Latino subcultures.[43,44] When Latinos immigrate to the US, they retain these predominant beliefs. With education and acculturation in the US, previous practices may be used less; however, this change may not be evident until the second-generation.[44]

Religion, through prayers and rituals, helps Latinos cope. Religious objects such as rosary beads, cross, and statues, can be blessed and used during rituals. Santeria is a combination of Christianity and African Voodoo and is practiced predominantly by Caribbean Latinos, Cubans, Dominicans, and Puerto Ricans. Santeria serves as both a religion and a health care system. In Santeria, health is seen as balance and illness as imbalance. Santeria integrates mind, body, and spirit while attempting to explain and control health.[45] Santeria priests may use spells and magic to ward off disease, help regain health, and keep evil spirits at bay. Unfortunately, the media may create a perception that Santeria is evil. White Santeria practices good magic and works with benevolent spirits.

Espiritismo is seen in Caribbean Latinos and is a blend of Indian, African, and Catholic beliefs. Like Santeria, Espiritismo uses spirits to affect health. Espiritismo differs in that it is viewed more as a practice than a religion. Some beliefs of Espiritismo include *mal del ojo* (evil eye), where bad sentiments or jealousy can bring on ill health. *Impachos* are intestinal blockages that are believed to occur if an individual drinks a beverage that had a spell on it. Another idea is that evil spirits cause mental illness. Individuals who hold this tenet do not believe these symptoms can be resolved with traditional medicine. Espiritistos are individuals who have the power to contact the spirit world, heal, analyze dreams, and foretell the future.

Other shamanic healers in the Latino cultures are *curanders* (i.e., healers believed to have been chosen by God) who have special healing powers, *sobadores*, masseuses, and *yerbalistas*, or herbalists.[44] Marlene Dobkin deRios,[46] a medical anthropologist who has spent almost two decades conducting research in Latin America, suggests that when caring for Latino immigrants, who have strong shamanic roots, psychologic interventions will most likely have benefit if the interventions are culturally sensitive.

Studies have shown that Latinos do use herbal therapies for health maintenance. Further research must be conducted on what kinds of herbs are used, where these herbs are obtained, and what their impact on cancer care is. In the late 1980's two Los Angeles county hospitals reported an increase of *Salmonella arizona* infections in Latino patients.[47] On further investigation the majority of the infections were found to be caused by the ingestion of rattlesnake capsules in patients with underlying autoimmune disease, cancer, diabetes, and arthritis. The capsules were obtained from Mexico and were found in the pharmacies of Latino neighborhoods.

The above is an example on how the use of herbal remedies must not be treated lightly. Dialogue on the use of folk remedies must be conducted as part of the patient's assessment and care. In predominantly Latino neighborhoods, outreach initiatives to pharmacies, *botanicas* (herbal shops), and folk healers can assist the

Box 28-2 Latino Cancer Report Research Initiatives

ACCESS TO CANCER SCREENING AND CARE:

- Study quality of cancer services provided to Hispanics/Latinos as compared to those received by other ethnic/racial groups by various health care settings and providers.
- Study the mediators or moderators that might help explain the differences in quality of care.
- Study the factors that contribute to adherence by Hispanics/Latinos to mammogram screening guidelines.
- Study prostate cancer screening, treatment, and outcomes for Hispanics/Latinos. Focus on how Hispanic/Latino men make decisions on screening and treatment options and what kind of outcomes they experience as a result.

TOBACCO USE AND CANCER:

- Study adolescent smoking onset and continuation.
- Study the adoption, continuation, and cessation of smoking in Hispanic/Latino men and women.
- Study parent-child communication strategies and the use of peers for smoking prevention in children and adolescents.
- Evaluate attitudes and behaviors of the Hispanic/Latino population regarding involuntary smoking.
- Evaluate advocacy skills and empowerment strategies for tobacco control in the Hispanic/Latino population.
- Study the use of pharmacotherapy in the Hispanic/Latino population.

STATUS OF COMMUNICATION OF CANCER RISK:

- Study how to communicate cancer risk to Hispanic/Latino patients.
- Provide training of risk communication and decision making among culturally distinct Hispanic/Latino groups.

ENVIRONMENT:

- Assess exposure to environmental pollutants/toxicants in Hispanic/Latino communities.
- Identify high-risk occupations and environments for Hispanics/Latinos by using geographic information systems (GIS) techniques.
- Study cancer risks of migrant farm workers and their families.

PATIENT-CLINICIAN:

- Study strategies to improve communications, decision making, and behavioral skills among Hispanic/Latino patients.
- Study cultural and gender factors that affect patient/health care provider communication in the Hispanic/Latino community.
- Study the effects of limited English proficiency among some Hispanics/Latinos on the quality of health care in various settings, such as health maintenance organizations (HMOs) and Medicaid programs.

INFECTIOUS AGENTS:

- Conduct cancer-related studies looking at human papillomavirus (HPV), hepatitis B virus (HBV), hepatitis B virus (HCV), and *Helicobacter pylori* among Hispanic/Latino population subgroups.
- Study the role of HPV in cervical cancer in Hispanics/Latinos. Correlate the sexual norms and beliefs to the incidence of HPV. Consider the validity of current Pap smear guidelines for Latinos in light of the epidemiology. Include Latinos in clinical trials and at-risk protocols for the new HPV vaccine.
- Study the role of HBV and HCV and other known risk factors in liver cancer among Hispanics/Latinos.
- Study the role of *H. pylori* in Hispanic/Latino stomach cancer risk. Investigate treatment of *H. pylori* infection among Hispanics/Latinos.

Box 28-2 LATINO CANCER REPORT RESEARCH INITIATIVES[48]—CONT'D

CANCER SURVIVORSHIP AND HEALTH-RELATED QUALITY OF LIFE:

- Conduct follow-up studies to determine the biologic and psychosocial factors that influence cancer survival rates among Hispanics/Latinos.
- Conduct qualitative and quantitative research using culturally appropriate instruments to assess qualify of life among Hispanics/Latinos with cancer.
- Assess the adaptability or suitability of existing quality-of-life measures for Hispanics/Latinos with cancer.
- Study the effectiveness of breast cancer treatments, factors that affect adherence to them, and the effects of the treatments on quality of life in Latinos.

EDUCATION AND TRAINING RECOMMENDATIONS:

- Increase the number of Hispanic/Latino health care professionals and Spanish-speaking health care providers, improve the Spanish language skills of providers who work with the Hispanic/Latino population, and make Spanish interpreter programs more effective; offer cultural competency and communications training to health care providers and researchers.
- Develop specially targeted cancer prevention and control programs and ensure that health professionals are fluent in them; encourage greater participation by Latino clinicians in clinical research activities.

OUTREACH COMMENTS:

- Pursue culturally targeted personal, print, electronic, and other forms of outreach to and education for the Hispanic/Latino public about cancer risk conceptions, misconceptions, prevention, screening, treatment, and research.

From *Redes En Acción Latino Cancer Report,* An NCI-funded project—Grant #5 UOI CA86117-05—Developed by Redes En Acción, San Antonio, Texas. Permission to use granted by Amelie G. Ramirez, DrPH, Principal Investigator.

health care provider in becoming informed about the variety of herbal medicines that are being used by the community.

Many of the traditional folk medicine practices of Latino subgroups are very similar to those practiced in Western Medicine. These include aromatherapy, therapeutic touch, herbal therapy, and meditative prayer. The key is knowing how to incorporate these beliefs to promote health, healing, and increase use of proven medical technology. The objective should be to enhance trust so that Latinos will be comfortable in sharing their beliefs and traditions.

THE LATINO CANCER REPORT

The Latino Cancer Report was published on March 1, 2004[48] at www.saludenaccion.org by the National Hispanic/Latino Cancer Network, as part of a mandate from the National Cancer Institute to develop a national agenda for cancer research, training, education, and outreach for the Latino community and to provide research, guidelines for policy makers. The process began in 2000. Data were collected from 624 key opinion leaders of the Latino community by means of surveys. Topics included access to care, tobacco use, status of communication of cancer risk, occupational and environment risk, infectious agents, cancer survivorship, and quality of life. Major cancer sites of concern were identified, and the information was assessed and presented to the National Steering Committee. The Latino cancer report provides information and recommendations that will be useful for individuals and organizations providing cancer care for this generation of Latinos and for the generations to follow.

The Latino Cancer Report identified cancer of the breast, cervix, lung, colon and rectum, prostate, liver, and stomach as key areas of concern (Box 28-2).

The Unequal Burden of Cancer

Another resource that has not been used to its fullest potential is the "The Unequal Burden of Cancer: an Assessment of NIH Research and Programs for Ethnic Minorities and the Medically Underserved."[49] This is an extensive study that was conducted to address the concern for ethnic minorities and the medically underserved. The project began early in 1998 and was completed later that year. This report discusses the cancer burden, research, accrual, treatment, and survivorship issues, along with priority setting initiatives, for ethnic minorities and the medically underserved.

Recommendations included expanding the SEER program coverage to incorporate a wider range of demographic and social characteristics, and emphasizing ethnicity rather than race. Both of these recommendations would assist in identifying and capturing necessary data for a diverse population. Outreach and research initiatives can be enhanced by this information, and outcomes may be improved. Increasing participation of ethnic minorities in clinical trials and identifying research needs within the context of cancer for this population were also among the suggestions made.

SUMMARY

As the Latino community continues to grow and age, issues with cancer and cancer care will continue to develop, and cancer incidence and mortality rates will soar. Issues that increase vulnerability such as educational status, insurance coverage, socioeconomic status, and acculturation must be on the forefront of policy makers' agendas. Policy change should begin with a comprehensive method to identify Latinos. Being able to identify this population on the national, regional, and local levels will allow for more accurate data collection, which in turn will provide information that will assist in targeting the urgent need areas. Research is required throughout the continuum of care from prevention, screening, and treatment to end-of-life care. The Latino Cancer and the Unequal Burden of Cancer reports provide direction for research on all levels.

REFERENCES

1. Guzman B: The Hispanic Population Census 2000 Brief, Washington, D.C., 2000, U.S. Census Bureau.
2. DePaula T, Lagana K, Gonzalez-Ramirez L: In Lipson JG, Dibble SL, Minarik PA, editors: *Culture and nursing care: a pocket guide,* ed 2, San Francisco, 1997, UCSF Nursing Press.
3. Oncology Nursing Society Multicultural Outcomes: *Guidelines for Cultural Competence,* Pittsburgh, Pa, 2000, Oncology Nursing Press.
4. Aday LA: Who are the vulnerable?. In Aday LA, editor: *At risk in America: the health and health care needs of vulnerable populations in the United States,* ed 2, San Francisco, 2001, Jossey-Bass.
5. O'Malley AS, Johnson AE, Mandelblatt J: Acculturation and breast cancer screening among Hispanic women in New York City, *Am J Public Health* 89(2):219-227, 1999.
6. Cohen MZ: Culturally competent care, *Semin Oncol Nurs* 17(4):153-156, 2001.
7. Huerta EE: Cancer Statistics for Hispanics, 2003: Good news, bad news, and the need for a health system paradigm change, *CA Cancer J Clin* 53:205-207, 2003.
8. Houts PS, Lenhard RE Jr, Varricchio C: The front page. Hispanic and Black Americans disproportionately uninsured. Cancer practice, *Multidisc J Cancer Care* 8(6):261-262, 2000.
9. National Cancer Institute: *An overview of the SEER Cancer Statistics Review,* 2002; available online at: http://cis.nci.gov/fact/1 10.htm.
10. American Cancer Society: Cancer Facts and Figures for Hispanics 2003-2005, Atlanta Ga., 2003-2005, The Society.
11. American Cancer Society: Cancer Facts and Figures, Atlanta Ga., 2003, The Society.
12. Hedeen A, White E: Breast cancer size and stage in Hispanic American women, by birthplace: 1992-1995, *Am J Public Health* 91(1):122-126, 2001.
13. Centers for Disease Control and Prevention: Invasive cervical cancer among Hispanic and non-Hispanic women: United States 1992-1999, *Morbidity Mortal Weekly Rep* 51:1067-1069, 2002.
14. Ferlay J and others: GLOBOCAN 2000: Cancer incidence, mortality and prevalence worldwide, Version 1.0, IARC Cancer Base No. 5, Lyon, 2000, IARC Press.
15. O'Brien K and others: Cancer statistics for Hispanics, 2003, *CA Cancer J Clin* 53:208-226, 2003.
16. Hunt LM and others: Abnormal Pap screening among Mexican-American women: impediments to receiving and reporting follow-up care, *Oncol Nurs Forum* 25(10): 1743-1749, 1998. Retrieved 10/28/04 from www.ons.org/xp6/ ONS/Library.
17. Ramirez Smiley M and others: Comparison of Florida Hispanic and Non-Hispanic Caucasian women in their health belief related to breast cancer and health locus of control, *Oncol Nurs Forum* 27(6):975-984, 2000. Retrieved 10/28/04 from www.ons.org/xp6/ONS/Library.

18. Otero-Sabogal R and others: Access and attitudinal factors related to breast and cervical cancer screening: Why are Latinos still under screened? *Health Ed Behav* 30(3):337-59, 2003.
19. Bastani R, Gallardo NY, Maxwell AE: Barriers to colorectal screening among ethnically diverse high and average risk individuals, *J Psychosoc Oncol* 19(3/4):65-84, 2001.
20. Selvin E, Brett KM: Breast and cervical cancer screening: sociodemographic predictors among white, black, and Hispanic women, *Am J Public Health* 93(4):618-623, 2003.
21. Laws MB, Mayo SJ: The Latino Breast Cancer Control Study, year one: factors predicting screening, mammography utilization by urban Latino women in Massachusetts, *J Community Health* 23(4J):251-267, 1998.
22. Catalano RA, Satariano WA: Unemployment and the likelihood of detecting early stage breast cancer, *Am J Public Health* 88(4):586-589, 1998.
23. Scarinci IC and others: An examination of sociocultural factors associated with cervical cancer screening low-income Latino immigrants of reproductive age, *J Immigrant Health* 5(3):199-128, 2003.
24. Reed SD and others: Knowledge and attitudes regarding routine health screening and prevention in Somal Vietnamese, and Latino women, *Clin J Womens Health* 2(3):105-111, 2002.
25. Blewett LA and others: Healthcare needs of the growing Latino population in rural America: focus group findings in one midwestern state, *J Rural Health* 19(1):33-41, 2003.
26. Ward B, Bertera EM, Hoge P: Developing and evaluating a Spanish TEL-MED message on breast cancer, *J Community Health* 22(2):127-135, 1997.
27. Cohen R: Cancer prevention and screening amoung Hispanic populations. In Frank-Stromborg M, Olsen SJ, editors: *Cancer prevention in diverse populations,* ed 2, Pittsburgh, 2001, Oncology Nursing Society.
28. Brice A: Access to health service delivery for Hispanics: a communication issue, *J Multicult Nurs Health* 6(2):7-17, 2001.
29. Navarro AM and others: Community-based education in nutrition and cancer: the Por La Vida Cuidandome curriculum, *J Cancer Ed* 15(3):168-172, 2000.
30. Dengelis NL and others: Two community outreach strategies to increase breast cancer screenings in low-income women, *J Cancer Ed* 16(1):55-58, 2001.
31. DePaula T, Lagana K, Gonzalez-Ramirez L: Mexican Americans. In Lipson JG, Dibble SL, Minarik PA, editors: *Culture and nursing care: a pocket guide,* ed 2, San Francisco, 1997, UCSF Nursing Press.
32. Juarbe T: Puerto Ricans. In Lipson JG, Dibble SL, Minarik PA, editors: *Culture and nursing care: a pocket guide,* ed 2, San Francisco, 1997, UCSF Nursing Press.
33. Varela L: Cubans. In Lipson JG, Dibble SL, Minarik PA, editors: *Culture and nursing care: a pocket guide,* ed 2, San Francisco, 1997, UCSF Nursing Press.
34. Nail LM: I'm coping as fast as I can: psychosocial adjustment to cancer and cancer treatment, *Oncol Nurs Forum* 28(6): 967-974, 2001; available online at www.ons.org/xp6/ONS/Library. Accessed April 16, 2002.
35. Aziz NM, Rowland JH: Cancer survivorship research among ethnic minority and medically underserved groups. Oncology Nursing Forum. 29(5), 2002. Retrieved 4/28/04 from http://journals.ons.org/xp6/ONS/Library.
36. Juarez G, Ferrell B, Borneman T: Perceptions of quality of life in Hispanic patients with cancer, *Cancer Pract Multidisc J Cancer Care* 6(6):318-324, 1998.
37. Dirksen SR, Reed-Erickson J: Well-being in Hispanic and Non-Hispanic white survivors of breast cancer, *Oncol Nurs Forum* 29(5):820-826, 2002.
38. Jetten J, Postmes T, Mcauliff B.J,: We're all individuals: group norms of individualism and collectivism, levels of identification and identity threat, *Eur J Soc Psychol* 32:189-207, 2002.
39. Triandis HC: The psychological measurement of cultural syndromes, *Psychologist,* 51(4):407-416, 1996.
40. Shkodriani GM, Gibbons JL: Individualism and collectivism among university students in Mexico and the United States, *J Soc Psychol* 135(6):765-772. 1995.
41. Tagliaferr M, Cohen I, Tripathy D: Complementary and alternative medicine in early stage breast cancer, *Semin Oncol* 28:121-134, 2001.
42. Lengacher CA and others: Design and testing of the use of complementary and alternative therapies survey in women with breast cancer, *Oncol Nurs Forum,* 30(5):811-822, 2003. Retrieved 4/27/04 from http://journals,ons.org/xp6/ONS/Library.
43. Taylor EJ: Spirituality, culture and cancer care, *Semin Oncol Nurs* 17(3):137-205, 2001.
44. Owens B, Dirksen SA: Review and critique of the literature of complementary and alternative use among Hispanic/Latino women with breast cancer, *Clin J Oncol Nurs* 8(2):151-156, 2004.
45. Pasquali EA: Santeria, *J Holistic Nurs* 12(4):380-390, 1994.
46. deRios, MD: What we can learn from shamanic healing: brief psychotherapy with Latino immigrant clients, *Am J Public Health* 92(10):1576-1578, 2002.
47. Waterman SH and others: Salmonella arizona infections in Latinos associated with rattlesnake folk medicine, *Am J Public Health* 80(3):286-289, 1990.
48. National Hispanic/Latino Cancer Network, Mandate From the National Cancer Institute: The Latino Cancer report; available online at www.saludenaccion.org/publications/latinocancerreportRptsummary.pdf.
49 Haynes MA, Smedley BD, editors: *The unequal burden of cancer: an assessment of NIH research and programs for ethnic minorities and the medically underserved,* Washington, D.C., 1998, Institute of Medicine National Academy Press.

CHAPTER

29 Rural Women and Cancer

Angeline Bushy

INTRODUCTION

During the past 2 decades a great deal of attention has been devoted to the plight of residents in rural communities and their health care systems.[1] However, not much has been written about the health concerns of certain rural subgroups living across the 50 states, in particular women with the diagnosis of cancer. This chapter includes an overview of rural demographic, social, economic, and cultural characteristics; highlights features of rural health care delivery systems; and presents general information about America's rural women. This is followed by a discussion about the experiences of women having a diagnosis of cancer who live in a rural setting.

The health status of a woman, regardless of the setting, affects everyone in her environment, particularly family members, and in rural settings oftentimes the community as a whole. Cancer in women is an infinitely broad topic to which justice cannot be done in one text chapter about residents in diverse rural settings. This purpose of this chapter is to expose health care professionals to factors in the rural context that can affect the manner in which services are rendered to consumers in those settings. Urban-based health care professionals often question the need to learn about rural perspectives, as evidenced by this comment: "I do not live or practice in a rural area; why is that information relevant to me?" One reason for needing this information is that rural residents often seek care and are referred to providers located in urban areas. Oncology care providers, in particular, must be aware of rural perspectives in order to plan, deliver, and evaluate interventions for clients who live and work in a more austere and remote community.

BACKGROUND

What Does "Rural" Mean?

Rural residents are not an insignificant group. Demographically, there are about 65 million Americans living in more than 75% of the US landmass; of these, about 52% are women. Rural and urban alike, population shifts throughout the last decade have led to significant changes in the racial and ethnic makeup of communities across the US. Increasing diversity is partly associated with changing immigration patterns relative to employment opportunities in rural areas, and partly to urban residents relocating to areas with natural amenities for recreation and retirement.

It is important to stress that rural communities are highly diverse; however, there are some regional population patterns. For instance, according to recent census reports, non-Hispanic African Americans account for more than 18% of the population in the Southeast. In some western states, American Indians and Alaska Natives constitute nearly 9% of the population. Increasingly, Asians, many of whom are refugees from Southeast Asia, are resettling in Midwestern states and along the Pacific coast to work in agriculture production. Similarly to urban areas across the nation, persons of Hispanic origin account for more than 11% of the population in many rural counties.[1-4]

Rural is not easy to define because it means different things to different people. Before proceeding to discuss characteristics of the rural lifestyle, it is important to consider what is meant by the term *rural* as it has been used in reference to individuals living in a variety of living situations and locations. Most people include geographic and population dimensions along with subjective perceptions when comparing rural with urban residency. Common definitions for rural usually include geographic size relative to population density; for example, number of persons living in a square mile. Table 29-1 lists defining terms for rural and urban.

Policy-makers and researchers often make use of the distinction between *metropolitan* and *nonmetropolitan*. A standard metropolitan statistical area (SMSA) is defined as a city or adjacent area having a total of 50,000 or more residents. Based on the 2000 census of the total US population, about 80% lived in a metropolitan area, and 20% resided in non-SMSAs. For others, rural refers to a community having fewer than 20,000 residents; still others use fewer than 10,000 residents; and a few use 2,500 or fewer residents as their delineator for *rural-urban*. Occasionally, one notes "farm residency" as the definition for *rural*. As a point of reference, of the total US population, about 5% live in towns of 2,500 residents; and less than 2% live on a farm. Another set of definitions distinguishes *urban*, having more 99 or more persons per square mile, from *rural*, having fewer than 99 persons per square mile.

Frontier and suburban are subclassifications of the general concept of rural. The term "frontier" is used in reference to regions having fewer than six people per square mile. Conversely, a few researchers use suburban residents for rural-focused studies.[5-7] Even though these areas may have a low(er) population density, suburban areas are adjacent to, and part of, a metropolis and generally do not reflect rural perspectives. Still another definition considers distance to services and/or "time to access services" (e.g., more than 30 minutes or more than 20 miles). The notion of time to access health care also may be applicable to residents who live in an inner city or suburban area, who must contend with transportation challenges in their day-to-day activities including accessing health care.[8-10]

Arriving at a common definition becomes more problematic because of stereotypical perceptions of rural residency. Some perceive rural life as idyllic, peaceful, and health-promoting; however, health care professionals must be aware of other, less favorable, living situations; for example, Indian reservations, most of which are located in rural areas and where the level of poverty is comparable to that of third-world countries.[11,12] Or, consider migrant camps, some

Table **29-1** Terms/Definitions of Rural and Urban

Term	Definition
Metropolitan (Standard Metropolitan Statistical Area [SMSA]) (Bureau of Census)	Population centers having 50,000 or more residents
Nonmetropolitan (non-Standard Metropolitan Statistical Area [non-SMSA]) (Bureau of Census)	Population centers having fewer than 50,000 residents; or, all areas that do not meet SMSA criteria
Urban (Office of Rural Health Policy)	Area having 99 or more persons per square mile
Rural (Office of Rural Health Policy)	Area having fewer than 99 persons per square mile
Frontier (Office of Rural Health Policy)	Area having 6 persons or fewer per square mile
Farm residence (Bureau of Census)	Residence outside of city limits; residents generally involved in a agriculture
Suburban (Bureau of Census)	Population centers adjacent to a metropolis

of which are situated in the midst of large fields and consist of one-room shanties, sheltering two or more large and intergenerational Mexican-American families.[13,14] Box 29-1 lists general characteristics of life in a rural community. When diagnosed with a chronic illness such as cancer, those living in impoverished rural communities experience even greater challenges than other rural women in accessing primary care, much less recommended screening programs and state-of-the-art treatments.[15,16]

Box 29-1 General Characteristics of Life in Rural Community*

- Greater distances between residents and services
- Informal social and professional interactions
- Overlapping relationships
- More immediate access to extended family networks
- Slower-paced lifestyle
- Preference for interacting with insiders (local residents)
- Social structures can pose threats to maintaining anonymity and confidentiality
- Mistrust of outsiders (newcomers) to the community
- Sense of geographic and/or social isolation (for some residents)
- Greater number of small enterprises (oftentimes family-owned); few large industries
- Economic industries extractive in nature, often oriented to land and nature and high-risk occupations (e.g., agriculture, mining, lumbering, fishing)
- Greater proportion of elderly and young residents, and intergenerational households
- Higher proportion of working poor and uninsured residents
- Residents more likely to report having a usual provider of health care; usually are sicker when seeking professional care
- Creatively rely on informal support systems (when formal services are not available)

**It is important to stress that there is wide diversity between and among rural settings; some of these items may not be characteristic of every community.*

As for the typical rural town: these are hard to describe because of their wide population and geographic diversity.[1,8] A rural town in South Dakota, for instance, is very different from one located in Louisiana, Maine, or Indiana. In fact, there can be significant variations among communities in the same state. In respect to rural policy, legislators' understanding of rural usually is based on the district they represent, which in turn is reflected in their pattern of decision making. As for available health care resources, that too is a relative concept. For instance, a community with 20,000 residents often has services that one expects to find in a large city; and residents in a community of 2,500 people often perceive one with a population of 10,000 as a "city," since certain types of medical specialists can be accessed there. By contrast, families living in a region viewed by the public as a remote frontier may not feel isolated. For them, urban-based health care services are relatively easy to access because of telecommunication possibilities and dependable transportation, along with having adequate health insurance.

Imprecise definitions of *rural* raise serious concern among policy-makers, researchers, and health care providers alike. Lack of a common language hampers a coordinated approach to understanding demographic, epidemiologic, cultural, and health-related problems of rural communities. A standardized definition of rural is critically needed for a more coordinated approach to describe clinical problems, monitor intervention outcomes, and evaluate health care delivery in those settings, particularly to women having a diagnosis of cancer.[9,17-19]

Characteristics of the Rural Lifestyle

In spite of wide diversity, there are certain features that are common to many rural communities. For example, compared to urban-metro areas, rural regions have a low(er) population density in relation to geographic area. Likewise, in small towns one notes a certain familiarity among residents. While listening to their conversations, one frequently overhears resident allude to extended travel time and distance to access certain services, in particular health care. Another theme that permeates many conversations is many rural residents' perceived high quality of life in nonmaterial terms and a preference for a slower-paced lifestyle.[8,20,21]

Oftentimes, rural residents have an extended community history, tracing family origins to ancestors who homesteaded in the area. There is a sense of community "rootedness and connectedness" among small-town residents that may not be as evident among urban populations. Having a shared intergenerational history implies small-town residents are well acquainted, if not related. They interact with neighbors and relatives, oftentimes on a daily basis, in a variety of settings in their community such as at church and school functions, when shopping at the grocery store, buying gas at the service station, going to the barber or beauty shop, as well as at the local hospital and doctors' offices. More than likely, a rural woman with a diagnosis of cancer knows most, if not all, of the employees who work in local government offices, social service agencies, and health care facilities.[8,20-25]

Overlapping relationships and familiarity can be a benefit and can also pose challenges to residents of small towns. On the one hand, face-to-face interactions can enhance both natural and official support networks, and the local grapevine is an information source, albeit not always accurate in nature. On the other hand, overfamiliarity can pose threats to anonymity and confidentiality for the individual or family experiencing a sensitive issue such as severe financial problems, an unplanned pregnancy, domestic abuse, behavioral health problems, or a diagnosis of cancer. Cultural, religious, social, economic, and geographic factors directly and indirectly affect the lifestyle choices and health status of a particular community. Rural people, for instance, are reported to be more conservative in their political preferences, religious beliefs, and gender role expectations. Many prefer to interact with people similar to themselves and are somewhat reluctant to establish close ties with outsiders, including urban-based health care professionals who provide outreach services in their community. Very little is available in the professional literature relative to rural health belief systems and the impact of these on women with cancer.[26,27]

Rural Economic and Social Structures

Economic structures are also diverse, but those in rural areas have some common features that can affect residents' lifestyle, health status, and care-seeking behaviors. In many instances, small towns are primarily dependent on one industry, perhaps two, which for the most part drive the local economy. When that enterprise is not faring well the entire town is affected, even residents who are indirectly associated with that economic infrastructure; for example, grocery stores, restaurants, and health care providers. Industries in rural settings tend to be predominately extractive in nature, including logging, agricultural, mining, and fishing. Jobs in these industries mostly are male-dominated: they are associated with demanding physical labor, seasonal in nature, and among the most hazardous occupations.[28]

In rural America, one also finds numerous small enterprises such as family farms, implement and automobile dealerships, grocery stores, service stations, banks, restaurants, and on occasion a drug store. Small enterprises usually provide full-time work for the owner's family; and, in some cases part-time or seasonal work for a few. Small businesses often do not provide benefits to employees, in particular health insurance. Two other typical major employers are the school system and, if one exists, the local hospital with its associated health care entities. Since most residents in a small town are acquainted, they usually know who works where, and when they are on the job. In turn, familiarity and overlapping relationships can have an impact on rural consumers health care-seeking behaviors.[9,26-29]

On the one hand, small entrepreneurial ventures can promote cohesiveness, autonomy, and flexibility for employees. Conversely, a family enterprise can place additional stress on those whose income is directly dependent on the success of the business. Sometimes certain individuals are expected to assume additional demands for the success of the business or subjugate his or her goals for the sake of family. In other cases, some members must seek outside employment to augment or sustain the business. As for rural women and their families, economic structures directly influence their employment options and care-seeking behaviors; for example, whether or not an individual participates in recommended cancer screenings and other kinds of health-promoting activities.[30,31]

It is important to stress that there is great diversity among rural women in regard to cultural, social, and economic status; thus one must look critically at national demographic information. Nevertheless, large national data sets can provide some useful information in making general comparisons between and among rural and urban women. Compared to their metropolitan counterparts, for instance, contemporary rural women have less access to advanced education, have fewer job opportunities, and receive lower salaries for similar employment. Regardless of setting, child care is a major problem for most women, especially those who are single parents or where both parents are working. In rural communities, child care providers are few and far between. For rural women, child care can pose an even greater challenge than accessing a health care provider. In association with fewer employment opportunities, there is a very low turnover in existing jobs, especially in the school system and within local health care facilities. Consequently, college-educated women may not be able to find work commensurate with their skills in rural towns. A few elect to commute to an urban area to work, and others accept the only available job in town even if it means being underemployed and not having health insurance benefits.[16,30-32]

Rural communities have higher rates of poverty than urban areas, which has a disproportionate impact on women and children. Child poverty rates exceed 35% in pockets throughout rural America. More than 50% of rural children in female-headed households live in poverty. The rate of rural women living in poverty is higher than for rural men. Across rural America, one finds a higher proportion of families who are among the working poor; that is, employed people who do not have health insurance benefits and cannot afford to purchase it. About 40% of all rural families fall into this category even though the adults may be working in two or more jobs. For families who are fortunate enough to have it, their insurance coverage often is inadequate and/or carries prohibitive deductibles and copayments. Along with having above-poverty status, the working poor do not qualify for public assistance such as Medicaid benefits.[9,17,18,32]

Economic and social infrastructures indirectly influence the health of women—sometimes for the

Box 29-2 Barriers to Health Care in Rural Areas*

- Fewer health care providers located at a greater distance from each other
- Unavailable outreach services
- Transportation challenges (no public transportation; not having access to personal transportation; not being able to drive)
- Lack of telephone services and/or access to the Internet
- Unpredictable weather and/or travel conditions
- Inability to pay for care and/or not having health insurance
- Lack of "know-how" or not having the ability to enroll in entitlement programs
- Lack of knowledge regarding health-promoting or illness-preventive interventions
- Inequitable reimbursement policies for rural providers
- Inadequate understanding on the part of providers about rural populations and their lifestyle
- Language barriers (caregivers not culturally and linguistically competent)
- Care and services not culturally appropriate
- Health/illness–related information not available locally (i.e., primary, secondary, and tertiary prevention; state-of-the-art interventions for specific diseases)
- Sparse resources (materials, professionals, equipment, information, fiscal)

**It is important to stress that there is wide diversity between and among rural settings; some or none of these barriers may exist in every community.*

better, sometimes for the worse—and in particular, of those with a diagnosis of cancer. The relationship between having adequate income, good nutrition, and strong social networks and health status makes it mandatory to have effective coordination among health care providers and social service agencies in medically underserved communities. It also is important to stress that historically rural women are known to be creative and self-reliant and to offer significant (most often uncompensated) contributions to their family and community. They have a critical role in transmitting community values to subsequent generations as well as in caring for those among them who are sick. Out of necessity, rural women relied on self-care and alternative healing practices to promote health, prevent illness, treat the sick, and support community members who are going through "tough times." Unfortunately, the contributions and strengths of rural women are underestimated and often overlooked by sociologists and health care professionals alike, in particular when planning and delivering health care to this population.[20-24] Box 29-2 identifies barriers to health care in rural areas.

RURAL AMERICA AND THE WOMEN WHO LIVE THERE

Demographically, there are similarities and regional variations among rural and urban women in the US. Figure 29-1 shows rural

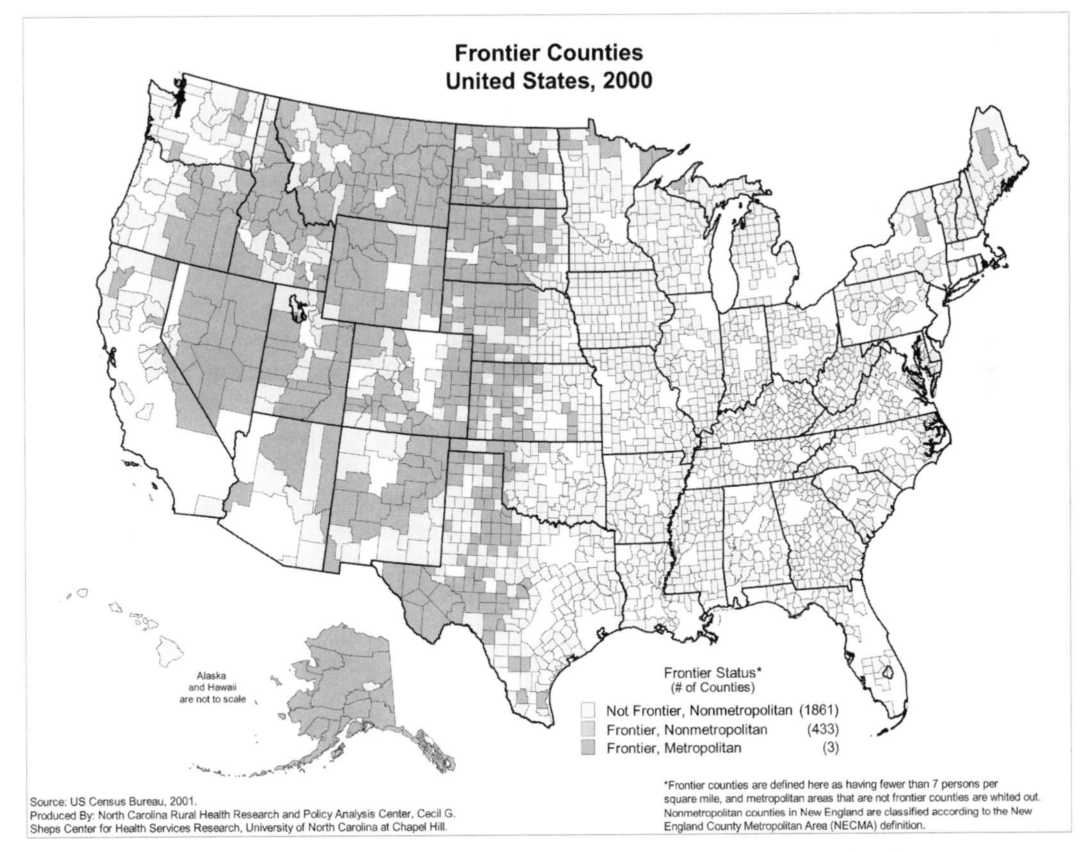

FIGURE 29-1 Frontier Counties, United States, 2000. (From North Carolina Rural Health Research and Policy Analysis Center, Cecil G. Shape Center for Health Services Research, University of North Carolina at Chapel Hill. Data from the US Census Bureau, 2001.)

counties in the US. For both, birth rates have declined while death rates remained the same. Both groups have experienced increases in age at marriage and rates of divorce, whereas fertility rates and household size have declined. Rural women, in particular, have fewer years of formal education, are more likely to be married, marry younger, have more children, live in larger families, and complete their families earlier. Rural households, too, are larger in number compared to urban, oftentimes comprised of several generations. Multigenerational living arrangements frequently emerge out of economic need. While such living arrangements can afford better access to kinship support systems, extended family households have the potential for familial conflicts. Living arrangements are an important consideration when planning care for women with a diagnosis of cancer, particularly those in high-risk groups such as the elderly, farm residents, lesbians, and minorities.[31-33]

The Elderly

More elderly women live in rural communities than in urban areas. Of the rural elderly, about 43% live in the South, 33% live in the Midwest, and the remaining 24% in other areas across the 50 states. Compared to urban elderly, rural elderly experience a high incidence of chronic health problems, but have fewer resources along with restricted access to essential services. The illness experiences and health care needs of the rural elderly often are misunderstood and neglected, perhaps as a corollary to the isolation and poverty found in rural communities. Societal values that emphasize productivity and adherence to a work ethic further diminish feelings of self-worth among the elderly. In respect to care-seeking behaviors, compared to urban elderly those in rural settings are more likely to self-treat with over-the-counter medications because they cannot either get to the doctor or afford medical services, or both. Rural elderly women are more likely to enter extended-care institutions and be admitted at earlier ages with fewer disabilities. Partially this finding is attributable to changes in the economic system, which leads to adults of working age moving away from rural communities to find work elsewhere. Traditionally this generation provided support and care to aging parents; their departure further contributes to the changing demographic profile of small town America. Isolation is exacerbated by the fact that rural towns often do not have essential health care and social services to support the elderly, in particular home health care, hospice services, and assisted living facilities.[9,17,18,34]

Farm Residents

Even though it may seem idyllic, farm residency has inherent risks and stressors for women similar to those described for a family business. Most often farms are a family venture. However, health care providers should understand that there is a growing number of women who are farm owners as the result of the death of a spouse or other family member. These women bear the day-to-day burdens of farming activities along with the financial burdens of the business. As for women living on farms, some may express feelings of emotional and geographic isolation, lacking the time and financial resources to adequately fulfill their multiple roles. They may experience chronic fatigue, feel helpless, and be frustrated because they are not able to take a vacation or pursue a personal career. Financial returns may be poor as an result of the numerous federal and state regulations coupled with the uncertainty of weather and growing conditions, both of which are unremitting concerns. Health care providers should not be surprised to find that farm women may not participate in cancer screening programs and experience disparities associated with diagnoses of cancer compared to rural women in general.[8,27,28,31]

Lesbians

Lesbians living in a rural setting are another subgroup of women about which little has been written, in particular those having a diagnosis of cancer. Anecdotal reports from these women indicate homophobia as one of their major concerns, especially on the part of rural health care professionals. Some speculate that traditional rural attitudes regarding women's roles and the preponderance of male physicians in small towns, coupled with lack of anonymity and threats to confidentiality, all contribute to unacceptable and oftentimes inadequate care for women with alternative sexual preferences. Since the literature is nonexistent, one can only speculate about the experiences of lesbians living in a rural setting who are diagnosed with cancer.[31]

Racial and Ethnic Minorities

Although the US is highly industrialized, some rural regions reflect conditions found only in developing countries. In rural counties with persistent poverty, for instance, some households do not have even the most basic utilities including electricity, indoor plumbing, and telephone services. Regardless of the setting, people of color have shorter life expectancies and poorer overall health. For those living in impoverished and medically underserved regions, access to health care may be limited to crisis events and illness prevention services and cancer screening may be nonexistent.[9,17,18,29,32,34]

In recent years, information about rural African Americans has become more available, and in turn, more is known about their health concerns. For instance, 95% of rural blacks live in the South; of these, 97% are considered poor. African American women are in the lowest-paying and least desirable jobs, and have poor perinatal outcomes and high rates of chronic problems related to obesity, hypertension, and diabetes. They also have a higher cancer mortality rate, particularly from breast cancer. Human immunodeficiency virus (HIV) infection is an emerging problem among heterosexual rural black women, but precise data are unavailable on the prevalence and incidence in this highly vulnerable group.[35-39]

Although they share a common language, Hispanics represent many distinct cultures. The largest segment of Hispanics in rural regions is comprised of Mexican-Americans working in agricultural production. The actual number of Hispanic migrants in the US is not available, since many are undocumented immigrants from Mexico. Families of migrant farm workers often live in substandard housing without access to potable water and toilet facilities. These women are at risk for domestic abuse, machinery-related accidents, exposure to cancer-inducing agricultural chemicals, and infectious diseases. As with African American women, HIV infection is on the increase among heterosexual Hispanic migrant women. Tracking the prevalence and incidence of certain diseases such as HIV or cancer is especially challenging, since migrants continuously travel from state-to-state with crop production. Of all rural women, migrants are least likely to receive prenatal care, illness-prevention interventions, and cancer screening. The disparity between rural and urban Hispanic women is even greater than the gap between blacks and whites.[13,14,40,41] Of note is that low-income Hispanics in urban areas are more likely to live near federally qualified health clinics (FQHC), and these are more likely to have bilingual staff than FQHC located in a rural setting that target rural migrant workers.[42,43] Availability of services, along with language, correlates positively with rates of prenatal care and cancer screening. Consequently, linguistically competent providers have a significant role in the success or failure of cancer prevention and screening initiatives targeting Hispanic migrant workers.

Despite government and tribal interventions, Native Americans have the poorest overall health status of all racial minorities.[9,11,12,17,18,29] This is a young population; 51% of Native Americans are female, with a median age 25.3 years; the median age for men is about 21.1 years. Early mortality and high birth rates influence the demographic profile of this population. The Native American birth rate is about 68% higher than all other races, with poor perinatal outcomes and a high neonatal mortality rate. Native American women have a lower life expectancy than other women, but they live longer than native men and men of other racial groups. More Indian women than men are divorced, separated, or widowed. About one fourth of all Native Americans live on reservations, predominantly located in more isolated rural regions. For many, the time required to reach the nearest Indian Health Service (IHS) facility can range anywhere from 30 minutes to 150 minutes, or more, depending on inclement weather and road conditions, and assuming the family has access to transportation at all.

Unemployment is rampant on reservations, the rate ranging from 45% to 95%. Native American women are employed in all salary levels except the highest. These women experience extreme poverty, illiteracy, cultural isolation, and racial discrimination. Native Americans have a very high prevalence of frostbite, tuberculosis, sexually transmitted diseases, diabetes, cancer of the cervix, and cirrhosis of the liver, along with a high incidence of abuse, accidents, violence, and suicide. Many of these chronic conditions could be prevented though improved socioeconomic status, education, and lifestyle. IHS offers cancer prevention and screening programs, but only to women who are enrolled members of federally recognized tribes.

In general, rural women are at higher risk of developing certain types of cancer because of environmental and behavioral factors, and they experience more negative outcomes as a consequence of the disease process. An example concerns cancer staging, which refers to the degree of tumor extension and growth at first diagnosis. Early staging is considered an indicator of quality medical care and improves outcomes for many cancer types. Disparities exist between urban and rural populations, with the rural population being at risk for late-stage diagnosis. Variations in diagnosis and treatment may be attributable to the disproportionately high percentage of high-risk groups in rural settings. However, it is important to note that definitions of rural are not consistent among studies focusing on cancer in rural women. An older population along with more high-risk groups, fewer health care providers, and greater distances to services are contributing factors to cancer-related disparities among nonmetropolitan women.[39]

CHARACTERISTICS OF RURAL HEALTH CARE SYSTEMS

Much has been written about access to care, or the lack thereof, in rural and remote regions of the US. According to *Rural Healthy People 2010,* access to quality health services including primary care is a priority for rural areas in all four geographic regions of the nation.[9,17,18] Health professional shortages, in particular the recruitment and retention of primary care providers, are major concerns among all state offices of rural health. Even though nearly a quarter of the US population lives in rural regions, only 10% of physicians practice there, and many rural hospitals are in an ongoing struggle to survive financial uncertainty.

When it comes to care-seeking behaviors, having a usual provider of care is viewed as a favorable factor in health status. About 15% of all adults in the US do not have a preferred doctor's office, clinic, or any other place in which they receive care. Comparatively, rural residents are more likely to identify a regular primary care provider. Partly, this finding is attributable to rural environments having a very low number of doctors. Sometimes one physician, or perhaps two, have lived and worked in the same community for decades. This physician provides care to families in the community from one generation to the next. There is an interesting dichotomy in respect to rural residents. On the one hand they make fewer doctor visits than their urban counterparts; and, when they do so they are sicker and more likely to be hospitalized. Rural people have a preference for interacting with people they know and hence may not trust health care providers who provide outreach services in their region. The working poor may not seek professional care unless they are seriously ill or in an emergency. For them, consulting a physician for illness prevention and health promotion care may not be a priority, given their financial situation. Any or all of these factors can deter care-seeking behaviors even if a service is available in the local area, including cancer-screening programs.[8,21,22]

CANCER IN RURAL WOMEN

Using the Boolean terms "rural women and cancer," a PubMed search produced several hundred citations. Of these, a significant proportion focused on international perspectives and a number of others described rural-urban treatment outcomes. Another large group described model programs to improve access to cancer screening that targeted specific minorities. There was a paucity of information describing the day-to-day issues confronting women in a rural context with a general diagnosis of cancer.[9,17,18,39]

Compared to urban communities, rural communities report a higher prevalence of chronic diseases including heart disease and cancer. The disproportionate prevalence of chronic disease is reflected in the higher crude all-causes mortality rates reported for rural areas. As for cancer, adjusting the data for age, race, and sex distributions effectively eliminates any rural disadvantage for cancer. Notable exceptions exist among select rural subpopulations in cancer, in particular the incidence and mortality rates for the Appalachian region. The death rate in rural Appalachia (176.3 per 100,000) for all cancers is higher than for all of Appalachia (173.1 per 100,000), and significantly higher than the national cancer death rate (166.7 per 100,000). Skin and lip cancer mortality rates are also higher in some rural regions and may be related to increased sun exposure, particularly among those working in agricultural production, which generally does not fall under Occupational Safety and Health Administration (OSHA) mandates. Certain behavioral and social factors are also associated with increased risk for certain types of cancer among rural populations; for example, smoking, alcohol use, and exposure to agricultural chemicals.

Some barriers to accessing cancer services are particularly salient in rural settings. Two of the most often cited barriers to access to both primary care and specialists are great geographic distances along with transportation challenges. Limited knowledge of the importance of early detection through regular screening and the high cost of screening are additional barriers for rural as well as urban women. Socioeconomic factors such as living in poverty and having limited education and limited employment options are barriers that can be more difficult to address but may be significant in terms of contributing to rural-urban cancer disparities. Being older, poorer, and less educated, coupled with limited knowledge about the importance of early detection and regular screening, all contribute to morbidity and mortality rates. In brief, failure to fully address both cancer prevention and treatment among rural populations is a significant obstacle to diminishing cancer mortality at a national level.[34-39]

A number of citations are available describing collaborative models in which rural and urban providers exhibited extraordinary creativity, resourcefulness, and resilience to offer education, cancer screening, and follow-up care to underserved communities. Most of the solutions advanced in the literature are highly dependent on access to primary care and clinical preventive services. Community initiatives that promote changes in high-risk behavior such as encouraging the use of sun block, wearing a hat, and staying inside or in shaded areas during peak sun hours have proven successful to reduce the incidence of skin cancer. Likewise, smoking cessation programs have reduced the incidence of other types of cancer in rural and urban settings alike. Five-year survival rates vary considerably depending on cancer type and the age of the individual at diagnosis. Rural residents typically are poorer, older, less well educated, and of minority origins, and they use fewer screening services, all of which contributes to late-stage diagnosis and poorer survival rates.

It is important to note that rural residents may experience variation in the quality, availability, and accessibility of services when evaluated against urban counterparts.[1,41-43] Limited access to quality medical care facilities, particularly cancer prevention programs, has a negative impact on the outcome of someone who is diagnosed with cancer. In particular, those receiving Medicaid and the uninsured are at a greater risk of late-stage cancer diagnosis. A diagnosis of cancer is difficult regardless of where one lives; in particular, rural women may be disadvantaged compared to urban counterparts. In oncology (cancer) centers, one usually finds an array of resources, programs, and services designed to meet the information and support needs relative to various types of cancer. These services can be a lifeline to help a woman navigate the complex health care system from initial diagnosis to the end of treatment, as well as for appropriate long-term follow-up care. For various reasons, women who live a great distance from an oncology center may not have access to this array of coordinated services. Consequently there is a critical need for patient care coordination (e.g., discharge planning, case management) between urban-based specialists and health care professionals located in rural, oftentimes medically underserved settings.

Considering the paucity of information on the topic, women as well as men who are cancer survivors have important insights and are in a position to make important contributions to oncology care in remote and underserved regions. Two international studies, one from Canada[44] and another from Australia[45,46] specifically focused on rural women with cancer. While the health care systems in these two nations are different than that of the US, the findings hold for the rural environment in general, and also to the rural context of the US in particular.

A comprehensive report produced by the Canadian Breast Cancer Network, a national network of breast cancer survivors, describes an ambitious study with focus groups to learn about the experiences of rural women with a diagnosis of breast cancer.[44] The insights may potentially apply also to other types of cancer. The focus groups varied in terms of the depth and breadth relative to living in a very remote setting and informal rural social structures.

The Canadian study also reflects the experiences of US women with a serious chronic illness, in particular cancer, who live in remote and sometimes isolated areas of the US.[8,21,22]

Analysis of the Canadian focus groups revealed one predominant theme; that is, becoming aware of and/or gaining access to health care information, support and services. There were four highly interrelated subthemes, as well: dealing with isolation, having to travel, feeling the financial burden, and coping with changing work. The next few paragraphs examine the interrelated themes in relation to the author's personal and professional experiences in rural contexts.

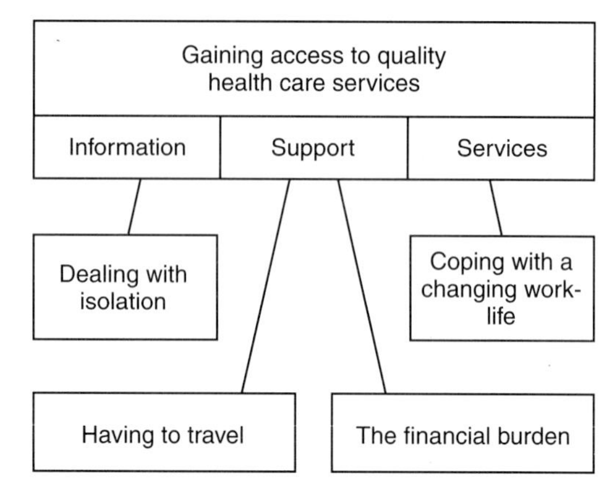

FIGURE 29-2 A conceptual Framework of distinct rural themes. (From: Canadian Breast Cancer Network (CBCN): *Perspectives of rural women with breast cancer,* 2001. For information, call 1-800-685-8820, or go to www.cbcn.ca. Accessed on February 24, 2005.)

Access to Health Care Information, Support, and Services

Regardless of the setting, becoming aware of available programs and services is a gradual process. Usually, the process for someone diagnosed with cancer, be it male or female, entails extensive, time-consuming and stressful searching. In a small town, information about prevention, screening, resources, and services relative to a particular type of cancer often is nonexistent, and when available it probably is dated. The Canadian women expressed disappointment about the types and levels of services offered in their locale and compared their situations negatively with that of urban women.[44] For most of them, a family physician, an oncologist, or a nurse practitioner was their primary resource to learn about potential health care and social services. For persons with a chronic illness living in some rural regions of the US, especially frontier areas, a comprehensive span of services and providers to meet their needs either does not exist; is fragmented, or is difficult to use. Not having the financial resources to pay for care, travel-related challenges such as no public transportation, not having a dependable vehicle, inclement weather, poor road conditions, and great distances to providers are the most often cited barriers for rural Americans as well as in the Canadian report.[8,20-22] Rural factors such as these can hinder a family from accessing information on a particular disease as well as health care and support services.

When available, health-related information is often culturally and linguistically inappropriate and written at a level that cannot be understood by the woman or her family, especially the elderly and members of ethnic minorities. Recent immigrants in particular may not be able to speak, much less read, English. In some cases, they are not able to read even basic texts in their native language, much less complex medical information that was translated from American English.

Generally, public libraries are a place where one expects to find information related to a variety of health topics. In a small town, however, if a library even exists it may not have Internet services. In cases where Internet service is available, usage time for each customer may be limited in order to equitably meet local needs. Sometimes a patron may find information relating to a particular diagnosis, but it is usually in an outdated medical or nursing text that was donated to the library by a local health care professional. Rarely does a small town library have state-of-the-science information on the prevention, diagnosis, and treatment for specific types of cancer. To address this information deficit, cancer centers should have standardized resources for various types of cancer that can be provided at the point of diagnosis. Such materials should be sensitive to the rural context and prepared in several formats (video, pamphlets, books, web sites, etc.) to address the needs of family members, including children of various ages. To assist rural women, in particular, it is important to provide detailed information on social services within the market area along with contact information for cancer support groups.[8,22,24,39]

The Canadians elaborated on their struggles to find the support they and their families needed. Among the barriers they cited were physical obstacles for those with disabilities, language barriers for those who could not speak or read English, and threats to confidentiality associated with overlapping relationships, familiarity, and lack of anonymity among small-town residents. Regardless of the setting, friends and family can have a significant role in sharing information and providing support for a woman with the diagnosis of cancer. A tight-knit community can also be a source of support to one of its members when experiencing life-crises. The Canadian women stressed the importance of being able to talk with caring others about what they were going through. Residing in a rural setting enhanced access to their extended family, friends, and neighbors who could provide the woman with more immediate and ongoing support. For some but not all of the women, family and friends most often provided such support. Conversely, extended kinship networks were identified as a source of additional stress, especially among women who were more private about their diagnosis and life situation.[23-27,44]

Cancer survivor support groups can be very helpful to a woman and her family system. However, establishing and sustaining a convenient support group of any type in a sparsely populated area can be a challenge; very few individuals may want to join one at any particular time. In other words, there may be only one, or maybe two, individuals in an entire county with a particular condition or diagnosis during any given period. In turn, those individuals may not be aware of the other person(s) with a similar diagnosis. Even though support groups are less likely to be available in rural settings, many of the Canadian women had attended one at some point. The challenges in sustaining support groups in small towns include not having a suitable meeting facility and leaders not having the background and knowledge to facilitate such a group. Leaders of cancer support groups should have a background in working with grief and loss, as well as current information about cancer treatments and resources.

Be it rural or urban, most women experience stress with running a home and parenting while coping with a diagnosis of cancer. Canadian women described the pressures placed on other individuals in the environment because of their illness and elaborated on the difficulties in finding the resources to meet family needs. For example, when they were gone from home for extended periods of time for treatment at the distant cancer center, family problems and needs were gravely exacerbated. In particular, they needed assistance with preparing meals, buying groceries, and taking children to school activities and day care, and in some cases they actually need transportation to and from medical care.

Travel-Related Challenges

It can be extremely difficult to access a local primary care provider, much less an oncology specialist located hundreds of miles from one's home. Traveling to obtain care from a specialist can be time-consuming, extremely exhausting for someone with a chronic illness, and particularly costly considering the cost of fuel, meals, lodging, and medical services. It is not unusual for someone who is poor or with a debilitating condition to not own a vehicle. Since few rural communities have public transportation, not having a vehicle or not being able to drive means the person must make arrangements for someone to transport them to obtain medical care, and this may pose real problems for some. When making appointments, it is important that health care providers be sensitive to travel challenges that patients are forced to contend with to obtain care. Sometimes services are provided on an outreach bases by cancer centers to select rural communities at scheduled intervals, for example monthly or once every 6 weeks. Outreach services and telehealth medicine can significantly improve access to specialty services, and usually they are greatly appreciated by rural residents regardless of the diagnosis. It is important to stress that members of the outreach team should be consistent for the sake of continuity of patient care and because rural residents prefer to interact with people they know.[20-22,32,34,39,47,48]

Collaboration among urban and rural health care providers is essential. Rural women rely heavily on local physicians for information and support. Upon discharge from the cancer center and the return to their rural home, it is not unusual for the patient to feel excluded from the specialist-driven cancer care system. Urban-based specialists must make every effort to include rural providers in the communication loop so they can better assist their patients. The Canadian women elaborated on the consequences of poor communication from cancer treatment centers to local physicians and how this hindered obtaining appropriate and timely information. In some cases a treatment could have been provided to the patient in her community but local physicians were not aware of those capabilities. In other words, the women were referred to a cancer center, when the local hospital and doctors could have worked with the oncologist to provide and monitor those treatments in her own community.[22,44]

Additional stressors are placed on rural residents as a result of the waiting for diagnostic tests that must be sent to a larger laboratory for analysis. The manner in which the findings are relayed to the woman by her doctor also can present problems, especially those living a great distance from the cancer center. How should the specialist communicate the report to her? For instance, must she again drive to the cancer center to see her specialist? Or, could the results be provided to her over the phone? Or, could a physician in the rural community be included on the oncology team and be able to share information with the patient and her family?

It is also stressful for those with a chronic illness who live in less populated areas simply to obtain pharmaceutical products and durable equipment. Pharmacists are far and few between in rural America! When available in a small town, privately owned drug stores usually do not stock costly and rarely used medications and durable medical equipment. Obtaining such products can be even more problematic for farm residents when refrigerated or express delivery is involved, or when roads are not in good travel condition.

A higher proportion of rural women with breast cancer choose mastectomy over lumpectomy, believing they have fewer treatment options such as reconstruction, prosthetics, and chemotherapy. Reasons given by rural women for pursuing a mastectomy most often related to the distance and time involved in traveling for radiation treatment, with the subsequent impact on child care, family responsibilities, finances, and work. Home health care services also may be limited or unavailable, which further limits nursing care for women who could benefit from such support.[39,44]

Ideally, cancer centers should collaborate with a rural nurse with a specialty, or at least an interest, in oncology care to coordinate care for patients in their own community. This nurse could serve as an advocate for patients with a diagnosis of cancer, help them navigate the complex cancer care system, and coordinate formal with informal services at the local level. A nursing case management model of care delivery would do much to reduce stress and anxiety among rural women having a diagnosis of cancer. Nurses who live within a particular community usually have insights about local preferences and the rural context and are thus in a better position to provide culturally sensitive care for patients in their care.[22,25,31,39]

Isolation

Canadians further elaborated on feelings of isolation when in their own community, as well as when in the city to obtain care at the cancer center. Isolation was especially profound when they had to be gone from home for an extended period of time for chemotherapy and radiation treatments. They described their sense of isolation when staying in a hotel room in an unfamiliar city without family and friends, with nothing to do, while trying to deal with treatment side effects. They greatly missed children, spouses, and the extended family support systems. Over time, most connected with other cancer patients at the cancer center. Upon returning home, they longed for their recently established support network of individuals who had a similar diagnosis. Feelings of isolation intensified when they were not able to find much-needed support in their own community. For some, the isolation was perceived to be a lack of interest from others. In other instances, the women isolated herself to avoid having to go into detail about her condition and being the topic of gossip for the local grapevine.

A common misunderstanding about rural life is an assumed connection among all residents. Small-town residence does not necessarily mean that all residents are connected to neighbors or family. Some do not want other residents, or even certain family members, to know much about them, much less about their cancer diagnosis, treatment, or disease progression. This preference can exacerbate feelings of loneliness and isolation.[22-28]

Financial and Job-Related Issues

Financial concerns are common among most who use the health care system. However, local economic structures can create additional problems for rural women with a diagnosis of cancer. Most often cited among rural women is the financial strain of not being able to work for an extended period of time coupled with the costs for travel, and in some cases child care as well as the actual cost of medical services. The Canadian women described the uniqueness of rural employment practices as discussed earlier in this chapter, with work options that rarely include a full-time salary in a single organization. Many worked at multiple part-time jobs, all without benefits and job security. A few were self-employed. In both cases the women were left without options when needing time off because of illness or for traveling to the specialist for care. With a part-time position, employers may be reluctant to keep someone with diagnosis of cancer on their payroll—someone who is perceived as unreliable as a consequence of the illness.[21,22,44]

The Australian study further elaborates on the social and economic difficulties of women with cancer who lived in rural settings.[45,46] These women faced significant financial burdens related to travel, child care responsibilities, and changes in work patterns. Compared with other rural women in general, those who worked on farms and were self-employed experienced exacerbated financial concerns. They expressed concerns about being a financial and emotional burden on partners and other family members when living in intergenerational households. In particular, findings from the Australian study are relevant to women with a diagnosis of cancer who live in more remote and frontier regions of the US.

IMPLICATIONS AND RECOMMENDATIONS

While the Canadian Breast Cancer Network study focused on women with breast cancer and their illness experiences, US-based specialists in oncology can find those perspectives highly relevant for rural men and for women with other types of cancer. As highlighted in this chapter, families of rural cancer patients have many unmet needs and additional burdens related to access and distance from services. Essentially, the more remote the community in which the survivor lives, the more difficult access becomes; this is especially true for residents living in regions designated as frontier. Box 29-3 lists online resources for those in rural areas.

Health care professionals in general, and oncology nurses in particular, must become informed about rural regions in their catchment areas and be sensitive to rural residents' care-seeking behaviors. For example, nurses should be aware that some women who live in rural areas are less likely to receive screening mammograms; more likely to be diagnosed at a more advanced stage; and have a poorer 5-year survival than urban women. In addition, rural women in general receive less tissue-conserving surgery and

Box 29-3 On-Line Resources

BUREAU OF PRIMARY HEALTH CARE

www.bphc.hrsa.gov

This site provides access to databases, resources, and links to information for vulnerable rural populations.

CANADIAN BREAST CANCER NETWORK

www.cbcn.ca

1-800-685-8820

National Voice of Canadian Breast Cancer Survivors; site has relevant information that includes the rural perspective

DIRECTORY OF STATE OFFICES OF RURAL HEALTH

www.ruralhealth.hrsa.gov/funding/50sorh.htm

An up-to-date listing of state rural health offices and associations including complete mailing addresses, phone and fax numbers, and Internet addresses. This online resource is a production of the Office of Rural Health Policy, Health Resources and Services Administration (HRSA).

INDIAN HEALTH SERVICES

www.ihs.gov

Site devoted to American Indian and Alaska Native health services and health statistics

NATIONAL RURAL HEALTH ASSOCIATION (NRHA)

www.nrharural.org

The National Rural Health Association (NRHA) is a membership organization dedicated to the improvement of health care services in rural areas. NRHA acts as a clearinghouse for information on rural health issues and an advocate for rural positions with policymakers. NRHA sponsors the nation's largest annual conference on rural health.

Box 29-3 On-Line Resources—cont'd

OFFICE OF RURAL HEALTH POLICY (ORHP)
www.ruralhealth.hrsa.gov
Mission is to promote better health care service in rural America. Established in August 1987 by the Administration, the office was subsequently authorized by Congress in December 1987 and located in the Health Resources and Services Administration. Congress charged the office with informing and advising the Department of Health and Human Services on matters affecting rural hospitals and health care, coordinating activities within the department that relate to rural health care, and maintaining a national information clearinghouse.

RURAL ASSISTANCE CENTER (RAC)
www.raconline.org
Product of the US Department of Health and Human Services' Rural Initiative, the Rural Assistance Center (RAC) was established in December 2002 as a rural health and human services "information portal." RAC helps rural communities and other rural stakeholders access the full range of available programs, funding, and research that can enable them to provide quality health and human services to rural residents.

RURAL HEALTH FINDER
www.healthfinder.gov/scripts/SearchContext.asp?topic=759&refine=1
Comprehensive site with URL links to numerous agencies and information related to rural topics

RURAL INFORMATION CENTER
www.nal.usda.gov/ric
Under the auspices of the US Department of Agriculture, the Rural Information Center (RIC) provides information services for rural communities, officials, organizations, and citizens; it provides over 3,000 links to current and reliable information on a wide variety of rural resources and funding sources; there is an extensive publication list.

RURAL NURSES ORGANIZATION (RNO)
www.rno.org
Official organization for nurses having an interest in rural areas; includes On line Journal of Rural Nursing

RURAL POLICY RESEARCH INSTITUTE (RUPRI)
www.rupri.org
RUPRI conducts policy-relevant research and facilitates public dialogue to assist policymakers in understanding the rural impacts of public policies and programs. Many policies that are not explicitly "rural policies" nevertheless have substantial implications for rural areas, and RUPRI is dedicated to understanding and articulating these implications. The site includes links to other policy and research entities.

have fewer treatment options because of their need to travel for radiotherapy and chemotherapy. For them, financial, social, family, and business-related burdens can be significant. Economic factors must always be a consideration when designing programs targeting a rural population and planning a continuum of care for a particular patient with a diagnosis of cancer.

There are many implications for research needs and policy recommendations associated with the rural social and economic factors discussed in this chapter. Imprecise definitions of rural have hindered the identification of the support needs of women with cancer, then assessing whether these needs are being met and deciding how best to improve their circumstances. Likewise, not much is documented about quality of life issues of women in these circumstances with a diagnosis of cancer. Even less is known about subgroups such as the elderly, ethnic minorities, lesbians, farm women, and other highly vulnerable rural populations.

Quality of life issues are reflected in an individual's day-to-day activities: transportation challenges to access services, time away from the home, child care and housekeeping duties, as well lacking of access to health care information, support and other types of services, having to travel for treatment, feelings of isolation, and the costs incurred for treatments. Then, too, there are job-related issues associated with the idiosyncrasies of rural economic infrastructures. Lifestyle factors along with care-seeking preferences and coping mechanisms of rural populations all are topics about which little is known relative to women having a diagnosis of cancer. In spite of their many challenges, rural residents are known for resourcefulness and creativity in dealing with day-to-day situations as well as crises that occur at various times. Researchers must attempt to learn about the resilience and hardiness that is evident in many rural communities. In turn, federal policy relative to health care delivery, reimbursement, and the education of health care professionals must take into consideration the rural perspective.

SUMMARY

This chapter presented a snapshot of rural women with a diagnosis of cancer. Mortality rates for various cancers vary by demographic attributes including age, race, sex, and residence, creating a diverse pattern of cancer survival not reflected in mortality rates. Based on the literature, rural residents demonstrate a lower adjusted rate of cancer than urban residents. However, their comparative advantage may be offset by the higher death rates due to being diagnosed at later stages of disease. Even though the adjusted incidence rate of cancer may be lower in some rural areas (compared with urban), the barriers to care may increase the likelihood of negative outcomes. Urban and rural America alike are faced with meeting the health care needs of an aging population. Along with limited resources the impact may be especially challenging for small communities having a disproportionate number of elderly and members of other high-risk groups. Ultimately, combating cancer requires a multidimensional approach aimed at improving access to health care services, including cancer screening, detection, and modifying risk factors. To enhance limited services and build on natural support systems, health care professionals must learn about the rural context. Clinicians must then integrate these findings into the care plans of women with a diagnosis of cancer who live in rural and medically underserved regions of the US.

REFERENCES

1. Office of Rural Health Policy (ORHP). *One department serving rural America—HHS Rural Task Force Report to the Secretary,* Washington, DC. 2002, The Office. Retrieved 2/25/05 from www.ruralhealth.hrsa.gov/PublicReport.htm.
2. Eberhardt M and others: *Urban and rural health chartbook. Health, United States, 2001.* Hyattsville, Md., 2001, National Center for Health Statistics. Retrieved 2/25/05 from www.cdc.gov/nchs/pressroom/01news/hus01.htm.
3. Bureau of the Census: *Census 2000: Briefs and special reports, 2003.* Retrieved 2/24/05 from www.census.gov/population/www/cen2000/briefs.html.
4. U.S. Department of Agriculture (USDA): *Briefing room—rural population and migration,* 2003. Retrieved 2/24/05 from http://ers.usda.gov/briefing/population.
5. U.S. Department of Agriculture (USDA): *Key topics—measuring rurality, 2003.* Retrieved 2/25/05 from http://ers.usda.gov/Topics/view.asp?T=104018.
6. Bureau of the Census: *Urban and rural classification,* 2000. Retrieved 2/24/05 from www.census.gov/geo/www/ua/ua_2k.html.
7. Jolfe D: *Rural poverty at a glance,* Washington, D.C., 2004, USDA. Retrieved 2/24/05 from http://ers.usda.gov/publications/rdrr100.
8. Bushy A: *Orientation to nursing in the rural community,* Thousand Oaks, Calif., 2000, Sage.
9. Gamm L and others: *Rural healthy people 2010: a companion document to healthy people 2010* (Vol. I), College Station, Tex., 2003, Texas A&M University. Retrieved 2/24/05 from www.srph.tamhsc.edu/centers/rhp2010/publications.htm.
10. Randolph R, Gual K, Slokfin R: *Rural populations and health care providers: a map book.* Chapel Hill, N.C., 2002, U. of North Carolina. Retrieved 2/24/05 from www.shepscenter.unc.edu/research_programs/rural_program/mapbook2003/index.html.
11. Indian Health Services (IHS): *IHS Fact sheet,* 2002. Retrieved 2/24/05 from www.ihs.gov/PublicInfo/PublicAffairs/ Welcome_Info/ThisFacts.asp.

12. Indian Health Services (IHS): *Regional differences in Indian Health,* Rockville, Md., 2002, The Service. Retrieved 2/24/05 from www.ihs.gov/PublicInfo/Publications/trends98/ region98.asp.
13. National Center for Farmworker Health (NCFH): *Overview of America's farm worker,* Buda, Tex., 2002, The Center. Retrieved 2/24/05 from www.ncfh.org/aaf_01.php.
14. Bureau of Primary Health Care (BPHC). *Migrant Health Program: National Advisory Council on Migrant Health Recommendations,* 2000. Retrieved 2/24/05 from http://bphc.hrsa.gov/migrant/NACMHRecommendations.htm
15. Health Resources Services Administration (HRSA): *United States health personnel fact book,* Washington, D.C., 2003, The Administration. Retrieved 2/24/05 from http://ask.hrsa.gov/detail.cfm?id=HRS00323.
16. Kaiser Foundation: *Key facts: Race, ethnicity and medical care,* 1999. Retrieved 2/24/05 from www.kff.org/minorityhealth/1523-index.cfm.
17. Gamm L and others: Rural healthy people 2010: identifying rural health priorities and models for practice, *J Rural Health* 18(1):9-14, 2002.
18. Gamm L and others: *Rural healthy people 2010: a companion document to healthy people 2010* (Vol. II), College Station, Tex., 2003, Texas A&M University. Retrieved 2/24/05 from www.srph.tamhsc.edu/centers/rhp2010/publications.htm.
19. Gamm L, Hutchison L, Dabney B, Dorsey A. *Rural healthy people 2010: a companion document to healthy people 2010* (Vol. III), College Station, Tex., 2003, Texas A&M University. Retrieved 2/24/05 from www.srph.tamhsc.edu/centers/rhp2010/publications.htm.
20. Long K, Weinert C: Rural nursing: Developing a theory base, *Sch Inq Nurs Pract* 3:113-127, 1989.
21. Stein H: The annual cycle and the cultural nexus of health care behavior among Oklahoma wheat farming families, *Cult Med Psy* 6:81-89, 1989.
22. Sullivan T, Weinert C, Cudney S: Management of chronic illness: voices of rural women, *J Adv Nurs* 44:566-574, 2003.
23. Roberts L and others: Personal health care attitudes of rural clinicians: a preliminary study of 127 multidisciplinary health care providers in Alaska and New Mexico, *Rural Ment Health* 28:30-36, 2003.
24. Casey M, Thiede C, Klinger J: Are rural residents less likely to obtain recommended preventive healthcare services? *Am J Prevent Med* 21:182-188, 2001.
25. Lambert D and others: *Rural mental health outreach: promising practices in rural areas,* Washington, D.C., 2003, Substance Abuse and Mental Health Services Administration. Retrieved 2/24/05 from http://muskie.usm.maine.edu/research/publications.jsp.
26. Huttlinger K and others: Suffering it out: meeting the needs of health care delivery in a rural area, *Online J Rural Nur Health Care* 1(2):2003. Retrieved 2/24/05 from www.rno.org/journal/issues/Vol-3/issue-2/Huttlinger_article.htm.
27. Ladner C, Cuellar N: Depression in rural hospice family caregivers, *Online J Rural Nursing Health Care* 3(1):2003. Retrieved 2/24/05 from www.rno.org/journal/issues/Vol-3/issue-1/TOC.htm.
28. Occupational Health and Safety (OSHA): *Safety and health topics: agricultural operations,* 2003. Retrieved 2/24/05 from www.osha.gov/SLTC/agriculturaloperations/index.html.
29. Bushy A: *Rural minority health resource book,* Kansas City, Mo., 2002, National Rural Health Association.
30. National Center for Health Statistics: *Health United States 2004,* Hyattsville, Md., 2004, U.S. Public Health Service. Retrieved 2/24/05 from www.cdc.gov/nchs/hus.htm.
31. Bushy A: Health issues of women in rural environments, *JOWMA* 53:53-56, 1998.
32. Probst J and others: *Minorities in rural America: an overview of population characteristics,* Columbia, SC, 2002, University of South Carolina. Retrieved 2/24/05 from http://rhr.sph.sc.edu/report/MinoritiesInRuralAmerica.pdf.
33. U.S. Department of Health and Human Services (DHHS): *Healthy People 2010,* Washington, D.C., 2001, U.S. Government Printing Office. Retrieved 2/24/05 from www.healthypeople.gov/34.
34. Probst J and others: *Access to care among rural minorities: older adults,* Columbia, SC, 2003, University of South Carolina. Retrieved 2/24/05 from http://rhr.sph.sc.edu/report.
35. Green L, Lewis R, Bediako S: Reducing and eliminating health disparities: a targeted approach, *J National Med Ass* 97:25-30, 2005.
36. Chilton J, Jones L: Rural health and women of color. Impact of breast cancer on African American women, *Am J Pub Health* 92:539-542, 2002.
37. Lane A, Martin M; Logic model use for breast health in rural communities, *Oncol Nurs Forum* 32:105-110, 2005.
38. Elliot T and others: Lake Superior Rural Cancer Care Project, Part I: an intervention trial. *Cancer Pract* 9:27-36, 2000.
39. Gosschalk A, Carozza S: Cancer in rural areas. *Rural Healthy People 2010: A companion document to Healthy People 2010,* (Vol 2), College Station, Tex., 2003, Texas A&M University System Health Science Center, School of Rural Public Health, Southwest Rural Health Research Center. Retrieved 2/24/05 from www.srph.tamhsc.edu/centers/ rhp2010/publications.htm.
40. Stewart K, Cianfrini L, Walker J: Stress, social support, and housing are related to health status among HIV-positive persons in the deep South of the United States, *AIDS Care* 17:350-358, 2005.
41. Bureau of Health Professions (BHPR): *Health professional shortage areas.* Retrieved 2/24/05 from http://bhpr.hrsa.gov/shortage.
42. Centers for Medicare and Medicaid Services (CMMS): *Federally qualified health centers.* Retrieved 2/24/05 from www.cms.hhs.gov/providerupdate/newfqhcregs.asp?
43. Centers for Medicare and Medicaid Services (CMMS); *Rural health clinics.* Retrieved 2/26/05 from www.cms.hhs.gov/providerupdate/oldrhcregs.asp.
44. Canadian Breast Cancer Network (CBCN): *Perspectives of rural women with breast cancer,* 2001. Retrieved 2/24/05 from www.cbcn.ca/english/publications.php?display&en&21.
45. McGrath P and others: A study of postdiagnosis breast cancer concerns for women living in rural and remote

Queensland. Part 1: personal concerns, *Aust J Rural Health* 7:34-42, 1999.

46. McGrath P and others: A study of postdiagnosis breast cancer concerns for women living in rural and remote Queensland. Part II: support issues, *Aust J Rural Health* 7:43-52, 1999.
47. Agency for Health Care Research and Quality (AHRQ): *Creating partnerships, improving health: the role of community based participatory research, 2003,* AHRQ Pub. No. 03-0037. Retrieved 2/24/05 from www.ahrq.gov/research/cbprrole.htm.
48. Johnson R: *Rural health response to domestic violence: policy and practice issues emerging public policy issues and best practices,* Washington, D.C., 2000, Federal Office of Rural Health. Retrieved 2/24/05 from http://ruralhealth.hrsa.gov/pub/domviol.htm.

APPENDIX

A Commonly Used Medications for Women with Cancer

ANTIANXIETY AGENTS

Uses

Treatment of anxiety. In addition, some benzodiazepines are used as hypnotics, as anticonvulsants to prevent delirium tremors during alcohol withdrawal, and as adjunctive therapy for relaxation of skeletal muscle spasms.

Action

Benzodiazepines are the largest and most frequently prescribed group of antianxiety agents. The exact mechanism is unknown.

ANTIANXIETY AGENTS

Name	Availability	Uses	Dosage Range (per day)	Side Effects
BENZODIAZEPINE ANTIANXIETY AGENTS				
Alprazolam (Xanax, Xanax XR, Niravam)	T: 0.25 mg, 0.5 mg, 1 mg, 2 mg T (DT): 0.25 mg, 0.5 mg, 1 mg, 2 mg S: 0.5 mg/5 ml, 1 mg/ml T: (ER): 0.5 mg, 1 mg, 2 mg, 3 mg	Anxiety, panic disorder	0.75-10 mg	Drowsiness, weakness, or fatigue; ataxia, slurred speech, confusion, lack of coordination, impaired memory, paradoxical agitation, dizziness, nausea
Chlordiazepoxide (Librium, Libritabs)	C: 5 mg, 10 mg, 25 mg T: 10 mg, 25 mg	Anxiety, alcohol withdrawal	5-300 mg	Same as alprazolam
Clorazepate (Tranxene)	C: 3.75 mg, 7.5 mg, 15 mg SD: 11.25 mg, 22.5 mg	Anxiety, alcohol withdrawal, anticonvulsant	7.5-90 mg	Same as alprazolam

Continued

All drug information for this adapted with permission from Hodgson B, Kizior R: Saunders Nursing Drug Handbook 2004, St. Louis, 2004, Saunders.

Antianxiety Agents—cont'd

Name	Availability	Uses	Dosage Range (per day)	Side Effects
Diazepam (Valium)	T: 2.5 mg, 5 mg, 10 mg S: 5 mg/5 ml, 5 mg/ml I: 5 mg/ml	Anxiety, alcohol withdrawal, anticonvulsant, muscle relaxant	2-40 mg	Same as alprazolam
Lorazepam (Ativan)	T: 0.5 mg, 1 mg, 2 mg S: 2 mg/ml I: 2 mg/ml, 4 mg/ml	Anxiety	0.5-10 mg	Same as alprazolam
Oxazepam (Serax)	C: 10 mg, 15 mg, 30 mg T: 15 mg	Anxiety, alcohol withdrawal	30-120 mg	Same as alprazolam
NONBENZODIAZEPINE ANTIANXIETY AGENTS				
Buspirone (BuSpar)	T: 5 mg, 10 mg, 15 mg, 30 mg	Anxiety	7.5-60 mg	Dizziness, lightheadedness, headache, nausea, restlessness
Hydroxyzine (Atarax, Vistaril)	T: 10 mg, 25 mg, 50 mg, 100 mg	Anxiety, rhinitis, pruritus, urticaria, nausea or vomiting	100-400 mg	Drowsiness; dry mouth, nose, and throat
Paroxetine (Paxil)	S: 10 mg/5 ml T: 10 mg, 20 mg, 30 mg, 40 mg T(CR): 12.5 mg, 25 mg, 37.5 mg	Anxiety, depression, obsessive-compulsive disorder, panic disorder	10-50 mg	Drowsiness; dry mouth, nose, and throat; dizziness, diarrhea, increased sweating, constipation, vomiting, tremors
Trazodone (Desyrel)	T: 50 mg, 100 mg, 150 mg, 300 mg	Anxiety, depression	100-400 mg	Drowsiness, dizziness, headache, dry mouth, nausea, vomiting, unpleasant taste
Venlafaxine (Effexor)	C: 37.5 mg, 75 mg, 150 mg	Anxiety, depression	37.5-225 mg	Drowsiness, nausea, headache, dry mouth

C, Capsules; *CR,* controlled release; *DT,* disintegrating tablets; *ER,* extended release; *I,* injection; *S,* solution; *SD,* single dose; *T,* tablets.

ANTIBIOTICS

Uses

Treatment of wide range of gram-positive or gram-negative bacterial infections; suppression of intestinal flora before surgery; control of acne; prophylactically to prevent rheumatic fever; prophylactically in high-risk situations (e.g., some surgical procedures or medical states) to prevent bacterial infection.

Action

Antibiotics (antimicrobial agents) are natural or synthetic compounds that have the ability to kill or suppress the growth of microorganisms.

Selection of Antimicrobial Agents

The goal of therapy is to produce a favorable therapeutic result by achieving antimicrobial action at the site of infection sufficient to inhibit the growth of the microorganism. The agent selected should be the most active against the most likely infecting organism, least likely to cause toxicity or allergic reaction. Factors to consider in selection of an antimicrobial agent include the following:

- Sensitivity pattern of the infecting microorganism
- Location and severity of infection (may determine route of administration)
- Patient's ability to eliminate the drug (status of renal and liver functions)
- Patient's defense mechanisms (includes both cellular and humoral immunity)
- Patient's age, whether pregnant, genetic factors, allergies, presence of a central nervous system disorder, preexisting medical problems

Categorization of Organisms by Gram Staining

Gram-Positive Cocci	Gram-Negative Cocci	Gram-Positive Bacilli	Gram-Negative Bacilli
AEROBIC			
Staphylococcus aureus	*Neisseria gonorrhoeae*	*Listeria monocytogenes*	*Escherichia coli*
Staphylococcus epidermidis	*Neisseria meningitidis*	*Bacillus antrocis*	*Klebsiella pneumoniae*
Streptococcus pneumoniae	*Moraxella catarrhalis*	*Corynebacterium diphtheriae*	*Proteus mirabilis*
Streptococcus pyogenes		*Anaerobic*	*Serratia marcescens*
Viridans streptococci		*Clostridium difficile*	*Pseudomonas aeruginosa*
Enterococcus faecalis		*Clostridium perfringens*	*Enterobacter spp.*
Enterococcus faecium		*Clostridium tetani*	*Haemophilus influenzae*
		Actinomyces spp.	*Legionella pneumophila*
ANAEROBIC			
Peptostreptococcus spp.			*Bacteroides fragilis*
Peptococcus spp.			*Fusobacterium* spp.

ANTIBIOTICS: AMINOGLYCOSIDES

Uses

Treatment of serious infections when other, less toxic, agents are not effective, are contraindicated, or necessitate adjunctive therapy (e.g., with penicillins or cephalosporins). Used primarily in the treatment of infections caused by gram-negative microorganisms such as those caused by *Proteus, Klebsiella, Pseudomonas, Escherichia coli, Serratia, and Enterobacter.*

Action

Bactericidal. Transported across bacterial cell membrane; irreversibly binds to specific receptor proteins of bacterial ribosomes. Interfere with protein synthesis, preventing cell reproduction and eventually causing cell death.

Antibiotics: Aminoglycosides

Name	Availability	Dosage Range	Side Effects
Amikacin (Amikin)	I: 250 mg/ml, 50 mg/ml	A: 15 mg/kg/day C: 15 mg/kg/day	Nephrotoxicity, neurotoxicity, ototoxicity (both auditory and vestibular), hypersensitivity (skin itching, redness, rash, swelling)
Gentamicin (Garamycin)	I: 40 mg/ml, 10 mg/ml	A: 3-5 mg/kg/day C: 6-7.5 mg/kg/day	Same as amikacin
Neomycin	T: 500 mg	A: 1 g for 3 doses as preoperative regimen	Nausea, vomiting, diarrhea
Netilimicin (Netromycin)	I: 100 mg/ml	A: 3-6.5 mg/kg/day C: 5.5-8 mg/kg/day	Same as amikacin
Streptomycin	I: 1 g	A: 15 mg/kg/day C: 20-40 mg/kg/day Max: 1 g	Same as amikacin Peripheral neuritis (numbness), optic neuritis (any vision loss)
Tobramycin (Nebcin)	I: 40 mg/ml, 10 mg/ml	A: 3-5 mg/kg/day C: 6-7.5 mg/kg/day	Same as amikacin

A, Adults; *C,* children; *I,* injection; *T,* tablets.

ANTIBIOTICS: CEPHALOSPORINS

Uses

Broad-spectrum antibiotics, which, like penicillins, may be used in a number of diseases including respiratory diseases, skin and soft tissue infection, bone/joint infections, and gastric ulcer infections, and prophylactically in some surgical procedures.

First-generation cephalosporins have good activity against gram-positive organisms and moderate activity against gram-negative organisms.

Second-generation cephalosporins have increased activity against gram-negative organisms.

Third-generation cephalosporins are less active against gram-positive organisms but more active against the Enterobacteriaceae, with some activity against *Pseudomonas aeruginosa.*

Fourth-generation cephalosporins have good activity against gram-positive organisms and gram-negative organisms.

Action

Cephalosporins inhibit cell wall synthesis or activate enzymes that disrupt the cell wall, causing a weakening in the cell wall, cell lysis, and cell death. May be bacteriostatic or bactericidal. Most effective against rapidly dividing cells.

ANTIBIOTICS: CEPHALOSPORINS

Name	Availability	Dosage Range	Side Effects
FIRST-GENERATION			
Cefadroxil (Duricef)	C: 500 mg T: 1 g S: 125 mg/5 ml, 250 mg/5 ml, 500 mg/5 ml	A: 1-2 g/day C: 30 mg/kg/day	Abdominal or stomach cramps/pain, fever, nausea, vomiting, diarrhea, headaches, oral/vaginal candidiasis
Cefazolin (Ancef, Kefzol)	I: 500 mg, 1 g, 2 g	A: 0.75-6 g/day C: 25-100 mg/kg/day	Same as cefadroxil
Cephalexin (Keftab)	C: 250 mg, 500 mg T: 250 mg, 500 mg, 1 g	A: 1-4 g/day C: 25-100 mg/kg/day	Same as cefadroxil
SECOND-GENERATION			
Cefaclor (Ceclor)	C: 250 mg, 500 mg T (ER): 375 mg, 500 mg S: 125 mg/5 ml, 187 mg/5 ml, 250 mg/5 ml, 375 mg/5 ml	A: 250-500 mg q8h C: 20-40 mg/kg/day	Same as cefadroxil May have serum sickness–like reaction
Cefmetazole (Zefazone)	I: 1 g, 2 g	A: 4-8 g/day	Same as cefadroxil
Cefotetan (Cefotan)	I: 1 g, 2 g	A: 1-6 g/day	Same as cefadroxil May cause unusual bleeding/bruising
Cefoxitin (Mefoxin)	I: 1 g, 2 g	A: 3-12 g/day	Same as cefadroxil
Cefpodoxime (Vantin)	T: 100 mg, 200 mg S: 50 mg/5 ml, 100 mg/5 ml	A: 200-800 mg/day C: 10 mg/kg/day	Same as cefadroxil
Cefprozil (Cefzil)	T: 250 mg, 500 mg S: 125 mg/5 ml, 250 mg/5 ml	A: 0.5-1 g/day C: 30 mg/kg/day	Same as cefadroxil

Continued

Antibiotics: Cephalosporins—cont'd

Name	Availability	Dosage Range	Side Effects
Cefuroxime (Ceftin, Kefurox, Zinacef)	T: 125 mg, 250 mg, 500 mg S: 125 mg/5 ml, 250 mg/5 ml I: 750 mg, 1.5 g	A (PO): 0.25-1 g/day; (IM/IV): 2.25-9 g/day C (PO): 250-500 mg/day; (IM/IV): 50-100 mg/kg/day	Same as cefadroxil
Loracarbef (Lorabid)	C: 200 mg, 400 mg S: 100 mg/5 ml, 200 mg/5 ml	A: 200-800 mg/day C: 15-30 mg/kg/day	Same as cefadroxil
THIRD-GENERATION			
Cefdinir (Omnicef)	C: 300 mg S: 125 mg/5 ml	A: 600 mg/day C: 14 mg/kg/day	Same as cefadroxil
Cefditoren (Spectracef)	T: 200 mg	A: 400-800 mg/day	Same as cefadroxil
Cefotaxime (Claforan)	I: 500 mg, 1 g, 2 g	A: 2-12 g/day C: 100-200 mg/kg/day	Same as cefadroxil
Ceftazidime (Fortaz, Tazicef, Tazidime)	I: 500 mg, 1 g, 2 g	A: 0.5-6 g/day C: 90-150 mg/kg/day	Same as cefadroxil
Ceftibuten (Cedax)	C: 400 mg S: 90 mg/5 ml, 180 mg/5 ml	A: 400 mg/day C: 9 mg/kg/day	Same as cefadroxil
Ceftizoxime (Cefizox)	I: 500 mg, 1 g, 2 g	A: 1-12 g/day C: 150-200 mg/kg/day	Same as cefadroxil
Ceftriaxone (Rocephin)	I: 250 mg, 500 mg, 1 g, 2 g	A: 1-4 g/day C: 50-100 mg/kg/day	Same as cefadroxil
FOURTH-GENERATION			
Cefepime (Maxipime)	I: 500 mg, 1 g, 2 g	A: 1-6 g/day	Same as cefadroxil

A, Adults; *C*, capsules; *C*, (dosage), children; *ER*, extended release; *I*, injection; *IM*, intramuscularly; *IV*, intravenously; *PO*, by mouth; *S*, suspension; *T*, tablets.

ANTIBIOTICS: FLUOROQUINOLONES

Uses

Fluoroquinolones act against a wide range of gram-negative and gram-positive organisms. They are used primarily in the treatment of lower respiratory infections, skin/skin structure infection, urinary tract infections, and sexually transmitted diseases.

Action

Bactericidal. Inhibit DNA gyrase in susceptible microorganisms, interfering with bacterial DNA replication and repair.

Antibiotics: Fluoroquinolones

Name	Availability	Dosage Range	Side Effects
Ciprofloxacin (Cipro, Cipro XR, Proquin XR)	T: 250 mg, 500 mg, 750 mg S: 5 g/100 ml I: 200 mg, 400 mg ER: 500 mg, 1000 mg	A (PO): 250-750 mg q12h; (IV): 200-400 mg q12h A (ER PO): 500-1000 mg q24h	Dizziness, headaches, nervousness, drowsiness, insomnia, abdominal pain, nausea, diarrhea, vomiting, phlebitis (parenteral), photosensitivity
Enoxacin (Penetrex)	T: 200 mg, 400 mg	A: 200-400 mg q12h	Same as ciprofloxacin
Gatifloxacin (Tequin)	T: 200 mg, 400 mg I: 200 mg, 400 mg S: 200 mg	A: 200-400 mg q12h	Same as ciprofloxacin
Gemifloxacin (Factive)	T: 320 mg	A: 320 mg daily	Same as ciprofloxacin
Levofloxacin (Levaquin)	T: 250 mg, 500 mg, 750 mg I: 250 mg, 500 mg, 750 mg OS: 250 mg/10 ml	A (PO/IV): 250-750 mg/day as single dose	Same as ciprofloxacin
Lomefloxacin (Maxaquin)	T: 400 mg	A: 400 mg/day	Same as ciprofloxacin
Moxifloxacin (Avelox)	T: 400 mg I: 400 mg	A: 400 mg/day	Same as ciprofloxacin; may prolong QT interval
Norfloxacin (Noroxin)	T: 400 mg	A: 400 mg q12h	Same as ciprofloxacin
Ofloxacin (Floxin)	T: 200 mg, 300 mg, 400 mg	A: 200-400 mg q12h	Same as ciprofloxacin
Sparfloxacin (Zagam)	T: 200 mg	A: 400 mg once, then 200 mg/day	Same as ciprofloxacin; QT prolongation, vaginitis

A, Adults; *ER*, extended release; *I*, injection; *IV*, intravenously; *OS*, oral solution; *PO*, by mouth; *S*, suspension; *T*, tablets.

ANTIBIOTICS: MACROLIDES

Uses

Macrolides act primarily against gram-positive microorganisms and gram-negative cocci. Macrolides are used in the treatment of pharyngitis/tonsillitis, sinusitis, chronic bronchitis, pneumonia, and uncomplicated skin/skin structure infections.

Action

Bacteriostatic or bactericidal. Reversibly bind to the P site of the 50S ribosomal subunit of susceptible organisms, inhibiting RNA-dependent protein synthesis.

ANTIBIOTICS: MACROLIDES

Name	Availability	Dosage Range	Side Effects
Azithromycin (Zithromax)	T: 250 mg, 500 mg, 600 mg S: 100 mg/5 ml, 200 mg/5 ml, 1 g packet I: 500 mg	A (PO): 500 mg once, then 250 mg days 2-5; (IV): 500 mg/day C (PO): 10 mg/kg once, then 5 mg/kg/day on days 2-5	PO: Nausea, diarrhea, vomiting, abdominal pain IV: Pain, redness, swelling at injection site
Clarithromycin (Biaxin)	T: 250 mg, 500 mg T (XL): 500 mg S: 125 mg/5 ml	A: 250-500 mg q12h C: 7.5 mg/kg q12h	Headaches, loss of taste, nausea, vomiting, diarrhea, abdominal pain/discomfort
Dirithromycin (Dynabec)	T: 250 mg	A, C (>12 yrs): 500 mg/day as a single daily dose	Dizziness, nausea, vomiting, diarrhea, abdominal pain, headaches, weakness
Erythromycin (Erytab, PCE, Eryc, EES, Eryped, Erythrocin)	T: 200 mg, 250 mg, 333 mg, 400 mg, 500 mg C: 250 mg S: 125 mg/5 ml, 200 mg/5 ml, 250 mg/5 ml, 400 mg/5 ml, 100 mg/2.5 ml	A (PO): 250-500 mg q6h C (PO): 30-50 mg/kg/day A, C (IV): 15-20 mg/kg/day Max: 4 g/day	PO: Nausea, vomiting, diarrhea, abdominal pain IV: Inflammation, phlebitis at injection site

A, Adults; *C*, capsules; *C* (dosage), children; *I*, injection; *IV*, intravenously; *PO*, by mouth; *S*, suspension; *T*, tablets; *XL*, long-acting.

ANTIBIOTICS: PENICILLINS

Uses

Penicillins may be used to treat a large number of infections, including pneumonia and other respiratory diseases, urinary tract infections, septicemia, meningitis, intraabdominal infections, gonorrhea and syphilis, and bone/joint infections.

Penicillins are classified based on an antimicrobial spectrum:

Natural penicillins are very active against gram-positive cocci but ineffective against most strains of *Staphylococcus aureus* (inactivated by enzyme penicillinase).

Penicillinase-resistant penicillins are effective against penicillinase-producing *Staphylococcus aureus* but are less effective against gram-positive cocci than the natural penicillins.

Broad-spectrum penicillins are effective against gram-positive cocci and some gram-negative bacteria (e.g., *Haemophilus influenzae, Escherichia coli, Proteus mirabilis*).

Extended-spectrum penicillins are effective against *Pseudomonas aeruginosa, Enterobacter, Proteus species, Klebsiella,* and some other gram-negative microorganisms.

Action

Penicillins inhibit cell wall synthesis or activate enzymes that disrupt the bacterial cell wall, causing a weakening in the cell wall, cell lysis, and cell death.

May be bacteriostatic or bactericidal. Most effective against bacteria undergoing active growth and division.

Antibiotics: Penicillins

Name	Availability	Dosage Range	Side Effects
NATURAL			
Penicillin G benzathine (Bicillin)	I: 600,000 units, 1.2 million units, 2.4 million units	A: 1.2 million units/day C: 0.3-1.2 million units/day	Mild diarrhea, nausea, vomiting, headaches, sore mouth/tongue, vaginal itching/discharge, allergic reaction (including anaphylaxis, skin rash, hives, itching)
Penicillin G potassium (Pfizerpen)	I: 1-, 2-, 3-, and 5-million unit vials	A: 2-24 million units/day C: 100-250,000 units/kg/day	Same as penicillin G benzathine
Penicillin G procaine (Wycillin)	I: 600,000 units, 1.2 million units, 2.4 million units	A, C: 0.6-1.2 million units/day	Same as penicillin G benzathine; increased risk of mental disturbances
Penicillin V (Pen-Vee K, V-Cillin-K)	T: 250 mg, 500 mg S: 125 mg/5 ml, 250 mg/5 ml	A: 0.5-2 g/day C: 25-50 mg/kg/day	Same as penicillin G benzathine
PENICILLINASE-RESISTANT			
Cloxacillin (Tegopen)	C: 250 mg, 500 mg S: 125 mg/5 ml	A: 1-2 g/day C: 50-100 mg/kg/day	Same as penicillin G benzathine; increased risk of liver toxicity
Dicloxacillin (Dynapen, Pathocil)	C: 125 mg, 250 mg, 500 mg S: 62.5 mg/5 ml	A: 1-2 g/day C: 12.5-25 mg/kg/day	Same as penicillin G benzathine Increased risk of liver toxicity

Continued

Antibiotics: Penicillins—cont'd

Name	Availability	Dosage Range	Side Effects
Nafcillin (Nafcil, Unipen)	C: 250 mg I: 500 mg, 1 g, 2 g	A (PO): 1-6 g/day; (IV): 2-6 g/day C (PO): 25-50 mg/kg/day; (IV): 50 mg/kg/day	Same as penicillin G benzathine; increased risk of interstitial nephritis
Oxacillin (Bactocill)	C: 250 mg, 500 mg S: 250 mg/5 ml I: 250 mg, 500 mg, 1 g, 2 g	A (PO/IV): 2-6 g/day C (PO/IV): 50-100 mg/kg/day	Same as penicillin G benzathine; increased risk of liver toxicity, interstitial nephritis
BROAD-SPECTRUM			
Amoxicillin (Amoxil, Polymox, Trimox)	T: 125 mg, 250 mg, 500 mg, 875 mg C: 250 mg, 500 mg S: 50 mg/ml, 125 mg/5 ml, 250 mg/5 ml	A: 0.75-1.5 g/day C: 20-40 mg/kg/day	Same as penicillin G benzathine
Amoxicillin/clavulanate (Augmentin)	T: 250 mg, 500 mg, 875 mg T (chewable): 125 mg, 200 mg, 250 mg, 400 mg S: 125 mg/5 ml, 200 mg/5 ml, 250 mg/5 ml, 400 mg/5 ml	A: 0.75-1.5 g/day C: 20-40 mg/kg/day	Same as penicillin G benzathine
Ampicillin (Omnipen, Polycillin, Principen)	C: 250 mg, 500 mg S: 125 mg/5 ml, 250 mg/5 ml I: 125 mg, 250 mg, 500 mg, 1 g, 2 g	A: 1-12 g/day C: 50-200 mg/kg/day	Same as penicillin G benzathine
Ampicillin/sulbactam (Unasyn)	I: 1.5 g, 3 g	A: 6-12 g/day C: 100-200 mg/kg/day	Same as penicillin G benzathine
Bacampicillin (Spectrobid)	T: 400 mg	A: 800-1-600 mg/day C: 25-50 mg/kg/day	Same as penicillin G benzathine
EXTENDED-SPECTRUM			
Carbenicillin (Geocillin)	T: 382 mg	A: 382-764 mg qid	Same as penicillin G benzathine
Piperacillin/tazobactam (Zosyn)	I: 2.25 g, 3.375 g, 4.5 g	A: 2.25-4.5 g q6-8h C: 200-400 mg/kg/day	Same as penicillin G benzathine
Ticarcillin/clavulanate (Timentin)	I: 3.1 g	A: 3.1 g q4-6h C: 200-300 mg/kg/day	Same as penicillin G benzathine (Timentin)

A, Adults; *C*, capsules; *C* (dosage), children; *I*, injection; *IV*, intravenously; *PO*, by mouth; *S*, suspension; *T*, tablets.

ANTIBIOTICS: SULFONAMIDES

Uses

The combination of sulfamethoxazole and trimethoprim is active against many bacteria except anaerobes, *Pseudomonas aeruginosa*, and many *Streptococcus faecalis* spp. It is also highly active and effective against *Pneumocystis carinii.*

Action

Sulfamethoxazole is a synthetic analogue of paraaminobenzoic acid, which competitively inhibits the synthesis of dihydropteric acid from PABA in microorganisms. Trimethoprim acts at a later step to inhibit the enzymatic reduction of dihydrofolic acid to tetrahydrofolic acid.

Antibiotics: Sulfonamides

Name	Availability	Usual Dosage Range	Side Effects
Sulfamethoxazole (SMX)/Trimethoprim (TMP) (Septra, Bactrim, Sulfatrim, others)	I: 80 mg/ml SMX + 16 mg/ml TMP T: 400 mg SMX + 80 mg TMP, 800 mg SMX + 160 mg TMP OS: 200 mg/5 ml SMX + 40 mg/5 ml TMP	8-10 mg/kg/day IV divided q6h or q8h or q12h 1 DS tablet PO bid or 2 ss tablets PO bid or 20 ml PO bid	Anorexia, nausea, vomiting, rash, urticaria, severe allergic reactions, fulminant hepatic necrosis, aplastic anemia, agranulocytosis, other blood dyscrasias

I, Injection; *DS,* double-strength; *IV,* intravenously; *OS,* oral suspension; *PO,* by mouth; *ss,* single-strength; *T,* tablets.

ANTIBIOTICS: TETRACYCLINES

Uses

Tetracyclines are broad-spectrum antibiotics that act against gram-negative, aerobic, and anaerobic bacteria, as well as spirochetes, mycoplasmas, rickettsiae, chlamydiae, and some protozoa.

Action

Bacteriostatic. Inhibit protein synthesis at the 30S ribosomal subunit.

ANTIBIOTICS: TETRACYCLINES

Name	Availability	Usual Dosage Range	Side Effects
Doxycycline (Doryx, Monodox, Vibra-Tabs, Vibramycin)	I: 100 mg/vial, 200 mg/vial T: 50 mg, 75 mg, 100 mg, 150 mg T (DR): 75 mg, 100 mg C: 50 mg, 75 mg, 100 mg, 150 mg OS: 25 mg/5 ml, 50 mg/5 ml	100mg IV/PO q12h	Gastrointestinal distress, photosensitivity, increased BUN, bulging fontanels, benign intracranial hypertension (rare)
Minocycline (Minocin, Vectrin)	T: 50 mg, 75 mg, 100 mg C: 50 mg, 75 mg, 100 mg	200 mg initially, then 100 mg PO q12h	Dizziness, light-headedness, vertigo, bulging fontanels, benign intracranial hypertension (rare)
Tetracycline (Bristacycline, Sumycin,	T: 250 mg, 500 mg C: 100 mg, 250 mg, 500 mg OS: 125 mg/5 ml	1-2 g/day PO in 2-4 divided doses	Diarrhea, nausea, vomiting, photosensitivity, rash, bulging fontanels, benign intracranial hypertension (rare)

BUN, Blood urea nitrogen; *C,* capsules; *DR,* delayed release; *I,* Injection; *OS,* oral suspension; *PO,* by mouth; *T,* tablets.

ANTIBIOTICS: METRONIDAZOLE

Uses

Metronidazole is a synthetic nitroimidazole active against *Trichomonas vaginalis*, *Entamoeba histolytica*, and *Giardia lamblia*.

Action

Bactericidal against nearly all obligate anaerobic bacteria including *Bacteroides fragilis*. It is inactive against aerobic bacteria and requires microbial reduction by a nitroreductase enzyme to form highly reactive intermediates that disrupt bacterial DNA and inhibit nucleic acid synthesis, leading to cell death.

ANTIBIOTICS: METRONIDAZOLE

Name	Availability	Usual Dosage Range	Side Effects
Metronidazole (Flagyl, Metro I.V., Metromidol)	I: 500 mg/vial, 500 mg/100 ml T: 250 mg, 500 mg R (ER): 750 mg C: 375 mg	7.5 mg/kg IV/PO q6h (max. 4.0 g/day), 500-750 mg PO tid	Ataxia, dizziness, headache, peripheral neuropathy, seizures, anorexia, GI discomfort, metallic taste perversion, nausea, vomiting, symptomatic candida cervicitis/vaginitis, vaginal discharge, disulfiram-like reaction, herheimer reaction, leukopenia, thrombocytopenia (rare), ototoxicity (rare)

I, Injection; *ER*, extended release; *IV*, intravenously; PO, by mouth; *R*, rectal; *T*, tablets.
NOTE: Dosages are usual adult dosage ranges. For specific dosages, please refer to the appropriate indications for which the antibiotic is used.

ANTIDEPRESSANTS

Uses

Used primarily for the treatment of depression. Imipramine is also used for childhood enuresis. Clomipramine is used only for obsessive-compulsive disorder (OCD). Monoamine oxidase (MAO) inhibitors are rarely used as initial therapy except for patients unresponsive to other therapy or when other therapy is contraindicated.

Action

Antidepressants are classified as tricyclic, MAO inhibitors, or second-generation antidepressants (further subdivided into selective serotonin reuptake inhibitors [SSRIs] and atypical antidepressants).

Antidepressants block metabolism, increase amount/effects of monoamine neurotransmitters, and act at receptor sites.

Antidepressants

Name	Availability	Uses	Dosage Range (per day)	Side Effects
TRICYCLICS				
Amitriptyline (Elavil)	T: 10 mg, 25 mg, 50 mg, 75 mg, 100 mg, 150 mg	Depression	40-300 mg	Drowsiness, blurred vision, constipation, confusion, postural hypotension, conduction defects, weight gain, seizure tendency
Clomipramine (Anafranil)	C: 25 mg, 50 mg, 75 mg	OCD	25-250 mg	Same as amitriptyline
Desipramine (Norpramin, Pertofrane)	T: 10 mg, 25 mg, 50 mg, 75 mg, 100 mg, 150 mg	Depression	25-100 mg	Same as amitriptyline
Doxepin (Sinequan)	C: 10 mg, 25 mg, 50 mg, 75 mg, 100 mg, 150 mg OC: 10 mg/ml	Depression	25-300 mg	Same as amitriptyline
Imipramine (Janimine, Tofranil)	T: 10 mg, 25 mg, 50 mg C: 75 mg, 100 mg, 125 mg, 150 mg	Depression, enuresis	30-300 mg	Same as amitriptyline
Nortriptyline (Aventyl, Pamelor)	C: 10 mg, 25 mg, 50 mg, 75 mg S: 10 mg/5 ml	Depression	25-100 mg	Same as amitriptyline
Protriptyline (Vivactil)	T: 5 mg, 10 mg	Depression	15-60 mg	Same as amitriptyline
MONOAMINE OXIDASE INHIBITORS (MAOIs)				
Phenelzine (Nardil)	T: 15 mg	Depression	15-90 mg	Sedation, hypertensive crisis, weight gain, orthostatic hypotension
Tranylcypromine (Parnate)	T: 10 mg	Depression	30-60 mg	Same as amitriptyline

Antidepressants—cont'd

Name	Availability	Uses	Dosage Range (per day)	Side Effects
SELECTIVE SEROTONIN REUPTAKE INHIBITORS (SSRIs)				
Citalopram (Celexa)	T: 20 mg, 40 mg S: 10 mg/5 ml	Depression	25-60 mg	Insomnia or sedation, nausea, agitation, headaches
Escitalopram (Lexapro)	T: 5 mg, 10 mg, 20 mg	Depression	10-20 mg	Insomnia or sedation, nausea, agitation, headaches
Fluoxetine (Prozac)	C: 10 mg, 20 mg, 40 mg T: 10 mg S: 20 mg/5 ml	Depression, OCD, bulimia	10-80 mg	Akathisia, sexual dysfunction, skin rash, hives, itching, decreased appetite, asthenia, diarrhea, drowsiness, headache, increased sweating, insomnia, nausea, tremors
Fluvoxamine (Luvox)	T: 25 mg, 50 mg, 100 mg	OCD	100-300 mg	Sexual dysfunction, fatigue, constipation, dizziness, drowsiness, headache, insomnia, nausea, vomiting
Paroxetine (Paxil)	T: 10 mg, 20 mg, 30 mg, 40 mg S: 10 mg/5 ml	Depression, OCD, panic attack, social anxiety disorder	20-50 mg	Asthenia, constipation, diarrhea, sweating, insomnia, nausea, sexual dysfunction, tremor, vomiting, urinary frequency or retention
Sertraline (Zoloft)	T: 25 mg, 50 mg, 100 mg S: 20 mg/ml	Depression, OCD, panic attack	50-200 mg	Sexual dysfunction, dizziness, drowsiness, anorexia, diarrhea, nausea, dry mouth, stomach cramps, decreased weight, headache, increased sweating, tremor, insomnia
ATYPICAL				
Bupropion (Wellbutrin, Wellbutrin SR, Wellbutrin XL)	T: 75 mg, 100 mg SR: 50 mg, 100 mg, 150 mg, 200 mg	Depression XL: 150 mg, 300 mg	150-450 mg	Insomnia, irritability, seizures
Mirtazapine (Remeron)	T: 15 mg, 30 mg, 45 mg	Depression	15-45 mg	Sedation, dry mouth, weight gain, agranulocytosis, liver toxicity
Nefazodone (Serzone)	T: 50 mg, 100 mg, 150 mg, 200 mg, 250 mg	Depression	200-600 mg	Sedation, orthostatic hypotension, nausea

Continued

ANTIDEPRESSANTS—CONT'D

Name	Availability	Uses	Dosage Range (per day)	Side Effects
Trazodone (Desyrel)	T: 50 mg, 100 mg, 150 mg, 300 mg	Depression	50-600 mg	Sedation, orthostatic hypotension, priapism
Venlafaxine (Effexor)	T: 25 mg, 37.5 mg, 50 mg, 75 mg, 100 mg C (ER): 37.5 mg, 75 mg, 150 mg	Depression, anxiety	75-375 mg	Increased blood pressure, agitation, sedation, insomnia, nausea
Duloxetine (Cymbalta)	C: 20 mg, 30 mg, 60 mg C (DR): 20 mg, 30 mg, 60 mg	Depression	4-60 mg	Nausea, dry mouth, constipation, decreased appetite, fatigue, somnolence, increased sweating

C, Capsules; *DR,* delayed release; *ER,* extended release; *OC,* oral concentrate; *OCD,* obsessive-compulsive disorder; *S,* suspension; *SR,* sustained release; *T,* tablets; *XL,* extended release.

ANTIDIABETIC AGENTS

Uses

Management of diabetes.

Action

Sulfonylureas: Interact with ATP-sensitive potassium channels in the beta cell membrane to increase secretion of insulin.

Non-Sulfonylurea Secretagogues: Bind to ATP-sensitive potassium channels on beta cells and increase insulin release.

Biguanides: Acts mainly by decreasing hepatic glucose output and, to a lesser extent, by increasing peripheral glucose utilization.

Thiazolidinediones: Increase the insulin sensitivity of adipose tissue, skeletal muscle, and the liver.

Alpha-Glucosidase Inhibitors: Inhibit the alpha-glucosidase enzymes that line the brush border of the small intestine, interfering with hydrolysis of carbohydrates and delaying absorption of glucose and other monosaccharides.

Antidiabetic Agents

Name	Availability	Dosage Range	Side Effects
SULFONYLUREAS (FIRST GENERATION)			
Chlorpropamide (Diabenese)	T: 100 mg, 250 mg	250-375 mg/day	Hypoglycemia particularly in elderly patients with impaired renal or hepatic function. Glyburide appears to cause a higher incidence of hypoglycemia than chlorpropamide, glipizide, or glimepiride Mild weight gain
Tolazamide (Tolinase)	T: 100 mg, 250 mg	250-500 mg/day	
Tolbutamide	T: 500 mg	1000-2000 mg/day	
SULFONYLUREAS (SECOND GENERATION)			
Glimepiride (Amaryl)	T: 1 mg, 2 mg, 4 mg	1-4 mg/day	
Glipizide (Glucotrol, Glucotrol XL)	T: 5 mg, 10 mg T (ER): 2.5 mg, 5 mg, 10 mg	5-20 mg/day	
Glyburide (DiaBeta, Micronase, Glynase Prestab)	T: 1.25 mg, 2.5 mg, 5 mg 5 mgT (micronized): 1.5 mg, 3 mg, 6 mg	5-20 mg/day 3-12 mg/day	
NON-SULFONYLUREA SECRETAGOGUES			
Nateglinide (Starlix)	T: 60 mg, 120 mg	60-120 mg tid before meals	Hypoglycemia may be less frequent with Nateglinide and Repaglinide than with Sulfonylureas
Repaglinide(Prandin)	T: 0.5 mg, 1 mg, 2 mg	1-4 mg tid before meals	
BIGUANIDES			
Metformin (Glucophage, Glucophage XR, Fortamet, Riomet)	T: 500 mg, 850 mg, 1000 mg T: (ER): 500 mg, 750 mg, 1000 mg Oral liquid: 500 mg/5 ml	1500-2550 mg/day	Does not cause hypoglycemia when used alone, does not cause weight gain when used either alone or in combination, may even produce a modest weight loss of 2 to 3 kg, metallic taste, nausea, diarrhea, abdominal pain, lactic acidosis (rare but potentially fatal)

Continued

Antidiabetic Agents—cont'd

Name	Availability	Dosage Range	Side Effects
THIAZOLIDINEDIONES			
Pioglitazone (Actos)	T: 15 mg, 30 mg, 45 mg	15-45 mg	Hepatotoxicity (a few well-documentated cases but rare), weight gain and fluid retention (can rarely lead to congestive heart failure)
Rosiglitazone (Avandia)	T: 2 mg, 4 mg, 8 mg	4-8 mg	
ALPHA-GLUCOSIDASE INHIBITORS			
Acarbose (Precose)	T: 25 mg, 50 mg, 100 mg	50-100 mg tid with meals	Abdominal pain, diarrhea, flatulence Acarbose in high doses has been associated rarely with moderate elevations in hepatic enzymes; fatal hepatic failure has been reported with acarbose Does not cause hypoglycemia when given alone
Miglitol (Glyset)	T: 25 mg, 50 mg, 100 mg	50-100 mg tid with meals	
OTHER			
Exenatide (Byetta)	I: 250 mcg/ml (prefilled pen)	5-10 mcg subQ bid before breakfast and dinner	Nausea, vomiting, diarrhea, increased risk of mild to moderate hypoglycemia when used in combination with a sulfonylurea
Pramlintide (Symlin)	I: 3 mg/5 ml vial (0.6 mg/ml)	60-120 mcg subQ tid before main meals	Headache, dizziness, fatigue, increased risk of insulin-induced severe hypoglycemia, nausea, vomiting, anorexia, abdominal pain, coughing, pharyngitis, systemic allergic reactions

ER, Extended release; *subQ*, subcutaneously; *T*, tablets.

Insulin Products

Name	Availability	Onset	Peak	Duration
Rapid-Acting		10-30 min	30-60 min	3-5 h
Insulin aspart (Novolog)	Vial: 10 ml Cartridge: 3 ml			
Insulin lispro (Humalog)	Vial: 10 ml Cartridge: 1.5 ml, 3 ml			
Insulin glulisine (Apidra)	Vial: 10 ml			
Regular		30-60 min	1.5-2 hrs	5-12 h
Humulin R	Vial: 10 ml Cartridge: 1.5 ml			
Novolin R	Vial: 10 ml Cartridge: 1.5 ml, 3 ml Syringe: 1.5 ml, 3 ml			
Intermediate-Acting		1-2 h	4-8 h	10-20 h
NPH (Humulin N, Novolin N)	Vial (Humulin N): 10 ml Cartridge (Humulin N): 3 ml Vial (Novolin N): 10 ml Cartridge (Novolin N): 1.5 ml Syringe (Novolin N): 1.5 ml			
Lente (Humulin L)	Vial: 10 ml			
Long-Acting				
Insulin detemir (Levimir)		1 h	No peak	20 h
Insulin glargine (Lantus)		1-2 h	No peak	24 h
Ultralente (Humulin U)		2-4 h	8-20 h	16-24 h

ANTIDIARRHEALS

Uses

Acute diarrhea, chronic diarrhea of inflammatory bowel disease, reduction of fluid from ileostomies.

Action

Systemic agents: Disrupt peristaltic movements, decrease gastrointestinal motility, increase transit time of intestinal contents.

Local agents: Adsorb toxic substances and fluids to large surface areas of particles in the preparation.

Antidiarrheals

Name	Availability	Type	Dosage Range
Bismuth subsalicylate (Pepto-Bismol)	T: 262 mg C: 262 mg L: 130 mg/15 ml, 262 mg/15 ml, 524 mg/15 ml	Local	A: 2 T or 30 ml C (9-12 yrs): 1 T or 15 ml C (6-9 yrs): $^{2}/_{3}$ T or 10 ml C (3-6 yrs): $^{1}/_{3}$ T or 5 ml
Diphenoxylate (with atropine) (Lomotil)	T: 2.5 mg L: 2.5 mg/5 ml	Systemic	A: 5 mg qid C: 0.3-0.4 mg/kg/day in 4 divided doses (L)
Kaolin (with pectin) (Kaopectate)	Suspension	Local	A: 60-120 ml after each bowel movement C (6-12 yrs): 30-60 ml C (3-6 yrs): 15-30 ml
Loperamide (Imodium)	C: 2 mg T: 2 mg L: 1 mg/5 ml, 1 mg/ml	Systemic	A: Initially, 4 mg; 16 mg/day maximum C (8-12 yrs): 2 mg tid (5-8 yrs): 2 mg bid (2-5 yrs): 1 mg tid (L)

A, Adults; *C,* capsules; *C* (dosage), children; *L,* liquid; *T,* tablets.

ANTIEMETICS FOR CHEMOTHERAPY-INDUCED NAUSEA AND VOMITING

Uses

Prevention of chemotherapy-induced acute emesis (nausea and vomiting that occurs within the first 24 hours of chemotherapy). Prevention and treatment of chemotherapy-induced delayed emesis (nausea and vomiting that occurs after 24 hours after chemotherapy).

Action

Peripheral neuroreceptors and the chemoreceptor trigger zone (CTZ) are known to contain receptors for serotonin, histamine (H1 and H2), dopamine, acetylcholine, opioids, and other endogenous neurotransmitters. Many antiemetics act by competitively blocking receptors for these substances, thereby inhibiting stimulation of peripheral nerves at the CTZ, and perhaps at the vomiting center.

Antiemetics

Name	Availability	Usual Adult Dosage	Some Common or Serious Side Effects
5-HYDROXYTRYPTAMINE TYPE 3 RECEPTOR ANTAGONISTS (5-HT3 ANTAGONISTS)			
Ondansetron (Zofran)	I: 2 mg/ml, 0.64 mg/ml OS: 4 mg/5 ml T: 4 mg, 8 mg, 24 mg ODT: 4 mg, 8 mg	32 mg IV 30 min before chemotherapy *OR* 0.15 mg/kg IV 30 min before chemotherapy, repeated 4 and 8 h after the first dose Moderately emetogenic chemotherapy: 8 mg PO 30 min before chemotherapy and repeat in 8 h, then 8 mg PO q12h for 1-2 days after chemotherapy Highly emetogenic chemotherapy: 24 mg PO 30 min before chemotherapy	Constipation, diarrhea, dry mouth, elevated liver function enzymes, headache, malaise, fatigue, anaphylaxis (rare), arrhythmias (rare), bronchospasm
Granisetron (Kytril)	I: 1 mg/ml OS: 2 mg/10 ml T: 1 mg	2 mg PO 1 h before chemotherapy OR 1 mg PO 1 h before and 1 mg 12 h after chemotherapy 10 mcg/kg IV 30 min before chemotherapy	Abdominal pain, asthenia, constipation, diarrhea, headache, somnolence
Dolasetron (Anzemet)	I: 100 mg/5 ml T: 50 mg, 100 mg	100 mg PO 1 h before chemotherapy 1.8 mg/kg *OR* 100 mg IV 30 min before chemotherapy	Blurred vision, dizziness, drowsiness, fatigue, sedation, fever, chills, headache, increased liver function tests, pruritus, sleep disorders, urinary retention, arrhythmias, hypotension
Palonosetron (Aloxi)	I: 0.25 mg/5 ml	0.25 mg IV as a single dose 30 min before start of chemotherapy	Constipation (rare but may be severe), diarrhea, headache, dizziness, fatigue, abdominal pain, insomnia, arrhythmias (rare)

Continued

ANTIEMETICS—CONT'D

Name	Availability	Usual Adult Dosage	Some Common or Serious Side Effects
CORTICOSTEROIDS			
Dexamethasone (Decadron, Hexadrol, Mymethasone)	I: 4 mg/ml, 10 mg/ml Elixir: 0.5 mg/5 ml T: 0.25 mg, 0.5 mg, 0.75 mg, 1.5 mg, 4 mg, 6 mg	20 mg IV before chemotherapy, 8 mg IV/PO bid for 3 days after chemotherapy	Mood changes, increased appetite, GI irritation, ulceration, fluid retention, weight gain, may mask signs of infection
DOPAMINE ANTAGONISTS			
Metoclopramide (Reglan)	I: 5 mg/ml OS: 5 mg/5 ml T: 5 mg, 10 mg C (ER): ODT: 5 mg, 10 mg	2 mg/kg/dose PO/IV q2-4h for 2 to 5 doses	Sedation, dose-related diarrhea, extrapyramidal effects
PHENOTHIAZINES			
Prochlorperazine (Compazine, Compro)	I: 5 mg/ml Syrup: 5 mg/5ml T: 5 mg, 10 mg, 25 mg C (ER): 10 mg, 15 mg Suppository: 2.5 mg, 5 mg, 25 mg	10 mg IV/PO q3-6h	Sedation, dry mouth, blurred vision, constipation, nasal congestion, urinary retention, extrapyramidal effects, hypotension, hypersensitivity, rare pancytopenia
ANTIHISTAMINES			
Diphenhydramine (Benadryl, others)	I: 50 mg/ml C: 25 mg, 50 mg Elixir: 12.5 mg/5 ml	Used to decrease side effects from other antiemetics (not effective as an antiemetic when used alone): 50 mg PO q4h prn for restlessness or acute dystonic reactions	Dizziness, dry mouth/nose/throat, dyskinesias, sedation, sleepiness, thickening of bronchial secretions
CANNABINIOIDS			
Dronabinol (Marinol)	C: 2.5 mg, 5 mg, 10 mg	5 mg/m(2) PO 1-3h before chemotherapy, 5 mg/m(2) PO q2-4h after chemotherapy for a total of 4-6 doses/day, may increase dose by 2.5 mg/(2) increments to a max dose of 15 mg/m^2/dose	Abnormal thinking, depersonalization, euphoria, paranoid reactions, confusion, depression, dizziness, drowsiness, ataxia, impaired coordination, vertigo, dry mouth, nausea, vomiting, hypertension, hypotension, palpitations, tachycardia, vasodilation/flushing
SUBSTANCE P ANTAGONISTS (NK-1 RECEPTOR ANTAGONISTS)			
Aprepitant (Emend)	C: 80 mg, 125 mg	125 mg PO 1 h before chemotherapy on day 1, 80 mg on day 2 and day 3	Somnolence, fatigue, hiccups

C, capsules; *ER*, extended release; *GI*, gastrointestinal; *I*, injection; *IV*, intravenously; *ODT*, orally disintegrating tablets; *OS*, oral suspension; *PO*, by mouth; *prn*, as needed; *T*, tablets.

ANTIHYPERTENSIVE AGENTS

Uses

Used for control of hypertension. Long-term treatment with antihypertensives may decrease morbidity and mortality attributable to high blood pressure, such as in cases of stroke, cardiovascular disease, and kidney disease.

Action

Thiazides: Act at the cortical diluting segment of nephron, block reabsorption of Na, Cl, and water; promote excretion of Na, Cl, K, and water.

Loop: Act primarily at the thick ascending limb of Henle's loop to inhibit Na, Cl, and water absorption.

Potassium-Sparing: Spironolactone blocks aldosterone action on distal nephron (causes K retention, Na excretion). Triamterene, amiloride act on distal nephron, decreasing Na reuptake and reducing K secretion.

Angiotensin-Converting Enzyme Inhibitors: Block the enzyme responsible for conversion of angiotensin I to angiotensin II, a powerful vasoconstrictor.

Angiotensin Receptor Blockers: Block the angiotensin II, subtype 1 receptor.

Beta Adrenergic Blockers: The exact mechanism of action is unclear. Bisoprolol, atenolol, metoprolol, acebutolol, and betaxolol are cardioselective in low doses. They have a greater effect on cardiac ($beta_1$) adrenergic receptors than on $beta_2$-adrenergic receptors in bronchi and blood vessels. They become less selective as their dosage is increased. Propranolol, timolol, nadolol, pindolol, penbutolol, and carteolol are nonselective.

Calcium Channel Blockers: All cause vasodilation, which decreases peripheral resistance. They exert differing effects on vascular smooth muscle, cardiac myocytes, and cardiac conducting tissues.

Alpha Adrenergic Blockers: Block postsynaptic $alpha_1$ adrenergic receptors.

Central Alpha-Adrenergic Agonists: Exert central $alpha_2$-adrenergic agonist effect that reduce sympathetic drive to the peripheral vasculature.

ANTIHYPERTENSIVE AGENTS

		Diuretics	
Name	Availability (Oral Formulations)	Dosage Range (per day)	Side Effects
THIAZIDE-TYPE			
Chlorothiazide (Diuril)	T: 250 mg, 200 mg	125-500 mg	
Hydrochlorothiazide (Microzide)	C: 12.5 mg T: 25 mg, 50 mg	12.5-50 mg	Hyperuricemia, hypokalemia, hypomagnesemia, hyperglycemia, hyponatremia, hypercalcemia, hypercholesterolemia, hypertriglyceridemia, pancreatitis, rashes and other allergic reactions, sexual dysfunction in men, photosensitivity reactions
Chlorthalidone (Thalitone)	T: 15 mg, 25 mg, 50 mg	12.5-50 mg	
Indapamide (Lozol)	T: 1.25 mg, 2.5 mg	1.25-5 mg	
Metolazone (Zaroxolyn)	T: 2.5 mg, 5 mg, 10 mg	1.25-5 mg	
Polythiazide (Renese)	T: 1 mg, 2 mg, 4 mg	2-4 mg	
LOOP			
Bumetanide (Bumex)	T: 0.5 mg, 1 mg, 2 mg	0.5-2 mg	Dehydration, circulatory collapse hypokalemia, hyponatremia, hypomagnesemia, hyperglycemia, metabolic alkalosis, hyperuricemia, blood dyscrasias, rashes, hypercholesterolemia, hypertriglyceridemia
Ethacrynic acid (Edecrin)	T: 25 mg, 50 mg	25-100 mg	
Furosemide (Lasix)	T: 20 mg, 40 mg, 80 mg	20-80 mg	
Torsemide (Demadex)	T: 5 mg, 10 mg, 20 mg, 100 mg	2.5-10 mg	

Continued

Antihypertensive Agents—cont'd

		Diuretics	
Name	Availability (Oral Formulations)	Dosage Range (per day)	Side Effects
POTASSIUM-SPARING			
Amiloride (Midamor)	T: 5 mg	5-10 mg	Hyperkalemia, GI disturbances, rash, headache
Eplerenone (Inspra)	T: 25 mg, 50 mg	25-100 mg	Hyperkalemia, hyponatremia
Spironoloactone (Aldactone)	T: 25 mg, 50 mg, 100 mg	12.5-100 mg	Hyperkalemia, hyponatremia, mastodynia, gynecomastia, menstrual abnormalities, GI disturbances, rash
Triamterene (Dyrenium)	C: 50 mg, 100 mg	50-150 mg	Hyperkalemia, GI disturbances, nephrolithiasis
		Angiotension-Converting Enzyme (ACE) Inhibitors	
Benazepril (Lotensin)	T: 5 mg, 10 mg, 20 mg, 40 mg	10-80 mg	Cough, hypotension (particularly with diuretic use or volume depletions), rash, acute renal failure in patients with bilateral renal artery stenosis or stenosis of the artery to a solitary kidney, angioedema, hyperkalemia particularly if also taking potassium supplements or potassium-sparing diuretics, mild-to-moderate loss of taste, hepatotoxicity, pancreatitis Blood dyscrasias and renal damage rare except in patients with renal dysfunction Increased fetal mortality with second- and third-trimester exposure
Captopril (Capoten)	T: 12.5 mg, 25 mg, 50 mg, 100 mg	12.5-150 mg	
Enalapril (Vasotec)	T: 2.5 mg, 5 mg, 10 mg, 20 mg	2.5-40 mg	
Fosinopril (Monopril)	T: 10 mg, 20 mg, 40 mg	10-80 mg	
Lisinopril (Prinivil, Zestril)	T: 2.5 mg, 5 mg, 10 mg, 20 mg, 30 mg, 40 mg	5-40 mg	
Moexipril (Univasc)	T: 7.5 mg, 15 mg	7.5-30 mg	
Perindopril (Aceon)	T: 2 mg, 4 mg, 8 mg	4-8 mg	
Quinapril (Accupril)	T: 5 mg, 10 mg, 20 mg, 40 mg	5-80 mg	
Ramipril (Altace)	C: 1.25 mg, 2.5 mg, 5 mg, 10 mg	1.25-20 mg	
Trandolapril (Mavik)	T: 1 mg, 2 mg, 4 mg	1-8 mg	
		Angiotensin Receptor Blockers (ARBS)	
Candesartan (Atacand)	T: 4 mg, 8 mg, 16 mg, 32 mg	8-32 mg	Similar to ACE inhibitors, including increased fetal mortality with second- and third-trimester exposure, but do not cause cough and rarely cause angioedema, loss of taste, hepatic dysfunction; rarely cause rhabdomyolysis
Eprosartan (Teveten)	T: 400 mg, 600 mg	400-800 mg	
Irbesartan (Avapro)	T: 75 mg, 150 mg, 300 mg	150-300 mg	
Losartan (Cozaar)	T: 25 mg, 50 mg, 100 mg	25-100 mg	
Olmesartan (Benicar)	T: 5 mg, 20 mg, 40 mg	20-40 mg	
Telmisartan (Micardis)	T: 20 mg, 40 mg, 80 mg	20-80 mg	
Valsartan (Diovan)	T: 40 mg, 80 mg, 160 mg, 320 mg	80-320 mg	

Antihypertensive Agents—cont'd

Beta Adrenergic Blockers			
Name	Availability (Oral Formulations	Dosage Range (per day)	Side Effects
Atenolol (Tenormin)	T: 25 mg, 50 mg, 100 mg	25-100 mg	Fatigue, depression, bradycardia, impotence, decreased exercise tolerance, congestive heart failure, worsening of peripheral arterial insufficiency May aggravate allergic reactions, bronchospasm May mask symptoms of and delay recovery from hypoglycemia, Raynaud's phenomenon, insomnia, vivid dreams or hallucinations, acute mental disorder, increased serum triglycerides, decreased HDL cholesterol Sudden withdrawal may lead to exacerbation of angina and myocardial infarction
Betaxolol (Kerlone)	T: 10 mg, 20 mg	4-40 mg	
Bisoprolol (Zebeta)	T: 5 mg, 10 mg	5-20 mg	
Metoprolol (Lopressor, (Toprol-XL))	T: 25 mg, 50 mg, 100 mg T (ER): 25 mg, 50 mg, 100 mg, 200 mg	50-200 mg 25-400 mg	
Nadolol (Corgard)	T: 20 mg, 40 mg, 80 mg, 120 mg, 160 mg	20-320 mg	
Propranolol (Inderal, Inderal-LA, InnoPran XL)	T: 10 mg, 20 mg, 40 mg, 60 mg, 80 mg C (ER): 60 mg, 80 mg, 120 mg, 160 mg	40-240 mg 60-240 mg	
Timolol (Blocadren)	T: 5 mg, 10 mg, 20 mg	10-60 mg	
BETA BLOCKERS WITH INTRINSIC SYMPATHOMIMETIC ACTIVITY			
Acebutolol (Sectral)	C: 200 mg, 400 mg	200-1200 mg	Similar to other beta adrenergic–blocking drugs, but with less resting bradycardia and lipid changes Acebutolol has been associated with a positive antinuclear antibody test and occasional drug-induced lupus
Carteolol (Cartrol)	T: 2.5 mg, 5 mg	2.5-10 mg	
Penbutolol (Levatol)	T: 20 mg	10-80 mg	
Pindolol	T: 5 mg, 10 mg	10-60 mg	
BETA BLOCKERS WITH ALPHA-BLOCKING ACTIVITY			
Carvedilol (Coreg)	T: 3.125 mg, 6.25 mg, 12.5 mg, 25 mg	12.5-50 mg	Similar to other beta adrenergic–blocking drugs, but more orthostatic hypotension, hepatotoxicity
Labetalol (Normodyne, Trandate)	T: 100 mg, 200 mg, 300 mg	200-1200 mg	

Continued

Antihypertensive Agents—cont'd

Calcium-Channel Blockers			
Name	Availability (Oral Formulations)	Dosage Range (per day)	Side Effects
Diltiazem (Cardizem CD, Cardizem LA, Cartia XT, Dilacor XR, Diltia XT, Tiazac, generics)	C (ER, once/day): 120 mg, 180 mg, 240 mg, 300 mg, 360 mg, 420 mg C (ER, bid): 60 mg, 90 mg, 120 mg, 180 mg, 240 mg, 300 mg	120-540 mg (once/day) 120-360 mg (in divided doses bid)	
Verapamil (Calan, Calan SR, Isoptin SR, Covera-HS, Verelan, Verelan PM, generics)	T: 40 mg, 80 mg, 120 mg T (ER): 120 mg, 180 mg, 240 mg T (ER, once/day): 180 mg, 240 mg C (ER): 120 mg, 180 mg, 240 mg, 360 mg C (ER): 100 mg, 200 mg, 300 mg	120-480 mg (in divided doses bid or tid) 120-480 mg (once/day or in divided doses bid) 180-240 mg (once/day) 120-480 mg (once/day) 100-400 mg (once/day)	Dizziness, headache, edema, constipation (especially verapamil), AV block, bradycardia, heart failure, lupus-like rash with diltiazem
DIHYDROPYRIDINES			
Amlodipine (Norvasc)	T: 2.5 mg, 5 mg, 10 mg	2.5-10 mg	Dizziness, headache, peripheral edema (more than with verapamil and diltiazem, more common in women), flushing, tachycardia, rash, gingival hyperplasia
Felodipine (Plendil)	T (ER): 2.5 mg, 5 mg, 10 mg	2.5-10 mg	
Isradipine (DynaCirc, DynaCirc CR)	C: 2.5 mg, 5 mg T (ER): 5 mg, 10 mg	5-10 mg	
Nicardipine (Cardene, Cardene SR)	C: 20 mg, 30 mg C (ER): 30 mg, 45 mg, 60 mg	60-120 mg	
Nifdedipine (Adalat CC, Procardia XL)	T (ER): 30 mg, 60 mg, 90 mg	30-90 mg	
Nisoldipine (Sular)	T (ER): 10 mg, 20 mg, 30 mg, 40 mg	10-60 mg	

Antihypertensive Agents—cont'd

Alpha Adrenergic Blockers			
Name	Availability (Oral Formulations)	Dosage Range (per day)	Side Effects
Prazosin (Minipress)	C: 1 mg, 2 mg, 5 mg	1-20 mg	Syncope with first dose (less likely with terazosin and doxazosin), dizziness and vertigo, headache, palpitations, fluid retention, drowsiness, weakness, anticholinergic effects, priapism, thrombocytopenia, atrial fibrillation
Terazosin (Hytrin)	C: 1 mg, 2 mg, 5 mg, 10 mg	1-20 mg	
Doxazosin (Cardura)	T: 1 mg, 2 mg, 4 mg, 8 mg	1-16 mg	
CENTRAL ALPHA ADRENERGIC AGONISTS			
Clonidine (Catapres)	T: 0.1 mg, 0.2 mg, 0.3 mg	0.1-0.6 mg	CNS reactions similar to methyldopa, but more sedation and dry mouth, bradycardia, heart block, rebound hypertension
Guanabenz	T: 4 mg, 8 mg	4-64 mg	Similar to clonidine
Guanfacine (Tenex)	T: 1 mg, 2 mg	1-3 mg	Similar to clonidine but milder
Methyldopa (Aldomet)	T: 125 mg, 250 mg, 500 mg	250 mg-2 g	Sedation, fatigue, depression, dry mouth, orthostatic hypotension, bradycardia, heart block, autoimmune disorders including colitis, hepatitis, hepatic necrosis, Coombs'-positive hemolytic anemia, lupuslike syndrome, thrombocytopenia, red cell aplasia, impotence
DIRECT VASODILATORS			
Hydralazine (Apresoline)	T: 10 mg, 25 mg, 50 mg, 100 mg	40-200 mg	Tachycardia, aggravation of angina, headache, dizziness, fluid retention, nasal congestion, lupus-like syndrome, hepatitis
Minoxidil	T: 2.5 mg, 10 mg	2.5-40 mg	Tachycardia, aggravation of angina, marked fluid retention, pericardial effusion, hair growth on face and body
Hydralazine (Apresoline)	T: 10 mg, 25 mg, 50 mg, 100 mg	40-200 mg	Tachycardia, aggravation of angina, headache, dizziness, fluid retention, nasal congestion, lupus-like syndrome, hepatitis
PERIPHERAL ADRENERGIC NEURON ANTAGONISTS			
Reserpine	T: 0.1 mg, 0.25 mg	0.1-0.25 mg	Nasal stuffiness, drowsiness, GI disturbances, bradycardia, psychic depression, nightmare with high doses, tardive dyskinesia

AV, Atrioventricular; *C,* capsules; *CNS,* central nervous system; *ER,* extended release; *GI,* gastrointestinal; *T,* tablets.

ANTIVIRALS

Uses

Treatment of human immunodeficiency virus (HIV) infection. Treatment of cytomegalovirus (CMV) retinitis in patients with AIDS, acute herpes zoster (shingles), genital herpes (recurrent), mucosal and cutaneous herpes simplex virus, chickenpox, and influenza A viral illness.

Action

Possible mechanisms of action of antivirals used for non-HIV infection may include interference with viral DNA synthesis and viral replication, inactivation of viral DNA polymerases, incorporation and termination of the growing viral DNA chain, prevention of release of viral nucleic acid into the host cell, or interference with viral penetration into cells.

Antivirals

Name	Availability	Uses	Side Effects
Acyclovir (Zovirax)	T: 400 mg, 800 mg C: 200 mg I: 50 mg/ml	Mucosal/cutaneous HSV-1 and HSV-2, varicella zoster (shingles), genital herpes, herpes simplex, encephalitis, chickenpox	Malaise, anorexia, nausea, vomiting, light-headedness
Amantadine (Symmetrel)	C: 100 mg S: 50 mg/5 ml	Influenza A	Anxiety, dizziness, light-headedness, headaches, nausea, loss of appetite
Cidofovir (Vistide)	I: 75 mg/ml	CMV retinitis	Decreased urination, fever, chills, diarrhea, nausea, vomiting, headaches, loss of appetite
Famciclovir (Famvir)	T: 125 mg, 250 mg, 500 mg	Herpes zoster, genital herpes	Headaches
Foscarnet (Foscavir)	I: 24 mg/ml	CMV retinitis, HSV infections	Decreased urination, abdominal pain, nausea, vomiting, dizziness, fatigue, headaches
Ganciclovir (Cytovene)	C: 250 mg, 500 mg I: 500 mg	CMV retinitis, CMV disease	Sore throat, fever, unusual bleeding/bruising
Oseltamivir (Tamiflu)	C: 75 mg S: 12 mg/ml	Influenza	Diarrhea, nausea, vomiting
Ribavirin (Virazole)	Aerosol: 6 g	Lowers respiratory infections in infants, children due to respiratory syncytial virus (RSV)	Anemia
Valacyclovir (Valtrex)	T: 500 mg	Herpes zoster, genital herpes	Headaches, nausea
Valganciclovir (Valcyte)	T: 450 mg	CMV retinitis	Anemia, abdominal pain, diarrhea, headaches, nausea, vomiting, numbness in hands/feet
Zanamivir (Relenza)	Inhalation: 5 mg	Influenza	Cough, diarrhea, dizziness, headaches, nausea, vomiting
Zidovudine (Retrovir)	T: 300 mg C: 100 mg S: 50 mg/5 ml	HIV infection	Unusual tiredness, fever, chills, headaches, nausea, muscle pain

AIDS, Acquired immune deficiency syndrome; *C,* capsules; *CMV,* cytomegalovirus; *HIV,* human immunodeficiency virus; *HSV-1,* herpes simplex virus type 1; *HSV-2,* herpes simplex virus type 2; *I,* injection; *OS,* oral solution; *S,* syrup; *T,* tablets.

CANCER CHEMOTHERAPEUTIC AGENTS

Uses

Treatment of a variety of cancers; may be palliative or curative. Treatment of choice in hematologic cancers. Frequently used as adjunctive therapy (e.g., with surgery, irradiation); most effective when tumor mass has been removed or reduced by radiation. Frequently used in combinations to increase therapeutic results, decrease toxic effects. Certain agents may be used in nonmalignant conditions; polycythemia vera, psoriasis, rheumatoid arthritis, or immunosuppression in organ transplantation.

Action

Most antineoplastics inhibit cell replication by interfering with the supply of nutrients or genetic components of the cell (DNA or RNA). Some antineoplastics, referred to as *cell cycle–specific* (CCS), are particularly effective during a specific phase of cell reproduction (e.g., antimetabolites and plant alkaloids). Other antineoplastics, referred to as *cell cycle–nonspecific*, act independently of a specific phase of cell division (e.g., alkylating agents and antibiotics). Some hormones are also classified as antineoplastics.

Anticancer Agents

Name	Availability	Side Effects
Abarelix (Plenaxis)	I: 100 mg	Serious or life-threatening reactions, allergic skin reactions, prolong QT interval, changes in liver function, loss in bone mineral density, hot flashes, problems sleeping, pain, breast enlargement/pain, constipation
Aldesleukin (Proleukin)	I: 22 million units Powder	Hypotension, sinus tachycardia, nausea, vomiting, diarrhea, renal impairment, anemia, rash, fatigue, agitation, pulmonary congestion, dyspnea, fever, chills, oliguria, weight gain, dizziness
Alemtuzumab (Campath)	I: 30 mg/3 ml	Rigors, fever, fatigue, hypotension, neutropenia, anemia, sepsis, dyspnea, bronchitis, pneumonia, urticaria
Alitretinoin (Panretin)	Gel: 0.1%	Burning, pain, edema, dermatitis, rash, skin disorders
Altretamine (Hexalen)	C: 50 mg	Nausea, vomiting, myelosuppression, peripheral neuropathy, altered mood, ataxia, dizziness, nervousness, vertigo
Aminoglutethimide (Cytadren)	T: 250 mg	Orthostatic hypotension, hypothyroidism, vomiting, anorexia, rash, drowsiness, headaches, fever, myalgia
Anastrozole (Arimidex)	T: 1 mg	Peripheral edema, chest pain, nausea, vomiting, diarrhea, constipation, abdominal pain, anorexia, pharyngitis, vaginal hemorrhage, anemia, leukopenia, rash, weight gain, sweating, increased appetite, pain, headaches, dizziness, depression, paresthesias, hot flashes, increased cough, dry mouth, asthenia, dyspnea, phlebitis
Arsenic trioxide (Trisenox)	I: 10 mg/ml	Atrioventricular block, GI hemorrhage, hypertension, hypoglycemia, hypokalemia, hypomagnesemia, neutropenia, oliguria, prolonged QT interval, seizures, sepsis, thrombocytopenia

Continued

Anticancer Agents—cont'd

Name	Availability	Side Effects
Asparaginase (Elspar)	I: 10,000 units	Anorexia, nausea, vomiting, liver toxicity, pancreatitis, nephrotoxicity, clotting factor abnormalities, malaise, confusion, lethargy, EEG changes, respiratory distress, fever, hyperglycemia, depression, stomatitis, allergic reactions, drowsiness
Azacitidine (Vidaza)	I: 100 mg	Nausea, anemia, thrombocytopenia, vomiting, pyrexia, leukopenia, diarrhea, fatigue, injection site erythema, constipation, neutropenia, ecchymosis
BCG (Tice BCG, TheraCys)	I: 50 mg, 81 mg	Nausea, vomiting, anorexia, diarrhea, dysuria, hematuria, cystitis, urinary urgency, anemia, malaise, fever, chills
Bevacizumab (Avastin)	I: 100 mg, 400 mg	Asthenia, pain, hypertension, diarrhea, leukopenia, abdominal pain, headache, nausea, vomiting, anorexia, stomatitis, constipation, upper respiratory infection, epistaxis, dyspnea, exfoliative dermatitis, proteinuria
Bexarotene (Targretin)	C: 75 mg Gel: 1%	Anemia, dermatitis, fever, hypercholesterolemia, infection, leukopenia, peripheral edema
Bicalutamide (Casodex)	T: 50 mg	Gynecomastia, hot flashes, breast pain, nausea, diarrhea, constipation, nocturia, impotence, pain, muscle pain, asthenia, abdominal pain
Bleomycin (Blenoxane)	I: 15 units, 30 units	Nausea, vomiting, anorexia, stomatitis, hyperpigmentation, nail changes, alopecia, pruritus, hyperkeratosis, urticaria, pneumonitis progression to fibrosis, decreased weight, rash
Bortezomib (Velcade)	I: 3.5 mg	Asthenia, diarrhea, nausea, constipation, peripheral neuropathy, vomiting, pyrexia, thrombocytopenia, psychiatric disorders, anorexia, decreased appetite, paresthesia, dysesthesia, anemia, headache, cough, dyspnea, pneumonia
Busulfan (Myleran)	T: 2 mg	Nausea, vomiting, hyperuricemia, myelosuppression, skin hyperpigmentation, alopecia, anorexia, decreased weight, diarrhea, stomatitis
Capecitabine (Xeloda)	T: 150 mg, 300 mg	Nausea, vomiting, diarrhea, stomatitis, bone marrow depression, hand-and-foot syndrome, dermatitis, fatigue, anorexia
Carboplatin (Paraplatin)	I: 50 mg, 150 mg, 450 mg, 50 mg/5 ml, 150 mg/15 ml, 450 mg/45 ml, 600 mg/60 ml	Nausea, vomiting, nephrotoxicity, bone marrow suppression, alopecia, peripheral neuropathy, hypersensitivity, ototoxicity, asthenia, diarrhea, constipation
Carmustine (BiCNU)	I: 100 mg	Anorexia, nausea, vomiting, bone marrow depression, pulmonary fibrosis, pain at injection site, diarrhea, skin discoloration
Carmustine (Gliadel Wafer)	Intracranial implant: 7.7 mg	Abnormal healing, see BiCNU

Anticancer Agents—cont'd

Name	Availability	Side Effects
Cetuximab (Erbitux)	I: 100 mg	Rash, acne, dry skin, tiredness/weakness, fever, constipation, abdominal pain, difficulty breathing, low blood pressure
Chlorambucil (Leukeran)	T: 2 mg	Bone marrow suppression, dermatitis, nausea, vomiting, liver toxicity, anorexia, diarrhea, abdominal discomfort, rash
Cisplatin (Platinol)	I: 50 mg, 100 mg	Nausea, vomiting, nephrotoxicity, bone marrow depression, neuropathies, ototoxicity, anaphylactic-like reactions, hyperuricemia, hypomagnesemia, hypophosphatemia, hypokalemia, hypocalcemia, pain at injection site
Cladribine (Leustatin)	I: 1 mg/ml	Nausea, vomiting, diarrhea, bone marrow depression, chills, fatigue, rash, fever, headaches, anorexia, diaphoresis
Clofarabine (Clolar)	I: 1 mg/ml	Vomiting, nausea, diarrhea, anemia, leukopenia, thrombocytopenia, neutropenia, febrile neutropenia, infection
Cyclophosphamide (Cytoxan)	I: 100 mg, 200 mg, 500 mg, 1 g, 2 g T: 25 mg, 50 mg	Nausea, vomiting, hemorrhagic cystitis, bone marrow depression, alopecia, interstitial pulmonary fibrosis, amenorrhea, azoospermia, diarrhea, darkening skin/fingernails, headaches, diaphoresis
Cytarabine (Cytosar, Ara-C)	I: 100 mg, 500 mg, 1 g, 2 g	Anorexia, nausea, vomiting, stomatitis, esophagitis, diarrhea, bone marrow depression, alopecia, rash, fever, neuropathies, abdominal pain
Dacarbazine (DTIC)	I: 200 mg	Nausea, vomiting, anorexia, liver necrosis, bone marrow depression, alopecia, rash, facial flushing, photosensitivity, flulike syndrome, confusion, blurred vision
Dactinomycin (Cosmegen)	I: 0.5 mg vial	Nausea, vomiting, stomatitis, esophagitis, pharyngitis, GI ulceration, proctitis, diarrhea, bone marrow depression, alopecia, erythema, acne, skin eruptions, hypocalcemia, fever, fatigue, myalgia, anorexia
Daunorubicin (Cerubidine)	I: 20 mg	CHF, nausea, vomiting, stomatitis, mucositis, diarrhea, red urine, bone marrow depression, alopecia, fever, chills, abdominal pain
Daunorubicin (DaunoXome)	I: 50 mg	Nausea, diarrhea, abdominal pain, anorexia, vomiting, stomatitis, myelosuppression, rigors, back pain, headaches, neuropathy, depression, dyspnea, fatigue, fever, cough, allergic reactions, sweating
Denileukin (Ontak)	I: 300 μg/2 ml	Hypersensitivity reaction, back pain, dyspnea, rash, chest pain, tachycardia, asthenia, flulike syndrome, chills, nausea, vomiting, infection
Docetaxel (Taxotere)	I: 20 mg, 80 mg	Hypotension, nausea, vomiting, diarrhea, mucositis, bone marrow suppression, rash, paresthesia, hypersensitivity, fluid retention, alopecia, asthenia, stomatitis, fever

Continued

ANTICANCER AGENTS—CONT'D

Name	Availability	Side Effects
Doxorubicin (Adriamycin)	I: 10 mg, 20 mg, 50 mg, 75 mg, 150 mg, 200 mg	Cardiotoxicity; including; CHF; arrhythmias; nausea; vomiting; stomatitis; esophagitis; GI ulceration; diarrhea; anorexia; red urine; bone marrow depression; alopecia; hyperpigmentation of nail beds and skin; local inflammation at injection site; rash; fever; chills; urticaria; lacrimation; conjunctivitis
Doxorubicin (Doxil)	I: 20 mg, 50 mg	Neutropenia, palmoplantar erythrodysesthesia syndrome, cardiomyopathy, CHF
Epirubicin (Ellence)	I: 2 mg/ml	Anemia, leukopenia, neutropenia, infection, mucositis
Erlotinib (Tarceva)	T: 25 mg, 100 mg, 150 mg	Rash, diarrhea, loss of appetite, tiredness, shortness of breath or trouble breathing, cough, nausea, infection, vomiting, inflammation of the mouth, itching, dry skin, eye problems, abdominal pain
Estramustine (Emcyt)	C: 140 mg	Increased risk of thrombosis, gynecomastia, nausea, vomiting, diarrhea, thrombocytopenia, peripheral edema
Etoposide (VePesid)	I: 20 mg/ml C: 50 mg	Nausea, vomiting, anorexia, bone marrow depression, alopecia, diarrhea, somnolence, peripheral neuropathies
Exemestane (Aromasin)	T: 25 mg	Dyspnea, edema, hypertension, mental depression
Floxuridine (FUDR)	I: 500-mg vial	Aphthosis, stomatitis, enteritis
Fludarabine (Fludara)	I: 50 mg	Nausea, diarrhea, stomatitis, bleeding, anemia, bone marrow depression, skin rash, weakness, confusion, visual disturbances, peripheral neuropathy, coma, pneumonia, peripheral edema, anorexia
Fluorouracil	I: 50 mg/ml Cream: 1%, 5% Solution: 1%, 2%, 5%	Nausea, vomiting, stomatitis, GI ulceration, diarrhea, anorexia, bone marrow depression, alopecia, skin hyperpigmentation, nail changes, headaches, drowsiness, blurred vision, fever
Flutamide (Eulexin)	C: 125 mg	Hot flashes, nausea, vomiting, diarrhea, hepatitis, impotence, decreased libido, rash, anorexia
Fulvestrant (Faslodex)	I: 250 mg/5 ml, 125 mg/2.5 ml syringes	Asthenia, pain, headache, injection site pain, flulike symptoms, fever, nausea, vomiting, constipation, anorexia, diarrhea, peripheral edema, dizziness, depression, anxiety, rash, increased cough, UTI
Gefitinib (Iressa)	T: 250 mg	Diarrhea, rash, dry skin, nausea, vomiting, pruritus, anorexia, asthenia, weight loss
Gemcitabine (Gemzar)	I: 200 mg, 1 g	Increased LFTs, nausea, vomiting, diarrhea, stomatitis, hematuria, myelosuppression, rash, mild paresthesias, dyspnea, fever, edema, flulike symptoms, constipation

Anticancer Agents—cont'd

Name	Availability	Side Effects
Gemtuzumab (Mylotarg)	I: 5 mg/20 ml	Anemia, hematuria, liver toxicity, pneumonia, herpes simplex, nausea, vomiting, dyspnea, headaches, hypotension, hypoxia, mucositis, myelosuppression, peripheral edema, tachycardia, thrombocytopenia
Goserelin (Zoladex)	I: 3.6 mg, 10.8 mg	Hot flashes, sexual dysfunction, decreased erections, gynecomastia, breast swelling, lethargy, pain, lower urinary tract symptoms, headaches, nausea, depression, sweating
Histrelin (Vantas)	SubQ implant: 50 mg	Hot flashes, asthenia, implant site reaction, testicular atrophy, renal impairment, bruising, pain/soreness/tenderness
Hydroxyurea (Hydrea)	C: 500 mg	Anorexia, nausea, vomiting, stomatitis, diarrhea, constipation, bone marrow depression, fever, chills, malaise
Ibritumomab (Zevalin)	Injection kit	Neutropenia, thrombocytopenia, anemia, infection, asthenia, abdominal pain, fever, pain, headache, nausea, peripheral edema, allergic reaction, GI hemorrhage, apnea
Idarubicin (Idamycin)	I: 5 mg, 10 mg, 20 mg	CHF, arrhythmias, nausea, vomiting, stomatitis, bone marrow depression, alopecia, rash, urticaria, hyperuricemia, abdominal pain, diarrhea, esophagitis, anorexia
Ifosfamide (Ifex)	I: 1 g, 3 g	Nausea, vomiting, hemorrhagic cystitis, bone marrow depression, alopecia, lethargy, somnolence, confusion, hallucinations, hematuria
Imatinib (Gleevec)	C: 100 mg T: 10 mg, 400 mg	Nausea, fluid retention, hemorrhage, musculoskeletal pain, arthralgia, weight gain, pyrexia, abdominal pain, dyspnea, pneumonia
Imiquimod (Aldara)	Topical cream: 5%	Skin reactions, erosion, flaking, edema, erythema
Interferon alfa 2a (Roferon-A)	I: 3 million units, 6 million units, 9 million units, 18 million units	Anorexia, nausea, diarrhea, bone marrow depression, pruritus, myalgia, dizziness, headaches, paresthesias, numbness, fatigue, fever, chills, dyspnea, flulike symptoms, vomiting, coughing, altered taste
Interferon alfa 2b (Intron-A)	I: 3 million units, 5 million units, 10 million units, 18 million units, 25 million units, 50 million units	Mild hypotension, hypertension, tachycardia with high fever, nausea, diarrhea, altered taste, weight loss, thrombocytopenia, bone marrow depression, rash, pruritus, myalgia, arthralgia associated with flulike syndromes
Irinotecan (Camptosar)	I: 40 mg, 100 mg	Diarrhea, nausea, vomiting, abdominal cramping, anorexia, stomatitis, increased SGOT (AST), severe myelosuppression, alopecia, sweating, rash, decreased weight, dehydration, increased alkaline phosphatase, headaches, insomnia, dizziness, dyspnea, cough, asthenia, rhinitis, fever, pain, back pain, chills

Continued

Anticancer Agents—cont'd

Name	Availability	Side Effects
Letrozole (Femara)	T: 2.5 mg	Hypertension, nausea, vomiting, constipation, diarrhea, abdominal pain, anorexia, rash, pruritus, musculoskeletal pain, back pain, arm/leg pain, arthralgia, fatigue, headaches, dyspnea, coughing, hot flashes
Leuprolide (Lupron, Eligard)	I: 3.75 mg, 5 mg, 7.5 mg, 11.25 mg, 15 mg, 22.5 mg, 30 mg, 45 mg	Hot flashes, gynecomastia, nausea, vomiting, constipation, anorexia, dizziness, headaches, insomnia, paresthesias, bone pain
Lomustine (CeeNU)	C: 10 mg, 40 mg, 100 mg	Anorexia, nausea, vomiting, stomatitis, liver toxicity, nephrotoxicity, bone marrow depression, alopecia, confusion, slurred speech
Mechlorethamine (Mustargen)	I: 10 mg/ml	Severe nausea and vomiting, metallic taste, diarrhea, bone marrow depression, alopecia, phlebitis, vertigo, tinnitus, hyperuricemia, infertility, azoospermia, anorexia, headaches, drowsiness, fever
Megestrol (Megace, Megace ES)	T: 20 mg, 40 mg Suspension: 40 mg/ml, 125 mg/ml	Deep vein thrombosis, Cushings-like syndrome, alopecia, carpal tunnel syndrome, weight gain, nausea
Melphalan (Alkeran)	T: 2 mg	Anorexia, nausea, vomiting, bone marrow depression, diarrhea, stomatitis
Mercaptopurine (Purinethol)	T: 50 mg	Anorexia, nausea, vomiting, stomatitis, liver toxicity, bone marrow depression, hyperuricemia, diarrhea, rash
Methotrexate	T: 2.5 mg, 5 mg, 7.5 mg, 10 mg, 15 mg I: 5 mg, 50 mg, 100 mg, 200 mg, 250 mg	Nausea, vomiting, stomatitis, GI ulceration, diarrhea, liver toxicity, renal failure, cystitis, bone marrow suppression, alopecia, urticaria, acne, photosensitivity, interstitial pneumonitis, fever, malaise, chills, anorexia
Mitomycin-C (Mutamycin)	I: 20 mg, 40 mg	Anorexia, nausea, vomiting, stomatitis, diarrhea, renal toxicity, bone marrow depression, alopecia, pruritus, fever, hemolytic uremic syndrome, weakness
Mitotane (Lysodren)	T: 500 mg	Anorexia, nausea, vomiting, diarrhea, skin rashes, depression, lethargy, somnolence, dizziness, adrenal insufficiency, blurred vision, decreased hearing
Mitoxantrone (Novantrone)	I: 20 mg, 25 mg, 30 mg	CHF, tachycardia, ECG changes, chest pain, nausea, vomiting, stomatitis, mucositis, myelosuppression, rash, alopecia, urine color change to bluish green, phlebitis, diarrhea, cough, headaches, fever
Nilutamide (Nilandron)	T: 50 mg	Hypertension, angina, hot flashes, nausea, anorexia, increased liver enzymes, dizziness, dyspnea, visual disturbances, impaired adaptation to dark, constipation, loss of libido

Anticancer Agents—cont'd

Name	Availability	Side Effects
Oxaliplatin (Eloxatin)	I: 50 mg, 100 mg, 50 mg/10 ml, 100 mg/20 ml	Fatigue, neuropathy, abdominal pain, dyspnea, diarrhea, nausea, vomiting, anorexia, fever, edema, chest pain, anemia, thrombocytopenia, thromboembolism, altered LFTs
Paclitaxel (Taxol)	I: 30 mg, 100 mg	Hypertension, bradycardia, ECG changes, nausea, vomiting, diarrhea, mucositis, bone marrow depression, alopecia, peripheral neuropathies, hypersensitivity reaction, arthralgia, myalgia
Pegaspargase (Oncaspar)	I: 750 units/ml	Hypotension, anorexia, nausea, vomiting, liver toxicity, pancreatitis, depression of clotting factors, malaise, confusion, lethargy, EEG changes, respiratory distress, hypersensitivity reaction, fever, hyperglycemia, stomatitis
Pemetrexed disodium (Alimta)	I: 500 mg	Stomach upset, nausea, vomiting, diarrhea, anemia, thrombocytopenia, neutropenia, tiredness, stomatitis, pharyngitis, loss of appetite, rash
Pentostatin (Nipent)	I: 10 mg	Nausea, vomiting, liver disorder, elevated LFTs, leukopenia, anemia, thrombocytopenia, rash, fever, upper respiratory infection, fatigue, hematuria, headaches, myalgia, arthralgia, diarrhea, anorexia
Plicamycin (Mithracin)	I: 2.5 mg	Anorexia, nausea, vomiting, stomatitis, diarrhea, clotting factor disorders, facial flushing, mental depression, confusion, fever, hypocalcemia, hypophosphatemia, hypokalemia, headaches, dizziness, rash
Procarbazine (Matulane)	C: 50 mg	Nausea, vomiting, stomatitis, diarrhea, constipation, bone marrow depression, pruritus, hyperpigmentation, alopecia, myalgia, paresthesias, confusion, lethargy, mental depression, fever, liver toxicity, arthralgia, respiratory disorders
Paclitaxel protein-bound particles (Abraxane)	I: 100 mg	Neutropenia, thrombocytopenia, anemia, hypersensitivity reaction, bradycardia, hypotension, abnormal ECG, cough, dyspnea, sensory neuropathy, myalgia/arthralgia, asthenia, fluid retention/edema, nausea, vomiting, diarrhea, mucositis, alopecia, bilirubin elevations, alkaline phosphatase elevations, AST (SGOT) elevations, injection site reaction
Rituximab (Rituxan)	I: 100 mg, 500 mg	Hypotension, arrhythmias, peripheral edema, nausea, vomiting, abdominal pain, leukopenia, thrombocytopenia, neutropenia, rash, pruritus, urticaria, angioedema, myalgia, headaches, dizziness, throat irritation, rhinitis, bronchospasm, hypersensitivity reaction
Streptozocin (Zanosar)	I: 1 g	May lead to insulin-dependent diabetes, nausea, vomiting, nephrotoxicity, renal tubular acidosis, bone marrow depression, lethargy, diarrhea, confusion, depression

Continued

Anticancer Agents—cont'd

Name	Availability	Side Effects
Tamoxifen (Nolvadex)	T: 10 mg, 20 mg	Skin rash, nausea, vomiting, anorexia, menstrual irregularities, hot flashes, pruritus, vaginal discharge or bleeding, bone marrow depression, headaches, tumor or bone pain, ophthalmic changes, weight gain, confusion
Temozolomide (Temodar)	C: 5 mg, 20 mg, 100 mg, 250 mg	Amnesia, fever, infection, leukopenia, neutropenia, peripheral edema, seizures, thrombocytopenia
Teniposide (Vumon)	I: 50 mg/5 ml	Hypotension with rapid infusion, diarrhea, nausea, vomiting, mucositis, bone marrow depression, alopecia, anemia, rash, hypersensitivity reaction
Thioguanine	T: 40 mg	Anorexia, stomatitis, bone marrow depression, hyperuricemia, nausea, vomiting, diarrhea
Thiotepa (Thioplex)	I: 15 mg	Anorexia, nausea, vomiting, mucositis, bone marrow depression, amenorrhea, reduced spermatogenesis, fever, hypersensitivity reactions, pain at injection site, headaches, dizziness, alopecia
Topotecan (Hycamtin)	I: 4 mg	Nausea, vomiting, diarrhea, constipation, abdominal pain, stomatitis, anorexia, neutropenia, leukopenia, thrombocytopenia, anemia, alopecia, headaches, dyspnea, paresthesia
Toremifene (Fareston)	T: 60 mg	Elevated LFTs, nausea, vomiting, constipation, skin discoloration, dermatitis, dizziness, hot flashes, sweating, vaginal discharge or bleeding, ocular changes, cataracts, anxiety
Tositumomab	I: 14 mg/ml and 0.1-0.25 mg/ml, 1.1-2.5 mg/ml	Asthenia, headache, dizziness, somnolence, cough, pharyngitis, dyspnea, rhinitis, fever, chills, pain, infection, human antimurine antibodies, hypothyroidism, hypotension, nausea, vomiting, abdominal pain, diarrhea, anorexia, anemia, neutropenia, thrombocytopenia, pneumonia, pleural effusion, dehydration, secondary cancers (myelodysplastic syndrome and/or acute leukemia), severe hypersensitivity, anaphylaxis (possibly fatal)
Trastuzumab (Herceptin)	I: 440 mg	CHF, S_3 gallop, nausea, vomiting, diarrhea, abdominal pain, anorexia, rash, peripheral edema, back or bone pain, asthenia, headaches, insomnia, dizziness, cough, dyspnea, rhinitis, pharyngitis

Anticancer Agents—cont'd

Name	Availability	Side Effects
Tretinoin (Vesanoid)	C: 10 mg	Flushing, nausea, vomiting, diarrhea, constipation, dyspepsia, mucositis, leukocytosis, dry skin/mucous membranes, rash, itching, alopecia, dizziness, anxiety, insomnia, headaches, depression, confusion, intracranial hypertension, agitation, dyspnea, shivering, fever, visual changes, earaches, hearing loss, bone pain, myalgia, arthralgia
Valrubicin (Valstar)	I: 200 mg/5 ml	Dysuria, hematuria, urinary frequency/incontinence, red urine, urinary urgency
Vinblastine (Velban)	I: 10 mg	Nausea, vomiting, stomatitis, constipation, bone marrow depression, alopecia, peripheral neuropathy, loss of deep tendon refluxes, paresthesias, diarrhea
Vincristine (Oncovin)	I: 1 mg, 2 mg, 3 mg	Nausea, vomiting, stomatitis, constipation, pharyngitis, polyuria, bone marrow depression, alopecia, numbness, paresthesias, peripheral neuropathy, loss of deep tendon reflexes, headaches, abdominal pain
Vinorelbine (Navelbine)	I: 10 mg, 50 mg	Elevated LFTs, nausea, vomiting, constipation, ileus, anorexia, stomatitis, bone marrow suppression, alopecia, vein discoloration, venous pain, phlebitis, interstitial pulmonary changes, asthenia, fatigue, diarrhea, peripheral neuropathy, loss of deep tendon reflexes

AST, Aspartate transaminase; *C,* capsules; *CHF,* congestive heart failure; *ECG,* electrocardiogram; *EEG,* electroencephalogram; *GI,* gastrointestinal; *I,* injection; *LFT,* liver function test; *SGOT,* serum glutamic-oxaloacetic transaminase; *SubQ,* subcutaneous; *T,* tablets; *UTI,* urinary tract infection.

CORTICOSTEROIDS

Uses

Symptomatic treatment of multiorgan disease/conditions. Rheumatoid arthritis, osteoarthritis, severe psoriasis, ulcerative colitis, lupus erythematous, anaphylactic shock, status asthmaticus, organ transplant.

Action

Suppress migration of polymorphonuclear leukocytes (PML) and reverse increased capillary permeability by their antiinflammatory effect. Suppress immune system by decreasing activity of lymphatic system.

Corticosteroids

Name	Availability	Route of Administration	Side Effects
Beclomethasone (Beclovent, Beconase, Vanceril, Vancenase)	Inhalation, nasal: 42 mg/spray, 84 mg/spray	Inhalation, intranasal	I: cough, dry mouth/throat, headaches, throat irritation Nasal: headaches, sore throat, sores inside nose
Betamethasone (Celestone, Diprosone)	I: 4 mg/ml	IV, intralesional, intraarticular	Nausea, vomiting, increased appetite, weight gain, trouble sleeping
Budesonide (Rhinocort, Pulmicort)	Nasal: 32 mg/spray	Intranasal	Nasal: headaches, sore throat, sores inside nose
Cortisone (Cortone)	T: 5 mg, 10 mg, 25 mg	PO	Same as betamethasone
Dexamethasone (Decadron)	T: 0.5 mg, 1 mg, 4 mg, 6 mg OS: 0.5 mg/5 ml I: 4 mg/ml	PO, parenteral	Same as betamethasone
Fludrocortisone (Florinef)	T: 0.1 mg	PO	Same as betamethasone
Flunisolide (AeroBid, Nasalide)	Inhalation, nasal: 25 mcg/spray	Inhalation, intranasal	Same as beclomethasone
Fluticasone (Flonase, Flovent, Flovent HFA, Flovent Diskus)	Inhalation: 44 mcg, 110 mcg, 220 mcg DPI: 50 mcg, 100 mcg, 250 mcg Nasal: 50 mg, 100 mcg	Inhalation, intranasal	Same as beclomethasone
Hydrocortisone (Cortef, Solu-Cortef)	T: 5 mg, 10 mg, 25 mg I: 100 mg, 250 mg, 500 mg, 1 g	PO, parenteral	Same as betamethasone
Methylprednisolone (Solu-Medrol)	T: 4 mg I: 40 mg, 125 mg, 500 mg, 1 g, 2 g	PO, parenteral	Same as betamethasone
Mometasone Furoate (Asmanex Twisthaler, Nasonex)	Inhalation: 200 μg Nasal: 50 μg/spray	Inhalation, intranasal	Same as betamethasone
Prednisolone (Prelone)	T: 5 mg OS: 5 mg/5 ml, 15 mg/5 ml	PO	Same as betamethasone
Prednisone (Deltasone)	T: 1 mg, 2.5 mg, 5 mg, 10 mg, 20 mg, 50 mg	PO	Same as betamethasone
Triamcinolone (Azmacort, Kenalog)	T: 4 mg, 8 mg Inhalation: 100 mg	PO, inhalation	Same as betamethasone I: cough, dry mouth/throat, headaches, throat irritation

DPI, Dry powder inhalation; *I*, injection; *IV*, intravenously; *OS*, oral suspension; *PO*, by mouth; *T*, tablets.

H_2 ANTAGONISTS

Uses

Short-term treatment of duodenal ulcer (DU), active benign gastric ulcer (GU); maintenance therapy of DU; pathologic hypersecretory conditions (e.g., Zollinger-Ellison syndrome); gastroesophageal reflux disease (GERD); and prevention of upper gastrointestinal bleeding in critically ill patients.

Action

Inhibit gastric acid secretion by interfering with histamine at the histamine H_2 receptors in parietal cells. Also inhibit acid secretion caused by gastrin.

H_2 Antagonists

Name	Availability	Dosage Range	Side Effects
Cimetidine (Tagamet)	T: 200 mg, 300 mg, 400 mg, 800 mg L: 300 mg/5 ml I: 150 mg/ml	Treatment of DU: 800 mg at bedtime, 400 mg bid or 300 mg qid Maintenance of DU: 400 mg at bedtime Treatment of GU: 800 mg at bedtime or 300 mg qid GERD: 1600 mg/day Hypersecretory: 1200-2400 mg/day	Headaches, fatigue, dizziness, confusion, diarrhea, gynecomastia
Famotidine (Pepcid)	T: 10 mg, 20 mg, 40 mg T (chewable): 10 mg T (DT): 20 mg, 40 mg Gelcap: 10 mg OS: 40 mg/5 ml I: 10 mg/ml, 0.4 mg/ml	Treatment of DU: 40 mg/day Maintenance of DU: 20 mg/day Treatment of GU: 40 mg/day GERD: 40-80 mg/day Hypersecretory: 80-640 mg/day	Headaches, dizziness, diarrhea, constipation, abdominal pain, tinnitus
Nizatidine (Axid)	T: 75 mg C: 150 mg, 300 mg OS: 15 mg/ml	Treatment of DU: 300 mg/day Maintenance of DU: 150 mg/day	Fatigue, urticaria, abdominal pain, constipation, nausea
Ranitidine (Zantac)	T: 75 mg, 150 mg, 300 mg Syrup: 15 mg/ml Granules: 150 mg Effervescent T: 25 mg I: 1 mg/ml, 25 mg/ml	Treatment of DU: 300 mg/day Maintenance of DU: 150 mg/day Treatment of GU: 300 mg/day GERD: 300 mg/day Hypersecretory: 0.3-6 g/day	Blurred vision, constipation, nausea, abdominal pain

C, Capsules; *DT,* disintegrating tablets; *DU,* duodenal ulcer; *GERD,* gastroesophageal reflux disease; *GU,* gastric ulcer; *I,* injection; *L,* liquid; *OS,* oral solution/suspension; *T,* tablets.

HUMAN IMMUNODEFICIENCY VIRUS (HIV) INFECTION

Uses

Antiretroviral agents are used in the treatment of HIV infection.

Action

There are currently four classes of antiretroviral agents used in the treatment of HIV disease: nucleoside reverse transcriptase inhibitors (NRTIs), nucleotide reverse transcriptase inhibitors (NtRTIs), nonnucleoside reverse transcriptase inhibitors (NNRTIs), and protease inhibitors (PIs).

ANTIRETROVIRAL AGENTS FOR TREATMENT OF HIV INFECTION

Name	Availability	Dosage Range	Side Effects
NUCLEOSIDE ANALOGUES			
Abacavir (Ziagen)	T: 300 mg OS: 20 mg/ml	A: 300 mg bid	Nausea, vomiting, malaise, rash, fever, headaches, asthenia, fatigue
Didanosine (Videx)	T: 25 mg, 50 mg, 100 mg, 150 mg, 200 mg C: 125 mg, 200 mg, 250 mg, 400 mg OS: 100 mg, 167 mg, 250 mg	T (>60 kg): 200 mg bid; (<60 kg): 125 mg bid OS (>60 kg): 250 mg bid; (<60 kg): 167 mg bid	Peripheral neuropathy, pancreatitis diarrhea, nausea, vomiting, headaches, insomnia, rash, hepatitis, seizures
Emtricitabine (Emtriva, FTC)	C: 200 mg	A: 200 mg/day	Hyperpigmentation of palms, soles
Lamivudine (Epivir)	T: 100 mg, 150 mg OS: 5 mg/ml, 10 mg/ml	A: 150 mg bid C: 4 mg/kg bid	Diarrhea, malaise, fatigue, headaches, nausea, vomiting, abdominal pain, peripheral neuropathy, arthralgia, myalgia, skin rash
Stavudine (Zerit)	C: 15 mg, 20 mg, 30 mg, 40 mg OS: 1 mg/ml	A: 40 mg bid (20 mg bid if peripheral neuropathy occurs)	Peripheral neuropathy, anemia, leukopenia, neutropenia
Zalcitabine (Hivid)	T: 0.375 mg, 0.75 mg	A (>60 kg): 0.75 mg tid; (<60 kg): 0.375 mg tid	Peripheral neuropathy, stomatitis, granulocytopenia, leukopenia
Zidovudine (Retrovir)	C: 100 mg T: 300 mg Syrup: 50 mg/5 ml, 10 mg/ml	A: 500-600 mg/day (100 mg 5 times/day or 300 mg bid)	Anemia, granulocytopenia, myopathy, nausea, malaise, fatigue, insomnia
Zidovudine/lamivudine (AZT/3TC) (Combivir)	C: 300 mg AZT/150 mg 3TC	A: 1 capsule bid	Bone marrow suppression, peripheral neuropathy, pancreatitis

Antiretroviral Agents for Treatment of HIV Infection—cont'd

Name	Availability	Dosage Range	Side Effects
Abacavir/lamivudine (Epzicom)	T: 600 mg ABC/ 300 mg 3TC	A: 1 tablet daily	Drug hypersensitivity, insomnia, depression, headache/migraine, fatigue/malaise, dizziness/vertigo, nausea, diarrhea, rash, pyrexia, abdominal pain/gastritis, abnormal dreams, anxiety, lactic acidosis with hepatomegaly, changes in body fat
Zidovudine/lamivudine/ Abacavir (AZT/3TC/ABC) (Trizivir)	C: 300 mg AZT/150 mg 3TC/300 mg ABC	A: 1 capsule bid	Bone marrow suppression, peripheral neuropathy, anaphylactic reaction
NUCLEOTIDE ANALOGUES			
Tenofovir (Viread)	T: 300 mg	A: 300 mg/day	Nausea, vomiting, diarrhea
COMBINATIONS			
Emtricitabine/tenofovir (Truvada)	T: 200 mg emtricitabine/ 300 mg tenofovir A: 1 tablet/day		Dizziness, diarrhea, nausea, vomiting, headache, rash, gas, skin discoloration, lactic acidosis, hepatotoxicity, kidney problems, changes in bone mineral density
NONNUCLEOSIDE ANALOGUES			
Delavirdine (Rescriptor)	T: 100 mg, 200 mg	A: 200 mg tid for 14 days, then 400 mg tid	Rash, nausea, headaches, elevations in LFTs
Efavirenz (Sustiva)	C: 50 mg, 100 mg, 200 mg	A: 600 mg/day C: 200-600 mg/day based on weight	Headaches, dizziness, insomnia, fatigue, rash, nightmares
Nevirapine (Viramune)	T: 200 mg	A: 200 mg/day for 14 days, then 200 mg bid	Rash, nausea, fatigue, fever, headaches, abnormal LFTs
PROTEASE INHIBITORS			
Amprenavir (Agenerase)	C: 50 mg, 150 mg OS: 15 mg/ml	A: 1200 mg bid C (4-16 yrs, <50 kg): 20 mg/kg bid or 15 mg/kg tid	Rash, diarrhea, headaches, nausea, vomiting, numbness, abdominal pain, fatigue
Atazanavir (Reyataz)	C: 100 mg, 150 mg, 200 mg	A: 400 mg/day	Increased liver function tests, jaundice, scleral icterus

Continued

Antiretroviral Agents for Treatment of HIV Infection—cont'd

Name	Availability	Dosage Range	Side Effects
Fosamprenavir (Lexiva)	T: 700 mg	A: 700-1400 mg bid	Same as amprenavir
Indinavir (Crixivan)	C: 200 mg, 400 mg	A: 800 mg q8h	Nephrolithiasis, hyperbilirubinemia, abdominal pain, asthenia, fatigue, flank pain, nausea, vomiting, diarrhea, headaches, insomnia, dizziness, altered taste
Lopinavir/ritonavir (Kaletra)	C: 133/33 mg OS: 80/20 mg	A: 400/100 mg/day C (4-12 yrs): 10-13 mg/kg bid	Diarrhea, nausea, vomiting, abdominal pain, headaches, rash
Nelfinavir (Viracept)	T: 250 mg, 625 mg Oral Powder: 50 mg/g	A: 750 mg q8h C: 20-25 mg/kg q8h	Diarrhea, fatigue, asthenia, headaches, hypertension, decreased ability to concentrate
Ritonavir (Norvir)	C: 100 mg OS: 80 mg/ml	A: Titrate up to 600 mg bid	Nausea, vomiting, diarrhea, altered taste sensation, fatigue, elevated LFTs and triglyceride levels
Saquinavir (Invirase)	C: 200 mg T: 500 mg	A: 600 mg tid	Diarrhea; elevations in LFTs, hypertriglycerides, cholesterol; abnormal fat accumulation; hyperglycemia
Saquinavir (Fortovase)	C: 200 mg	A: 1200 mg tid	Diarrhea; elevations in LFTs, hypertriglycerides, cholesterol; abnormal fat accumulation; hyperglycemia
Tiorabavur (Aptivus)	C: 250 mg	A: 500 mg bid coadministered with ritonavir 200 mg	Diarrhea, nausea, vomiting, abdominal pain, tiredness, headache, liver problems, rash, thrombocytopenia, hyperglycemia, hypertriglycerides, hypercholesterolemia

A, Adults; *C*, capsules; *C* (dosage), children; *LFTs*, liver function tests; *OS*, oral solution; *T*, tablets.

LAXATIVES

Uses

Short-term treatment of constipation; colon evacuation before rectal/bowel examination; prevention of straining (e.g., after anorectal surgery, myocardial infarction); to reduce painful elimination (e.g., episiotomy, hemorrhoids, anorectal lesions); modification of effluent from ileostomy, colostomy; prevention of fecal impaction; removal of ingested poisons.

Action

Laxatives ease or stimulate defecation. Mechanisms by which this is accomplished include (1) attracting, retaining fluid in colonic contents as a result of hydrophilic or osmotic properties; (2) acting directly or indirectly on mucosa to decrease absorption of water and NaCl; or (3) increasing intestinal motility, and decreasing absorption of water and NaCl by virtue of decreased transit time.

Bulk-forming: Act primarily in small/large intestine. Produce soft stool in 1 to 3 days.

Lubricants: Promote stool passage by coating the fecal surface with an oil layer that retains fecal fluid and prevents absorption of fecal water by the colon.

Hyperosmotic agents: Act in colon. Produce soft stool in 1 to 3 days.

Saline: Acts in small/large intestine, colon (sodium phosphate). Produces watery stool in 2 to 6 h (small doses produce semifluid stool in 6 to 12 h).

Stimulants: Act in colon. Produce semifluid stool in 6 to 12 h.

Surfactants: Act in small/large intestine. Produce soft stool in 1-3 days.

Laxatives

Name	Onset of Action	Uses
BULK		
Psyllium (Metamucil, Konsyl)	12-24 h up to 3 days	First-line for postpartum women; elderly; patients with diverticulosis, irritable bowel syndrome, hemorrhoids Safe for chronic use
Methylcellulose (Citrucel)	12-24 h up to 3 days	First-line for postpartum women; elderly; patients with diverticulosis; irritable bowel syndrome, hemorrhoids Safe for chronic use
Polycarbophil (Fibercon, Mitrolan)	Same as above	Same as methylcellulose
SURFACTANT		
Docusate sodium (Colace)	1–3 days	Aids in passage of hard, painful feces; prevents straining
Docusate calcium (Surfak)	Same as above	Same as docusate sodium
Docusate potassium (Dialose)	Same as above	Same as docusate sodium
LUBRICANT		
Mineral oil (Kondremul)	6-8 h	Prevents straining
SALINE		
Magnesium citrate (Citro-Nesia)	30 min to 3 h	Bowel evacuation for colonic procedures/examinations, fecal impaction, hepatic coma

Continued

Laxatives—cont'd

Name	Onset of Action	Uses
Magnesium hydroxide	Same as above	Same as magnesium citrate
Sodium phosphate (Fleets Phospho-Soda)	5-15 min	Same as magnesium citrate
HYPEROSMOTIC		
Glycerin	<30 min	Short-term relief of constipation
Lactulose (Chronulac)	1-3 days	Hepatic comas
Polyethylene glycol-electrolyte solution (GoLYTELY)	30-60 min	Bowel evacuation for colonic procedures/ examinations
STIMULANT		
Bisacodyl (Dulcolax)	PO: 6-12 h Rectal: 15-60 min	Same as polyethylene glycol-electrolyte solution Acts in 15-60 min
Casanthranol (in Peri-Colace)	6-12 h	Same as polyethylene glycol-electrolyte solution
Cascara sagrada	6-12 h	Bowel evacuation for colonic procedures/ examinations
Castor oil	6-12 h	Same as polyethylene glycol-electrolyte solution
Senna (Senokot)	6-12 h	Same as polyethylene glycol-electrolyte solution

NONSTEROIDAL ANTIINFLAMMATORY DRUGS (NSAIDS)

Uses

Provide symptomatic relief from *pain/inflammation* in the treatment of musculoskeletal disorders (e.g., rheumatoid arthritis, osteoarthritis, ankylosing spondylitis); *analgesic* for low to moderate pain; *reduction in fever* (many agents not suited for routine/prolonged therapy because of toxicity).

Action

Exact mechanism for antiinflammatory, analgesic, antipyretic effects unknown. Inhibition of enzyme cyclooxygenase, the enzyme responsible for prostaglandin synthesis, appears to be a major mechanism of action. Direct action on hypothalamus heat-regulating center may contribute to antipyretic effect.

NSAIDs

Name	Availability	Dosage Range	Side Effects
Aspirin	T: 81 mg, 160 mg, 325 mg Suppository: 300 mg, 600 mg	P (A): 325-650 mg q4h as needed C: Up to 60-80 mg/kg/day Arthritis: 3.2-6 g/day JRA: 60-110 mg/kg/day RF (A): 5-8 g/day C: 75-100 mg/kg/day TIA: 1300 mg/day MI: 81-325 mg/day	GI upset, dizziness, headaches
Celecoxib (Celebrex)	C: 100 mg, 200 mg	OA: 200 mg/day RA: 100-200 mg bid FAP: 400 mg bid	Diarrhea, back pain, dizziness, heartburn, headaches, nausea, stomach pain
Diclofenac (Voltaren)	T: 25 mg, 50 mg, 75 mg, 100 mg	Arthritis: 100-200 mg/day	Indigestion, constipation, diarrhea, nausea, headaches, fluid retention, abdominal cramps
Diflunisal (Dolobid)	T: 250 mg, 500 mg	Arthritis: 0.5-1 g/day P: 0.5 g q8-12h	Headaches, abdominal cramps, indigestion, diarrhea, nausea
Etodolac (Lodine)	T: 400 mg, 500 mg T (ER): 400 mg, 500 mg, 600 mg C: 200 mg, 300 mg	Arthritis: 600-800 mg/day P: 200-400 mg q6-8h	Indigestion, dizziness, headaches, bloated feeling, diarrhea, nausea, weakness, abdominal cramps
Fenoprofen (Nalfon)	C: 200 mg, 300 mg T: 600 mg	Arthritis: 300-600 mg tid or qid P: 200 mg q4-6h as needed	Nausea, indigestion, nervousness, constipation, shortness of breath, heartburn
Flurbiprofen (Ansaid)	T: 50 mg, 100 mg	Arthritis: 200-300 mg/day	Indigestion, nausea, fluid retention, headaches, abdominal cramps, diarrhea

Continued

NSAIDs—cont'd

Name	Availability	Dosage Range	Side Effects
Ibuprofen (Motrin, Advil)	T: 100 mg, 200 mg, 400 mg, 600 mg, 800 mg T (chewable): 50 mg, 100 mg C: 200 mg S: 100 mg/5 ml, 100 mg/2.5 ml Drops: 40 mg/ml	Arthritis: 1.2-3.2 g/day P: 400 mg q4-6h as needed Fever: 200 mg q4-6h as needed JA: 30-40 mg/kg/day	Dizziness, abdominal cramps, stomach pain, heartburn, nausea
Indomethacin (Indocin)	C: 25 mg, 50 mg C (SR): 75 mg S: 25 mg/5 ml Suppository: 50 mg	Arthritis: 50-200 mg/day Bursitis/tendinitis: 75-150 mg/day GA: 150 mg/day	Fluid retention, dizziness, headaches, abdominal pain, indigestion, nausea
Ketoprofen (Orudis)	T: 12.5 mg C: 25 mg, 50 mg, 75 mg C (ER): 100 mg, 150 mg, 200 mg	Arthritis: 150-300 mg/day P: 25-50 mg q6-8h as needed	Headaches, nervousness, abdominal pain, bloated feeling, constipation, diarrhea, nausea
Ketorolac (Toradol)	T: 10 mg I: 15 mg/ml, 30 mg/ml	P (PO): 10 mg q4-6h as needed; (IM/IV): 60-120 mg/day	Fluid retention, abdominal pain, diarrhea, dizziness, headaches, nausea
Meloxicam (Mobic)	C: 7.5 mg, 15 mg OS: 7.g mg/5 ml	Arthritis: 7.5-15 mg/day	Heartburn, indigestion, nausea, diarrhea, headaches
Nabumetone (Relafen)	T: 500 mg, 750 mg	Arthritis: 1-2 g/day	Fluid retention, dizziness, headaches, abdominal pain, constipation, diarrhea, nausea
Naproxen (Anaprox, Naprosyn)	T: 200 mg, 250 mg, 375 mg, 500 mg T (CR): 375 mg S: 125 mg/5 ml	Arthritis: 250-550 mg/day P: 250 mg q6-8h JA: 10 mg/kg/day GA: 750 mg once, then 250 mg q8h	Tinnitus, fluid retention, shortness of breath, dizziness, drowsiness, headaches, abdominal pain, constipation, heartburn, nausea
Oxaprozin (Daypro)	C: 600 mg	Arthritis: 600-1800 mg/day	Constipation, diarrhea, nausea, indigestion
Piroxicam (Feldene)	C: 10 mg, 20 mg	Arthritis: 20 mg/day	Abdominal pain, stomach pain, nausea
Sulindac (Clinoril)	T: 150 mg, 200 mg	Arthritis: 300 mg/day GA: 400 mg/day	Dizziness, abdominal pain, constipation, diarrhea, nausea
Tolmetin (Tolectin)	T: 200 mg, 600 mg C: 400 mg	Arthritis: 600-1800 mg/day JA: 15-30 mg/kg/day	Fluid retention, dizziness, headaches, weakness, abdominal pain, diarrhea, indigestion, nausea, vomiting

A, Adults; *C,* capsules; *C* (dosage), children; *CR,* controlled release; *ER,* extended release; *FAP,* familial adenomatous polyposis; *GA,* gouty arthritis; *GI,* gastrointestinal; *I,* injection; *IM,* intramuscularly; *IV,* intravenously; *JA,* juvenile arthritis; *JRA,* juvenile rheumatoid arthritis; *MI,* myocardial infarction; *OA,* osteoarthritis; *OS,* oral suspension; *P,* pain; *PO,* by mouth; *RA,* rheumatoid arthritis; *RF,* rheumatic fever; *S,* suspension; *T,* tablets; *TIA,* transient ischemic attack.

NUTRITION: ENTERAL

Enteral nutrition (EN), also known as *tube feedings*, provides food/nutrients via the gastrointestinal (GI) tract using special formulas, delivery techniques, and equipment. All routes of EN consist of a tube through which liquid formula is infused.

General Indications

Tube feedings are used in patients with major trauma and burns; those undergoing radiation and/or chemotherapy; patients with liver failure, severe renal impairment, physical or neurologic impairment; preoperatively and postoperatively to promote anabolism; prevention of cachexia, and malnutrition.

Routes of Enteral Nutrition Delivery and Their Indications

Nasogastric (NG): Most common for short-term feeding in patients unable or unwilling to consume adequate nutrition by mouth. Requires at least a partially functioning GI tract.

Nasoduodenal (ND): Nasojejunal (NJ): Patients unable or unwilling to consume adequate nutrition by mouth. Requires at least a partially functioning GI tract.

Gastrostomy: Patients with esophageal obstruction or impaired swallowing; patients in whom NG, ND, or NJ not feasible; or, when long-term feeding indicated.

Jejunostomy: Patients with stomach or duodenal obstruction, impaired gastric motility; patients in whom NG, ND, or NJ not feasible or when long-term feeding is indicated.

Initiating Enteral Nutrition

With continuous feeding, initiation of isotonic (about 300 mOsm/L) or moderately hypertonic feeding (up to 495 mOsm/L) can be given full strength, usually at a slow rate (30 to 50 ml/h) and gradually increased (25 ml/h q6-24h). Formulas with osmolality of >500 mOsm/L are generally started at half strength and gradually increased in rate, then concentration. Tolerance is increased if the rate and concentration are not increased simultaneously.

Protein: Has many important physiologic roles and is the primary source of nitrogen in the body. Provides 4 kcal/g protein.

Carbohydrate (CHO): Provides energy for the body and heat to maintain body temperature. Provides 3.4 kcal/g carbohydrate.

Fat: Provides concentrated source of energy. Referred to as kilocalorie-dense or protein-sparing. Provides 9 kcal/g fat.

Electrolytes, vitamins, trace elements: Contained in formulas (not found in specialized products for renal and hepatic insufficiency).

Complications

Mechanical: Usually associated with some aspect of the feeding tube.

Aspiration pneumonia: Caused by delayed gastric emptying, gastroparesis, gastroesophageal reflux, or decreased gag reflex. May be prevented or treated by reducing infusion rate, using lower-fat formula, feeding beyond pylorus, checking residuals, using small-bore feeding tubes, elevating head of bed 30° to 45° during and for 30 to 60 min after intermittent feeding, and regularly checking tube placement.

Esophageal, mucosal, pharyngeal irritation, otitis: Caused by using large-bore NG tube. Prevented by use of small bore whenever possible.

Irritation, leakage at ostomy site: Caused by drainage of digestive juices from site. Prevented by close attention to skin/stoma care.

Tube, lumen obstruction: Caused by thickened formula residue, formation of formula-medication complexes. Prevented by frequently irrigating tube with clear water (also before and after giving formulas/medication), avoiding instilling medication if possible.

Gastrointestinal: Usually associated with formula, rate of delivery, unsanitary handling of solutions, or delivery system.

Diarrhea: Caused by low-residue formulas, rapid delivery, use of hyperosmolar formula, hypoalbuminemia, malabsorption, microbial contamination, or rapid GI transit time. Prevented by using fiber-supplemented formulas, decreasing rate of delivery, using dilute formula, and gradually increasing strength.

Cramping, gas, abdominal distention: Caused by nutrient malabsorption, rapid delivery of refrigerated formula. Prevented by delivering formula by continuous methods, giving formulas at room temperature, decreasing rate of delivery.

Nausea, vomiting: Caused by rapid delivery of formula, gastric retention. Prevented by reducing rate of delivery, using dilute formulas, selecting low-fat formulas.

Constipation: Caused by inadequate fluid intake, reduced bulk, inactivity. Prevented by supplementing fluid intake, using fiber-supplemented formula, encouraging ambulation.

Metabolic: Fluid/electrolyte status should be monitored. Refer to monitoring section. In addition, the very young and very old are at greater risk of developing complications such as dehydration or overhydration.

Monitoring

Daily: Estimate nutrient intake, fluid intake/output, weight of patient, clinical observations.

Weekly: Electrolytes (potassium, sodium, magnesium, calcium, phosphorus), blood glucose, blood urea nitrogen (BUN), creatinine, liver function tests (e.g., serum glutamic-oxaloacetic transaminase/aspartate transaminase [SGOT/AST], alkaline phosphatase), 24-hour urea and creatinine excretion, total iron-binding capacity (TIBC) or serum transferrin, triglycerides, cholesterol.

Monthly: Serum albumin.

Other: Urine glucose, acetone (when blood glucose >250), vital signs (temperature, respirations, pulse, blood pressure) q8h.

NUTRITION: PARENTERAL

Parenteral nutrition (PN), also known as *total parenteral nutrition* (TPN) or *hyperalimentation* (HAL), provides required nutrients to patients by intravenous (IV) route of administration. The goal of PN is to maintain or restore nutritional status caused by disease, injury, or inability to consume nutrients by other means.

Indications

Conditions when patient is unable to use alimentary tract via oral, gastrostomy, or jejunostomy routes. Impaired absorption of protein caused by obstruction, inflammation, or antineoplastic therapy. Bowel rest necessary because of gastrointestinal (GI) surgery or ileus, fistulas, or anastomotic leaks. Conditions with increased metabolic requirements (e.g., burns, infection, trauma). Preserve tissue reserves as in acute renal failure. Inadequate nutrition from tube feeding methods.

Components of Parenteral Nutrition

Protein: In the form of crystalline amino acids (CAA), primarily used for protein synthesis. Several products are designed to meet specific needs for patients with renal failure (e.g., NephrAmine), liver disease (e.g., HepatAmine), and stress/trauma (e.g., Aminosyn HBC), and for use in neonates and pediatrics (e.g., Aminosyn PF, TrophAmine). Calories: 4 kcal/g protein.

Energy: In the form of dextrose, available in concentrations of 5% to 70%. Dextrose <10% may be given peripherally; concentrations >10% must be given centrally. Calories: 3.4 kcal/g dextrose.

IV fat emulsion: Available in the form of 10% or 20% concentrations. Provides a concentrated source of energy/calories (9 kcal/g fat) and is a source of essential fatty acids. May be administered peripherally or centrally.

Electrolytes: Major electrolytes (calcium, magnesium, potassium, sodium; also acetate, chloride, phosphate). Doses of electrolytes are individualized, based on many factors (e.g., kidney and/or liver function, fluid status).

Vitamins: Essential components in maintaining metabolism and cellular function; widely used in PN.

Trace elements: Necessary in long-term PN administration. Trace elements include zinc, copper, chromium, manganese, selenium, molybdenum, and iodine.

Miscellaneous: Additives include insulin, albumin, heparin, and histamine$_2$–blockers (e.g., cimetidine, ranitidine, famotidine). Other medication may be included, but compatibility for admixture should be checked on an individual basis.

Routes of Administration

PN is administered via either peripheral or central vein.

Peripheral: Usually involves 2-3 L/day of 5% to 10% dextrose with 3% to 5% amino acid solution along with IV fat emulsion. Electrolytes, vitamins, trace elements are added according to pt needs. Peripheral solutions provide about 2000 kcal/day and 60-90 g protein/day.

Central: Usually uses hypertonic dextrose (concentration range of 15% to 35%) and amino acid solution of 3% to 7% with IV fat emulsion. Electrolytes, vitamins, trace elements are added according to patient needs. Central solutions provide 2000-4000 kcal/day. Must be given through large central vein with high blood flow, allowing rapid dilution, avoiding phlebitis/thrombosis.

Monitoring

Baseline: Complete blood count (CBC), platelet count, prothrombin time, weight, body length/head circumference (in infants), electrolytes, glucose, blood urea nitrogen (BUN), creatinine, uric acid, total protein, cholesterol, triglycerides, bilirubin, alkaline phosphatase, lactate dehydrogenase (LDH), SGOT (AST), albumin, other tests as needed.

Daily: Weight, vital signs (TPR), nutritional intake (kcal, protein, fat), electrolytes (potassium, sodium chloride), glucose (serum, urine), acetone, BUN, osmolarity, other tests as needed.

2–3 times/wk: CBC, coagulation studies (PT, PTT), creatinine, calcium, magnesium, phosphorus, acid-base status, other tests as needed.

Weekly: Nitrogen balance, total protein, albumin, prealbumin, transferrin, liver function tests (serum glutamic-oxaloacetic transaminase/aspartate transaminase [SGOT/AST], serum glutamate pyruvate transaminase SGPT [ALT]), alkaline phosphatase, LDH, bilirubin, hemoglobin (Hgb), uric acid, cholesterol, triglycerides, and other tests as needed.

Complications

Mechanical: Malfunction in system for IV delivery (e.g., pump failure; problems with lines, tubing, administration sets, catheter). Pneumothorax, catheter misdirection, arterial puncture, bleeding, hematoma formation may occur with catheter placement.

Infectious: Infections (patients often more susceptible to infections), catheter sepsis (e.g., fever, shaking chills, glucose intolerance) where no other site of infection is identified.

Metabolic: Includes hyperglycemia, elevated cholesterol and triglycerides, abnormal liver function tests.

Fluid, electrolyte, acid-base disturbances: May alter potassium, sodium, phosphate, magnesium levels.

Nutritional: Clinical effects seen may be caused by lack of adequate vitamins, trace elements, essential fatty acids.

OPIOID ANALGESICS

Uses

Relief of moderate to severe pain associated with surgical procedures, myocardial infarction, burns, cancer, or other conditions. May be used as an adjunct to anesthesia, either as a preoperative medication or intraoperatively as a supplement to anesthesia. Codeine and hydrocodone have an antitussive effect. Opium tinctures, such as paregoric, are used for severe diarrhea. Methadone relieves severe pain but is used primarily as part of heroin detoxification.

Action

Opioids refer to all drugs having actions similar to morphine and to receptors combining with these agents. Major effects are on the central nervous system (produce analgesia, drowsiness, mood changes, mental clouding, analgesia without loss of consciousness, nausea and vomiting) and GI tract (decrease HCl secretion; diminish biliary, pancreatic, and intestinal secretions; diminish propulsive peristalsis). Also affect respiration (depressed) and cardiovascular system (peripheral vasodilation, decrease peripheral resistance, inhibit baroreceptor reflexes).

OPIOID ANALGESICS

		Analgesic Effects			
Names	Availability	Onset (min)	Peak (min)	Duration (h)	Dosage Range
Butorphanol (Stadol)	I: 1 mg/ml, 2 mg/ml	IM: 10-30 IV: 2-3	IM: 30-60 IV: 30	IM: 3-4 IV: 2-4	IM: 1-4 mg q3-4h IV: 0.5-2 mg q3-4h
Codeine	I: 30 mg, 60 mg T: 30 mg, 60 mg	IM: 10-30 PO: 30-45	IM: 30-60 PO: 60-120	IM/PO: 4-6	IM/PO (A): 15-60 mg q4-6h; (C): 0.5 mg/kg q4-6h
Fentanyl (Sublimaze, Duragesic, Atiq)	I: 50 mcg/ml Patch: 12.5 mcg, 25 mcg, 50 mcg, 75 mcg, 100 mcg,	IM: 7-15 IV: 1-2 Patch: 24 hours Troche/Lozenge: 0.2 mg, 0.4 mg, 0.6 mg, 0.8 mg, 1.2 mg, 1.6 mg	IM: 20-30 IV: 3-5	IM: 1-2 IV: 0.5-1 Patch: 72 hours	IM: 50-100 mcg q1-2h
Hydrocodone	Combination oral	10-30	30-60	4-6	5-10 mg q4-6h
Hydromorphone (Dilaudid)	T: 1 mg, 2 mg, 3 mg, 4 mg, 8 mg S: 3 mg I: 1 mg/ml, 2 mg/ml, 3 mg/ml, 4 mg/ml, 10 mg/ml	PO: 30 IM: 15 IV: 10-15	PO: 90-120 IM: 30-60 IV: 15-30	PO: 4-5 IM: 4-5 IV: 4	PO: 1-4 mg q3-6h IM: 1-4 mg q3-6h IV: 0.5-1 mg q3h ER: 3 mg q4-8h
Levorphanol (Levo-Dromoran)	T: 2 mg I: 2 mg/ml	PO: 10-60 IM: —	PO: 90-120 IM: 60	4-5	PO: 2-4 mg q4h IM: 2-3 mg q4h
Meperidine (Demerol)	T: 50 mg, 100 mg I: 25 mg/ml, 50 mg/ml, 75 mg/ml, 100 mg/ml	PO: 15 IM: 10-15 IV: 1	PO: 60-90 IM: 30-60 IV: 5-7	2-4	PO/IM (A): 50-150 mg q3-4h (C): 1-1.8 mg/kg q3-4h IM/PO: 2.5-10 mg q3-4h
Methadone (Dolophine)	T: 5 mg, 10 mg OS: 5 mg/5 ml, 10 mg/5 ml I: 10 mg/ml	PO: 30-60 IM: 10-20 IV: —	PO: 90-120 IM: 60-120 IV: 15-30	PO: 4-6 IM: 4-5 IV: 3-4	

Opioid Analgesics—cont'd

Names	Availability	Analgesic Effects: Onset (min)	Analgesic Effects: Peak (min)	Analgesic Effects: Duration (h)	Dosage Range
Morphine (Roxanol, MS Contin, Kadian, Depodur, Astramorph PF, Avinza, Duramorph, Infumorph)	T (ER): 15 mg, 30 mg, 60 mg, 100 mg, 200 mg C (ER Kadian): 20 mg, 30 mg, 50 mg, 60 mg, 100 mg OS: 10 mg/5 ml, 20 mg/5 ml, 20 mg/ml I: 0.5 mg/ml, 1 mg/ml, 2 mg/ml, 4 mg/ml, 10 mg/ml, 15 mg/ml, 25 mg C (ER Avinza): 30 mg, 60 mg, 90 mg, 120 mg	PO: 30-60 IM: 10-30 IV: —	PO: 90 IM: 30-60 IV: 20	PO: 4 IM/IV: 4-5	PO: 10-30 mg q4h IM: 5-20 mg q4h IV: 0.05-0.1 mg/kg q4h
Nalbuphine (Nubain)	I: 10 mg/ml, 20 mg/ml	IM: 2-15 IV: 2-3	IM: 60 IV: 30	IM: 3-6 IV: 3-4	IM/IV: 10-20 mg q3-6h
Oxycodone (Roxicodone)	T: 15 mg, 30 mg				
	OS: 5 mg/5 ml, 20 mg/ml T (ER): 10 mg, 20 mg, 40 mg, 80 mg, 160 mg	30	60	3-4	5-15 mg or 5 ml q4-6h (ER): q12h (dose titrated)
Propoxyphene (Darvon)	T: 100 mg	15-60	60-120	4-6	PO: 100 mg q4-6h
Tramadol (Ultram)	T: 50 mg T (DT): 50 mg	30-60	120	4-6	PO: 50-100 mg q4-6h

A, Adults; *C*, children; *DT*, disintegrating tablets; *ER*, extended release; *I*, injection; *IM*, intramuscularly; *IV*, intravenously; *OS*, oral solution; *PO*, by mouth; *S*, supplement; *T*, tablets.

OPIOID ANTAGONISTS

Uses

Primarily used to reverse respiratory depression induced by narcotic overdosage.

Action

Prevents/reverses effects of mu (μ) receptor opioid agonists (e.g., increases respiration, reverses sedative effect).

Opioid Antagonists

Name	Availability	Dosage Range	Side Effects
Nalmefene (Revex)	I: 100 mcg /ml, 1 mg/ml	IV/IM/SubQ: Titrated individually	Nausea, vomiting, tachycardia, hypertension
Naloxone (Narcan)	I: 0.02 mg/ml, 0.4 mg/ml, 1 mg/ml	IV/IM/SubQ (A): 0.4-2 mg May repeat at 2- to 3-min intervals; (C): 0.01 mg/kg May give subsequent doses of 0.1 mg/kg	Same as nalmefene
Naltrexone (Depade, ReVia)	T: 50 mg	PO: 50 mg/day or 100 mg every other day or 150 mg every third day	Abdominal pain, anxiety, diarrhea, tachycardia, increased sweating, loss of appetite, nausea

A, Adults; *C* (dosage), children; *I*, injection; *SubQ*, subcutaneously; *T*, tablets.

SEDATIVE-HYPNOTICS

Uses

Treatment of insomnia (e.g., difficulty falling asleep initially, frequent awakening, awakening too early).

Action

Sedatives decrease activity, moderate excitement, and have calming effects. Hypnotics produce drowsiness, enhance onset/maintenance of sleep (resembling natural sleep). Benzodiazepines are the most widely used agents (largely replace barbiturates): greater safety, lower incidence of drug dependence.

Sedative-Hypnotics

Name	Availability	Dosage Range	Side Effects
BENZODIAZEPINES			
Estazolam (ProSom)	T: 1 mg, 2 mg	A: 1-2 mg E: 0.5-1 mg	Daytime sedation, memory and psychomotor impairment, tolerance, withdrawal reactions, rebound insomnia, dependence
Flurazepam (Dalmane)	C: 15 mg, 30 mg	A/E: 15-30 mg	Same as estazolam
Quazepam (Doral)	T: 7.5 mg, 15 mg	A: 7.5-15 mg E: 7.5 mg	Same as estazolam
Temazepam (Restoril)	C: 7.5 mg, 15 mg, 30 mg	A: 15-30 mg E: 7.5-15 mg	Same as estazolam
Triazolam (Halcion)	T: 0.125 mg, 0.25 mg	A: 0.125-0.25 mg E: 0.125 mg	Same as estazolam
NONBENZODIAZEPINES			
Zaleplon (Sonata)	C: 5 mg, 10 mg	A: 5-10 mg E: 5 mg	Headaches, dizziness, myalgia, somnolence, asthenia, abdominal pain
Zolpidem (Ambien)	T: 5 mg, 10 mg	A: 10 mg E: 5 mg	Dizziness, daytime drowsiness, headaches, confusion, depression, hangover, asthenia
Eszopicline (Lunesta)	T: 1 mg, 2 mg, 3 mg	A: 2-3 mg E: 1-2 mg	Headache, dry mouth, dyspepsia, nausea, depression, dizziness, somnolence, respiratory tract infection, rash, unpleasant taste
Ramelteon (Rozerem)	T: 8 mg	A: 8 mg	Headache, somnolence, fatigue, dizziness, nausea, exacerbated insomnia, respiratory tract infection

A, Adults; *C*, capsules; *E*, elderly; *T*, tablets.

APPENDIX

B Assessment Tools

CONTENTS

MINI-MENTAL STATE EXAMINATION (MMSE)

The Mini-Mental State Examination (MMSE) is a widely used method for assessing cognitive mental status. The evaluation of cognitive functioning is important in clinical settings because of the recognized high prevalence of cognitive impairment in medical patients. As a clinical instrument, the MMSE has been used to detect impairment, follow the course of an illness, and monitor response to treatment. The MMSE has also been used as a research tool to screen for cognitive disorders in epidemiologic studies and follow cognitive changes in clinical trials.

MMSE Sample Items

1. Orientation to time
   "What is the date?"
2. Registration
   "Listen carefully; I am going to say three words. You say them back after I stop. Ready? Here they are...
   APPLE (pause), PENNY (pause), TABLE (pause). Now repeat those words back to me."
   (Repeat up to 5 times, but score only the first trial.)
3. Naming
   "What is this?" *(Point to a pencil or pen.)*
4. Reading
   "Please read this and do what it says." *(Show examinee the words on the stimulus form.)*
   CLOSE YOUR EYES

PAIN, SUFFERING, AND SPIRITUAL ASSESSMENT

Pain is a complex subjective experience that involves both neurophysiologic and emotional aspects. Many individual factors can affect individuals' experiences of pain and subsequent responses to treatment including their past experiences with pain, the meaning they assign to their current pain, and underlying mood disorders (e.g., anxiety, depression, anger). At times, affective and cognitive dimensions of pain along with psychosocial and spiritual issues can produce an overwhelming amount of suffering. However, pain and suffering are not inextricably linked. That is, some patients with pain report no suffering.

Attending to suffering, by listening and offering empathy, is a critical nonpharmacologic intervention. Obtaining a spiritual history can help patients and their caregivers further understand and attend to the suffering aspects of pain.

Obtaining a Spiritual History

S = Spiritual belief system	Do you have a spiritual life that is important to you? Do you have a formal religious affiliation? What is your clearest sense of the meaning of your life at this time?
P = Personal spirituality	When you are afraid or in pain, how do you find comfort? Describe the beliefs and practices of your religion that you personally accept. In what ways is your spirituality/religion meaningful to you in your daily life?
I = Integration with spiritual community	Do you belong to any religious or spiritual groups? How do you participate in this group? In what ways is this group a source of support to you?
R = Ritualized practices and restrictions	What lifestyle activities or practices does your religion encourage, discourage, or forbid? What meaning do these practices hold for you? To what extent do you follow these practices?
I = Implications for medical care	Would you like to discuss religious/spiritual implications of health care? Are there specific elements of medical care that your beliefs/religion discourage/forbid? Are there any persons you would like us to include in your spiritual care planning?
T = Terminal events planning	Are there any unresolved areas of your life at this point that you would like us to assist you with addressing? Are there practices or rituals you would like available in the hospital or home? For what in your life do you still feel gratitude even though you are in pain?

Hints for conversations about suffering and faith:

- Let the patient set the agenda; you don't need to ask about fear, unless they open the door to it.
- **Don't underestimate the power of silence. Sometimes the best support is simply listening.**
- A person generally isn't looking for advice, just someone to listen and affirm that fear, anger, sadness, etc., are normal.

REFERENCES:

Ambuel B, Weissman D: *Fast fact and concept #19: taking a spiritual history*, 2000, EPERC; available online at www.epercmcw.edu; Byock L: *Dying well: The prospect for growth at the end of life*, Riverhead, 1997, Putnam; Cassell EJ: Diagnose suffering, *Ann Intern Med* 131(7):531-534, 1991; Paice JA: Managing psychological conditions in palliative care, *Am J Nurs* 102(11):36-43.

PSYCHOSOCIAL PAIN ASSESSMENT FORM

Patient: ______________________________ Age: ________ Date: ______________
Med. Record #: ________________ Significant Other: ______________________
Diagnosis: ______________________ Primary Physician: ____________________
Pain Syndrome: ____
Duration of Pain: __________________ Assessed by: ________________________

Please circle appropriate descriptors.

1. **Build:** Cachectic Thin Medium Heavy Obese
2. **Attire:** Disheveled Hospitalized Casual Professional
3. **Eye Contact:** Avoided Appropriate Stared
4. **Attention:** Distracted <..................................l..................................> Hypervigilant
   Focused
5. **Manner:**

Flat	Depressed	Distant	Cooperative
Engaging	Humorous	Dramatic	Agitated
Anxious	Tearful	Sobbing	Defensive
Sarcastic	Argumentative	Angry	Hostile

6. **Verbal Expression:** Terse Vague Average Articulate Verbose
7. **Reasoning Ability:** Impaired Age-Appropriate Advanced
8. **Overall Perspective:** Pessimistic <...> Optimistic
   Unrealistic <...> Realistic
9. **Impressions:**
   ____
   ____
   ____
10. **Interventions:**
   ____
   ____
   ____
11. **Recommendations:**
   ____
   ____
   ____

RATING (0-10)

(0 = no concern, 10 = greatest concern)

	Interviewer	Patient	Significant Other
Economic			
Social support			
Activities of daily living			
Emotional issues			
Coping			

Introduction

We recognize that people are often concerned about the impact of pain on many areas of their lives. Unrelieved pain can cause economic, emotional, spiritual, and social problems, in addition to medical and physical ones. We will be looking at the overall impact of pain in your life and asking several questions to help the Pain Team better understand your personal concerns. The first area we will be addressing is the economic impact of your pain.

Economic

1. How are you supporting yourself financially?
   Work________________ Family________________ Disability ________________
   Partner________________ Retirement/Pensions________________ Other________________
   Friends________________ Savings ________________
2. Some people we see are concerned about meeting their economic needs. Which of these are worrisome to you?
   None ________________
   Housing ________________ Clothing ________________ Prescriptions________________
   Food________________ Childcare________________ Insurance________________
   Transportation________________ Medical bills________________ Other ________________
3. How has your economic situation changed? Better ________________ Worse ________________
   Describe:
   ____
   ____
   ____
4. How upsetting have these changes been to you?
   Describe:
   ____
   ____
   ____
5. What would be different in your life if you could afford to change it?
   Describe:
   ____
   ____
   ____
6. Please rate your overall level of concern regarding these economic issues.

RATING (0-10)

(0 = no concern; 10 = greatest concern)

	Interviewer	Patient	Significant Other
Economic			

Social Support

We believe that pain affects not just you, but your entire family. We'd like to look at ways in which you've noticed this impact.

1. Who do you turn to when you're uncomfortable or in pain?
   Self ________________ Others ________________ God ________________

Continued

PSYCHOSOCIAL PAIN ASSESSMENT FORM—CONT'D

Name: ______________________ Relationship: ______________________
How accessible is this person to you?

____

How helpful is this to you?

____

2. How comfortable are you sharing your feelings/fears with your loved ones?
What makes this difficult for you?
Describe:
____
____
____
3. How satisfied are you with communication with your doctor/medical team?
Describe:
____
____
____
4. Losing people who are important to us affects us deeply. Have you suffered any recent losses?
Yes_____ **No**_____
Describe:
____
____
Breaking up ______________ Separation ______________
Divorce ______________ Death ______________
Moving away ______________ Other ______________
5. Please rate your overall level of concern regarding these social support issues.

RATING (0-10)

(0 = no concern; 10 = greatest concern)

	Interviewer	Patient	Significant Other
Social support			

Activities of Daily Living

Physical impact

Often unrelieved pain affects a person's daily routine. How is your pain affecting you in these activities of daily living?

1. Affecting your sleeping patterns? **Yes**_____ **No**_____
Frequent napping _____ Difficulty going to sleep _____
Nightmares _____ Difficulty staying asleep _____
Drowsiness _____ Difficulty waking up _____
Chronic fatigue _____ Other _____
2. Affecting your eating habits? **Yes**_____ **No**_____
Weight loss/gain _____ Special diet _____
Loss of appetite _____ Feeding tube _____
Nausea/vomiting _____ Difficulty swallowing _____
Changes in taste _____ Other _____

3. Affecting your hygiene/elimination habits? **Yes**_____ **No**_____
   Diarrhea _____ Constipation _____
   Catheter _____ Ostomy _____
   Difficulty grooming _____ Incontinence _____
   Difficulty bathing _____ Other _____
4. Affecting your ability to move? **Yes**_____ **No**_____
   Generalized weakness _____ Limited range of motion _____
   Bed bound _____ Wheel chair _____
   Crutches/walker/cane _____ Walking/standing _____
   Getting in/out of car _____ Climbing stairs _____
   Lifting/carrying _____ Other _____
   No longer athletic _____ Shortness of breath _____
5. Affecting your roles in your family? **Yes**_____ **No**_____
   In what ways?
   ____
6. Affecting your sexual functioning? **Yes**_____ **No**_____
   In what ways?
   ____
7. Affecting your physical appearance? **Yes**_____ **No**_____
   In what ways?
   ____
8. How has your energy level changed? **Less**_____ **Same**_____ **Improved**_____
9. Please rate your overall level of concern regarding these physical changes.

RATING (0-10)

(0 = no concern; 10 = greatest concern)

	Interviewer	Patient	Significant Other
Activities of daily living			

Emotional

Pain affects our emotions. These questions will help us better understand your pain's impact upon you emotionally.

1. Have you been troubled by any of these feelings:
   Depression **Yes**_____ **No**_____ *Describe:* ______________________
   Frustration/Anger **Yes**_____ **No**_____ *Describe:* ______________________
   Anxiety **Yes**_____ **No**_____ *Describe:* ______________________
   Panic Attacks **Yes**_____ **No**_____ *Describe:* ______________________
   Mood Swings **Yes**_____ **No**_____ *Describe:* ______________________
   Difficulty Concentrating **Yes**_____ **No**_____ *Describe:* ______________________
   Loss of Motivation **Yes**_____ **No**_____ *Describe:* ______________________
2. Do you ever see or hear things that others don't? **Yes**_____ **No**_____
   Describe:
   ____
   ____

Continued

PSYCHOSOCIAL PAIN ASSESSMENT FORM—CONT'D

3. Are there any medical tests or procedures that frighten you? **Yes**_____ **No**_____
   Describe:
   ____
   ____
4. Have you ever thought about hurting yourself or taking your life? **Yes**_____ **No**_____
   Describe:
   ____
   ____
5. Please rate your overall level of concern regarding these emotional issues.

RATING (0-10)

(0 = no concern; 10 = greatest concern)

	Interviewer	Patient	Significant Other
Emotional issues			

Coping

People handle pain and distress in many ways. These questions will help us better understand how you cope with upsetting situations.

1. Sometimes, doing things we enjoy distracts us from our pain. What activities are you able to do that you enjoy?
   None _____
   Family _____ Friends _____ Hobbies _____ Reading _____
   Religion _____ Gardening _____ Traveling _____ Exercise _____
   Art/Music _____ TV _____ Pets _____ Other: _____
2. Some people find comfort in spirituality that helps them cope with difficult situations. What role does spirituality have in helping you?
   Describe:
   ____
   ____
3. Many people in your situation ask, "Why did this happen to me?" How have you attempted to "make sense" of your painful experiences?
   Describe:
   ____
   ____
4. Past stressful events can affect us in the present. What kinds of stress have you had to handle before?
   Describe:
   ____
   ____
   Child abuse? **Yes**_____ **No**_____ *Describe:* ______________________
   Sexual abuse? **Yes**_____ **No**_____ *Describe:* ______________________
   Family violence? **Yes**_____ **No**_____ *Describe:* ______________________
5. Some people find that counseling sessions or attending support groups can help them cope with stressful situations.
   Have you ever been in counseling? **Yes**_____ **No**_____
   What was the focus of your therapy? ___________

Have you ever attended a support group? **Yes**_____ **No**_____
What kind? ___________________________
How helpful was this? ____

____

6. Some people are prescribed medications to help them cope. Which of these have you been prescribed?
None_____ Other: ____
Antianxiety medications? **Yes**_____ **No**_____ *Describe:* ____________________________
Antidepressant medications? **Yes**_____ **No**_____ *Describe:* __________________________
Pain medications? **Yes**_____ **No**_____ *Describe:* ___________________________________
Do you ever take your prescriptions differently than ordered? **Yes**_____ **No**_____
Describe: ____
7. Some people use chemicals to help them cope. Which of these do you use?
Tobacco? **Yes**_____ **No**_____ *Describe:* _____________________________________
Alcohol? **Yes**_____ **No**_____ *Describe:* ______________________________________
Recreational drugs? **Yes**_____ **No**_____ *Describe:* ______________________________
Have you ever tried to stop using these? **Yes**_____ **No**_____ *Describe:* _______________
Do you worry about your usage of these? **Yes**_____ **No**_____ *Describe:* _______________
Has your family worried about your usage of these? **Yes**_____ **No**_____ *Describe:* __________
8. What changes do you expect in your future?
Describe: ____
9. Overall, how satisfied are you with your present quality of life?
Describe: ____
10. Please rate your overall level of concern regarding your ability to cope or manage your pain.

RATING (0-10)

(0 = no concern; 10 = greatest concern)

	Interviewer	Patient	Significant Other
Coping			

Used with permission from Shirley Otis-Green, City of Hope National Medical Center.

SPIRITUAL WELL-BEING SCALE

For each of the following statements circle the choice that best indicates the extent of your agreement or disagreement as it describes your personal experience:

SA = Strongly Agree
MA = Moderately Agree
A = Agree
D = Disagree
MD = Moderately Disagree
SD = Strongly Disagree

1. I don't find much satisfaction in private prayer with God. SA MA A D MD SD
2. I don't know who I am, where I came from, or where I am going. SA MA A D MD SD
3. I believe that God loves me and cares about me. SA MA A D MD SD
4. I feel that life is a positive experience. SA MA A D MD SD
5. I believe that God is impersonal and not interested in my daily situations. SA MA A D MD SD
6. I feel unsettled about my future. SA MA A D MD SD
7. I have a personally meaningful relationship with God. SA MA A D MD SD
8. I feel very fulfilled and satisfied with life. SA MA A D MD SD
9. I don't get much personal strength and support from my God. SA MA A D MD SD
10. I feel a sense of well-being about the direction my life is headed in. SA MA A D MD SD
11. I believe that God is concerned about my problems. SA MA A D MD SD
12. I don't enjoy much about life. SA MA A D MD SD
13. I don't have a personally satisfying relationship with God. SA MA A D MD SD
14. I feel good about my future. SA MA A D MD SD
15. My relationship with God helps me not to feel lonely. SA MA A D MD SD
16. I feel that life is full of conflict and unhappiness. SA MA A D MD SD
17. I feel most fulfilled when I'm in close communion with God. SA MA A D MD SD
18. Life doesn't have much meaning. SA MA A D MD SD
19. My relation with God contributes to my sense of well-being. SA MA A D MD SD
20. I believe there is some real purpose for my life. SA MA A D MD SD

APPENDIX

C Other Resources

The Lung Cancer Alliance
www.lungcanceralliance.org

American Cancer Society (ACS)
www.cancer.org

American Cancer Society: Tobacco and Cancer
www.cancer.org/quittobacco

American Lung Association (ALA)
www.lungusa.org

American Society of Clinical Oncology
www.asco.org

BRCAPRO: estimates the risk of *BRCA1* and *BRCA2* genetic mutations for women who have a strong family history of breast or ovarian cancer (or both)
http://astor.som.jhmi.edu/BayesMendel/brcapro.html

Cancer Care, Inc.
www.cancercare.org

Coalition of Cancer Cooperative Groups
www.cancertrialshelp.org

Colorectal Cancer Network
www.colorectal-cancer.net

Conversations! The International Newsletter for Those Fighting Ovarian Cancer
www.Ovarian-News.org

fertileHOPE
www.fertilehope.org

Gilda Radner Familial Ovarian Cancer Registry
www.OvarianCancer.com

Gilda's Club Worldwide
www.GildasClub.org

Gynecologic Cancer Foundation
www.wcn.org/gcf

Harvard's Center for Cancer Prevention: your disease risk – Cancer
www.yourdiseaserisk.harvard.edu/hccpquiz.pl?lang=english&func=home&=cancer_index

International Association For the Study of Lung Cancer (IASLC)
www.iaslc.org

Lance Armstrong Foundation
www.livestrong.org

Living Beyond Breast Cancer
www.lbbc.org

Leukemia and Lymphoma Society
www.leukemia.org

Lung Cancer Online Foundation (LCOF)
www.lungcanceronline.org/foundation

Lymphoma Research Foundation
www.lymphoma.org

National Breast Cancer Coalition
www.natlbcc.org

National Cancer Institute Genetics of Breast and Ovarian Cancer (includes comparison of Gail and Claus models)
www.nci.nih.gov

National Cancer Institute: Genetics of Breast and Ovarian Cancer (includes comparison of Gail and Claus models)
www.cancer.gov/cancertopic/pdg/genetics/breast-and-ovarian/healthprofessional#Reference/.53

National Coalition for Cancer Survivorship
www.canceradvocacy.org

National Comprehensive Cancer Network (NCCN)
www.nccn.org

National Directory of Trained Genetics Professionals
www.cancer.gov/search/genetics_services

National Familial Lung Cancer Registry (NFLCR)
www.path.jhu.edu/nfltr

National Ovarian Cancer Association (NOCA)
www.OvarianCanada.org

National Ovarian Cancer Coalition (NOCC)
www.Ovarian.org

Native American Cancer Research
www.natamcancer.org

Oncology Nursing Society
www.ons.org

OncoLink
www.oncolink.upenn.edu

Ovarian Cancer National Alliance (OCNA)
www.OvarianCancer.org

Ovarian Cancer Research Fund, Inc. (OCRF)
www.ocrf.org

SHARE: Self-help for Women with Breast or Ovarian Cancer
www.sharecancersupport.org

Society of Gynecologic Oncologists (SGO)
www.sgo.org

Susan G. Komen Breast Cancer Foundation
www.komen.org

Women Against Lung Cancer (WALC)
www.4walc.org

Y-Me National Breast Cancer Organization
www.y-me.org

Young survival coalition
www.youngsurvival.org

Index

A

Page numbers followed by *f* indicate figures; *t*, tables; *b*, boxes.

C

F

G

H

I

J

K

L

M

N

O

P

Q

R

S